AF545028

Obstetric Care

Obstetric Care

Edited by
Martin Olsen
East Tennessee State University

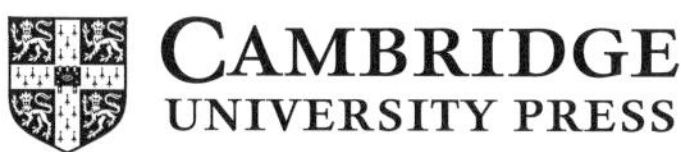

CAMBRIDGE
UNIVERSITY PRESS

University Printing House, Cambridge CB2 8BS, United Kingdom

One Liberty Plaza, 20th Floor, New York, NY 10006, USA

477 Williamstown Road, Port Melbourne, VIC 3207, Australia

4843/24, 2nd Floor, Ansari Road, Daryaganj, Delhi – 110002, India

79 Anson Road, #06-04/06, Singapore 079906

Cambridge University Press is part of the University of Cambridge.

It furthers the University's mission by disseminating knowledge in the pursuit of education, learning, and research at the highest international levels of excellence.

www.cambridge.org
Information on this title: www.cambridge.org/9781107158047
DOI: 10.1017/9781316662571

First published 2017

Printed in the United Kingdom by TJ International Ltd. Padstow Cornwall

A catalogue record for this publication is available from the British Library.

Library of Congress Cataloging-in-Publication Data
Names: Olsen, Martin, editor.
Title: Obstetric care / edited by Martin Olsen.
Description: Cambridge, United Kingdom; New York, NY, USA: Cambridge University Press, 2017. | Includes bibliographical references and index.
Identifiers: LCCN 2017008241 | ISBN 9781107158047 (hardback)
Subjects: | MESH: Pregnancy Complications | Labor, Obstetric | Delivery, Obstetric
Classification: LCC RG525 | NLM WQ 240 | DDC 618.2–dc23
LC record available at https://lccn.loc.gov/2017008241

ISBN 978-1-107-15804-7 Hardback

Every effort has been made in preparing this book to provide accurate and up-to-date information that is in accord with accepted standards and practice at the time of publication. The authors, editors, and publishers can make no warranties that the information contained herein is totally free from error, not least because clinical standards are constantly changing through research and regulation. The authors, editors, and publishers therefore disclaim all liability for direct or consequential damages resulting from the use of material contained in this book. Readers are strongly advised to pay careful attention to information provided by the manufacturer of any drugs or equipment that they plan to use.

To those physicians who have taken stands against medical corruption; may you look in your mirrors with pride.

Contents

Contributors

Olukayode Akinlaja, MD, MBA
Assistant Professor
Department of Obstetrics and Gynecology
University of Tennessee College of Medicine
Chattanooga, TN

Melanie D. Altizer, MD
Assistant Professor
Department of OB/GYN
Virginia Tech-Carilion School of Medicine

Heather Anaya, DO
Clinical Assistant Professor
Division of Maternal-Fetal Medicine
Department of Obstetrics and Gynecology
University of Iowa Carver College of Medicine

Leah W. Antoniewicz, MD
Assistant Professor
Department of OB/GYN
Baylor College of Medicine

Isaac Babarinsa, MBBS, MSc, MRCOG, FWACS
Senior Attending Physician
Department of Obstetrics and Gynecology
Sidra Medical and Research Center, Doha, Qatar

Anitra Beasley, MD, MPH
Department of Obstetrics & Gynecology
Baylor College of Medicine
Houston, TX

Jasjit K. Beausang, MD
Assistant Professor
Department of Obstetrics and Gynecology
Drexel University College of Medicine

Alexandria Betz, DO
Maternal Fetal Medicine Fellow Associate
Division of Maternal-Fetal Medicine
Department of Obstetrics and Gynecology
University of Iowa Carver College of Medicine

Natalie Bowersox, MD, FACOG
Clinical Assistant Professor of Surgery
Cleveland Clinic Foundation

Phillip L. Bressman, MD
Affiliated Assistant Professor
University of Tennessee College of Medicine
Nashville, TN

Jeremy P. Campbell, MB ChB (Hons.), MRCSEd, FRCA
Consultant Anaesthetist
Queen Charlotte's and Chelsea Hospital
Imperial College Healthcare NHS Trust
London, UK

Christinne Canela, MD, FACOG
Attending Physician
Department of Obstetrics and Gynecology
Carilion Clinic
and
Assistant Professor
Virginia Tech-Carilion School of Medicine

Frances Casey, MD, MPH
Assistant Professor
VCU Medical Center

Kenneth K. Chen, MD
Assistant Professor of Medicine & Assistant Professor of ObGyn
Alpert Medical School of Brown University

David Churchill, MD, FRCOG
Consultant Obstetrician
The Royal Wolverhampton NHS Trust,
New Cross Hospital Wolverhampton, UK

Shontreal M. Cooper, MD
Resident Physician
Department of Obstetrics and Gynecology
Hahnemann University Hospital

Lauren Coyne, MD
Clinical Assistant Professor
University of Iowa Hospitals and Clinics
Department of Obstetrics and Gynecology

Charles Cox
The Royal Wolverhampton NHS Trust, New Cross Hospital Wolverhampton, UK

George H. Davis, DO, FACOOG
Professor of Obstetrics and Gynecology
Division of Maternal-Fetal Medicine
Quillen College of Medicine
East Tennessee State University

Julie DeCesare, MD, FACOG
Associate Professor
Department of Obstetrics and Gynecology
University of Florida College of Medicine Pensacola

Marygrace Elson, MD, MME
Clinical Professor Obstetrics and Gynecology
University of Iowa Carver College of Medicine
Iowa City, IA

Georgia Ferrell, MD
Instructor
University of Tennessee, Nashville

Heather Frey, MD
Assistant Professor, Clinical
Department of Maternal Fetal Medicine
Ohio State University Wexner Medical Center

Etoi A. Garrison, MD, PhD
Associate Professor
Division of Maternal Fetal Medicine
Department Obstetrics and Gynecology
Vanderbilt University

William Gist, MD
Assistant Professor and Program Director
Department of Obstetrics and Gynecology
University of Tennessee College of Medicine
Chattanooga, TN

Aaron Goldberg, MD
Assistant Professor
Department Obstetrics and Gynecology
Medical College of Virginia

William Goodnight, MD
Associate Professor
University North Carolina Dept. Ob/Gyn

Cornelia R. Graves, MD
Medical Director, Tennessee Maternal Fetal Medicine
Medical Director, Perinatal Services, St. Thomas Health Systems
Professor, University of Tennessee
Clinical Professor, Vanderbilt University
Adjunct Professor, Meharry Medical College

Gareen Hamalian, MD, MPH
Department of Psychiatry
University of Colorado School of Medicine

Mohamad Hamdi, MD
Assistant Professor of Obstetrics and Gynecology (Clinical)
The Alpert Medical School of Brown University
Providence, RI

M. Camille Hoffman, MD, MSCS
Department of Obstetrics & Gynecology
Division of Maternal Fetal Medicine and Department of Psychiatry
University of Colorado School of Medicine

Jessica R. Jackson, MD, MSBS
University of Florida
Gainesville, FL

Sonia Jackson, MD
Resident
Department of Obstetrics and Gynecology, Meharry Medical College Nashville, TN

Zachary C. Kuhlmann, DO
Clinical Associate Professor
Program Director
Department of Obstetrics and Gynecology
University of Kansas School of Medicine — Wichita

Gwinnett M. Ladson, MD
Professor
Department of Obstetrics and Gynecology, Meharry Medical College
Nashville, TN

Julia Lagow, DO, FACOG
University of Florida, Department of OB/GYN
Obstetrics and Gynecology Residency Program
Sacred Heart Health System

Heidi Leftwich, DO
Assistant Professor of Obstetrics and Gynecology
Division of Maternal-Fetal Medicine

University of Massachusetts
Medical School/UMASS
Memorial Medical Center
Worcester, MA

Kimberly R. Looney, MD
Assistant Professor
Department of Obstetrics and Gynecology, Meharry Medical College Nashville, TN

Anjali Martinez, MD
Obstetrics and Gynecology
The George Washington University
Washington DC

Sarina Martini, MD
Clinical Assistant Professor
University of Iowa Hospitals and Clinics
Department of Obstetrics and Gynecology
Iowa City, IA

Gene La Monica, MD, FACOG
Adjunct Assistant Professor and Attending in Maternal-Fetal Medicine
Department of Obstetrics and Gynecology
Weill-Cornell Medicine — Qatar, Sidra Medical and Research Center, Doha, Qatar

Mahmoud Moussa, MD, MRCOG
Clinical Fellow
The Royal Wolverhampton NHS Trust,
New Cross Hospital
Wolverhampton, UK

Loriana Newman, MD
Assistant Professor
Clinical Dept. of Obstetrics and Gynecology
Ohio State University Wexner Medical Center

Martin Olsen, MD
Professor
East Tennessee State University
Department of Ob/Gyn

Damali Campbell Oparaji, MD
Assistant Professor
Department of Obstetrics, Gynecology and Women's Health
Rutgers, the State University of New Jersey
Rutgers New Jersey Medical School
Newark, NJ

Stephen K. Patrick, MD
Associate Professor
Department of Obstetrics and Gynecology
Baylor College of Medicine
Houston, TX

Joseph E. Peterson, MD
Clinical Associate Professor
Department of Health Sciences
University of Florida

Sara Petruska, MD
Associate Professor
University of Louisville

Felicity Plaat, BA, MBBS, FRCA
Consultant Anaesthetist
Queen Charlotte's and Chelsea Hospital
Imperial College Healthcare NHS Trust
London, UK

Moune Jabre Raughley, MD, FACOG
Assistant Professor and Attending in Obstetrics and Gynecology
Department of Obstetrics and Gynecology
Weill-Cornell Medicine — Qatar, Sidra Medical and Research Center, Doha, Qatar

Erin C. Rebele, MD
Assistant Professor of Obstetrics and Gynecology
Vanderbilt University
Vanderbilt University School of Medicine
Nashville, TN

Scott D. Richard, MD
Associate Professor
Drexel University College of Medicine
Department of Obstetrics and Gynecology
Division of Gynecologic Oncology
Philadelphia, PA

Fidelma B. Rigby, MD
Associate Professor Maternal Fetal Medicine
Department OB/GYN
VCUHS
Richmond, VA

Natalie E. Roche, MD
Assistant Professor
Department of Obstetrics, Gynecology and Women's Health
Rutgers, the State University of New Jersey
Rutgers New Jersey Medical School
Newark, NJ

Stephen Rotholz, MD
Assistant Professor
Department of Obstetrics and Gynecology

University of Colorado School of Medicine
Colorado Institute for Maternal &
Fetal Health

Karen M. Schneider, MD
Associate Professor
Department of Obstetrics and Gynecology
Baylor College of Medicine
Houston, TX

Sarah Shaffer, DO
Clinical Assistant Professor
Department of Obstetrics & Gynecology
University of Iowa

Joseph Shumway, MD, MPH, FACOG
Senior Consulting Physician
Director of Education
Department of Obstetrics and Gynecology
Sidra Medical and Research Center
Doha, Qatar
Weill Cornell School of Medicine, Qatar

Rolanda Standifer, MD
Assistant Professor
Division of Maternal Fetal Medicine
Department Obstetrics and Gynecology
Vanderbilt University

Colleen K. Stockdale, MD, MS
Clinical Associate Professor
Department of Obstetrics & Gynecology
University of Iowa
Iowa City, IA

Theodore Tsaltas, MD
Assistant Professor
Department Ob/Gyn
University of Tennessee College of Medicine
at Chattanooga

Clinton A. Veselis, MD
Instructor
Drexel University College of Medicine
Department of Obstetrics and Gynecology
Division of Gynecologic Oncology
Philadelphia, PA

Roxanne A. Vrees, MD
Assistant Professor of Obstetrics and Gynecology
Warren Alpert Medical School of Brown University
Women & Infants Hospital
Providence, RI

Selman I. Welt, MD, RDMS
Professor
East Tennessee University
Department of OB/GYN

Denise Willers, MD
Associate Professor
Dept. Obstetrics and Gynecology
Washington University School of Medicine
in St. Louis

Ann E. Williford, MD
Instructor- Department of Clinical Medical Education
University of Tennessee Health Science Center
Nashville, TN

Preface

Practitioners of obstetrics and gynecology must have a thorough understanding of the breadth of the subject matter while also accepting the challenge of comprehending the depth of information required to give outstanding patient care to women. *Obstetric Care* is the second book in a series of three texts that cover the breadth of the Ob/Gyn specialty. Modern Ob/Gyn leaders divide our specialty into three divisions: office practice, obstetrics, and gynecology. *Office Care of Women* was the first book in this series and *Gynecologic Care* rounds out the subject matter. After a thorough understanding of the specialty, readers can then move on to literature review or subspecialty texts to further their knowledge on the depth of obstetrics and gynecology.

The care of pregnant patients is uniquely satisfying. The practice of obstetrics combines the need for outstanding technical skills with the intellectual challenges of medical management for both maternal and fetal conditions. Outstanding psychosocial skills combined with crisis management abilities are also essential. The volume of material covering these and other topics within the discipline of obstetrics is vast. This book is tightly written and is designed to be read in its entirety. The basic information provided here can be used as a review or as a springboard to a more knowledgeable review of the literature in depth.

Advances in the care of obstetric patients and their fetuses have created dramatic improvements in maternal and newborn health in most, but not all, areas of the world. Obstetric care is critically important to the families that are served by each maternal care provider since the loss of a mother has a devastating impact on each member of that family. Entire societies benefit when maternal and child healthcare improvements occur. I hope this book inspires excellence in the practice of obstetrics.

Normal Labor

Etoi A. Garrison

Introduction

Term labor begins as result of complex signaling cascade between the mother, placenta, and fetus. Labor is the process by which uterine contractions result in progressive cervical dilation and delivery of the fetus. The inciting event for human labor remains unclear. Human labor is influenced by maternal, fetal, and placental hormones, which alter myometrial responsiveness and facilitate organized uterine contractions in response to oxytocin, prostaglandins, and inflammatory mediators.[1–3] The first stage of labor is characterized by two phases: the latent phase and the active phase. The latent phase of labor has a slower rate of dilation. An evaluation of contemporary labor management challenges our historical understanding of labor progress and indicates that the transition from the latent phase to active phase occurs at a more advanced cervical dilation than previously thought. The duration of labor can be influenced by maternal factors, fetal factors, and labor practices. This chapter will review labor physiology, present a description of labor mechanics, and review contemporary evidence to support normal labor progress.

Scope of the Problem

Why is it important to understand normal labor? Successful inpatient management of women in labor depends upon the obstetric provider's ability to recognize normal labor from abnormal labor and above all "to do no harm" should there be a need for medical intervention. In 2014, the combined primary and repeat cesarean section rate for the United States averaged 32.2%.[4] The primary cesarean section rate for term nulliparous low-risk women with a singleton vertex fetus averaged 26%.[4] Evidence describes significant variability for the primary cesarean section rate at the state and hospital level. In 2009, the primary cesarean section rate for nulliparous term low-risk women ranged from 2.4% to 36.5% depending upon hospital type and location.[5] Regional practice patterns, patient demographics, hospital characteristics, and local resources can influence clinical decision making with regard to the route of delivery.[6] A basic understanding of normal labor is important in order to deliver safe healthcare to our patients and minimize the risk of adverse outcomes for mother and baby.

Labor Hormonal Physiology

Activation of the fetal hypothalamic pituitary axis, progesterone withdrawal, and estradiol synthesis have each been identified as the triggering mechanism for labor in several species. [7] In humans, however, the identification of one inciting event for term labor remains controversial. Corticotropin-releasing hormone (CRH), estradiol precursors, progesterone, and prostaglandins are all believed to play an important role in facilitating myometrial contractility.[1–3,8]

In humans, the fetal hypothalamic pituitary axis is activated by placental production of CRH. CRH stimulates the production of dehydroepiandrostenedione (DHEAS) by the fetal adrenal gland, which is subsequently converted by the placenta to estradiol and estriol. The estrogen precursors, in turn, promote transcription of gap junction proteins and receptors for oxytocin, PGF2α, and PGE_2.[7–9] Unlike other species, human concentrations of progesterone remain stable toward the end of pregnancy and there is no evidence of a decline near term.[7,8,10,11] There is, however, evidence in humans that labor is associated with increased expression of myometrial and amniotic fluid membrane progesterone receptor isoforms, which increase intracellular calcium and transcription of contraction associated proteins.

In humans, myometrial prostaglandin receptors are upregulated toward the latter half of pregnancy.[8]

Prostaglandins directly enhance uterine contractility by increasing the intracellular calcium concentration. Prostaglandins stimulate the release of calcium from the sarcoplasmic reticulum and promote the influx of extracellular calcium into cells via activation of transmembrane calcium channels.[1,2,7,8]

A review of the hormonal mediators of labor would be incomplete without a brief review of oxytocin and its mechanism of action. Oxytocin is a polypeptide of hypothalamic origin, which is stored and released intermittently from the posterior pituitary. Oxytocin is secreted in a pulsatile fashion and undergoes hepatic and renal degradation. During pregnancy, it is inactivated by placental oxytocinase. There is evidence that the maternal oxytocin concentration remains relatively unchanged during the antepartum period; however, maternal oxytocin concentrations increase during the second stage of labor.[12–14] Near term, there is an increase in myometrial responsiveness to oxytocin, which is largely mediated by an increase in the number of oxytocin receptors, their distribution within the myometrium, and relative affinity to oxytocin. The number of oxytocin receptors has been demonstrated to increase 100- to 200-fold during pregnancy with a peak concentration in early labor.[12,15,16] Evidence shows a greater number and distribution of oxytocin receptors within the uterine fundus compared to the lower uterine segment.[12] Receptor sensitivity to oxytocin also increases near term. High-affinity oxytocin receptors have been identified in the decidua and amnion. It is postulated that receptor activation in these tissues may play a role in the production of prostaglandins, which also promote uterine contractility.[12,15] Oxytocin is a potent uterotonic agent capable of stimulating uterine contractions with concentrations as low as 1–2 mIU/min.[15] Higher doses may be required, however, in order to generate contractions of sufficient frequency and intensity to facilitate cervical dilation. Intravenous oxytocin is rapidly degraded and has a biologic half-life of 3–4 min.

Labor Mechanics

Successful labor depends upon many factors. The three most important of which are the uterus, the fetus, and the pelvis. A popular mnemonic to describe these three is the "power," "passenger," and "pelvis."[17] Alterations in any of these variables can affect the duration of labor and its success.

Power

Uterus

Uterine contractions may be characterized by their frequency, intensity, and duration. Objective methods of assessing uterine activity include direct palpation, measurement via external tocodynamometer, and measurement through an intrauterine pressure catheter (IUPC). Direct palpation can be used to estimate frequency and duration of contractions although it is less exact with regard to duration and intensity compared to the external tocodynamometer. The external tocodynamometer measures changes in abdominal wall tension, which can occur as a result of uterine contractions, maternal repositioning, fetal movement, or increased intra-abdominal pressure due to maternal factors such as coughing or laughter. Uterine contractions produce a slow increase in abdominal wall tension, which will peak and then return to baseline. Neither external tocodynamometer nor palpation will permit an assessment of baseline uterine tone or contraction intensity. An IUPC provides the most accurate evaluation of uterine tone, contraction intensity, and contraction frequency. Because the IUPC must traverse the vagina and cervix prior to intrauterine placement, its use is associated with a theoretical risk of ascending infection. In randomized controlled trials (RCTs) of internal and external monitor use, internal monitors were not associated with a significant reduction in cesarean section or an increase in intrauterine infection.[18] A recent retrospective cohort study, however, reports a twofold higher risk of fever for women with an IUPC compared to women without (11.7 versus 4.5%, adjusted odds ratio (AOR) 2.0, 95% confidence interval (CI) 1.6–2.5), there was no significant difference in composite neonatal morbidity.[19] Use of the IUPC can be especially beneficial for women with a high body mass index (BMI) with a body habitus that does not permit adequate external evaluation of uterine tone. Additional studies are needed in order to determine the risks and benefits of this device with regard to maternal infection.

The minimum frequency of uterine contractions necessary to result in cervical change is variable and poorly defined. The American Congress of Obstetrics and Gynecology (ACOG) and the National Institute of Child Health and Human Development (NICHD) have defined the upper limit of normal uterine contraction frequency as less than or equal to five contractions in 10 min, averaged over a 30 min window.[20,21] Tachysystole is a term used to define abnormal uterine contraction frequency of more than five contractions in 10 min averaged over 30 min. Any documentation of tachysystole should also include the presence or absence of fetal heart rate decelerations.

After placing the IUPC, the Montevideo unit (MVU) can be used as an objective estimate of uterine activity. The MVU is a measure of the average strength of uterine contractions (peak amplitude minus basal amplitude in mmHg) multiplied by the number of contractions over 10 min. ACOG recommends a threshold of ≥200 MVU to define adequate labor in the active phase.[22,23] The MVU threshold associated with adequate labor in the latent phase has not been determined.

Definitions for several fetal characteristics that may affect the duration of labor are detailed below.

Passenger

Fetal Size

Relative disproportion between fetal weight and maternal pelvic dimensions can increase the risk for prolonged labor, cesarean section, and shoulder dystocia.[24] In the third trimester, ultrasound-derived estimates of fetal weight have an average range of error of 15%. The superiority of ultrasound-derived estimates of fetal weight over clinical estimates has not been established.[25] Among parous post-term women with fetal estimated fetal weight (EFW) > 4,000 g, the mean standard error of the patient's estimate of fetal weight was not significantly different from the standard error of the estimation of fetal weight by her obstetric provider.[26]

Fetal Lie

The term fetal lie refers to the long axis of the fetus in relation to the long axis of the mother. Fetal lie can be longitudinal, transverse, or oblique. In a singleton gestation, delivery of a fetus in a transverse or oblique lie is not recommended due to higher risk of risk of cord prolapse and greater risk of neonatal morbidity. Delivery of a fetus with a longitudinal lie can be attempted.

Fetal Presentation

The expression fetal presentation refers to the fetal part above or within the pelvic inlet. In a fetus with a longitudinal lie, the presentation can be either vertex, breech, brow, or chin (mentum). The term compound presentation refers a fetus that has two body parts within the pelvic inlet. A funic presentation occurs when a fetus has its umbilical cord within the pelvic inlet below the level of a fetal part. With a funic presentation, the umbilical cord will deliver or "present" before a fetal part.

Fetal Attitude

The term fetal attitude refers to the degree of flexion or extension of the fetal head in relation to the spine. The fetal attitude can be either flexed (fetal chin in close proximity to the chest), extended (fetal chin extended superiorly such that the occiput is in closer approximation to the base of the posterior neck), or military (fetal head is neither flexed nor extended, the coronal and sagittal planes of the head are contiguous with the coronal and sagittal planes of the body). The degree of extension will determine the presenting bony part and the largest presenting diameter of the fetal head. With a brow presentation, the head is extended and will present the larger diameter through the pelvic inlet (vertex to mentum 13.5 cm). With a face presentation, the head is hyperextended with an average presenting diameter of 9.5 cm (submentum to bregma). Labor arrest is more common when larger diameters present through the pelvic inlet. The architecture of the pelvic floor may help to either maintain flexion or exert corrective forces on an extended head in the early stages of labor.

Fetal Position

The expression fetal position refers to the relationship of the fetal presenting part to the maternal pelvis and is detailed in Table 1.1. Persistent occiput transverse and occiput posterior position can affect the duration of labor and the likelihood of vaginal delivery success.

Fetal Station

The term fetal station refers to the location of bony presenting part above or below the level of the ischial spines. Station is measured in centimeters above (+1 to +5) or below (−1 to −5) the ischial spine, which is designated by 0 station. During a pelvic examination, a right-handed person will most easily palpate the ischial spine on the maternal right at approximately 8 o'clock position. A left-handed examiner will most easily palpate the ischial spine on the maternal left at 4 o'clock position.

Table 1.1 Fetal Presentations and Positions in Labor

Lie	Presentation	Leading Fetal Part	Attitude	Diameters (average cm)	Position
Longitudinal	Breech	Sacrum			Sacrum anterior Sacrum posterior Sacrum transverse
	Cephalic	Occiput	Military	Occipital-frontal (11 cm)	Occiput anterior Occiput posterior Occiput transverse
			Flexed	Suboccipital bregmatic (9.5 cm)	Occiput anterior Occiput posterior Occiput transverse
	Brow	Frontal bone	Extended	Verticomental (13.5 cm)	Frontoanterior Frontoposterior Frontotransverse
	Face	Mentum(chin)	Hyperextended	Submental bregmatic (9.5 cm)	Mentum anterior Mentum posterior Mentum transverse
	Compound	Variable			
	Funic	None-Umbilical cord presents			

Pelvis

Primer on Pelvic Assessment

Normal labor at term requires (1) an appropriate match between the fetal head size and the size of the pelvis, (2) effective uterine propulsive forces, and (3) normal positioning of the presenting fetal part as it traverses the pelvis and pelvic floor. The pelvis is an important component of this triad, which is often overlooked.

Definitions for pelvic diameters, pelvic planes, and pelvic types are detailed below. A comparative evaluation of pelvic types is detailed in Table 1.2. Historically, Coldwell and Malloy are credited with identifying and characterizing four basic female pelvic types, which are named according to the shape of the pelvic inlet.[27] Gynecoid (female) and anthropoid (elongated oval) shaped pelvises have more favorable pelvic diameters for vaginal delivery while android (male) and platypelloid (transverse oval) have shorter anteroposterior and transverse pelvic diameters respectively. These types are seen in Figure 22.1 in Chapter 22. In actual practice, a female pelvis may combine characteristics from several pelvic types.[28] Descriptions of specific components of the boney pelvis are seen in Box 1.1.

An argument can be made that detailed evaluation of the pelvic inlet, mid-pelvis, and pelvic outlet is slowly becoming a lost art. This is in part due to the fact that radiographic attempts to determine threshold pelvic diameters indicative of cephalopelvic disproportion (CPD) have low sensitivity and specificity for the prediction of cesarean section. Neither X-ray pelvimetry, computed tomography, nor magnetic resonance imaging have been proven to have sufficient sensitivity and specificity to predict cesarean section due to CPD prior to the onset of labor.[29,30] It has been said that there is no pelvic shape in which labor is absolutely contraindicated. Fetal weight and head size are important variables as is the ability of the head to “mold” within the pelvis overtime. Clinical evaluation of the pelvis can, however, be a useful adjunct to the maternal assessment and should be used to identify those women who are at risk for a prolonged or protracted labor course due to pelvic dimensions relative to fetal size.

Cardinal Movements of Labor

The fetal head performs a series of movements in order to present its smallest diameter as it traverses inferiorly through the pelvis and vagina. Fetal movement during labor is a continuous process that is

Table 1.2 Comparative Evaluation of Pelvic Characteristics According to Pelvic Type

	Gynecoid (Female)	Android (Male)	Anthropoid	Platypelloid
Pelvic shape of inlet	Oval – round	Heart shaped	Elongated oval	Transverse oval
Pelvic inlet diameters – Diagonal conjugate (Average)	(12.5 cm)	Average to short	Very long	Very short
– Transverse diameter (Average)	(13.5 cm)	Average	Average to Narrow	Wide
Posterior capacity	Deep, broad	Shallow	Long, narrow	Shallow
Anterior capacity (forepelvis)	Rounded, broad	Narrow, angled	Long, rounded	Shallow
Midpelvis characteristics				
– Sidewalls	Straight	Convergent (funnel)	Straight	Straight-divergent
– Ischial spines	Not prominent	Prominent	Variable	Variable
– Interspinous diameter (Average)	10.5 cm	Narrow (9.5 cm)	Average-narrow	Wide
Pelvic outlet				
Subpubic arch	Wide, >90	Angular		
Theoretical risk of malpresentation	none	Possible occiput posterior	Possible occiput posterior	Possible deep transverse arrest

Modified from Caldwell W, Moloy H. Anatomical variations in the female pelvis and their effect in labor, with a suggested classification. *Am J Obstet Gynecol*. 1933;26:479; Whitley 1985.

Box 1.1 Components of the female boney pelvis

Pelvic inlet Boundaries for the bony pelvic inlet are the sacral promontory, bilateral iliopectineal line, and the symphysis pubis.

Diagonal conjugate Distance from sacral promontory to the inferior border of the symphysis pubis. Can be assessed clinically in order to estimate the true anteroposterior diameter of the pelvic inlet.

Obstetric conjugate Distance from the superior border of the symphysis pubis to the sacral promontory. Can only be measured radiographically. A clinical estimation of this diameter can be determined by subtracting 1.5 cm from the diagonal conjugate.

Midpelvis The midpelvis is bounded anteriorly by the inferior border of the symphysis pubis, laterally by the ischial spines, posteriorly by the sacrum. It is considered the pelvic plane with the smallest pelvic dimension.

Pelvic Outlet Most inferior boundary of the bony pelvis. It is defined by the pubic arch, pubic rami, ischial tuberosities, and tip of the coccyx. The pelvic outlet is of less clinical significance. It can be described by the angle of the subpubic arch and the distance between the ischial tuberosities. The average pubic angle is > 90° and can accommodate two fingers.

characterized by seven discrete events. The fetus may perform these sequentially or the fetus may perform several simultaneously during its descent through the birth canal.[17] The events are described in Box 1.2.

Labor Progress

Labor is defined as the process by which regular uterine contractions result in cervical dilation and effacement. Labor is divided into three discreet stages. The first stage of labor begins with the onset of labor and ends with complete cervical dilation. The second stage of labor begins with complete cervical dilation and ends with delivery of the fetus. The third stage of labor begins with delivery of the fetus and ends with delivery of the placenta. The first stage of labor is divided into two phases: (i) the latent phase, which is characterized by a slow rate of cervical dilation, and (ii) the active phase, which has a more rapid rate of dilation. Skilled evaluation of the cervix with regard to dilation and effacement are necessary in order to track labor progress. Effacement refers to the ability of the cervix to decrease in thickness and length over time as labor progresses. Effacement can be reported as an absolute length or as a percentage. A cervix that is 0% effaced is thick, is typically at least 2 cm long, and has not begun

Box 1.2 Cardinal movements of labor

1. **Engagement** occurs when the widest diameter of the presenting part passes through the pelvic inlet. With a cephalic presentation, the largest anteroposterior and transverse diameters of the fetal head entering the pelvic inlet will depend upon the attitude of flexion. In a fully flexed head, the biparietal diameter (BPD) (average length at term 9.5 cm) is the widest diameter to traverse the pelvic inlet and the suboccipitobregmatic diameter is the longest anterior posterior diameter (average length at term 9.5 cm). Engagement typically occurs when the leading fetal part reaches the level of the ischial spines (O station) and is an appropriate test of the size of the pelvic inlet relative to fetal dimensions.
2. **Descent** refers to downward movement of the fetus through the pelvic inlet, midpelvis, and pelvic outlet onto the pelvic floor. This is a continuous process. The rate of descent is affected by maternal parity, uterine contractile forces, pelvic dimensions, fetal size, and maternal pushing effort prior to delivery.
3. **Flexion** of the fetal head is believed to begin before the onset of labor. The degree of flexion increases passively during the course of labor as the fetus traverses the pelvis and encounters the pelvic floor.
4. **Internal Rotation.** Many fetuses will enter the pelvis in the occiput transverse position. Movement of the fetal head from occiput transverse to the occiput anterior (common) or occiput posterior (less common) occurs passively as the fetus encounters the symphysis pubis and inferior hollow of the sacrum.
5. **Extension** refers to upward movement of the chin away from the fetal chest as the occiput passes below the symphysis. The birth canal curves upward as the fetal presenting part begins to pass the inferior border of the sacrum and reaches the coccygeus and ileococcygeus muscles of the pelvic floor. Progressive extension of the fetal head occurs due to the downward force exerted by uterine contractions and the upward forces generated by resistance from the musculature of the pelvic floor.
6. **External Rotation** refers to passive lateral movement of the fetal head to its anatomically correct position. After the fetal head passes the vaginal introitus, resistance from the pelvic floor is no longer a determining factor in the direction of movement of the fetal head. Intrinsic tone within the musculature of the head and neck will facilitate passive lateral rotation of the head so that the face and anterior thorax are properly aligned within the same plane.
7. **Expulsion** refers to the delivery of the body below the level of the fetal head. The downward forces generated by uterine contractions and maternal pushing efforts and the upward resistance generated by the pelvic floor facilitate rotation of the anterior shoulder below the symphysis and out the vaginal introitus. The body follows the anterior shoulder in similar fashion.

to decrease in size due to labor forces. A cervix that is 100% effaced has no palpable length or thickness. An effacement of 80% or more is typically observed for women in the active phase of labor. There is a significant association between maternal parity and the rate of cervical dilation and effacement. Progressive descent of the fetal presenting part is expected as labor progresses. Like cervical dilation, fetal station can be affected by parity, uterine contractile forces, fetal size, and pelvic dimensions.

The onset of labor is hard to define as it is often made retrospectively in a patient with uterine contractions after documented evidence of cervical change is present. Exactly when a patient develops uterine contractions of sufficient intensity and frequency to begin the process of cervical change is difficult to determine with certainty. The latent phase of labor is characterized by a period of slow cervical change while the active phase of labor is characterized by a rapid rate of cervical dilation. Identification of the period in which the patient transitions from the latent phase to the active phase is often made retrospectively as it is dependent upon the timing and frequency of cervical examinations in labor.

Landmark data presented by Friedman has been used historically to define normal and abnormal rates of cervical dilation in labor. In the original study, the rate of cervical dilation during term labor at term for 500 primaparous and 500 multiparous women was used to generate a sigmoid shaped curve of average labor progress.[31,32] The plotting of the cervical dilation in cm (y-axis) against time in hours (x-axis) transforms the cervical examination from a static assessment performed at discrete intervals into a continuous process by which the average rate of change

Box 1.3 Average spontaneous labor characteristics in a study of 500 primaparous and 500 multiparous women at term in the 1950s

	Primipara[a]	95th percentile	Multipara[b]	95th percentile
Latent phase duration(mean, h)	8.6	20.6	5.3	13.6
Active phase duration (mean, h)	4.9	11.7	2.2	5.2
Maximum slope (cm/h)	3.0	1.2 (5th percentile)	5.7	1.5 (5th percentile)
Second stage duration (mean, h)	57 min	2.5	18 min	50 min

Data from: [a]Friedman E. Primigravid labor. *Obstet Gynecol.* 1955;6:567 and [b]Friedman E., Labor in multiparas: A graphicostatistical analysis. *Obstet Gynecol.* 1956;8:691.

can be determined. The latent phase of labor is characterized by a more flattened slope. The latent phase is followed by a brief acceleration phase in which the slope begins to increase. The active phase corresponds to a steep slope, which is characterized by the most rapid rate of cervical change (see Figure 1.1). The reported mean and 5th percentile of normal duration of the latent phase, active phase, first stage, and second stage of labor are listed in Box 1.3. It is important to note that the most rapid rate of cervical dilation begins after 4 cm cervical dilation is achieved and as a result 4 cm is used to signal the beginning of the active phase. The average rate of cervical dilation in the active phase for nulliparous women was 3.2 cm/h with 1.2 cm/h as the 5th percentile of normal.[31] From 1955 to 2000 as a result of the Freidman studies, a cervical dilation of 4 cm was used to denote the active phase of labor and a minimum rate of cervical dilation of 1 cm/h in the active phase was expected. In the studies published by Friedman, only 13.8% of the primparous women and 11.2% of the multiparous women were augmented with pitocin. Approximately 51.4% of the nulliparas and 20.2% for multiparas were delivered by low forceps. As expected in the 1950s, the cesarean section rate in the study population was very low (1.8% for nulliparas and 0.8% multiparas).[31,32]

Labor management options have changed significantly over the last five decades. Labor induction, epidural analgesia, oxytocin, and continuous fetal monitoring are readily available options for patients

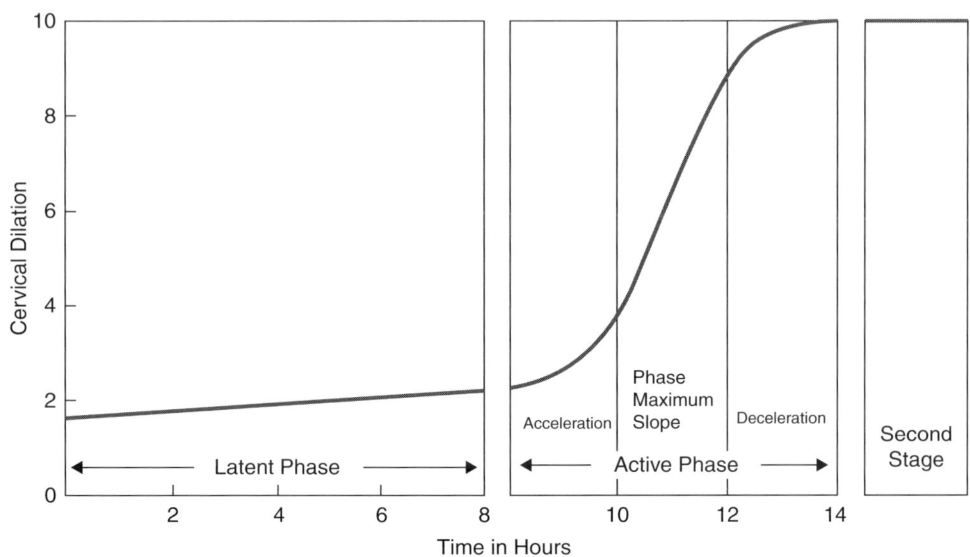

Figure 1.1 Friedman's curve.

and their obstetric providers. The obesity epidemic has resulted in an average BMI that is higher now than it was in the 1950s and as a result fetal macrosomia is more common now than it was five decades ago. More recent studies evaluating labor progress with a contemporary patient population have challenged traditionally held beliefs regarding the latent phase duration, active phase duration, and cervical dilation, which heralds the beginning of the active phase. The transition from latent to active labor was evaluated by Peisner and Rosen in 1986.[33] Approximately 1,600 nulliparous and multiparous women in spontaneous labor were evaluated. In this study, active labor was defined as a cervical dilation rate of 1.5 cm/h for multiparas and 1.2 cm/h for nulliparas; both of which are the 5th percentile of normal according to the original Friedman cohort.[33] With contemporary labor management, only 50% of women at 4 cm cervical dilation met active phase criteria. At 5 cm, 74% of women were in the active phase. At 6 cm, 89% of women met active phase criteria. This study suggests that a significant percentage of women who go on to have a vaginal delivery will still be in the latent phase of labor at 4 cm of cervical dilation. Review of data generated by the National Collaborative Perinatal Project from 1959 to 1966 similarly determined a slow rate of cervical change prior to 6 cm, regardless of parity.[34] Retrospective evaluation of contemporary spontaneous term labor data from the Consortium on Safe Labor further challenged historical assumptions regarding the duration and rate of dilation in the active phase.[35] In this study, detailed labor and delivery data from >62,000 women in 19 medical centers from 2002 to 2008 was evaluated. It was found that 71–84% of women received an epidural and 45–47% received oxytocin augmentation. Nulliparous and multiparous women were determined to have a similar slow rate of cervical change prior to 6 cm dilation. For nulliparas, a change in cervical dilation from 4 to 5 cm could take up to 6.4 h (95th percentile) and a change in cervical dilation from 5 to 6 cm could take up to 3.2 h (95th percentile). After achievement of dilation to 6 cm, the rate of cervical change increased regardless of parity although multiparas were noted to have a faster rate of change. Median and 95th percentile duration of incremental cervical change according to parity is detailed in Box 1.4. ACOG and the Society for Maternal Fetal Medicine (SMFM) issued a consensus statement in support of the recommendations generated by Zhang et al. and the Consortium on Safe Labor data.[36] With contemporary labor management, most women in term labor continue to have a slow rate of cervical change from 4 to 6 cm and as a result 6 cm and not 4 cm should be considered the threshold cervical dilation for the initiation of the active phase.[36]

Second Stage of Labor

With regard to the duration of the second stage of labor, the Consortium on Safe Labor data regarding the median and 95th percentile duration of the second stage of labor are detailed in Box 1.4. It should be

Box 1.4 Median duration (h) for each centimeter of change in cervical dilation for nulliparas and multiparas (parity =1) in spontaneous labor

Cervical dilation (cm)	Nullipara		Multipara	
	Median (h)	95th percentile (h)	Median (h)	95th percentile (h)
3–4	1.8	8.1	——	——
4–5	1.3	6.4	1.4	7.3
5–6	0.8	3.2	0.8	3.4
6–7	0.6	2.2	0.5	1.9
7–8	0.5	1.6	0.4	1.3
8–9	0.5	1.4	0.3	1.0
9–10	0.5	1.8	0.3	0.9

* An interval-censored regression model to estimate the distribution of time for progression from one centimeter to the next with the assumption of log normal distribution of the labor data.

Modified from Zhang J, Landy H, Branch D, et al. Consortium on safe labor: Contemporary patterns of spontaneous labor with normal neonatal outcomes. *Obstet Gynecol* 2010;116:1281.

noted that an epidural extended the median duration of the second stage by 1 h for nulliparous women.[35] In addition to epidural analgesia, there are a number factors that have been reported to influence the length of the second stage including fetal position, parity, fetal weight, maternal BMI, epidural analgesia, and maternal pushing efforts. With contemporary management and continuous fetal monitoring, an absolute maximum threshold duration for the second stage of labor, which is associated with an increased risk of neonatal morbidity has yet to be clearly defined.[36] While most women will have a second stage duration of less than 2 h, the ACOG/SMFM consensus document now considers at least 2 h of pushing for multiparas and 3 h of pushing for nulliparas without an epidural appropriate. For women with an epidural, at least 3 h of pushing for multiparas and 4 h of pushing for nulliparas are appropriate depending upon maternal and fetal status. There is no evidence that these time limits are associated with increased maternal or neonatal morbidity.[36]

Delivery of the Fetus

The obstetric provider is physically present during the second stage of labor in order to facilitate maternal pushing efforts, assess fetal position and station as the fetus navigates the pelvis, and to assure maternal and fetal stability prior to delivery. During the delivery process, the obstetric provider is responsible for leading a team that includes the patient, her support person(s), nursing staff, and pediatric staff if they are called to attend. It is not only the obstetric provider's hands but his or her voice that can play an important role in the facilitation of a safe delivery for mother and baby. Communication with the patient during the intrapartum period manages patient expectations enables the patient to be a proactive participant and facilitates nursing support during the birth process.

When delivery is imminent, the fetal head will extend through the vaginal introitus. The obstetric provider should place gentle pressure on the fetal head in order to minimize rapid extension of the head and reduce the risk of perineal and/or periurethral injury. The head will deliver over the perineum and then rotate laterally so that the face and body are in the anatomically correct orientation. Nuchal umbilical cord loops may be reduced if they are loose or the cord may be transected and cut if reduction over the head is not possible. The patient should then be asked to push while the obstetric provider applies gentle downward and outward traction in the axis of the pelvic curve on the fetal head in order to facilitate delivery of the anterior shoulder. The posterior shoulder is then delivered with upward traction. It is important to avoid injury to the maternal perineum and fetal brachial plexus during this process. Avoiding excessive use of force and excessive lateral traction are ways to reduce fetal and maternal risk.

Meconium staining of amniotic fluid is no longer an indication for intubation and suctioning below the level of the vocal cords if the fetus is vigorous at delivery. If the fetus is depressed, however, prompt evaluation is recommended per American Academy of Pediatrics (AAP) guidelines.[37] If the amniotic fluid is meconium stained and the fetus is vigorous, routine suctioning below the vocal cords is not indicated.

After delivery, holding the baby at or below the level of the placenta/maternal perineum will facilitate passive transfusion of blood from the cord to the baby. Passive transfusion will cease when the cord is clamped or when the umbilical veins begin the spasm and contract. There is evidence that a > 2 min delay in umbilical cord clamping for term infants after delivery results in a significant increase in hematocrit, ferritin, and stored iron at 2 to 6 months with no significant increase in the risk of maternal hemorrhage. Delayed cord clamp was associated, however, with an increased neonatal risk of jaundice and polycythemia.[38,39] In preterm infants <37 weeks gestation, a > 30 s delay was associated with a decreased risk of anemia requiring transfusion, 50% reduction in intraventricular hemorrhage, and decreased risk of necrotizing enterocolitis compared to infants with immediate cord clamping. A higher bilirubin was also identified in this population.[40] For preterm infants, ACOG supports the practice of delayed cord clamping (>30 s) compared to immediate cord clamping when clinically possible in a vigorous infant. For term infants, however, the data is insufficient to either confirm or refute the benefits of delayed cord clamping (>2 min).[41] Additional data is required in order to determine the neonatal benefits in term infants associated with a shorter duration of delay (>30 s) and or with "milking" of the umbilical cord prior to clamping.

After delivery, the infant should be placed on the mother's abdomen and dried. A blanket and hat may be placed on the neonate in order to assist with temperature regulation. The neonate should lay with its bare chest and abdomen exposed on the maternal skin near the patient's breast in order to facilitate bonding and attachment. Meta-analysis of data from 13 RCTs suggests that immediate or early "skin to skin contact" increases the likelihood of breastfeeding initiation at 1 to 4 months by 27% (RR 1.27; 95% CI, 1.06 to 1.53) and results in higher blood glucose at 75 to 90 min of life compared with standard care.[42]

Third Stage of Labor

The third stage of labor begins after delivery of the baby and ends with delivery of the placenta. The three signs of placental separation are: (1) change in shape of the uterine fundus as it begins to contract, (2) lengthening of the umbilical cord as the placenta descends through the cervix, and (3) a gush of blood from the vagina secondary to separation of the placenta from the uterine myometrium. Separation of the placenta can occur passively without manual manipulation of the placenta or uterus. Active management of the third stage of labor refers to: (1) administration of uterotonic medication after delivery of the baby in order to improve uterine tone, (2) controlled traction on the umbilical cord and counter traction against the fundus/lower uterine segment in order hasten placental separation and prevent uterine inversion, and (3) uterine massage after delivery of the placenta.[43,44] Active management of the third stage of labor has been proven in randomized controlled trials to significantly decrease the risk of postpartum hemorrhage and is recommended by ACOG as a universal measure to reduce the risk of postpartum hemorrhage due to uterine atony for all women regardless of the their pre-delivery hemorrhage risk.[45]

Concluding Remarks

Normal labor is a complex process that requires adequate uterine contractions, a fetus of sufficient size to navigate the maternal pelvis, and favorable pelvic dimensions relative to fetal size. Fetal presentation, position, and the attitude of flexion of the fetal vertex can affect the duration of labor, its likelihood of success, and the safety of a vaginal delivery attempt. Labor is not a passive process for the obstetric provider as it requires careful evaluation of the cervix over time, along with an assessment of uterine contractions and an assessment of fetal descent within the pelvis. These evaluations distinguish those women who would benefit from obstetric interventions from those who are progressing as expected. Abnormal labor can increase maternal and fetal risk of an adverse outcome. Chapter 2 will present the evidence supporting our current understanding of abnormal labor and review management strategies proven to reduce maternal and fetal morbidity once abnormal labor is identified.

References

1. Ravanos K, Dagklis T, Petousis S, Margioula-Siarkou C, Prapas Y, Prapas N. Factors implicated in the initiation of human parturition in term and preterm labor: a review. *Gynecol Endocrinol* 2015;31(9):679–83.
2. Norwitz ER, Robinson JN, Challis JR. The control of labor. *N Engl J Med* 1999;341:660–6.
3. Challis JRG, Matthews SG, Gibb W, Lye SJ. Endocrine and paracrine regulation of birth at term and preterm. *Endocr Rev* 2000;21:514–50.
4. Hamilton BE, Martin JA, Osterman MJ, Curtin SC, Matthews TJ. Births: Final Data for 2014. *Natl Vital Stat Rep* 2015 Dec;64(12):1–64.
5. Kozhimannil KB, Law MR, Virnig BA. Cesarean delivery rates vary tenfold among US hospitals: Reducing variation may address quality and cost issues. *Health Aff (Millwood)* 2013;32:527–35.
6. American College of Obstetricians and Gynecologists, Society for Maternal-Fetal Medicine. Obstetric care consensus no. 1: safe prevention of the primary cesarean delivery. *Obstet Gynecol* 2014;123(3):693–711.
7. Lockwood C. The initiation of parturition at term. *Obstet Gynecol Clin North Am* 2004;31(4):935.
8. Liao J, Buhimschi C, Norwitz E. Normal labor: mechanism and duration. *Obstet Gynecol Clin North Am* 2005;32:145.
9. Beshay V, Carr B, Rainey W. The human fetal adrenal gland, corticotropin releasing hormone, and parturition. *Semin Reprod Med* 2007;25(1):14.
10. Oh S, Kim C, Park I, et al. Progesterone receptor isoform (A/B) ratio of human fetal membranes increases during term parturition. *Am J Obstet Gynecol* 2005;193:1156.
11. Messano S. Myometrial progesterone responsiveness. *Semin Reprod Med* 2007;25:5–13.
12. Fuchs A, Fuchs F, Husslein P, Soloff M. Oxytocin receptors in the human uterus during pregnancy and parturition. *Am J Obstet Gynecol* 1984;150:734.
13. Fuchs A, Husslein P, Fuchs F. Oxytocin and the initiation of human parturition. II. Stimulation of prostaglandin production in human decidua by oxytocin. *Am J Obstet Gynecol* 1981;141:694.
14. Blanks AM, Thornton S. The role of oxytocin in parturition. *Br J Obstet Gynecol* 2003;110(suppl 20):46.

15. Zeeman G, Khan-Dawood F, Dawood M. Oxytocin and its receptor in pregnancy and parturition: Current concepts and clinical implications. *Obstet Gynecol* 1997;89:873.
16. Dawood M, Wang C, Gupta R, et al. Fetal contribution to oxytocin in human labor. *Obstet Gynecol* 1978;52:205.
17. Garrison EA, Kilpatrick SJ. Normal Labor. In: Gabbe SG, Niebyl JR, Simpson JL, Landon MB, Galan HL, Jauniaux ERM, Driscoll DA, eds. *Obstetrics: Normal and Problem Pregnancies*. Philadelphia: Saunders Elsevier, 6th ed.;2012.
18. Bakker JJ, Verhoeven CJ, Janssen PF, et al. Outcomes after internal versus external tocodynamometry for monitoring labor. *N Engl J Med* 2010;362:306–13.
19. Harper LM, Shanks AL, Tuuli MG, Roehl KA, Cahill AG. The Risks and Benefits of Internal Monitors in Laboring Patients. *Am J Obstet Gynecol.* 2013;209(1):38.e1–38.
20. Macones G, Hankins G, Spong C, et al. The 2008 National Institute of Child Health and Human Development workshop report on electronic fetal monitoring: update on definitions, interpretation, and research guidelines. *Obstet Gynecol* 2008;112:661.
21. American College of Obstetricians and Gynecologists. Induction of labor. ACOG Practice Bulletin No. 107. *Obstet Gynecol* 2009;114:386–97.
22. Caldeyro-Barcia R, Sica-Blanco Y, Poseiro J, et al. A quantitative study of the action of synthetic oxytocin on the pregnant human uterus. *J Pharmacol Exp Ther* 1957;121:18.
23. American College of Obstetricians and Gynecologists. Obstetric care consensus no. 1: Safe prevention of the primary cesarean delivery. *Obstet Gynecology* 2014;123(3):693–711.
24. Rossi A, Mullin P, Prefumo F. Prevention, management, and outcomes of macrosomia: A systematic review of literature and meta-analysis. *Obstet Gynecol Surv* 2013;68(10):702.
25. American College of Obstetricians and Gynecologists. *Fetal Macrosomia*. Washington, DC: American College of Obstetricians and Gynecologists;2000.
26. Chauhan SP, Sullivan CA, Lutton TC, Magann EF, Morrison JC. Parous patients' estimate of birth weight in postterm pregnancy. *J Perinatol* 1995. May–Jun;15(3):192–4.
27. Caldwell W, Moloy H. Anatomical variations in the female pelvis and their effect in labor, with a suggested classification. *Am J Obstet Gynecol* 1933; 26:479.
28. Whitley, N. ed. *A Manual of Clinical Obstetrics*. Baltimore: Lippincott;1985:162–7.
29. Maharaj D. Assessing cephalopelvic disproportion: back to the basics. *Obstet Gynecol Surv* 2010; 65(6):387.
30. Zaretsky M, Alexander J, McIntire D, et al. Magnetic resonance imaging pelvimetry and the prediction of labor dystocia. *Obstet Gynecol* 2005;106(5 Pt 1):919.
31. Friedman E. Primigravid labor. *Obstet Gynecol* 1955;6:567.
32. Friedman E. Labor in multiparas; a graphicostatistical analysis. *Obstet Gynecol* 1956;8:691.
33. Peisner DB, Rosen MG. Transition from latent to active labor. *Obstet Gynecol* 1986;68:441.
34. Zhang J, Troendle J, Mikolajczyk R, et al. The natural history of the normal first stage of labor. *Obstet Gynecol* 2010;115:705.
35. Zhang J, Landy H, Branch D, et al. Consortium on Safe Labor. Contemporary patterns of spontaneous labor with normal neonatal outcomes. *Obstet Gynecol* 2010;116:1281.
36. Obstetrics Care Consensus No. 1. Safe prevention of the primary cesarean delivery. *Obstet Gynecol* 2014;123(3):693.
37. Committee on Obstetric Practice, American College of Obstetricians and Gynecologists. (ACOG) Committee Opinion No. 379: Management of delivery of a newborn with meconium-stained amniotic fluid. *Obstet Gynecol* 2007;110(3):739.
38. Hutton E, Hassan E. Late vs early clamping of the umbilical cord in full term neonates: Systematic review and meta-analysis of controlled trials. *JAMA* 2007;297:1241.
39. McDonald S, Middleton P, Dowswell T, et al. Effect of timing of umbilical cord clamping of term infants on maternal and neonatal outcomes. *Cochrane Database Syst Rev* 2013;(7):CD004074.
40. Rabe H, Diaz-Rossello J, Duley L, et al. Effect of timing of umbilical cord clamping and other strategies to influence placental transfusion at preterm birth on maternal and infant outcomes. *Cochrane Database Syst Rev* 2012;(8):Art. No.: CD003248.
41. Committee on Obstetric Practice. American College of Obstetricians and Gynecologists. Committee Opinion No. 543: Timing of umbilical cord clamping after birth. *Obstet Gynecol* 2012;120:1522.
42. Moore ER, Anderson GC, Bergman N, Dowswell T. Early skin-to-skin contact for mothers and their healthy newborn infants. *Cochrane Database Syst Rev* 2012;(5):CD003519.
43. Rogers J, Wood J, McCandlish R, et al. Active versus expectant management of third stage of labour: The Hinchingbrooke randomised controlled trial. *Lancet.* 1998;351:693.

44. Begley M, Gyte G, Devane D, McGuire W, Weeks A. Active versus expectant management for women in the third stage of labour. *Cochrane Database Syst Rev* 2011;(11):CD007412.

45. Main, EK, Goffman, D, Scavone, BM, Low, LK, Bingham D, Fontaine, PL, Gorlin, JB, Lagrew, DC, Levy, BS. National Partnership for Maternal Safety: Consensus Bundle on Obstetric Hemorrhage. *Obstet Gynecol* 2015 July:126(1);155–62.

Abnormal Labor

Rolanda Standifer and Etoi A. Garrison

Introduction

Labor is a complex physiologic process by which regular uterine contractions lead to progressive cervical dilation, effacement, and fetal descent through the pelvis. Labor that results in vaginal birth involves three key factors commonly referred to as the "three Ps": the power, the passenger, and the pelvis.[1] The power refers to strength, duration, and frequency of uterine contractions. The passenger refers to the estimated fetal weight, fetal position, fetal lie, and fetal presentation. The pelvis refers to the maternal bony pelvis. For hospital-based deliveries, there is a fourth "P" that can significantly influence the likelihood of a successful vaginal birth – the obstetric provider.

A thorough understanding of normal and abnormal labor will enable the obstetrician to offer evidence-based interventions that can improve the odds of vaginal delivery and minimize maternal and fetal risk by determining when a cesarean section is indicated. While the term cephalopelvic disproportion (CPD) is often used in discussions of labor management, by itself the term CPD is imprecise. The six classic dysfunctional labor patterns are listed in Box 2.1. This chapter will present the evidence supporting our current understanding of abnormal labor, review maternal–fetal risk factors, and present evidence-based management options should abnormal labor occur.

Box 2.1 Classic dysfunctional labor patterns

Protracted latent phase	*Latent phase disorder*
Protracted dilation	*First stage disorder*
Arrest of dilation	*First stage disorder*
Prolonged deceleration phase	*First stage disorder*
Protracted descent	*Second stage disorder*
Arrest of descent	*Second stage disorder*

Scope of the Problem

Emanuel Friedman published studies evaluating the labor progress of 500 primigravid and nulligravid women in the 1950s, all of whom presented in spontaneous labor.[2,3] Our understanding of normal labor and the criteria for the diagnosis of labor dystocia (abnormal labor) were historically developed from the outer limits of the Friedman curve.[4] Friedman's work advanced previously published studies designed to characterize cervical dilation in labor with respect to time.[5] The validity and clinical utility of the sigmoid curve originally presented by Friedman has been corroborated by numerous studies since its original publication.[5–12] Friedman's curve is shown in Figure 1.1 of Chapter 1. Contemporary obstetric practice and the rising cesarean section rate has caused the traditional interpretation of the Friedman to be questioned.[13] Data from the Consortium on Safe Labor published by Zhang et al. present an evaluation of contemporary labor progress for over 62,000 nulliparous and multiparous women that challenges the threshold cervical dilation for the diagnosis of active labor and challenges our understanding of labor duration.[13,14] The American Congress of Obstetrics and Gynecology (ACOG) and the Society for Maternal-Fetal Medicine (SMFM) published a consensus document, which emphasized the importance of allowing adequate time for the first and second stages of labor to progress based upon the Consortium for Safe Labor data and other recent studies. This chapter will review the evidence that forms the basis for current recommendations.

Latent Phase

The first stage of labor begins with the onset of labor and ends with complete cervical dilation. It is characterized by two phases: a latent phase and an active phase. The latent phase of labor begins with the onset of labor and ends when there is a transition from a slow rate of dilation to a more rapid rate of cervical dilation. Clinically, maternal symptoms may include contractions of varying intensity with a very slow rate of accompanying cervical change. The duration of latent labor is difficult to determine with certainty because it is difficult to know exactly when cervical change begins in a woman who is contracting regularly. Labor can only be confirmed by a cervical examination after dilation has already occurred. As a result, reports of latent phase duration are highly variable. In Freidman's evaluation of labor for 500 nulliparous and multiparous women, the average duration of the latent phase was 6.4 h for nulliparous women and 4.8 h for multiparous women. The 95th percentile for women who went on to have a vaginal delivery was 20 and 14 h, respectively.[2,3] In Friedman's study populations, 13.8% of the primparous women and 11.2% of the multiparous women were augmented with pitocin. Approximately 51.4% of the nulliparas and 20.2% for multiparas were delivered by low forceps. The cesarean section rate was 1.8% for nulliparas and 0.8% multiparas.[2,3] Epidural analgesia was given to 8.4% of the nulliparas and 10.6% of the multiparas. With contemporary labor management, epidural analgesia, cesarean section, and pitocin administration have become increasingly more common.

Data generated by the Consortium on Safe Labor have been used to characterize contemporary labor progress. In studies published by Zhang et al., detailed labor and delivery data were collected from 2002 to 2008 in > 62,000 women at 19 medical centers.[14] In the study cohort, 71–84% of women received an epidural and 45–47% received oxytocin augmentation. A comparative evaluation of the first stage of labor data generated by Friedman and the Consortium on Safe Labor are presented in Table 2.1. The first stage of labor is shorter for nulliparas and multiparas in contemporary data presented by the Consortium on Safe labor compared that reported by Friedman. A direct comparison is made difficult, however, due to significant differences in study design. In the Consortium on Safe Labor cohort, all multiparas were admitted to the hospital with a 4 cm or more cervical dilation and as a result the complete duration of latent labor cannot be determined from the data presented. An admission cervical examination for the subjects in the Friedman study was not reported. The median rate of cervical dilation in the active phase for subjects in the Friedman study was 3.3 cm/h for nulliparas and 5.7cm/h for multiparas. The 5th percentile for nulliparas and multiparas was 1.2 cm/h and 1.5 cm/h respectively.[2,3] A median rate of cervical dilation in the active phase was not reported for subjects in the Zhang study. Detailed information regarding the median rate of cervical dilation according to centimeter was reported in the Zhang study. From 6–7 cm, the median and 95th percentile rates of cervical dilation for nulliparas and multiparas were 0.6 cm/h (95th percentile 2.2cm/h) and 0.5 cm/h (95th percentile 1.9 cm/h).[14]

Disorders and Treatment of Latent Phase

Based upon the original Friedman data, prolonged latent phase is defined as >20 h for the nulliparous woman and > 14 h for the multiparous women.[15]

The threshold durations above reflect the 95th percentile of the latent phase duration expected after admission in labor. Cervical dilation on admission can, however, affect latent phase duration. An evaluation of the literature is also complicated by the fact that there is disagreement regarding the cervical dilation used to designate the end of the latent phase and the beginning of the active phase. It has been estimated that, with in tact membranes, many women may be in latent phase for hours to days prior to hospital admission. If there are no maternal or fetal contraindications, observation and expectant management are recommended for women who are hospitalized with in tact membranes and have a prolonged latent phase. If there are clinical indications for an expedited delivery (i.e. pre-eclampsia, gestational hypertension, uncontrolled diabetes at term, ruptured membranes), augmentation with oxytocin, artificial rupture of membranes, or a cervical ripening agent may be employed.

Level I evidence to support latent phase management is limited. In a randomized controlled study of term nulliparous women with in tact membranes in labor for >18 h, the cesarean section rate for those women randomized to expectant management/therapeutic rest was not significantly different from those who were actively managed with a cervical ripening agent and amniotomy (expectant management 37.5% c-section rate vs cervical ripening/amniotomy 23%, p=0.07).[16] In a Cochrane review of early amniotomy/oxytocin for prevention or treatment of prolonged first stage labor compared with routine care, active management was associated with a minor reduction in the cesarean section rate relative to standard care. The studies evaluated did not assess women with a 20 h or more latent phase duration.[17,18]

Table 2.1 Comparative Evaluation of the Duration of Spontaneous Labor at Term using data from Friedman and the Consortium on Safe Labor

Parameter	Friedman		Consortium on Safe Labor	
	Mean or Median	Mean or Median of the 95th Percentile	Mean or Median	Mean or Median of the 95th Percentile
Nulliparas	**Admission cervix – unknown**		**Admission cervix 2–2.5cm (*n*=4, 247)**	
Total duration (h)	10.1	25.8		
Stages				
First (h)	9.7	24.7	8.5	20
Second (min)	33.0	117.5	36 66	168 -without epidural 216 -with epidural
Latent phase duration (h)	6.4	20.6		
Maximal dilation(rate), cm/h	3.3	1.2*		
Median time to dilate 1 cm in active phase (h)	–	–	0.5–0.6#	2.2
Multiparas	**Parity range 1–5 or more**	**Parity range 1–5 or more**	**Parity=1 (*n*=16,755) Admission cervix 4–5cm**	**95th percentile**
Total duration (h)	6.2	19.5		
Stages				
First (h)	8.0	18.8	3.7	15.8
Second (min)	8.5	46.5	24 30	80 -without epidural 120 -with epidural
Latent phase duration	4.8	13.6	–	–
Maximal Dilation(rate), cm/h	5.7	1.5*	–	–
Median time to dilate 1 cm in active phase (h)	–	–	0.3–0.5#	1.9

* 5th percentile, #time to dilate 1 cm in active phase (from 6 to 7 cm, 7 to 8 cm, 8 to 9 cm, and 9 to 10 cm). Modified from Friedman E. Primigravid labor. *Obstet Gynecol.* 1955;6:567, Friedman E. Labor in multiparas: a graphicostatistical analysis. *Obstet Gynecol.* 1956;8:69, and Zhang J, Landy H, Branch D et al. Consortium on safe labor: Contemporary patterns of spontaneous labor with normal neonatal outcomes. *Obstet Gynecol.* 2010;116: 1281.

For patients in whom delivery is not medically indicated, discharge to home versus a trial of therapeutic rest with an intravenous sedative can be used to reduce discomfort until the patient is demonstrated to have a more rapid rate of cervical change. In 1961, Freidman retrospectively evaluated a series of 957 nulliparas who were admitted in latent labor. Less than 10% remained in latent labor beyond 20 h of admission. Approximately half of the subjects were given therapeutic rest and half were given continuous oxytocin. Ninety percent of the women in the cohort delivered vaginally regardless of therapeutic intervention. Women with therapeutic rest may have had a slightly shorter latent phase compared to those who received oxytocin induction.[15] Theoretical benefits to therapeutic rest in the latent phase include decreased number of cervical examinations and reduced risk of chorioamnionitis, and a possible reduced risk of postpartum hemorrhage. Rigorous studies are needed, however, in order to substantiate these assertions. Due to the variable duration of latent phase, early amniotomy should not be performed in nulliparous women with prolonged latent phase. This may potentially lead to prolonged rupture of membranes and its associated infectious morbidity.

Active Phase Labor

The active phase of labor is denoted by regular uterine contractions and a more rapid rate of cervical change. The cervical dilation indicative of the beginning of the active phase and the minimum rate of dilation expected have recently become the subject of debate. Historical data evaluating spontaneous labor curves by Friedman and others determined that the cervical dilation associated with the transition from latent phase to active phase is likely between 3 and 5 cm.[2,3,19] Four centimeters was traditionally designated as the threshold for the initiation of the active phase. Minimum rates of 1.2 cm/h for nulliparas and 1.5 cm/h for multiparas were expected for women who reached 4 cm or more in labor based upon 95th percentile parameters achieved by women in the Friedman dataset. More recent reviews suggest that active phase can begin anywhere from 3 to 6 cm and will depend on variables affecting the individual labor.[5,11] These authors argue that an arbitrary cervical dilation cutoff to diagnose the active phase may sacrifice accuracy, oversimplify labor progress, and place the patient at risk for cesarean due to an incorrect diagnosis.[5] The ACOG and SMFM have utilized data from recent studies to recommend a cervical dilation threshold of 6 cm to indicate the beginning of the active phase. These organizations also argue for a longer duration of observation in active labor before a diagnosis of a labor arrest is made.[20]

Disorders and Treatment of the Active Phase of Labor

There are two main types of active phase disorders: protraction and arrest. Protracted labor refers to slower than normal progression of cervical dilation in the active phase. Arrest of labor is traditionally defined as a complete cessation of cervical dilatation for 2 h or more despite adequate uterine contractions. The traditional definition of protracted active phase is based upon Friedman's work and has been defined as a rate of cervical dilation of less than 1 cm/h, which would represent a rate of less than the 5th percentile in this study cohort.[21]

Data from the Consortium on Safe labor, however, support slower rates of cervical dilation in the active phase.[14] See Table 2.2. An evaluation of the duration of labor from 1 cm dilation to the next suggests that for nulliparous women admitted with a cervical dilation of 3 cm, it could take more than 6 h to progress from 4 to 5 cm (95th percentile). It could take more than 3 h to progress from 5 to 6 cm. For nulliparous women after 6 cm, the 95th percentile rate of change from one cm to the next ranged from 1.4 to 2.2 h per cm.

Table 2.2 Median Duration of Time Elapsed in Hours for Each Centimeter of Cervical Dilation in Spontaneous Labor According to Parity

Cervical Dilation (cm)	Parity 0 (95th Percentile)	Parity 1 (95th Percentile)
3–4	1.8 (8.1)	–
4–5	1.3 (6.4)	1.4 (7.3)
5–6	0.8 (3.2)	0.8 (3.4)
6–7	0.6 (2.2)	0.5 (1.9)
7–8	0.5 (1.6)	0.4 (1.3)
8–9	0.5 (1.2)	0.3 (1.0)
9–10	0.5 (1.8)	0.3 (0.9)

Median elapsed time, h (95th percentile).

Modified from Zhang J, Landy H, Branch D et al. Consortium on safe labor: Contemporary patterns of spontaneous labor with normal neonatal outcomes. *Obstet Gynecol*. 2010;116: 1281.

Prior to 6 cm, nulliparas and multiparas were found to have a similar slow rate of cervical change. After 6 cm, the rate of cervical change for both groups increased (median 0.3–0.5 cm/h); however, multiparas were noted to dilate at a faster rate than nulliparas. These data suggest that 6 cm should be used to designate the beginning of the active phase given the slow rate of cervical change documented prior to this point.

In 2011, a systematic analysis of 18 studies was published, which further supports our understanding of the duration of the active phase in nulliparous women.[21] In a study by Neal et al., active labor was diagnosed with a cervical dilation between 3 and 5 cm and patients were managed at the discretion of their providers. A mean cervical dilation rate of 1.2 cm/h was identified; however, a variance of 0.6 cm/h (2 SD) was noted. The mean and 95th percentile duration of labor were 6 and 13.4 h, values consistent with those identified in the Consortium on Safe Labor dataset.[5,21] In the evaluation of spontaneous labor by Zhang et al., for nulliparous women the median duration of labor from 4 cm cervical dilation to 10 cm was 4.2 h (95th percentile 16.1 h). For women with one prior vaginal delivery, the median duration of labor from 4 to 10 cm was 3.7 h (95th percentile 15.8 h).

Given the variable duration of the active phase and recent controversy regarding the cervical dilation at which it should begin, there is no consensus regarding an acceptable maximum active phase duration. Further, there is no consensus regarding the minimum rate of cervical change considered acceptable in the active phase. A review of the Consortium on Safe

Labor data and Level III evidence (expert opinion) would support a 95th percentile active phase labor duration > 13–15 h and a rate of change of <0.5 cm/h for a protracted labor diagnosis.[22] Slower rates of labor progress are not, however, an indication for cesarean section.[23] With appropriate fetal monitoring and contemporary management, a safe vaginal delivery remains possible and will depend upon the maternal/fetal assessment and uterine activity.

Treatment of Protraction of Labor in the Active Phase

The most common causes of protracted labor are inadequate uterine activity, abnormal position of the fetal presenting part, and relative CPD. A decrease in the frequency and/or intensity of uterine contractions can delay labor progress in the active phase. The use of external tocometers and intrauterine pressure catheter (IUPC) in order to assess uterine activity was described in Chapter 1. For women with active phase labor disorders, the IUPC can be used to obtain an objective measure of the frequency, intensity, and duration of uterine contractions. To place an IUPC, the cervix must be sufficiently dilated and an amniotomy must be performed (if the membranes were previously in tact), in order to allow access to the uterine cavity. After placing the IUPC, the Montevideo unit (MVU) can be used as an objective estimate of uterine activity as previously described in Chapter 1. The MVU is a measure of the average strength of uterine contractions [(average contraction peak amplitude (mmHg) – minus baseline (mmHg)] multiplied by the number of contractions over 10 min. ACOG recommends a threshold of ≥200 MVU to define adequate labor in the active phase. [22] Montevideo units of 200–250 have been described as being adequate to result in cervical change for women in the active phase of labor who ultimately delivered vaginally and in women with active phase arrest who ultimately delivered by cesarean.[24,25] A wide range of MVUs are sufficient to cause cervical change. Fetal monitoring during the active phase is required in order to determine fetal tolerance to the uterine contraction pattern and the MVUs generated. MVU >200 in active labor is associated with the lower limit of uterine contractility that has been demonstrated to result in active phase cervical change and normal Apgar scores.

When uterine underactivity is present, oxytocin may be administered. Oxytocin has a half-life of 3–4 min and can be titrated to achieve adequate contractions, every 2–4 min with goal duration of 60–90 s. Oxytocin is released from the posterior pituitary in a pulsatile fashion and is best administered intravenously by continuous infusion due to first pass effect with oral administration. High- and low-dose oxytocin protocols have been published.[26–28] Low-dose protocols begin at a concentration of 1–2 milliunits/min with dose adjustments made every 30–40 min. There is no universally accepted maximal dose of oxytocin; however, tachysystole is more common with higher doses. Many nursing protocols require separate physician orders once a concentration of 20 miliunits/min has been reached. Higher doses of oxytocin may be utilized if there is an indication and if fetal tolerance is assured.

Active Phase Arrest

Active phase labor arrest has traditionally been defined as the absence of cervical change for at least 2 h in the active phase of labor despite adequate uterine contractions. The "2 h rule" was established by National Institutes of Health (NIH) Cesarean Birth Task Force and ACOG in the 1980s in an effort to reduce the rising cesarean section rate due to abnormal labor or labor dystocia.[29,30] In 1989, ACOG recommended the following criteria prior to first stage labor arrest diagnosis: (1) Confirmation of active phase labor with a cervical dilation of 4 cm or more and (2) sufficient uterine activity as defined by >200 MVU in 10 min for 2 h without cervical change. Several more recent studies have challenged our understanding of the active phase and the duration of labor, which can be safely permitted prior to confirming labor arrest. Rouse et al. published several studies that demonstrate the efficacy and safety of at least 4 h of expectant management for women with active phase arrest.[31] In 1999, these authors evaluated 542 women who presented in term spontaneous labor with active phase arrest per NIH/ACOG criteria. Subjects were given 4 h of oxytocin augmentation at >200 MVUs or 6 h of oxytocin augmentation if >200 MVUs could not be sustained. When subjects were augmented with >2 h of oxytocin, 91% of multiparas and 74% of nulliparas delivered vaginally. When subjects were augmented with >4 h of oxytocin 88% of multiparas and 56% of nulliparas delivered vaginally.[31] This study was repeated in 2001 with a more contemporary cohort. Sixty-one percent of women with a labor arrest by ACOG criteria subsequently had a vaginal delivery when labor was allowed to continue. The 5th percentile rate of cervical dilation for women with oxytocin augmentation was 0.5cm/h. While there were no serious neonatal injuries reported, the risks of chorioamnionitis/endometritis (26%) and shoulder dystocia (13%) were higher than expected. The cesarean section rate in this cohort was 18% for nulliparas and 5% for multiparas.[32] The maternal and fetal risks associated with expectant management beyond 2 h for women with active phase arrest were evaluated by Henry et al. in 2008.[33] A cohort of 1,014 women with active phase arrest by ACOG criteria were identified and labor was allowed to continue for 2–6 h after the arrest diagnosis. In this retrospective evaluation, 33% of the women delivered vaginally. Subjects were less likely to have endomyometritis, chorioamnionitis, and postpartum hemorrhage compared to those with a labor arrest who were delivered by cesarean section. They were, however, more likely to have chorioamnionitis and shoulder dystocia compared to those women who delivered vaginally without a labor disorder. There was no evidence of increased neonatal risk for those with labor arrest and a subsequent vaginal delivery.[33]

ACOG recommendations regarding diagnostic criteria for active phase labor arrest were modified in 2014 due to studies by Rouse et al. and others supporting the likelihood of vaginal delivery with an extended period for observation for women in active labor who exhibit no cervical change despite adequate uterine contractions. Recommendations were modified: cervical dilation signaling the onset of the active phase of labor has been changed to 6 cm based upon a review of the Consortium on Safe Labor data and other studies.[14,20,23] ACOG recommends extension of the "2 h rule" as a result of recent studies, which support the safety of continued labor augmentation and expectant management in women with labor arrest. Active phase arrest is now defined as no cervical change in 4 h for women with ruptured membranes and MVU ≥ 200. If MVU ≥ 200 cannot be obtained, active phase arrest can be diagnosed after 6 h of active phase labor assuming oxytocin augmentation and membrane rupture.[23] It is hoped that revised guidelines will result in a greater likelihood of vaginal delivery and lower the cesarean section rate. Evidence detailing the maternal and neonatal risks associated with contemporary management of women using the new guidelines is limited.[5] It is uncertain if the new guidelines will result in a lowering of the cesarean section rate. The effect of labor prolongation according to the new guidelines on maternal infectious risks and neonatal morbidity are uncertain.

Disorders of the Second Stage

There are two disorders of the second stage: (1) protraction and (2) arrest or failure to descend. Protraction of the second stage is defined as fetal descent through the pelvis at less than the expected rate of 1 cm/h in nulliparous women and 2 cm/h in multiparous women based upon Friedman data.[2,3] Failure to descend was previously defined by ACOG as complete cessation of descent after 3 h of maternal pushing efforts in nulliparous women with an epidural, 2 h of pushing for nulliparous women without an epidural, 2 h of pushing for multiparous women with an epidural, and 1 h of pushing for multiparous women without an epidural.[34] Historically, extrapolation of Friedman's second stage duration data was limited due to common practice patterns in the 1950s. Approximately 10% of women received epidural analgesia, and a similarly small percentage of women were given pitocin augmentation. Operative vaginal delivery was more common after 2 h of maternal pushing despite reassuring fetal testing. With the advent of fetal monitoring in the second stage, it is incumbent upon the obstetric provider to know the maximum duration for second stage pushing that will permit a vaginal delivery and will not result in a significant increase in maternal or fetal risk. In a study by Kilpatrick et al., 6,991 women were retrospectively evaluated from 1976–1987, <10% were given regional anesthesia.[35] None of the subjects were augmented with pitocin and all delivered spontaneously. The 95th percentile second stage duration for nulliparous women with continuous fetal monitoring in spontaneous labor without an epidural was 132 min compared with 185 min for nulliparas with an epidural.[35] The median duration of the second stage in nulliparous women was 50 min and for multiparous women it was 20 min.

Prolonged second stage duration can increase maternal morbidity as it has been demonstrated to increase the risk of intraamniotic infection, post-partum hemorrhage, and perineal lacerations. Reported neonatal morbidities include sepsis, asphyxia, and birth trauma although the absolute risk of these morbidities remains quite low.[36] A positive correlation has been found between second-stage duration and adverse maternal outcomes (hemorrhage, infection, perineal lacerations), and a negative correlation has been identified between prolonged duration of the second stage and the likelihood of a successful vaginal delivery.[20] In a secondary analysis of a multicenter trial designed to evaluate the efficacy of fetal pulse oximetry by Rouse et al., maternal and neonatal outcomes following second stage labor for 4,126 nulliparous women were evaluated.[37] The study confirmed a decline in vaginal delivery rates with progressive duration of the second stage and increased risk of chorioamnionitis (overall rate, 3.9%), third- or fourth-degree perineal laceration (overall rate, 8.7%), and uterine atony (overall rate, 3.9%). Among individual adverse neonatal outcomes, only admission to a neonatal intensive care unit was significantly associated with second stage duration (odds ratio, 1.4). It is important to note that with second stage duration of 3 to <4 h, 27% of the participants delivered vaginally and with a second stage duration of 4 to <5 h, 24% of subjects delivered vaginally. This study is consistent with others in multiparous women who confirmed incremental increase in maternal risk and identified a significant likelihood of vaginal delivery success despite protracted second stage.[37–41] It remains unclear if the maternal risks associated with prolonged second stage of labor occur as a result of the labor duration or if dysfunctional labor occurs in women who are predisposed to hemorrhage and infection as a result of other factors. In the absence of randomized controlled trials, a second stage threshold duration, which would necessitate operative intervention in order to minimize maternal and fetal risk, has not been identified.[20]

Based upon the available evidence, a workshop convened by the Eunice Kennedy Shriver National Institute of Health Child Health and Human Development (NICHD), ACOG, and SMFM recommend prior to diagnosing second stage labor arrest that the following criteria be considered if maternal and fetal conditions permit, at least 2–3 h of pushing for multiparas with and without an epidural and 3–4 h of pushing for nulliparas with and without an epidural. See Table 2.3. Continued maternal pushing can be considered despite current recommendations if slow but incremental progress is made, if the fetal status remains reassuring, and if there is no suspicion of cephalopelvic disproportion or macrosomia. Maternal and fetal risk with second stage duration must be weighed against maternal and fetal risk should operative vaginal delivery or cesarean section be offered.

The common contributing factors for prolonged second stage include the use of regional anesthesia, fetal macrosomia, large maternal body habitus, inadequate maternal expulsive efforts, and occiput posterior presentation. Treatment of prolonged second stage depends on the underlying cause and requires an assessment of uterine activity, fetal weight, fetal position, and clinical pelvimetry. Expectant management is reasonable if the cause is likely due to regional analgesia. Maternal exhaustion leading to suboptimal expulsive efforts may require an assisted vaginal delivery with forceps or vacuum. In a manner similar to that with active labor, poor progress in the second stage may be related to inadequate contractile force. Titration of oxytocin may be required to facilitate descent if contraction frequency is diminished. Macrosomia and concern regarding cephalopelvic disproportion are a relative contraindication to an assisted second stage and warrant consideration of an abdominal delivery. Occiput posterior position contributes to a longer duration of active labor, may increase the duration of the second stage, and has a lower rate of vaginal delivery. Often, the occiput posterior position will rotate to occiput anterior as the labor progresses. However, if there is persistence of this positioning and a protracted active phase or labor arrest, manual rotation, an operative vaginal delivery, or abdominal delivery may be warranted.

Table 2.3 Recommended 95th Percentile Duration for the Second Stage of Labor

	95th Percentile
Nulliparas	
Second stage without an epidural	3 h
Second stage with an epidural	4 h
Multiparas	
Second stage without an epidural	2 h
Second stage with an epidural	3 h

Source: Modified from Spong C, Berghella V, Wenstrom K, et al. Preventing the first cesarean delivery: Summary of a joint Eunice Kennedy Shriver National Institute of Child Health and Human Development, Society for Maternal-Fetal Medicine, and American College of Obstetricians and Gynecologists Workshop. ***Obstet Gynecol***. 2012;120(5):1181.

Labor Practices That Can Affect the Duration of the First and Second Stages

The use of epidural analgesia is a common practice in contemporary obstetrics. It is associated with a significant reduction in pain due to uterine contractions and is a preferred option for pain relief for a large proportion of childbearing women. Controversy persists, however, regarding the effect of epidural dosing on the duration of labor and cesarean section risk.

A Cochrane meta-analysis of 38 studies was conducted to determine the effect of epidural analgesia compared to alternative options for pain control or no analgesia on several labor related outcomes.[42] Epidural analgesia was reported to provide superior pain relief compared to alternative options or no analgesia. The duration of the second stage was prolonged by 14 min for women with an epidural compared to controls [mean difference, 13.66 min; 95% CI, 6.67 to 20.66). The epidural was associated with an increased rate of operative vaginal delivery (OR, 1.42; 95% CI, 1.28 to 1.57) and cesarean section for fetal distress (RR 1.43, 95% CI 1.03 to 1.97). The overall risk of cesarean section, however, was unchanged (RR 1.10, 95% CI 0.97 to 1.25) as was the risk of cesarean section due to labor dystocia ((RR 0.90, 95% CI 0.73 to 1.12). The factors associated with an increased risk of operative vaginal delivery and cesarean section due to fetal distress are unclear and may be influenced by heterogeneity in study design or provider specific variables related to patient care. Epidural use during labor was noted to extend the second stage by 14 min in the randomized controlled trials (RCTs) selected for the meta-analysis. Retrospective studies of second stage duration, however, report a 60–90 min increase in second stage length.[14,43] In a retrospective cohort study by Worstell et al., 4,605 women were studied.[43] Nulliparas with an epidural were noted to have a 60-min increase in the median duration of second-stage labor compared to those without. The 95th percentile duration of the second stage was 95 min longer for nulliparas with an epidural and 101 min longer for multiparas with an epidural compared to those without an epidural ($p < .001$).

For women with a dense epidural in the second stage, delayed pushing is a temporary alternative to immediate pushing in the second stage. With delayed pushing, uterine contractions passively facilitate descent of the fetus through the pelvis until the maternal urge to push improves. Theoretical benefits of this approach include the ability to allow the patient to rest in order to better maximize maternal pushing efforts, reduce maternal exhaustion, and decrease the risk of operative vaginal delivery due to poor pushing efforts. A meta-analysis of 12 RCTs found that delayed pushing was associated with an increased rate of vaginal delivery compared to immediate pushing in the second stage (61.5% compared with 56.9%, pooled RR 1.09, 95% confidence interval [CI] 1.03–1.15).[44] However, this benefit was not statistically significant among the high-quality studies reviewed (59.0% compared with 54.9%, pooled RR 1.07, 95% CI 0.98–1.26). Further, no significant difference was identified in the operative vaginal delivery rate. Additional studies are needed in order to determine if delayed pushing is associated with improved maternal and fetal outcomes.[45,46]

Concluding Remarks

A careful evaluation of labor progress, maternal status, and the fetal heart rate are required before a diagnosis of dystocia can be made. Whenever maternal and fetal status permit, expectant management is recommended for women with in tact membranes in the latent phase and a labor duration of more than 20 h (nulliparas) and 14 h (multiparas). ACOG and SMFM recommend waiting until the patient has reached at least 6 cm of cervical dilation prior to entry into the active phase of labor. The adequacy of uterine contractions in the active phase should be assessed over 4–6 h before making a diagnosis of labor arrest if maternal and fetal status permit prolonged observation. It is important to assess labor progress within the context of maternal and fetal tolerance as the well-being of both will take precedence over set hourly thresholds for labor duration in the first or second stage.

References

1. Garrison EA, Kilpatrick SJ. Normal labor. In: Gabbe SG, Niebyl JR, Simpson JL, Landon MB, Galan HL, Jauniaux ERM, Driscoll DA, eds. *Obstetrics: Normal and Problem Pregnancies*. Philadelphia: Saunders Elsevier, 13th ed., 2012.
2. Friedman, EA. Primigravid labor: A graphicostatistical analysis. *Obstet Gynecol.* 1955;6:567–89.
3. Friedman, EA. Labor in multiparas; A graphicostatistical analysis. *Obstet Gynecol.* 1956;8: 686–703.
4. Battista LR, Wing DA. Abnormal labor and induction of labor. In: Gabbe SG, Niebyl JR, Simpson JL, Landon MB, Galan HL, Jauniaux ERM, Driscoll DA, eds. *Obstetrics: Normal and Problem Pregnancies*. Philadelphia: Saunders Elsevier, 13th ed., 2012.
5. Cohen WR, Friedman EA. Perils of the new labor management guidelines. *Am J Obstet Gynecol.* 2015; 212:420–7.

6. Hendricks CH, Brenner WE, Kraus G. Normal cervical dilatation pattern in late pregnancy and labor. *Am J Obstet Gynecol.* 1970;106:1065–82.

7. Ledger WJ. Monitoring of labor by graphs. *Obstet Gynecol.* 1969;34:174–81.

8. Kwast BE, Lennox CE, Farley TMM. World Health Organization partograph in management of labor. *Lancet.* 1994;343:1399–404.

9. Drouin P, Nkounawa F. The value of the partogram in the management of labor. *Obstet Gynecol.* 1979;53:741–5.

10. Cibils LA, Hendricks CH. Normal labor in vertex presentation. *Am J Obstet Gynecol.* 1965;91:385–95.

11. Peisner DB, Rosen MG. Transition from latent to active labor. *Obstet Gynecol.* 1986;68: 448–51.

12. Incerti M, Locatelli A, Ghidini A, Ciriello E, Consonni S, Pezzullo JC. Variability in rate of cervical dilatation in nulliparous women at term. *Birth.* 2011;38:30–5.

13. American College of Obstetricians and Gynecologists, Society for Maternal-Fetal Medicine. Obstetric care consensus no. 1: Safe prevention of the primary cesarean delivery. *Obstet Gynecol.* 2014;123(3):693–711.

14. Zhang J, Landy H, Branch D, et al. Consortium on Safe Labor. Contemporary patterns of spontaneous labor with normal neonatal outcomes. *Obstet Gynecol.* 2010;116:1281.

15. Friedman EA, Sachtleben MR. Dysfunctional labor. I. Prolonged latent phase in the nullipara. *Obstet Gynecol.* 1961;17:135–48.

16. Bräne E, Olsson A, Andolf E. A randomized controlled trial on early induction compared to expectant management of nulliparous women with prolonged latent phases. *Acta Obstet Gynecol Scand.* 2014; 93:1042–1049.

17. Nachum Z, Garmi G, Kadan Y, Zafran N, Shalev E, Salim R. Comparison between amniotomy, oxytocin or both for augmentation of labor in prolonged latent phase: a randomized controlled trial. *Reprod Biol Endocrinol.* 2010;8:136.

18. Wei S, Wo BL, Qi HP, Xu H, Luo ZC, Roy C, et al. Early amniotomy and early oxytocin for prevention of, or therapy for, delay in first stage spontaneous labor compared with routine care. *Cochrane Database Syst Rev* 2013;8:CD006794.

19. Hanley GE, Munro S, Greyson D, Gross MM, Hundley V, Spiby H, Janssen PA. Diagnosing onset of labor: A systematic review of definitions in the research literature. *BMC Preg Childbirth.* 2016;16:71.

20. American College of Obstetricians and Gynecologists, Society for Maternal-Fetal Medicine. Caughey A, Cahill A, Guise J, et al., eds. Obstetric care consensus no. 1: Safe prevention of the primary cesarean delivery. *Am J Obstet Gynecol.* 2014;210(3):179–193.

21. Neal JL, Lowe NK, Ahijevych KL, et al. "Active labor" duration and dilation rates among low-risk, nulliparous women with spontaneous labor onset: a systematic review. *J Midwifery Women Health.* 2010;55:308–318.

22. Millen KR, Kuo K, Zhao L, Gecsi K. Evidence-based guidelines in labor management. *Obstet Gynecol Surv.* 2014 Apr;69(4):209–17.

23. Spong CY, Berghella V, Wenstrom KD, et al. Preventing the first cesarean delivery: summary of a joint Eunice Kennedy Shriver National Institute of Child Health and Human Development, Society for Maternal-Fetal Medicine, and American College of Obstetricians and Gynecologists Workshop. *Obstet Gynecol.* 2012;120:1181–93.

24. Hauth JC, Hankins GDV, Gilstrap LC, Strickland DM, Vance P. Uterine contractions pressures with oxytocin induction/augmentation. *Obstet Gynecol.* 1986; 68:305.

25. Hauth JC, Hankins GCV, Gilstrap LC. Uterine contractions pressures achieved in parturients with active phase arrest. *Obstet Gynecol.* 1991;78: 344.

26. ACOG Committee on Practice Bulletins – Obstetrics. ACOG Practice Bulletin No. 107: Induction of labor. *Obstet Gynecol.* 2009;114:386.

27. Clark SL, Simpson KR, Knox GE, et al. Oxytocin: new perspectives on an old drug. *Am J Obstet Gynecol.* 2009;200:35.e1–35.e6.

28. Seitchik J, Amico J, Robinson AG, Castillo M. Oxytocin augmentation of dysfunctional labor. IV. Oxytocin pharmacokinetics. *Am J Obstet Gynecol.* 1984;150:225.

29. National Institutes of Health. Cesarean Birth Task Force Development Report. *Obstet Gynecol.* 1981;57:537–45.

30. American College of Obstetricians and Gynecologists. *Dystocia. ACOG Technical Bulletin no. 137.* Washington DC: American College of Obstetricians and Gynecologists, 1989.

31. Rouse DJ, Owen J, Hauth JC. Active phase labor arrest: oxytocin augmentation for at least 4 hours. *Obstet Gynecol.* 1999;93:323–8.

32. Rouse DJ, Owen J, Savage KG, Hauth JC. Active phase labor arrest: revisiting the 2-hour minimum. *Obstet Gynecol.* 2001;98:550–4.

33. Henry DE, Cheng YW, Shaffer BL, et al. Perinatal outcomes in the setting of active phase arrest of labor. *Obstet Gynecol.* 2008;112:1109–15.

34. Operative vaginal delivery: *ACOG Practice Bulletin No. 17.* Washington, DC: American

College of Obstetricians and Gynecologists, 2000. PMID: 13702000.

35. Kilpatrick, SJ, Laros RK, Jr. Characteristics of normal labor. *Obstet Gynecol.* 1989; 74, 85–7.
36. Laughon S, Berghella V, Reddy U, et al. Neonatal and maternal outcomes with prolonged second stage of labor. *Obstet Gynecol.* 2014;124(1):57.
37. Rouse D, Weiner S, Bloom S, et al. Second-stage labor duration in nulliparous women: relationship to maternal and perinatal outcomes. *Am J Obstet Gynecol.* 2009;201:357.
38. Cheng Y, Hopkins L, Laros R, et al. Duration of the second stage of labor in multiparous women: maternal and neonatal outcomes. *Am J Obstet Gynecol.* 2007;196(6):585.e1.
39. Allen V, Baskett T, O'Connell C, et al. Maternal and perinatal outcomes with increasing duration of the second stage of labor. *Obstet Gynecol.* 2009;113:1248.
40. Le Ray C, Audibert F, Goffinet F, et al. When to stop pushing: effects of duration of second-stage expulsion efforts on maternal and neonatal outcomes in nulliparous women with epidural analgesia. *Am J Obstet Gynecol.* 2009;201:361.e1.
41. Cheng YW, Hopkins LM, Caughey AB. How long is too long: Does a prolonged second stage of labor in nulliparous women affect maternal and neonatal outcomes? *Am J Obstet Gynecol.* 2004;191:933.
42. Anim-Somuah M, Smyth RM, Jones L. Epidural versus non-epidural or no analgesia in labour. *Cochrane Database Syst Rev.* 2011;(12):CD000331.
43. Worstell T, Ahsan AD, Cahill AG, Caughey AB. Length of the second stage of labor: What is the effect of an epidural? *Obstet Gynecol.* 2014;123(suppl 1):84S.
44. Tuuli M, Frey H, Odibo A, Macones G, Cahill A. Immediate compared with delayed pushing in the second stage of labor: A systematic review and meta-analysis. *Obstet Gynecol.* 2012;120(3):660.
45. Fraser W, Marcoux S, Krauss I, et al. Multicenter, randomized, controlled trial of delayed pushing for nulliparous women in the second stage of labor with continuous epidural analgesia. *Am J Obstet Gynecol.* 2000;182:1165.
46. Hansen S, Clark S, Foster J. Active pushing versus passive fetal descent in the second stage of labor: a randomized controlled trial. *Obstet Gynecol.* 2002;99:29.

Induction and Augmentation of Labor

Aaron Goldberg

Introduction

Induction of labor refers to initiation of labor, prior to the onset of spontaneous labor, using pharmacologic or mechanical methods, or a combination of them. The rate of induction of labor has increased since the 1990s, reaching a high of 23.8% in 2010. Recent efforts to decrease the rate of induction of labor have likely helped to decrease this rate to 23.3% in 2012, with the most drastic declines occurring with inductions of labor in the early term periods, especially those at 38 weeks gestation.[1]

The goal of induction is to initiate labor in women for whom the benefits to the mother or fetus of delivery outweigh the risk of continuing pregnancy. Ideally the process leads to vaginal delivery. If the cervical status is unfavorable, induction of labor with oxytocin alone can lead to an increased risk of cesarean section. To minimize this risk in women with an unfavorable cervix, cervical ripening is recommended involving a variety of methods.

While there are a many of appropriate indications to pursue induction of labor, contraindications include placenta previa, vasa previa, transverse fetal lie, breech presentation, umbilical cord prolapse, active genital herpes, prior classical cesarean and prior myomectomy when the endometrial cavity was entered.

Augmentation of labor occurs when medical interventions are used to supplement the ongoing process of labor. Augmentation is required only for obstetric indications; it is not done for convenience.

Scope of the Problem

The use of induction of labor has risen drastically in recent decades. According to the Centers for Disease Control and Prevention (CDC), induction of labor was used for 9.6% of all births and 8.1% of those occurring in the early term period in 1990. By 2010, induction of labor was used in 23.8% all births and 19.8% of early term births. Efforts across the past few years to reduce the rate of elective inductions of labor in late preterm and early term pregnancies have reversed this trend. A decline in inductions of labor has been noted since 2010, with the most significant decline occurring among early term deliveries. In 2012, the induction rate was 23.3% for all births.

The decision to induce labor requires an evaluation of the relative risks to both the mother and fetus of induction comparing the benefits and risks of earlier delivery to the benefits and risks associated with continuation of the pregnancy. In addition, given the well-known risks of cesarean delivery, efforts to maximize the likelihood of vaginal delivery are warranted.

In general, indications for induction of labor are not absolute and must take into account maternal and fetal status as well as gestational age. Decision regarding when to induce labor should be individualized and consultation with specialists in maternal-fetal medicine may be appropriate. Examples of maternal and neonatal conditions that may require induction of labor are seen in Box 3.1.

Induction of labor may be considered electively in women at term gestation (i.e., 37 weeks through 42 weeks gestation) without maternal or neonatal complications if the patients have a risk for rapid delivery, have difficulty with transportation, live a long distance from the hospital, or have other compelling psychosocial reasons for induction. However, given the increased risks of neonatal morbidity even in early term deliveries, the American Congress of Obstetricians and Gynecology (ACOG) states that it is inappropriate to deliver women at gestations less than 39 weeks unless there exists an appropriate medical indication for such early delivery.[2] Accurate assessment of gestational age is crucial in considering proceeding with induction of labor, especially when performed without medical indication. ACOG has

Box 3.1 Maternal and fetal conditions that may require induction of labor

- Chorioamnionitis
- Premature rupture of membranes
- Fetal demise
- Placental abruption
- Preeclampsia/eclampsia
- Gestational hypertension
- Post-term pregnancy
- Maternal medical conditions (including diabetes mellitus, hypertension, renal disease, chronic pulmonary disease)
- Evidence of fetal compromise (i.e. fetal growth restriction, oligohydramnios)

Box 3.2 Criteria for determining gestational age

- Ultrasound measurement at less than 20 weeks of gestation supports gestational age of 39 weeks or higher
- Fetal heart tones have been documented as present for 30 weeks by Doppler ultrasonography
- It has been 36 weeks since a positive serum or urine human chorionic gonadotropin pregnancy test result

proposed criteria for confirming gestational age of at least 39 weeks which are listed in Box 3.2.[3]

Induction of labor is contraindicated for a variety of reasons including placenta previa or vasa previa, transverse fetal lie, umbilical cord prolapse, active genital herpes infection, prior classical cesarean section, and prior myomectomy where the endometrial cavity was entered.

Maternal risks of induction include cesarean delivery, chorioamnionitis, uterine atony, and uterine rupture in patients with a prior cesarean or other uterine surgery. Fetal risks include fetal heart rate abnormalities resulting from tachysystole, which is defined as more than five contractions within a 10-minute period. Specific methods of induction pose unique risks and are described below.

Cervical Ripening

Prior to initiating induction of labor, the status of the cervix must be assessed. Women who have not experienced cervical changes such as dilation or effacement and softening of the cervix may have an "unfavorable cervix." These patients have a lower chance of successful induction of labor. In order to help predict success at induction of labor, the Bishop score has long been used to evaluate the "favorability" of the cervix for labor induction; this is presented in Table 3.1. A score >9 suggests a very high likelihood of success while a score <5 suggests an "unfavorable" cervix and the need for cervical ripening prior to stimulation of uterine contractions with oxytocin. Recent research has studied the role of evaluating the cervical length via transvaginal ultrasound to help predict success of induction of labor. This modality has not been found this to be a helpful predictor of outcomes from induction of labor.[4]

Methods of Cervical Ripening

Cervical ripening refers to changes in the cervix that allow for its softening, dilation, and thinning in response to uterine contractions leading to uterine contractions. In order to increase the success of induction in women with an unfavorable cervix, various methods of cervical ripening may be used prior to starting oxytocin to stimulate uterine contractions in an effort to increase the vaginal delivery rate. These methods are described below.

Prostaglandins

Two types of prostaglandins are available for use in cervical ripening: (1) prostaglandin E_2 (PGE2) and (2) prostaglandin E_1 (PGE1).

Use of either PGE1 or PGE2 for cervical ripening is associated with infrequent complications including uterine tachysystole. This can lead to fetal heart rate abnormalities, and uterine rupture when used with women with prior cesarean.[5] ACOG recommends against the use of prostaglandins for the induction of labor in patients with a prior cesarean delivery or other uterine surgery.

PGE2 (dinoprostone) is available commercially in two forms. The first is Prepidil®, which is formulated as a gel with 0.5 mg of dinoprostone in a 3 cc syringe. It is administered into the cervical canal to induce cervical ripening. Doses can be repeated every 6 hours for a total of three doses.

The second formulation of PGE2 is Cervidil®. This is a vaginal insert in which 10 mg of dinoprostone is embedded in a mesh sac connected to a tail. The

Table 3.1 Bishop Scoring System

Factor					
Score	Dilation (cm)	Position of Cervix	Effacement (%)	Station (-3 to +3)	Cervical Consistency
0	Closed	Posterior	0–30%	–3	Firm
1	1–2	Midposition	40–50%	–2	Medium
2	3–4	Anterior	60–70%	–1, 0	Soft
3	5–6	n/a	80%+	+1, +2	–

Source: Modified from Bishop EH. Pelvic scoring for elective induction. *Obstet Gynecol.* 1974; 24: 267.

mesh sac containing the medication is placed into the posterior vagina, where controlled release of the dinoprostone occurs at a rate of 0.3 mg/h. The insert is removed after 12 hours and dosing is not repeated. If uterine tachysystole or fetal heart rate abnormalities develop, the insert can easily be removed, generally leading to a cessation of the medication's effect. Other forms of prostaglandins cannot be removed and hence the medication effect is unable to be discontinued should such need arise.

In a meta-analysis including over 1,800 women, use of PGE2 was found to shorten induction to delivery times compared to the use of oxytocin alone, but did not change the cesarean rate.[6]

PGE1 (misoprostol) is available as Cytotec®. While its primary use is for treatment of gastric ulcers, it has been successfully used in an off-label manner for many years for cervical ripening and may be administered orally or vaginally. It is available as 100- or 200-microgram tablets, which are easily scored to facilitate the smaller doses needed for cervical ripening. When used vaginally, either 25 or 50 micrograms may be placed in the posterior vagina. Doses may be repeated in 4 to 6 hours if spontaneous labor has not started. Use of the higher 50-microgram dose is associated with increased risks of uterine tachysystole, as well as meconium passage and aspiration compared to PGE2. The lower dose was comparable to PGE2.[7,8]

Oral administration requires an increased dose. Studies suggest that a 100-microgram oral dose is equivalent to a 25-microgram vaginal dose.[9] In a small trial comparing the efficacy and safety of oral versus vaginal misoprostol, Cheng et al. randomized over 200 women between 34 and 42 weeks gestation with an unfavorable Bishop score to cervical ripening with either oral or vaginal misoprostol. The authors found that the oral route, while associated with a higher incidence of maternal nausea, had a lower incidence of uterine tachysystole and cesarean delivery compared to vaginal misoprostol.[10]

A comparison of the use of PGE1 with PGE2 shows variable data in terms of efficacy. Studies are limited somewhat by differing investigational designs and outcome measures. Austin et al. conducted a systematic review and meta-analysis to compare vaginal misoprostol with the vaginal dinoprostone insert. After identifying 11 randomized trials that met inclusion criteria with over 1,500 patients, these authors found that misoprostol use was associated with a higher incidence of vaginal delivery within 12 and 24 hours and a reduced need for oxytocin administration compared to the dinoprostone group. Cesarean section rates and neonatal outcomes were otherwise similar.[11]

Intracervical Foley Catheter

Use of an intracervical Foley catheter has been shown to be effective for cervical ripening and induction of labor.[12] A 16-french foley catheter is typically placed such that the balloon is within internal cervical canal. This can be done manually or during a speculum exam using ring forceps to insert the catheter into the cervix. The balloon is then filled with 30–50 cc of sterile saline to provide distension of the lower uterine segment. This leads to endogenous prostaglandins release and subsequent cervical ripening. Gentle downward traction is generally applied to the catheter as well; the catheter may be taped to the patient's thigh to keep it in place. The catheter is left in place for up to 12 hours or until it spontaneously is expulsed from the cervix in to the vagina.

Comparison of prostaglandin administration to the intracervical foley catheter for cervical ripening generally suggests similar rates of cesarean delivery with decreased rates of uterine tachysystole for the intracervical foley. A 2012 Cochrane review evaluating the use of mechanical methods of induction of labor including 71 randomized controlled trials totaling 9,722 women found that, compared with prostaglandins, use of the foley catheter is associated with a similar cesarean delivery rate, reduced incidence of uterine tachysystole, and similar maternal and neonatal complications. In addition, compared with oxytocin alone, the foley catheter is associated with a decreased cesarean delivery rate.[13]

Comparison of the standard foley catheter to a specially designed cervical balloon catheter produced by Cook Medical Systems specifically indicated for cervical ripening prior to induction of labor showed a significantly reduced time to delivery and lower costs for the standard foley.[14]

Previous research has examined combining the transcervical foley catheter with extra amniotic saline infusion. This procedure involves infusion of sterile saline through the input port of the foley to further enhance the effect. Karjane et al. performed a randomized trial involving 140 women being induced with a Bishop score less than 5 assigned to either foley alone or foley with extra-amnionic saline infusion. These authors found that time to delivery was significantly shorter in the extra-amnionic saline infusion arm without any differences in cesarean rates or other adverse events.[15] Conversely a similarly designed multicenter randomized trial involving 188 women found that the use of extra-amnionic saline infusion in conjunction with the transcervical foley catheter did not improve delivery interval.[16]

A variety of studies have evaluated the efficacy of cervical ripening with a combination of the foley catheter and misoprostol compared to either misoprostol or foley catheter alone, showing mixed results. A recent meta-analysis of eight studies involving 1,153 patients comparing cervical ripening with the foley catheter plus misoprostol versus misoprostol alone found that a combination of foley plus misoprostol resulted in a shorter time to delivery and reduced rates of tachysystole; however, the rate of chorioamnionitis was increased compared to both misoprostol or foley alone. The frequency of cesarean delivery was not different.[17] Another recent Cochrane review revealed similar conclusions.[18]

Hygroscopic Dilators

Several products exist that can be placed directly into the cervical os and slowly expand as they absorb water. Osmotic dilators include *Laminaria japonicum*, a natural product made from seaweed, and synthetic options such as Lamicel and Dilapan. They are narrow and rod-shaped, with a string on one end to facilitate later removal from the vaginal. In order to help ripen the cervix, as many as will comfortably fit into the cervical os are placed during a sterile speculum exam. They are then removed 12–24 hours later and augmentation may commence with oxytocin if spontaneous labor has not yet begun. They can be placed in an outpatient setting. These are more commonly used for cervical ripening prior to second trimester abortions than for induction of labor at term.

Membrane Stripping

A common obstetric practice, known as membrane stripping, has been thought to help induce labor and cervical ripening by causing disruption cervical–amnionic membrane interface. This is performed during the course of a cervix exam, where the examiner uses a finger to "sweep" the membranes at their interface with the cervix. The thinking is that doing this routinely in women at term will reduce the likelihood of requiring induction of labor and hasten spontaneous labor. While prior research suggests that the practice may reduce the need for induction of labor due to post term pregnancy, many of these trials have been small and suffered from bias. A review of 22 trials involving nearly 3,000 women evaluating the use of routine membrane stripping at term found little benefit. It was noted that routine membrane stripping may help reduce the need for induction of labor with a number needed to treat of eight, but posed risks of discomfort and other mild adverse effects.[19]

Nipple Stimulation

Obstetric providers have long suggested nipple or breast stimulation as a natural and cost-effective method of induction of labor. In low-risk pregnancies with a favorable cervix, this method may help hasten labor. In a systematic review of multiple studies involving 719 women, breast stimulation was compared with no intervention. Researchers concluded that nipple stimulation was associated with an increase in the rate of women in labor within 72 hours without differences in the cesarean delivery rate, or rate of meconium stained amnionic fluid.[23]

Nitric Oxide Donor Medications

Interest in the use of medications that increase nitric oxide has stemmed from the observation that nitric oxide may be involved in cervical ripening and uterine contractions.[20] While initial studies using isosorbide mononitrate and glyceryl trinitrate showed promising results, randomized controlled trials have produced mixed results. Schmitz et al. conducted a randomized trial including 1,300 women at 41 weeks gestation randomized to either isosorbide mononitrate or placebo and found no difference in the cesarean rate, but also worse side effects in the study group.[21] Similarly, a Cochrane Database review including 10 high-quality studies involving 1,889 patients found no role of nitric oxide donors for induction of labor when compared to various forms of prostaglandins for cervical ripening.[22] Until further research demonstrates efficacy, use of nitric oxide donors for cervical ripening should be considered experimental.

Labor Induction with Favorable Cervix

As noted, induction of labor in women with an unfavorable cervix typically starts with cervical ripening efforts as described previously. In many cases, this will lead to spontaneous uterine contractions. However, in those who have completed cervical ripening or who present with a favorable cervix prior to spontaneous labor, intravenous oxytocin or amniotomy may be used to stimulate uterine contractions or to help improve the rate of labor progression.

Oxytocin

Synthetic oxytocin, or Pitocin, is one of the most commonly used medications in modern obstetrics. Uterine response to oxytocin improves with greater gestational age, however, the response of individual patients is variable and unpredictable. Given this wide therapeutic index, various protocols have been developed to guide providers in titrating the oxytocin infusion to safely maintain regular uterine contractions. The goal is generally to mimic spontaneous labor with contractions occurring every 3–5 minutes and avoid tachysystole and associated fetal heart rate abnormalities. The half-life of the oxytocin is approximately 5 minutes, so that should tachysystole occur, decreasing or stopping the infusion usually quickly leads to reduction or even cessation of contractions.

ACOG recommends that each labor and delivery unit maintain protocols for oxytocin administration using precise infusion pumps and close monitoring of the maternal contraction pattern and the fetal heart rate tracing. Synthetic oxytocin, Pitocin, is typically diluted 10 units in 1,000 mL of saline for a concentration of 10 mU/ml.

Oxytocin infusion regimens may be of the "low-" or "high-dose" regimen. Either strategy is appropriate for labor augmentation. The low-dose regimen is associated with less uterine tachysystole and associated fetal heart rate abnormalities. High-dose regimens may lead to shorter intervals to delivery, but are associated with increased tachysystole and fetal heart rate changes.[3] Table 3.2 presents examples for typical oxytocin regimens.

It is important to note that the therapeutic window for oxytocin is wide with drastic differences in dose requirements between patients.

Due to a structural similarity to arginine vasopressin, oxytocin has an antidiuretic effect. At doses above 20mU/minute, oxytocin can lead to water intoxication due to reduced free water excretion, possibly leading to seizures, coma, and even death. Hence, extreme care should be undertaken when infusing such high doses of oxytocin.

Should tachysystole or fetal heart rate abnormalities, the infusion may be decreased or even stopped until the fetal heart rate improves and the contraction rate decreases.

Amniotomy

Another well-known obstetric practice is to artificially, or intentionally, rupture the amnionic membranes in

Table 3.2 Low- and High-Dose Oxytocin Infusion Regimens

	Starting Dose (mU/minute)	Incremental Increase (mU/minute)	Dosage Interval (minutes)
Low-dose	0.5–2	1–2	15–40
High-dose	6	3–6	15–40

Source: From ***Induction of Labor – Practice Bulletin***. American College of Obstetricians and Gynecologists. 2009.

hopes of accelerating spontaneous labor. Typically performed in the setting of a patient already laboring with a cervix at least partially dilated, it has been shown to shorten the length of labor without significant increases in the cesarean delivery rate. There does exist an increased risk of abnormal heart rate tracings and cesarean for fetal distress.

In a patient with a favorable cervix, this may also be performed in order to induce labor. It is usually combined with the use of oxytocin to help maintain labor progression. A trial involving 209 patients found that early amniotomy at 1 to 2 cm dilation was associated with a 4-hour decrease in labor duration compared to later amniotomy at 5 cm dilation. In addition, the rate of chorioamnionitis and umbilical cord compression was also higher in the early amniotomy group. Interestingly, the study found that when oxytocin infusion was adjusted in 30- vs. 60-minute increments, these risks were resolved.[24]

In Cochrane Database reviews of aminotomy for both labor augmentation and induction of labor, there was no clear benefit and studies often differed in methods so that comparisons were difficulty. Results were variable and did not always include a clinically significant outcome.[25–27] Based on the available evidence, the reviewers were unable to recommend routine amniotomy.

Risks of amniotomy include umbilical cord prolapse, chorioamnionitis, and the possible hemorrhage in a case of unanticipated vasa previa.

Special Situations

Elective Induction after 39 Weeks Gestation

As noted, recent efforts to reduce the rate of elective induction of labor in late preterm and early term deliveries have been successful. The neonatal risks of delivery before 39 weeks gestation are well documented. Controversy remains, however, regarding elective induction of labor at term after 39 weeks gestation. It has traditionally been thought that elective induction with an unfavorable cervix is associated with a higher cesarean rate. This was largely based on studies showing significantly increased cesarean delivery rates in nulliparous women undergoing electively induced labor compared to spontaneous labor.[28–30]

More recent research has compared induction of labor to expectant management in the belief that these comparison groups better reflect clinical practice. In a meta-analysis of five randomized trials including women with vertex singleton pregnancies without other indication for induction of labor between 39 and 41 weeks gestation, induction of labor compared with expectant management found that labor induction resulted in similar rates of cesarean delivery and operative vaginal delivery; a lower frequency of meconium-stained amnionic fluid and similar maternal morbidity were identified.[31] In addition, other meta-analyses that included patients with medical indications for labor induction at term showed a significant decrease in cesarean rates.[32,33] Darney et al. (2013) and Mishanina et al. (2014) similarly both found that even when controlling for cervical status and indication for induction of labor, the risk of cesarean delivery was lower among those with induced labor compared to expectant management at term.[34,35]

Prior Cesarean

The risk of uterine rupture is of paramount concern when considering induction of labor for women with a prior cesarean delivery. Studies have consistently shown an increased risk of uterine rupture in the setting of labor induction or augmentation.[36] Research investigating specific methods of labor induction remain limited in their ability to draw conclusions about the safest method of labor induction in the setting of prior cesarean delivery. According to ACOG, induction of labor may be performed in women with a prior low transverse cesarean section, but the use of prostaglandins in general should be avoided due to an increased risk of uterine rupture compared to other methods of labor induction and augmentation. The use of oxytocin and foley catheter induction is acceptable.[3,37] Induction of labor should not be undertaken in those for whom trial of labor after cesarean is otherwise contraindicated, for example those with a prior classical or T-incision, prior uterine rupture or prior extensive uterine surgery.[37]

Other risk factors that may be associated with decreased success for induction of labor after a prior cesarean are seen in Box 3.3.[38]

Premature Ruptured Membranes

It remains unclear what the optimal means of labor induction is preferred in the setting of ruptured membranes prior to spontaneous labor. While oxytocin has been shown to decrease the interval to delivery, if the cervix is unfavorable, vaginal prostaglandins may be

Box 3.3 Factors associated with decreased success for induction of labor

- Older maternal age
- Shorter maternal height
- Greater body mass index
- Greater weight gain during pregnancy
- Older gestational age
- Hypertension
- Diabetes mellitus
- Cervical dilation < 3 cm.

used. A study evaluating the use of misoprostol in this setting randomized 197 patients with premature rupture of membranes after 36 weeks gestation to either misoprostol or oxytocin found that misoprostol was a safe alternative to oxytocin with a similar rate of vaginal delivery and no increase in adverse events.[39]

The use of a foley catheter or other mechanical methods for labor induction in the setting of ruptured membranes is often avoided due to concerns regarding a possible increased risk of infection or umbilical cord prolapse; however, the available evidence is insufficient to make a conclusion regarding such methods.[3]

Intrauterine Fetal Demise

According to ACOG, when demise occurs after 28 weeks gestation, management should be similar to typical obstetric protocols for labor induction. Further, the use of misoprostol or oxytocin appears safe and effective when demise occurs in the mid-trimester between 24 and 28 weeks gestation.[3]

Augmentation in the Laboring Patient

When labor dysfunction, or protracted first stage of labor (as discussed in Chapter 2) is diagnosed, modern research has revised the traditional understanding of prolonged first and second stages of labor previously put forth by Friedman in the 1950s. In women with a dysfunctional labor pattern, in an effort to help augment labor to progress toward a vaginal delivery, clinicians may perform an amniotomy if the patient's amniotic membranes remain intact or use oxytocin to increase the strength and frequency of contractions. During latent labor, external monitoring of uterine contractions is typically sufficient to monitor the frequency and relative strength of contractions.

In the setting of arrest of the active phase of labor, an intrauterine pressure catheter (IUPC) may be used to help improve assessments of the contraction pattern. Placed internally into the uterine cavity after either artificial or spontaneous amniotomy, an IUPC is a plastic catheter with a pressure transducer at the tip. When connected to sensors at the patient bedside, the strength of uterine contractions are measured as mmHg above the baseline uterine pressure. Based on the work of Caldeyro-Barcia and colleagues, Montevideo units (MVUs) provide an objective measurement of uterine contractile strength during labor and are calculated by adding the total amplitude of each contraction over a 10-minute period. For example, three contractions in 10 minutes each measuring 50 mmHg above the baseline would equal 150 MVUs. In conjunction with a protocol similar to one of the aforementioned oxytocin regimens, oxytocin is increased in an effort to improve the contraction pattern and reduce the risk of cesarean section due to dysfunctional labor. In order to achieve adequate labor during a dysfunctional labor pattern, a goal of at least 200 MVUs is generally considered sufficient.

While IUPCs have become commonplace in modern obstetric care, research varies on the effectiveness of IUPCs compared to external uterine monitoring. A recent Cochrane Database review of three moderate quality studies including 1,945 women found no difference in maternal or neonatal outcomes when comparing standard external monitoring to internal monitoring[40] while another recent retrospective review suggested a increased risk of maternal infection when internal IUPCs were used with no difference in cesarean rates.[41]

Current recommendations for managing arrest of the active phase of labor suggest that at least 4 hours of adequate contractions of at least 200 MVUs or 6 hours of inadequate contractions with no cervical change be present before proceeding with cesarean delivery for the indication of active phase arrest.[42]

Concluding Remarks

Both induction and augmentation of labor are safe and effective methods to help initiate labor or improve progression of labor. When physicians consider induction of labor for their patients, they must weigh the risk of ongoing pregnancy with the risks of delivery, including the risk of cesarean delivery. Potential neonatal morbidity must be evaluated and relevant contraindications to induction of labor must be assessed. A variety of options for labor induction exist, including both pharmacologic and mechanical methods. Non-medically indicated induction of labor before 39 weeks gestation should generally be avoided. Ultimately, both the decision to induce a woman's labor, and the method with which to do so, should be individualized in consideration of each patient's maternal and neonatal risks and likely benefits.

References

1. Osterman MJK, Martin JA. *Recent Declines in Induction of Labor by Gestational Age. NCHS Data Brief, No. 155.* Hyattsville, MD: National Center for Health Statistics. 2014.
2. Nonmedically Indicated Early-Term Deliveries – Committee Opinion No. 561. American College of Obstetrician and Gynecologists. April 2013.
3. Induction of labor – Practice Bulletin, No. 107. American College of Obstetrician and Gynecologists. August 2009.
4. Hatfield AS, Sanchez-Ramos L, Kaunitz AM. Sonographic cervical assessment to predict the success of labor induction: A systematic review with metaanalysis. *Am J Obstet Gynecol* 2007;197:186–92.
5. Plaut MM, Schwartz ML, Lubarsky SL. Uterine rupture associated with the use of misoprostol in the gravid patient with a previous cesarean section. *Am J Obstet Gynecol* 1999;180:1535.
6. Owen J, et al. A randomized, double-blind trial of prostaglandin E2 gel for cervical ripening and meta-analysis. *Am J Obstet Gynecol* 1991;165:991.
7. Wing DA, et al. A comparison of misoprostol and prostaglandin E2 gel for preinduction cervical ripening and labor induction. *Am J Obstet Gynecol* 1995a; 172:1804.
8. Wing DA, et al. Misoprostol: An effective agent for cervical ripening and labor induction. *Am J Obstet Gynecol.* 1995b;172:1804.
9. Wing DA, Park MR, Paul RH. A randomized comparison of oral and intravaginal misoprostol for labor induction. *Obstet Gynecol* 2000;95:905.
10. Cheng SY, Ming H, Lee JC. Titrated oral compared with vaginal misoprostol for labor induction: A randomized controlled trial. *Obstet Gynecol* 2008;111:119–25.
11. Austin SC, Sanchez-Ramos L, Adair CD. Labor induction with intravaginal misoprostol compared with the dinoprostone vaginal insert: a systematic review and metaanalysis. *Am J Obstet Gynecol* 2010;202:624.e1–9.
12. Sherman DJ, et al. Ripening of the unfavorable cervix with extraamniotic catheter balloon: Clinical experience and review. *Obstet Gynecol Surv* 1996; 51:621–7.
13. Jozwiak M, et al. Mechanical methods for induction of labor (review). *The Cochrane Library* 2012;(3).
14. Mei-Dan E, et al. Comparison of two mechanical devices for cervical ripening: A prospective quasi-randomized trial. *J Matern Fetal Neonatal Med* 2012;25:723–7.
15. Karjanc NW, Brock EL, Walsh SW. Induction of labor using a foley balloon, with and without extra-amnionic saline infusion. *Obstet Gynecol* 2006;107:234–9.
16. Lin MG, et al. Transcervical foley catheter with and without extra-amnionic saline infusion for labor induction: a randomized controlled trial. *Obstet Gynecol* 2007;110:558–65.
17. Chen W, et al. Meta-analysis of Foley catheter plus misoprostol versus misoprostol alone for cervical ripening. *Int J Gynaecol Obstet* 2015;129:193–8.
18. Jozwiak M, et al. Mechanical methods for induction of labor. *Cochrane Database of Syst Rev* 2012;(3).
19. Boulvain M, Stan C, Irion O. Membrane sweeping for induction of labour. *Cochrane Database Syst Rev* 2005 Jan 25;(1).
20. Vaisanen-Tommiska M, et al. Nitric oxide metabolites in cervical fluid during pregnancy: Further evidence for the role of cervical nitric oxide in cervical ripening. *Am J Obstet Gynecol* 2003;188:779.
21. Schmitz T, et al. Outpatient cervical ripening by nitric oxide donors for prolonged pregnancy: a randomized controlled trial. *Obstet Gynecol.* 2014;124:1089–97.
22. Kelly AJ, Munson C, Minden L. Nitric oxide donors for cervical ripening and induction of labor. *Cochrane Database Syst Rev* 2011 Jun 15;(6).
23. Kavanagh J, Kelly AJ and Thomas J. Breast stimulation for cervical ripening and induction of labor. *Cochrane Database Syst Rev* 2005 Jul 20;(3):CD003392.
24. Mercer BM, et al. Early versus late amniotomy for labor induction: A randomized trial. *Am J Obstet Gynecol* 1995;173:1321–5.
25. Bricker L, Luckas M. Amniotomy alone for induction of labour. *Cochrane Database Syst Rev* 2000, Issue 4.
26. Howarth GR, Botha DJ. Amniotomy plus intravenous oxytocin for induction of labour. *Cochrane Database Syst Rev* 2001;(3).
27. Smyth RM, Allred SK and Markham C. Amniotomy for shortening spontaneous labour. *Cochrane Database Syst Rev* 2007 Oct 17; (4).

28. Luthy DA, Malmgren JA, Zingheim RW. Cesarean delivery after elective induction in nulliparous women: the physician effect. *Am J Obstet Gynecol* 2004; 191:1511–5.
29. Vrouenraets FP, et al. Bishop score and risk of cesarean delivery after induction of labor in nulliparous women. *Obstet Gynecol* 2005;105:690–7.
30. Vahratain A, et al. Labor progression and risk of cesarean delivery in electively inducted nulliparas. *Obstet Gynecol* 2005; 105:698–704.
31. Saccone G, Berghella V. Induction of labor at full term in uncomplicated singleton gestations: a systematic review and meta-analysis of randomized controlled trials. *Am J Obstet Gynecol* 2015; 11:629–36.
32. Caughey A, Sundaram V, Kaimal A, et al. Systematic review: elective induction of labor versus expectant management of pregnancy. *Ann Intern Med* 2009;151:252–63.
33. Wood S, Cooper S, Ross S. Does induction of labor increase the risk of cesarean section? A systematic review and meta-analysis of trials in women with intact membranes. *BJOG* 2014; 121:674–85.
34. Darney BG, Snowden JM, Cheng YW, et al. Elective induction of labor at term compared with expectant management: maternal and neonatal outcomes. *Obstet Gynecol* 2013;122:761–9.
35. Mishanina E, Rogozinksa E, Thatthi T, et al. use of labor induction and risk of cesarean delivery: a systematic review and meta-analysis. *CMAJ* 2014; 186:665–73.
36. Vaginal Birth After Previous Cesarean – Practice Bulletin No. 115. American College of Obstetrician and Gynecologists. 2010.
37. Tolcher MC, et al. Predicting Cesarean Delivery After Induction of Labor Among Nulliparous Women at Term. *Obstet Gynecol* 2015; 126: 1059–68.
38. Wing DA, Paul RH. Induction of labor with misoprostol for premature rupture of membranes beyond thirty-six weeks' gestation. *Am J Obstet Gynecol* 1998; 179:94–9.
39. Lin MG, et al. Misoprostol for labor induction in women with term premature rupture of membranes: a meta-analysis. *Obstet Gynecol* 2005; 106:593–601.
40. Bakker JJ, et al. Internal versus external tocodynamometry during increased or augmented labour. *Cochrane Database Syst Rev* 2012; 12.
41. Harper LM, et al. The risks and benefits of internal monitors in laboring patients. *Am J Obstet Gynecol* 2013; 209:38.e1–6.
42. *Safe Prevention of the Primary Cesarean Delivery.* American College of Obstetricians and Gynecologists. March 2014.

Placental Abnormalities

Loriana Newman and Heather Frey

Introduction

The placenta is a unique organ. Unlike other organs, which develop during embryogenesis and function throughout the lifetime of the organism, the placenta is only present during pregnancy. It serves as the maternal–fetal interface and its function is critical to the normal growth and development of the fetus. The placenta regulates the transfer of nutrients, enables respiratory gas exchange, secretes hormones, prevents rejection of the fetus by the maternal immune system, and eliminates fetal waste products[1]. It is important that obstetricians are familiar with the different types of abnormalities of the placenta, providing timely diagnosis and proper management of each condition, thereby minimizing the risk of adverse maternal and fetal outcomes.

Scope of Problem

Abnormalities of the placenta adversely affect fetal health and can lead to complications such as fetal growth restriction, fetal heart rate abnormalities, and even fetal death. Maternal health may also be adversely affected because abnormal placentation may increase such risks as intrapartum and postpartum hemorrhage, retained placenta, and infection.

General risk factors for placental abnormalities include multiparity, advanced maternal age, infertility treatment, smoking, and a history of cesarean delivery. The incidence of certain placental abnormalities, such as morbidly adherent placenta, has dramatically increased over the past 50 years with the rise of cesarean delivery rates, and as more women delay childbearing.[2,3] This condition is associated with an over 19-fold increase in adverse outcome, which results in a higher mean cost of inpatient care per hospitalization. It has been calculated that this rise has translated to over $115 million of additional spending for inpatient care for deliveries affected by placenta accreta between 2001 and 2011.[4]

Normal Placenta

The normal placenta is a discoid-shaped organ. The placenta starts to develop at the time of implantation of the blastocyst. The outer layer of the blastocyst, the trophoblast cell layer, separates into the inner cytotrophoblastic layer and the outer syncytiotrophoblastic mass. The syncytiotrophoblast develops into the outer layer of the chorionic villi. The connection with maternal blood supply is established by the extravillous trophoblasts, which are the cells that migrate into the decidua and myometrium to remodel uterine arteries and form the spiral arteries. The maternal aspect of the placenta attached to the endometrium is called the basal plate and the fetal aspect is called the chorionic plate. Within the intervillous space between these plates, the maternal blood bathes the chorionic villi and maternal-fetal exchange of gas and nutrients occurs.[1]

The placenta has a multitude of roles in gestation. It allows the exchange of gases (oxygen and carbon dioxide) and permits transfer of proteins, carbohydrates, lipids, electrolytes, and vitamins. It acts as a selective barrier in this role, protecting the fetus by reducing the transfer of many potentially toxic substances. The placenta is also an endocrine organ producing human chorionic gonadrotrophin, estrogen, progesterone, and other hormones.[5] Finally, it plays an immunologic role. Maternal antibodies of the IgG subclass are transported to the fetus, resulting in passive immunity to many infectious diseases, while acting as a barrier to protect the fetus from in utero infection with many organisms. Unfortunately, some viruses, protozoa, and bacteria can cross the placenta, potentially, resulting in significant morbidity and even mortality in the fetus and newborn.[1]

Abnormal Placenta

Abnormalities of the placenta can occur at the fetal interface where the umbilical cord inserts into the organ, the maternal interface where myometrial attachment occurs, or within the organ itself. There are specific risk factors, complications, and management recommendations for each of these abnormalities. The remainder of the chapter will focus on several of the most common placental abnormalities. Although placenta previa is one of the most common abnormalities of the placenta, it is not specifically covered in this chapter as it is included in Chapter 27, Antepartum Hemorrhage.

Velamentous Cord Insertion

A normal placenta is characterized by the central insertion of the umbilical cord into the chorionic plate. In contrast, a velamentous cord insertion inserts into the fetal membranes (Figure 4.1). As the umbilical cord vessels travel through the membranes toward the placental body, they lack protection from Wharton's jelly and thus are at risk for compression.[6] The overall incidence of velamentous cord insertion is 1%.[7] The prevalence is higher in multiple pregnancies, particularly monochorionic twins.[8] Other risk factors include nulliparity, obesity, infertility, placenta previa, and tobacco use.[9]

While definitive diagnosis of a velamentous cord insertion is made by gross examination of the placenta after delivery, ultrasound can be used to detect this condition in the antenatal period. The American Congress of Obstetricians and Gynecologists recommends that the placental cord insertion site should be documented when technically possible.[10] Diagnosis is possible as early as the late first trimester,[11] but cord insertion is typically evaluated in the mid trimester during performance of an anatomic fetal survey. The umbilical cord can be identified with gray-scale, with demonstration of entry of the umbilical vessel branches into the chorionic plate using color Doppler flow.[7] In one study, the sensitivity for antenatal detection at 18 weeks was 62.5%, with a specificity of 100%.[12]

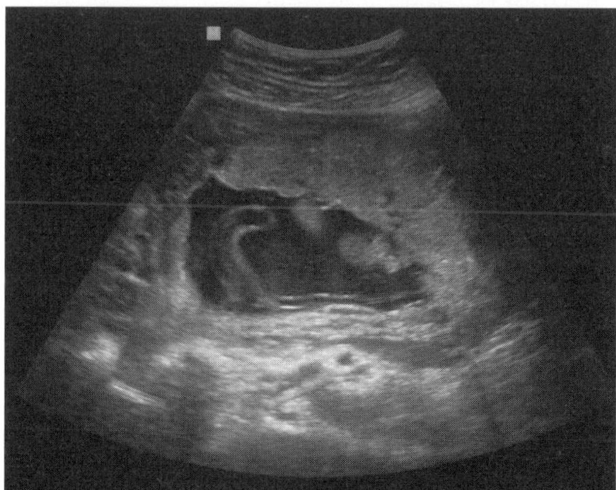

Figure 4.1 Velamentous cord insertion. On the posterior aspect of the uterus the umbilical cord is seen inserting into the membranes and traversing along the membranes to the anterior placenta.

Complications

The most catastrophic complications of velamentous cord occur when it is associated with vasa previa (see next section). However, pregnancies complicated by velamentous cord insertion are associated with other complications as well. Heinonen and colleagues performed a retrospective study of singleton pregnancies in Finland over four years and identified 216 pregnancies complicated by velamentous cord insertion. These pregnancies had a higher risk of low birth weight, pre-term delivery, low Apgar scores, and abnormal fetal heart rate patterns.[13] Fates of intrauterine fetal demise may also be increased, with one large cohort study showing a rate of 2.6% in pregnancies with velamentous cord insertions compared to 0.28% in the control group.[14] During labor, velamentous cord insertion is associated with fetal heart rate abnormalities, potentially resulting in the need for cesarean delivery.[10] Complications may occur after delivery as well including postpartum hemorrhage and need for manual removal of placenta or curettage.[14] See Figure 5.3 for an example of velamentous cord insertion.

Among monochorionic pregnancies that already have an elevated risk of complications, the finding of velamentous cord may further increase the risk of discordant fetal growth and fetal growth restriction.[8] The rate of twin-to-twin transfusion syndrome is increased in this setting as well[15]

Management

Prenatal management of velamentous cord insertion should include transvaginal ultrasonography with color Doppler flow in order to exclude vasa previa since velamentous cord insertion may be associated with suboptimal fetal growth. Serial assessment of fetal growth via ultrasound may be considered, with initiation of further antenatal testing if growth or fluid abnormalities develop. Some clinicians advocate for scheduled cesarean when the velamentous cord insertion is located in the lower uterine segment as this particular finding has been associated with increased risks of non-reassuring fetal heart rate tracings and emergency cesarean delivery.[10] Caution should be used after delivery due to the risk of postpartum hemorrhage, umbilical cord avulsion, and need for manual placental extraction or curettage.

Vasa Previa

Vasa previa occurs when umbilical cord vasculature is located close to or directly overlying the cervix (Figure 4.2). The incidence is estimated to be 1/2,500 deliveries,[16] and risk factors include velamentous cord insertion, accessory placental lobe, placenta previa, multiple gestation, and in-vitro fertilization.[17] An example of vasa previa is seen in Box 27.2.

In some cases, vasa previa may be diagnosed clinically with palpation of fetal vessels, fetal heart rate abnormalities, or vaginal bleeding at the time of rupture of membranes. Fortunately, this may be avoided with the use of ultrasound antenatally. As part of a midtrimester anatomy ultrasound, the placental location, cord insertion, and number of placental lobes is assessed. If the placenta is low-lying, multiple lobes are present, or velamentous cord insertion is identified, a targeted screening ultrasound for vasa previa with transvaginal ultrasound and Doppler color flow should be performed.[18] In a retrospective study by Bronsteen et al., all cases of vasa previa between 1990 and 2010 at a single institution were evaluated. Fifty-six of 58 cases of vasa were correctly diagnosed with ultrasound, corresponding to a sensitivity of 96.6%. Risk factors noted above were present in all but three vasa previa cases.[19]

Complications

Rupture of membranes in a pregnancy with vasa previa can lead to hemorrhage and fetal death. Vaginal bleeding and fetal heart rate abnormalities may require emergent delivery. In the Bronsteen study, the rate of emergent delivery was 11.7% and mortality rate was 4.5%. Preterm bleeding was a common complication of vasa previa, occurring in 42% of patients.[19]

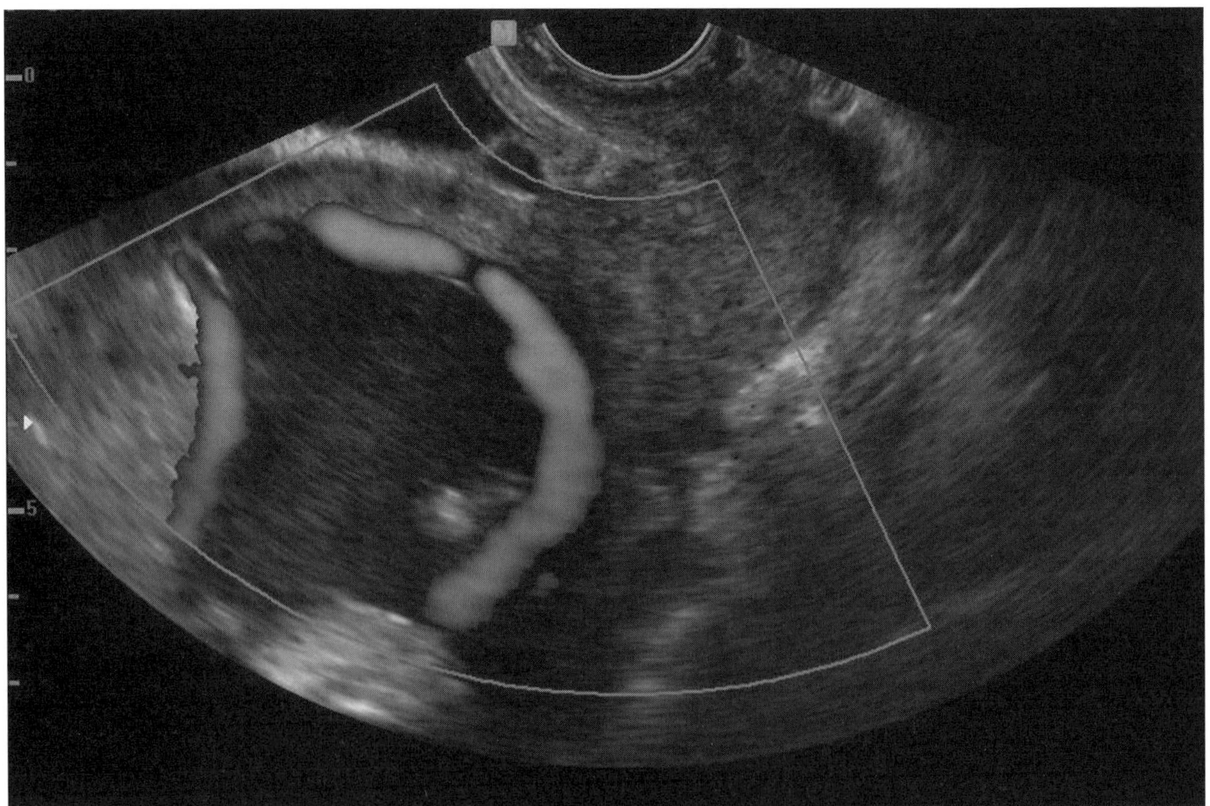

Figure 4.2 Vasa previa. On transvaginal ultrasound, color Doppler was utilized to identify the umbilical vessels overlying the cervix.

Undiagnosed vasa previa has a higher rate of perinatal mortality. It is associated with up to 60% rate of perinatal mortality.[16] Other complications arise from the increased risk of preterm delivery and associated complications of prematurity for the neonate.[18]

Management

If vasa previa is suspected at the time of midtrimester anatomy ultrasound, repeat ultrasound should be performed in the third trimester as some suspected vasa previas will resolve.[20] Generally delivery mode should be cesarean performed prior to labor or spontaneous rupture of membranes. The risk of perinatal death increases with advancing gestational age, while risks of prematurity decrease.[16] Some providers recommend outpatient care throughout the pregnancy while others recommend hospitalization in the third trimester. Recent recommendations from the Society of Maternal Fetal Medicine suggest that women with vasa previa should be offered antenatal corticosteroids between 28 and 32 weeks. Consideration should be made for preterm hospitalization at 30–34 weeks, and scheduled delivery at 34–37 weeks gestation by cesarean.[21] In cases of vaginal bleeding and suspected vasa previa, cesarean delivery should be completed urgently. Delivery should occur at an institution with appropriate resources for neonatal resuscitation, including blood transfusion. It has also been recommended that at the time of surgery, the provider should attempt to avoid lacerating the vessels, and ideally the fetus should be delivered en caul with intact membranes.[22]

Succenturate Lobe

A succenturate placental lobe is a small accessory lobe, which is connected to the main placenta by membranes and fetal vessels (Figure 4.3). It does not include bilobate or bipartite placentas, which have two lobes of equal size connected by a bridge of placental tissue. [23] The incidence ranges from 0.59 to 6%. Risk factors include multiparity, antenatal bleeding, placenta previa, advanced maternal age, and in vitro fertilization.[24,25]

Although the diagnosis often does not occur until birth, some cases may be diagnosed prenatally by ultrasound when a discrete lobe is found separate from the body of the placenta. In one study, only 13% of succenturate lobes were diagnosed prior to delivery.[24] An accurate diagnosis can be challenging because vessels may be misdiagnosed as an amniotic band. Color Doppler imaging can help improve diagnostic capability as it allows visualization of vessels crossing the membranes.[26] A posterior lobe is particularly difficult to identify with transabdominal imaging because ultrasound does not penetrate the fetal body satisfactorily.[27] For this reason, when a patient presents with vaginal bleeding of unknown etiology, transvaginal ultrasound should be considered to check for previa of a succenturate lobe even when transabdominal ultrasound shows that the main placenta is away from the cervical os.[28]

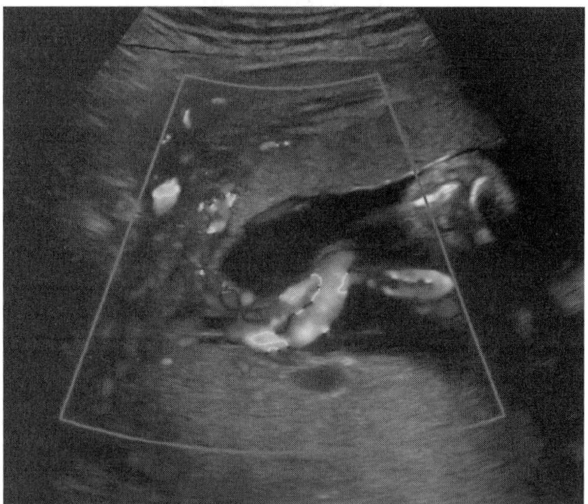

Figure 4.3 Succenturate lobe. In this image the placental insertion site was noted to be marginal and a succenturate lobe was also seen anteriorly.

Complications

Complications can arise from rupture of fetal vessels between the main placenta and the succenturate lobe, potentially resulting in fetal distress and even life threatening bleeding. When the succenturate lobe is not diagnosed antenatally, postpartum hemorrhage, retained placenta, and infection may occur.[24,27]

Management

If a succenturate lobe is suspected antenatally, transvaginal ultrasonography with color Doppler is recommended to evaluate for vasa previa. In the absence of vasa previa, the mode of delivery does not need to be altered.[26] Close attention is necessary during the third stage of labor to ensure that all placental lobes deliver in a timely fashion.

Morbidly Adherent Placenta

The term morbidly adherent placenta (MAP) refers to a group of conditions in which there is inappropriate invasion of the placenta into the uterus. MAP is generally classified into three categories based on the degree of invasion into the myometrium or serosa. In placenta accreta, the chorionic villi attach to the myometrium, while in placenta increta, the chorionic villi penetrate the myometrium. The most invasive form is placenta percreta, in which the chorionic villi penetrate through the myometrium to the uterine serosa or adjacent organs. The incidence of MAP has risen over time as the incidence of cesarean deliveries has increased. In 1950, the incidence was 1/30,000 compared to an incidence of 1/533 to 1/2,500 deliveries in more recent years.[2,3] Within the category of morbidly adherent placentas, accreta is most common (79%), followed by increta (14%) and percreta (7%).[3]

The most important risks factor for MAP are placenta previa in the current pregnancy and a history of prior cesarean delivery. The frequency of MAP increases with the number of prior cesarean deliveries, particularly in the setting of a concurrent previa. In a prospective cohort study of 30,132 women undergoing cesarean deliveries, women with a placenta previa had a 3% chance of accreta with no prior cesarean, 11%, 40%, 40%, 61%, and 67% with one, two, three, and four or more prior cesareans, respectively. In women *without* a placenta previa, the risk of accreta was 0.24% in the first cesarean delivery and up to 6.74% at the time of the sixth or more cesarean delivery.[3,29]

Other risk factors for MAP include advanced maternal age and multiparity,[2] history of other uterine surgeries, uterine irradiation, Asherman syndrome, uterine fibroids, uterine anomalies, hypertensive disorders of pregnancy, and smoking.[30]

Diagnosis of MAP may be suspected based on clinical history and imaging with ultrasound and possibly magnetic resonance imaging (MRI). A definitive diagnosis is made when pathologic examination identifies chorionic villi embedded in the myometrium without an intervening decidual layer. Ultrasound has been found to be more accurate when a patient's history and risk factors for MAP are known, with a sensitivity of 77–87%, specificity of 96–98%, positive predictive value of 65–93%, and negative predictive value of 98%.[31,32] Sensitivity decreases to 53.3% and specificity to 88% when physicians are blinded to a patient's clinical status.[33] Concerning ultrasound findings include multiple vascular lacunae within the placenta, as well as loss of normal hypoechoic retroplacental zone or retroplacental myometrial thickness < 1 mm. There may be a loss of the typical uterine serosa–bladder interface. Blood vessels or placenta may also be seen extending past the uterine–placental margin, the uterine serosa, and even into the bladder or other neighboring organs.[34] (Figure 4.4). Ultrasound should be the first line diagnostic tool, with the more expensive MRI used as an adjunctive diagnostic tool if ultrasound is inconclusive, the placenta is posterior, or there is concern for invasion into neighboring organs.[35]

Complications

The peripartum maternal complications of morbidly adherent placenta are well-described, and include hemorrhage, need for blood transfusion, cesarean hysterectomy, and admission to intensive care unit.[36] In addition, when percreta is present, there is risk of massive transfusion > 10 units, infection, maternal or perinatal death, and ureteral ligation or fistula formation.[37] A case–control study conducted by Gielchinsky et al. showed that preterm birth and small for gestational age infants are also more common among women with placenta accreta.[36]

Management

Antenatal management may include antenatal corticosteroid administration in preterm pregnancies

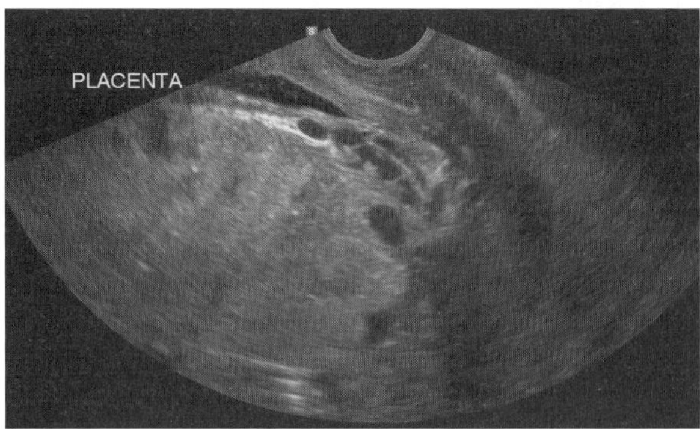

Figure 4.4 Placenta increta. This image was obtained at 21 weeks gestation from a woman who was found to have placenta increta at the time of delivery. Multiple large lacunae are seen and there was concern for invasion into the bladder wall. The myometrium adjacent to the bladder appears thin.

if delivery is likely within 7 days. Rhogam should be given if vaginal bleeding occurs in an Rh negative patient, and supplementation with iron and folic acid may help prevent anemia.[38] The most important management steps involve delivery planning. Patients must be counseled regarding possible complications that may occur at the time of delivery, and be consented for possible hysterectomy. Patients with MAP are best managed in a tertiary care center with a multidisciplinary approach including collaboration with maternal fetal medicine, anesthesiology, neonatology, and gynecologic oncology. A retrospective study found that patients cared for by a multidisciplinary team were less likely to require large volume blood transfusion, repeat surgery for bleeding complications, and maternal admission to the intensive care unit. A type and screen should be up-to-date to ensure the patient does not have rare red blood cell antibodies, and delivery should be planned in a hospital with an adequate supply of blood products.[39,40]

Decisions regarding timing of delivery should be individualized after discussion with the patient and the multidisciplinary team. The goal is to deliver in a controlled setting with planning for cesarean hysterectomy if needed. There should, however, be a contingency plan in the event that the patient requires an emergent delivery, and some physicians recommend pre-term delivery at 34 to 35 weeks in order to decrease this possibility. A decision analysis by Robinson and Grobman supported planned delivery at 34 weeks gestation in order to optimize maternal and neonatal outcomes.[41] Practitioners and patients can consider later preterm delivery in the absence of antepartum bleeding, suspected percreta, or other complications.

Particularly in suspected cases of increta or percreta, most deliveries are completed by a planned cesarean hysterectomy with the placenta left in situ. Both general and regional anesthesia techniques are safe for most cesarean deliveries. General anesthesia may be the more appropriate choice if severe hemorrhage is anticipated or encountered.[42] The blood bank should be alerted of the potential for massive transfusion requirements and packed red blood cells as well as fresh frozen plasma should be available. Large bore venous access and use of pneumatic compression devices are recommended, and care should be taken in positioning and padding the patient to prevent injury or nerve damage. The dorsal lithotomy position may be used to allow vaginal access for packing or cystoscopy. Physicians can consider preoperative cystoscopy with placement of ureteral stents and/or use of a three-way Foley catheter for irrigation, drainage, or distension of the bladder. The skin incision should be individualized based on the patient's characteristics including her prior surgical history and body habitus. A vertical skin incision generally provides greater access and visualization for hysterectomy, and a classical or posterior uterine incision may be necessary to avoid the placenta when making the uterine incision. If the patient desires fertility and the preoperative suspicion for MAP is low, physicians can await spontaneous placental separation. On the other hand, if a cesarean hysterectomy is planned, the placenta should be left in situ with closure of the hysterotomy incision before proceeding with removal of the uterus. If the bladder is adherent to the uterus or there is concern for bladder involvement with placenta percreta, a portion of the bladder may need to be excised to prevent massive hemorrhage. Supracervical hysterectomy is possible in some cases; however, persistent bleeding may necessitate total hysterectomy. Prophylactic antibiotics should be repeated after 2–3 hours of 1500 ml blood loss. Finally, the patient care team should anticipate potential need for postoperative recovery in the intensive care unit.[30,35]

If a patient strongly desires future fertility, she can be counseled on the possibility of conservative management. This requires that the patient is hemodynamically stable with a normal coagulation status. The patient should be counseled that the outcome of this management is unpredictable. Complications can arise such as hemorrhage, infection, intensive care admission, and need for additional treatment (uterine artery ligation or embolization, methotrexate, hysterectomy at a later time). There are rare case reports of successful subsequent pregnancy after conservative management. In a retrospective study of 26 patients who were treated with conservative management at one tertiary care center, 21 patients (80.7%) avoided hysterectomy but the majority required additional treatment including arterial embolization, methotrexate, blood transfusion, hypogastric artery ligation, antibiotics, or curettage. Three of the patients (11.5%) had a successful pregnancy in the follow-up period of the study.[43] A larger multicenter retrospective study was completed with 167 patients in whom conservative management was attempted. The success rate for avoidance of hysterectomy was 78.4%. Of the 36 patients who required hysterectomy, 18 were treated with primary hysterectomy within 24 hours of delivery, and the other 18 with delayed hysterectomy (performed a median of 22 days after delivery). Severe maternal morbidity was encountered in 6% of the patients. These morbidities included sepsis, peritonitis,uterine necrosis, postpartum uterine rupture, fistula, injury to adjacent organs, acute pulmonary edema, acute renal failure, venous thromboembolic events, or maternal death. Other possible complications included blood transfusion (41.9%), infection (28%), and transfer to intensive care unit (25.7%). Spontaneous resorption of the placenta was verified in 75% of patients, and the remaining 25% required hysteroscopic resection or curettage to remove retained placenta.[44]

Circumvallate Placenta

In a circumvallate placenta, the chorionic plate is smaller than the basal plate. As a result, the edges of the placenta roll inward and the chorionic membranes insert inward from the edge of the placenta toward the umbilical cord.[45] Estimates of the incidence range from 1 to 6%.[46] The only reported risk factor is that of multigravidity.[47]

Antenatal diagnosis is difficult, but ultrasound may show an irregular placental edge, uplifted margin, and/or a placental sheet or shelf (where the placental edge is thin or sheet like). Even when focused placental imaging is completed by experienced sonographers, most circumvallate placentas are not diagnosed antenatally.[48] In a study of 139 patients with pathologically confirmed circumvallate placenta in a Japanese hospital, the incidence was 1.8% and none of the cases were diagnosed prior to delivery.[45] Three-dimensional sonography may be helpful in diagnosis, allowing creation of a surface rendering of the placenta that can show the thick peripheral ring on the chorionic plate, coined the "tire" sign by one group.[49] Circumvallate placenta can be differentiated from amniotic sheets because amniotic sheets attach to the uterine wall while placental membranes do not.[50]

Complications

Circumvallate placenta is associated with a higher incidence of premature delivery, oligohydramnios, non-reassuring fetal status, requirement for emergency cesarean delivery, placental abruption, intrauterine fetal demise, and low Apgar scores.[45] Unlike with amniotic bands, there is not an increased risk of fetal deformity.[50] Vaginal bleeding is the most common symptom of circumvallate placenta. Women with circumvallate placenta may also have higher rates of postpartum complications including the need for manual removal of the placenta, hemorrhage, and endometritis.[51]

Management

If circumvallate placenta is suspected based on ultrasound findings, the placental margins should be reassessed in the third trimester. If circumvallation is present, a fetal growth scan is indicated. Routine obstetric care can be continued unless fetal growth restriction is suspected.[52]

Chorioangioma

Chorioangioma is an abnormal proliferation of vessels arising from chorionic tissue. It is the most common benign tumor of the placenta with an incidence of about 1%. The rate rises with maternal age such that most chorioangiomas are found in women older than 30 years. Other risk factors include hypertension, diabetes, and female fetuses.[53]

Most chorioangiomas are found postnatally after close pathologic evaluation,[54] but large chorioangiomas may be diagnosed antenatally. These lesions appear as well-circumscribed, solid masses on ultrasound that may bulge from the fetal surface of the placenta into the amniotic fluid (Figure 4.5). The appearance can be difficult to differentiate from placental hematomas,[55] but color Doppler imaging can identify vessels.[56]

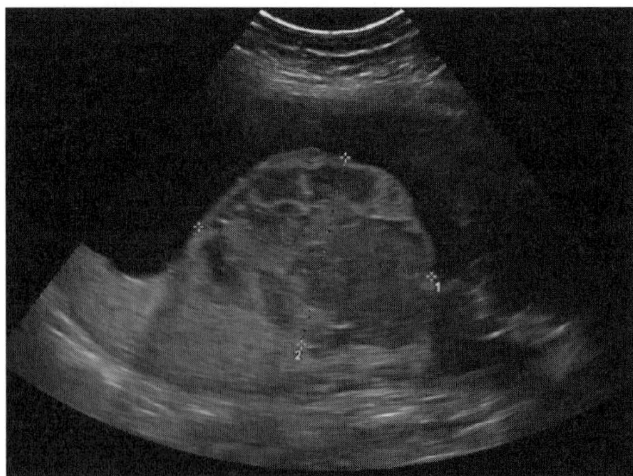

Figure 4.5 Chorioangioma. In this image, the placental mass is well circumscribed and bulging from the fetal side of the placenta into the amniotic fluid.

Complications

Small tumors are usually asymptomatic, but larger tumors larger than 4 cm in diameter are associated with complications. Polyhydramnios and preterm labor are the most common complications, but other adverse events include non-immune hydrops, fetal anemia and/or thrombocytopenia, fetal heart failure, fetal growth restriction, pre-eclampsia, placental abruption, and perinatal death. Postpartum hemorrhage is also more common in women with large lesions.[54,57]

Management

Pregnancies with chorioangioma should be managed with close antenatal surveillance. This may include serial growth ultrasounds and consideration of non-stress testing. Complications may necessitate early delivery depending on severity of complications, fetal surveillance, gestational age, and neonatal facilities.[58] When complications arise early in gestation, intervention may be considered. Serial fetal transfusions for fetal anemia may be used as a temporizing measure,[56] and alcohol slerosis or fetoscopic laser coagulation of vessels supplying the tumor may be employed as more definitive treatment.[59] While successful pregnancies resulting in term deliveries have been described with the use of endoscopic laser coagulation of feeding vessels, this treatment can result in significant complications including fetal bleeding, preterm delivery, and even fetal death.[60]

Concluding Remarks

Placental abnormalities play an important role in prenatal care. Close surveillance is often necessary if placental abnormalities are diagnosed. They cannot all be diagnosed during the antepartum period with ultrasound. Adjuvant use of color Doppler examination can often help in identifying these abnormalities. As the placenta plays a crucial role in nutrient and gas exchange, hormone regulation, and blood flow, it follows that many placental abnormalities can lead to growth restriction and poor fetal outcomes. Depending on the type of abnormality and fetal growth, antenatal surveillance with non-stress testing may be necessary. It is also important to take placental abnormalities into account when planning for delivery, as many of these conditions are associated with higher rates of peripartum complications such as hemorrhage, retained placenta, and infection.

References

1. N.M. Gude, C.T. Roberts, B. Kalionis, G. Roger. Growth and function of the normal human placenta. *Thrombosis Research* 2004; 114: 397–407.
2. S. Wu, M. Kocherginsky, J.U. Hibbard. Abnormal placentation: Twenty-year analysis. *Am J Obstet Gynecol* 2005; 192(5): 1458–1461.
3. D.A. Miller, J.A. Chollet, T.M. Goodwin. Clinical risk factors for placenta previa-placenta accrete. *Am J Obstet Gynecol* 1997; 177(1): 210–214.
4. M.F. Mogos, J.L. Salemi, M. Ashley et al. Recent trends in placenta accreta in the United States and its impact on maternal-fetal morbidity and healthcare-associated costs, 1998–2011. *J Matern Fetal Neonatal Med* 2016; 29(7): 1077–82.
5. J. Dancis. The placenta. *J Pediatr* 1959; 55 (1): 85–101.
6. J. Hasegawa, R. Matsuoka, K. Ichizuka, et al. Velamentous cord insertion: Significance of prenatal detection to predict perinatal complications. *Taiwanese J Obstet Gynecol* 2006; 45(1): 21–25.
7. W. Sepulveda, I. Rojas, J. A. Robert, et al. Prenatal detection of velamentous insertion of the umbilical cord: A prospective color Doppler study. *Ultrasound Obstet Gynecol* 2003; 21(6): 564–569.
8. E.M. Kent, F.M. Brethnach, J.E. Gillan, et al. Placental cord insertion and birthweight discordance in twin pregnancies: Results of the national prospective ESPRiT study. *Am J Obstet Gynecol* 2011; 205(4): 376.e1–376.e7.
9. S. Raisanen, L. Georgiadis, M. Harju, et al. Risk factors and adverse pregnancy outcomes among births affected by velamentous umbilical cord insertion: A retrospective population-based register study. *Eur J Obstet Gynecol Reproduc Biol* 2012; 165: 231–234.
10. ACR-ACOG-AIUM-SRU Practice Parameter for the performance of obstetrical ultrasound. 2014 (Resolution 39).
11. W. Sepulveda. Velamentous insertion of the umbilical cord: a first-trimester sonographic screening study. *J Ultrasound Med* 2006; 25 (8): 963–968.
12. J. Hasegawa, R. Matsuoka, K. Ichizuka, et al. Velamentous cord insertion into the lower third of the uterus is associated with intrapartum fetal heart rate abnormalities. *Ultrasound Obstet Gynecol* 2006; 27 (4): 425–429.
13. S. Heinonen, M. Ryynanen, P. Kirkinen, et al. Perinatal diagnostic evaluation of velamentous umbilical cord insertion: Clinical, Doppler, and ultrasonic findings. *Obstet Gynecol* 1996; 87(1): 112–117.
14. T.F. Esakoff, Y.W. Cheng, J.M. Snowden, et al. Velamentous cord insertion: Is it associated with

adverse perinatal outcomes? *J Matern Fetal Neonatal Med* 2015; 28(4): 409–412.

15. M.H. Fries, R.B. Goldstein, S.J. Kilpatrick, et al. The role of velamentous cord insertion in the etiology of twin-twin transfusion syndrome. *Obstet Gynecol* 1993; 81: 569–574.
16. O.K. Oyelese, M. Turner, C. Lees, S. Campbell. Vasa previa: An avoidable obstetric tragedy. *Obstet Gynecol Survey* 1999; 54 (2): 138–145.
17. S. Baulies, N. Maiz, A. Munoz, et al. Prenatal ultrasound diagnosis of vasa previa and analysis of risk factors. *Prenat Diagn* 2007; 27: 595–599.
18. M.R. Silver. Abnormal placentation: Placenta previa, vasa previa, and placenta accreta. *Obstet Gynecol* 2015; 125 (3): 654–668.
19. R. Bronsteen, A. Whitten, M. Balasubramanian, et al. Vasa previa: Clinical presentations, outcomes, and implications for management. *Obstet Gynecol* 2013; 122 (2 Pt 1): 352–357.
20. W. Lee, L. Virginia, S. Janet, et al. Vasa previa: Prenatal diagnosis, natural evolution, and clinical outcome. *Obstet Gynecol* 2000;95 (4): 572–576.
21. Society of Maternal-Fetal (SMFM) Publications Committee. #37: Diagnosis and management of vasa previa. *Am J Obstet Gynecol* 2015; 213(5): 615–619.
22. Y. Oyelese, J. Simulian. Placenta previa, placenta accreta, and vasa previa. *Obstet Gynecol* 2006; 107 (4): 927–941.
23. B.A. Spirt, E.H. Kaga, L.P. Gordon, L.S. Massad. Antepartum diagnosis of succenturiate lobe: Sonographic and pathologic correlation. *J Clin Ultrasound* 1981; 9 (3): 139–140.
24. S. Suzuki, M. Agarashi. Clinical significance of pregnancies with succenturiate lobes of placenta. *Arch Gynecol Obstet* 2008; 277(4): 299–301.
25. K. Bernischke, P. Kaufmann, R.N. Baergen, editors. Placental shape aberrations. In: *Pathology of the human placenta*. 5th ed. New York: Springer; 2005.
26. A.F. Cavaliere, P. Rosati, P. Ciliberti, et al. Succenturiate lobe of placenta with vessel anomaly: A case report of prenatal diagnosis and literature review. *Clin Imaging* 2014; 38(5): 747–750.
27. K. Hata, T. Hata, H. Aoki, et al. Succenturiate placenta diagnosed by ultrasound. *Gynecol Obstet Invest* 1988; 25: 572–576.
28. K. Shukunami, W. Tsunezawa, K. Hosokawa, F. Kotsuji. Placenta previa of a succenturiate lobe: A report of two cases. *Eur J Obstet Gynecol Reprod Biol* 2001; 99: 276–277.
29. R.M. Silver, M.B. Landon, D.J. Rouse, et al. Maternal morbidity associated with multiple repeat cesarean deliveries. *Obstet Gynecol* 2006; 107(6): 1226–1232.
30. Publications Committee, Society for Maternal-Fetal Medicine, M.A. Belfort. Placenta Accreta. *Am J Obstet Gynecol* 2010; 203(5): 430–439.
31. C.R. Warshak, R. Eskander, A.D. Hull, et al. Accuracy of ultrasonography and magnetic resonance imaging in the diagnosis of placenta accreta. *Obstet Gynecol* 2006; 108: 573–581.
32. C.H. Comstock, J.J. Love Jr, R.A. Bronsteen, et al. Sonographic detection of placenta accreta in the second and third trimesters of pregnancy. *Am J Obstet Gynecol* 2004; 190: 1135–1140.
33. E.M. Berkley, A.Z. Abuhamad. Prenatal diagnosis of placenta accreta: Is sonography all we need? *J Ultrasound Med* 2013; 32: 1345–1350.
34. R.M. Silver, K.A. Fox, J.R. Barton, et al. Center for excellence for placenta accreta. *Am J Obstet Gynecol* 2015; 212(5): 561–568.
35. American College of Obstetricians and Gynecologists. Placenta accreta: Committee opinion no. 529. *Obstet Gynecol* 2012; 120:207–211.
36. Y. Gielchinsky, D. Mankuta, N. Rojansky, et al. Perinatal outcome of pregnancies complicated by placenta accreta. *Obstet Gynecol* 2004; 104: 527–530.
37. J.M. O'Brien, J.R. Barton, E.S. Donaldson. The management of placenta percreta: Conservative and operative strategies. *Am J Obstet Gynecol* 1996; 175(6): 1632–1638.
38. A. Imdad, Z.A Bhutta. Routine iron/folate supplementation during pregnancy: Effect on maternal anaemia and birth outcomes. *Paediatr Perinat Epidemiol* 2012; 26: 168–177.
39. A.C. Wortman, J.M. Alexander. Placenta accreta, increta, and percreta. *Obstet Gynecol Clin* 2013; 40(1): 137–154.
40. A.G. Eller, M.A. Bennett, M. Sharshiner, et al. Maternal morbidity in cases of placenta accreta managed by a multidisciplinary care team compared with standard obstetric care. *Obstet Gynecol* 2011; 117: 331–337.
41. B.K. Robinson, W.A. Grobman. Effectiveness of timing strategies for delivery of individuals with placenta previa and accreta. *Obstet Gynecol* 2010; 115: 835–842.
42. American Society of Anesthesiologists Task Force on Obstetric Anesthesia. Practice guidelines for obstetric anesthesia: an updated report by the American Society of Anesthesiologists Task Force on Obstetric Anesthesia. *Anesthesiology* 2007; 106: 843–863.
43. F. Bretelle, B. Courbiere, C. Mazouni, et al. Management of placenta accreta: Morbidity and outcome. *Eur J Obstet Gynecol Reproduc Biol* 2007; 133(1): 34–39.
44. L. Sentilhes, C. Ambroselli, G. Kayem, et al. Maternal outcome after conservative treatment of placenta accreta. *Obstet Gynecol* 2010; 115 (3): 526–534.

45. S. Suzuki. Clinical significance of pregnancies with circumvallate placenta. *J Obstet Gynaecol Res* 2008; 34(1): 51–54.
46. K. Bernischke, P. Kaufmann. Placental shape aberrations: Circumvallate and circummarginate placentas. In: *Pathology of the human placenta*, 4th ed. Springer: New York, 2000; 211–214.
47. M. Maqueo-Topete, J. Chavez-Azuela, S. Valenzuela-Lopez, J. Espinosa-Hernandez. Placenta accreta and circumvallate (extrachorialis). *Obstet Gynecol* 1968; 32: 397–401.
48. R.D. Harris, W.A. Wells, W.C. Black, et al. Accuracy of prenatal sonography for detecting circumvallate placenta. *AJR Am J Roentgenol* 1997; 168(6): 1603–1608.
49. C. Arlicot, P. Herve, E. Simon, F. Perrotin. Three-dimensional surface rendering of the chorionic placental plate: The "Tire" sign for the diagnosis of a circumvallate placenta. *J Ultrasound Med* 2012; 31: 337–341.
50. C.L. Sistrom, J.E. Ferguson. Abnormal membranes in obstetrical ultrasound: Incidence and significance of amniotic sheets and circumvallate placenta. *Ultrasound Obstet Gynecol* 1993; 3: 249–255.
51. D. Wilson, R.J. Paalman. Clinical significance of circumvallate placenta. *Obstet Gynecol* 1967; 29(6): 774–778.
52. T.R. Moore. Placenta and umbilical cord imaging. In: R.K. Creasy, R. Resnik, J.D. Iams, et al. *Creasy and Resnik's maternal-fetal medicine: principles and practice*. Philadelphia: Saunders, 2014; 379–395.
53. M. Guschmann, W. Henrich,M. Entezami, J.W. Dudenhausen. Chorioangioma – new insights into a well-known problem. I. Results of a clinical and morphological study of 136 cases. *J Perinat Med* 2003; 31 (2): 163–169.
54. H.S. Wallenburg. Chorioangioma of the placenta. Thirteen new cases and a review of the literature from 1939 to 1970 with special reference to the clinical complications. *Obstet Gynecol Surv* 1971; 26: 411–425.
55. B. Bromley, B.R. Benacerraf. Solid masses on the fetal surface of the placenta: Differential diagnosis and clinical outcome. *J Ultrasound Med* 1994; 13: 883–886.
56. Y. Zalel, R. Gamzu, Y. Weiss, et al. Role of color Doppler imaging in diagnosing and managing pregnancies complicated by placental chorioangioma. *J Clin Ultrasound* 2002; 30 (50): 264–269.
57. K. Bernischke, P. Kaufmann. Benign tumors: Chorangiosis. In: *Pathology of the human placenta*, 4th ed. Springer: New York, 2000; 778–789.
58. W. Sepulveda, J.L. Alcalde, C. Schnapp, M. Bravo. Perinatal outcome after prenatal diagnosis of placental chorioangioma. *Obstet Gynecol* 2003; 102 (5 Pt 1): 1028–1033.
59. R.A. Quintero, H. Reich, R. Romero, et al. In utero endoscopic devascularization of a large chorioangioma. *Ultrasound Obstet Gynecol* 1996; 8(1): 48–52.
60. W. Sepulveda, A.E. Wong, L. Herrera, et al. Endoscopic laser coagulation of feeding vessels in large placental chorioangiomas: report of three cases and review of invasive treatment options. *Prenat Diagn* 2009; 29 (3): 201–206.

Management of Obstetric Umbilical Cord Complications

Phillip L. Bressman

Introduction

On June 3, 1965, Gemini 4 astronaut Ed White became the first American to walk in space. With that historic event the word "umbilical" became part of everyday vocabulary. Photos taken by fellow astronaut James McDivitt and now available from National Aeronautics and Space Administration (NASA) as high-definition (HD) images (see Figure 5.1) show a gold-wrapped umbilical line and tether serving as a lifeline connecting White to the mothership.

The videos of White rolling in space encircled by loops of his umbilical tether are eerily reminiscent of present-day ultrasound videos of fetuses "playing" with loops of umbilical cords in utero.

Before the umbilical tether, there was the umbilical cord, one vein and two arteries (most of the time) encased in Wharton's jelly. Soon after development of the fetal pole ultrasound imaging of the umbilical cord was possible. Growing to 50 to 60 cm in length, the umbilical cord is a true lifeline tethering the fetus to the placenta and the uterine mothership. Compression, occlusion, entanglement, malpresentation, or rupture of the cord may lead to fetal injury or death.

Scope of the Problem

Every laboring patient with a viable fetus also has an umbilical cord. Most cords are normal, some are abnormal, and some are normal but are in a position vulnerable to occlusion, compression, or rupture. Umbilical cord entanglement and its most common variation, the nuchal cord, have been considered for centuries as common causes of obstetric complication. Many incidences of neonatal depression or stillbirth have been attributed to cord compromise.

We now have technology to evaluate cord function and position. Electronic fetal monitoring records variable heart rate decelerations associated with cord compression. High-resolution ultrasound has allowed detection of cord position including malpresentations and nuchal umbilical cords. Umbilical artery Doppler velocimetry is used as a method of fetal surveillance. Unfortunately, the sometimes premature widespread use of testing has led to unnecessary intervention and has contributed to the rising cesarean section rate. Medical technology advances rapidly and it is incumbent upon every obstetrician to use best evidence to determine how to incorporate these advances into safe, quality patient care.

Umbilical Cord Entanglements and Nuchal Cords

Entanglement of the fetus in the umbilical cord may result in cord compression and cord occlusion. Variable fetal heart rate decelerations representing cord compression are the most common periodic changes seen on fetal heart rate monitors and fetal heart tracings suggestive of cord compression are among the leading causes of cesarean section. These cord compressions, if prolonged or severe, may lead to intrauterine fetal compromise or death. In the absence of other obvious causes, many cases of intrauterine fetal demise are attributed to these "umbilical cord accidents" [1].

The most common form of cord entanglement is the nuchal cord. Prenatal screening for fetal nuchal cords with ultrasound is possible but there is no consistent data that this is useful for management [2]. It therefore seems reasonable to view single nuchal cords found at ultrasound as incidental findings. The same may be said for multiple nuchal loops in that multiple loops appear to result in no adverse neonatal outcome. In one series, multiple loops numbering up to four, although associated with an increase in meconium stained fluid and abnormal fetal heart rate patterns, resulted in no long-term sequelae [2,3].

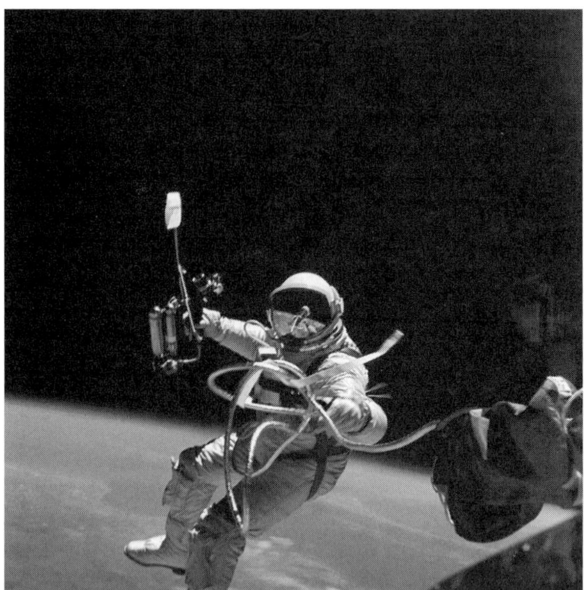

Figure 5.1 Astronaut with umbilical tether line. Image credit: NASA.

Nuchal cords have long been recognized as a complicating factor in vaginal deliveries. Classic teaching of nuchal cord management involves efforts to either (1) reduce a loose nuchal cord by slipping a loose loop over the fetal head or (2) double clamp and cut a tight nuchal cord to facilitate safe vaginal delivery [4]. Nuchal cords, however, are present in approximately 25% of deliveries but are not associated with statistically worse outcomes than the other 75% of deliveries [1]. Even tight nuchal cords do not appear to be associated with clinically significant adverse outcomes [5]. Conversely, manipulation of a nuchal cord has been recognized as a potentially catastrophic event when vigorous attempts to reduce result in cord rupture [6]. Also, cord reduction simply results in a loop of cord hanging outside the perineum. Some would describe this by its more common name, "cord prolapse." Finally, doubly clamping and cutting a tight nuchal cord could be devastating if done prior to delivering the shoulders when an unrecognized shoulder dystocia is present [7].

It is doubtful that these two time-honored practices, cord reduction and doubly clamping and cutting, will be abandoned but there are two other maneuvers which may be more appropriate to safe patient care. Both have been described in midwifery journals. The first, delivering through the cord, simply requires slipping loose loops of umbilical cord back over the shoulders and body as the infant is delivered [6]. The second, the somersault maneuver, is appropriate for all vertex deliveries and requires more description.

The somersault maneuver results in "somersaulting" the infant at the perineum without putting undue tension on a tight nuchal cord. Once the nuchal cord is recognized the infant's shoulders are slowly delivered without cord manipulation. The infant's head is flexed and kept close to the perineum while the body is somersaulted out to complete the delivery. The infant and cord are then disentangled and delayed cord clamping if appropriate is possible [6,8]. The somersault maneuver easily lends itself to simulation-based learning. An excellent online video produced by the East Carolina University College of Nursing demonstrates the technique and can be found at www.youtube.com/watch?v=WaJ6sZ4nfnQ.

Other less common varieties of umbilical cord entanglement occur. True knots are found in 1% of pregnancies and are difficult to detect prenatally. Knots have been reported as a cause of fetal demise and are associated with advanced maternal age, multiparty, long umbilical cords, and monoamniotic twins [9]. The cord entanglement seen in monoamniotic twins is often detected by ultrasound as early as the first trimester. A recent systematic literature review suggests that such cord entanglement is not a contributor to adverse prenatal events in these twin pregnancies [10]; this conclusion is different than classic teaching on the topic.

Thus, the most common cord entanglement that providers are likely to encounter is the nuchal cord, present in one out of four deliveries. A busy practitioner will therefore encounter this "complication" quite frequently. It is important to realize that nuchal cords rarely have a negative impact on outcome and prenatal diagnosis by ultrasound should not alter management. It is unlikely that practitioners will ever stop reducing or clamping and cutting nuchal cords, but these maneuvers optimally should be deferred until after the anterior shoulder has been delivered. Abandonment of these maneuvers in favor of delivering through the cord or somersaulting the infant as described above is recommended by the author.

Umbilical Cord Prolapse

Although the incidence of umbilical cord prolapse has remained essentially the same at 3 to 4 per 1,000 deliveries over the past 75 years, the perinatal mortality has fallen from nearly 50% to less than 10% [11–13]. Abandonment of complex obstetric procedures such as internal podalic version, breech extraction, funic reduction, and high forceps in favor of rapid cesarean section to accomplish delivery, coupled with advances in neonatal resuscitation, has greatly improved neonatal outcomes and decreased maternal morbidity [14]. Umbilical cord prolapse is a true obstetric emergency, which lends itself particularly well to coordinated team efforts by nurses, obstetricians, anesthesiologists, and neonatologists to achieve optimal outcomes [15].

Cord prolapse occurs when a length or coil of umbilical cord slips through the cervix and presents alongside or in front of the fetal presenting part. The loop may be visible in the vagina or at the introitus or may be palpated as a pulsatile mass on vaginal exam. If the cord is not visible or palpable, it is referred to as an occult prolapse. In such cases, the only presenting sign may be changes in electronic fetal heart rate tracings suggestive of cord compression [16].

Umbilical cord compression between the fetal-presenting part and the maternal pelvis results in decreased placental blood flow to the fetus. If left untreated, such cord compression may cause fetal hypoxia and fetal injury or death [15]. This diminished blood flow is seen as repetitive variable fetal heart rate decelerations, prolonged decelerations, or sudden bradycardia. Any of these fetal heart rate changes should prompt consideration of the diagnosis of cord prolapse, either overt or occult [16].

Risk factors for umbilical cord prolapse share two characteristics, rupture of membranes and a fetus that is not fully engaged in the pelvis or firmly applied to the cervix. Multiparous pregnancy, fetal malpresentation, polyhydramnios, multiple gestation, and low birth weight, either due to prematurity or growth restriction, are at risk for cord prolapse. It has been stated that anywhere from 10% to almost 50% of prolapse cases result from obstetric manipulation. Associated interventions include amniotomy, insertion of internal monitors, amnioinfusion, operative vaginal delivery, and external cephalic version [14–16]. Potentially any obstetric manipulation that elevates the presenting fetal part within the pelvis could cause umbilical cord prolapse.

If prolapse occurs when vaginal delivery is imminent, prompt continuation of vaginal delivery efforts is sometimes appropriate, but the treatment of choice for most cases of umbilical cord prolapse is rapid cesarean section. When prolapse is recognized, an examiner should place a hand in the vagina and elevate the presenting part to decompress the cord. Elevation of the presenting part should be maintained until delivery. This is a true emergency best managed by a prepared team. A call for help should mobilize anesthesia, the newborn intensive care unit (NICU) team, more nursing assistance, anoperating room (OR) team, and a laborist or another provider if available. Ancillary procedures such as maternal position change, intravenous (IV) fluid bolus, maternal oxygen administration, and tocolytics should be considered as preparations are being made for abdominal delivery [17,18]. A sample protocol for management [18] is seen in Box 5.1.

Fetal prognosis following cord prolapse is considerably better with prompt delivery, but there are times when cesarean section is not readily available. For example, a patient might rupture membranes at home and experience cord prolapse, or cord prolapse might occur in a health facility, such as a birthing center or small labor and delivery unit, without the capability to perform a rapid section. While preparations are made for section or for transport to an appropriate facility for section, temporizing measures for decompression of the cord should be instituted. As previously noted, the health care provider should lift the fetal presenting part higher in the pelvis away from the cord. Changing the maternal position to knee-chest or Trendelenburg should be considered. Replacing loops of prolapsed cord back into the vagina with a moist sponge to decrease the risk of vasospasm has also been suggested [17]. Because it may be difficult to maintain prolonged manual elevation of the fetus, a technique of catheterizing the bladder, retrofilling with 500–700 mL of saline, and then clamping the catheter has been described [19]. This method has been used both with and without short term tocolysis.

Funic reduction by instrument has largely been abandoned. Tapered instruments called bougies and specially designed hooked and grasping tools called cord repositors were once used to elevate and return the cord to an intrauterine position. Today these are only of historical interest [14].

More recently, a technique for funic reduction by manual replacement has been described. With this technique, an assistant applies "gentle abdominal pressure in the suprapubic area" while the delivering

Box 5.1 Sample umbilical cord prolapse management protocol

Umbilical Cord Prolapse

Purpose

To outline actions taken to alleviate or reduce compression of the umbilical cord due to prolapse until an emergency cesarean delivery can be performed.

Procedure

1. Assess patient for prolapsed cord by visualizing the introitus and palpating for umbilical cord with vaginal exam.
2. If cord is palpable, protect cord by placing it between the two examining fingers.
3. Apply gentle pressure against presenting part to release compression of cord. Continue to protect cord until delivery.
4. Call for assistance.
5. Notify provider and anesthesia immediately.
6. Initiate procedures for emergency cesarean delivery.
7. Call NICU team to attend delivery.
8. Educate and reassure patient/family.
9. Discontinue Pitocin if in use.
10. Administer bolus of Lactated Ringers solution or normal saline.
11. Give oxygen at 10 L/min by tight face mask.
12. Consider position changes to increase perfusion, such as knee-chest, Trendelenburg, or lateral positions.
13. Continue fetal monitoring.

Documentation

Document assessments, education, interventions, and communication with and attendance of physician and ancillary staff / teams.

practitioner elevates the fetal head with a vaginal hand and attempts to slip the prolapsed loop of cord above the widest part of the fetal head. The aim is to replace the cord into the nuchal area [20].

Finally, in cases of previable rupture of membranes with prolapse, it may be desirable to attempt conservative management until fetal viability has been reached. The cord should be replaced into the vagina with a moist sponge and the patient should be managed according to the guidelines recommended for premature rupture of membranes. There is insufficient data to evaluate the efficacy of this approach given that reported successes are rare [14].

Antepartum Funic Presentation

The term, funic presentation, refers to an umbilical cord presentation in the lower uterine segment below the fetal-presenting part with membranes intact. Antepartum diagnosis of funic presentation may be made by ultrasound. Many of these patients will have fetal malpresentations and delivery by cesarean section prior to labor is commonly indicated [21]. Some funic presentations resolve spontaneously prior to labor and have no obstetric sequelae [22]. Patients with persistent funic presentation who experience spontaneous rupture of membranes will be at increased risk of umbilical cord prolapse. All such patients should be counseled regarding early recognition of spontaneous labor or rupture of membranes and should be instructed to come to the hospital immediately when or if these conditions are suspected [15].

Many would suggest that cesarean section prior to labor in the term vertex fetus with funic presentation is a reasonable consideration after thorough patient counseling. Another option for labor management in these pregnancies is the careful use of fetal monitoring with delay of the rupture of membranes in the hope that the cord will spontaneously reduce as labor progresses and the fetal vertex engages. Signs of severe cord compression should prompt abdominal delivery [16].

In term patients with an unengaged vertex fetus and significant cervical dilation, controlled rupture of membranes may be considered by “needling” the amniotic membranes. This is a technique that has been utilized for decades in the unengaged fetus at risk for cord prolapse. The membranes are punctured under direct vision with a needle in an effort to slowly release fluid [16]. Success is variable and there are no published studies proving the safety of this technique.

Velamentous Cord Insertion and Vasa Previa

Velamentous cord insertions (see Figure 5.2) occur when umbilical vessels splay from the placental surface into the amniotic membranes without the protection of Wharton’s jelly. Velamentous cord insertions are found in 1–2% of singleton pregnancies but are

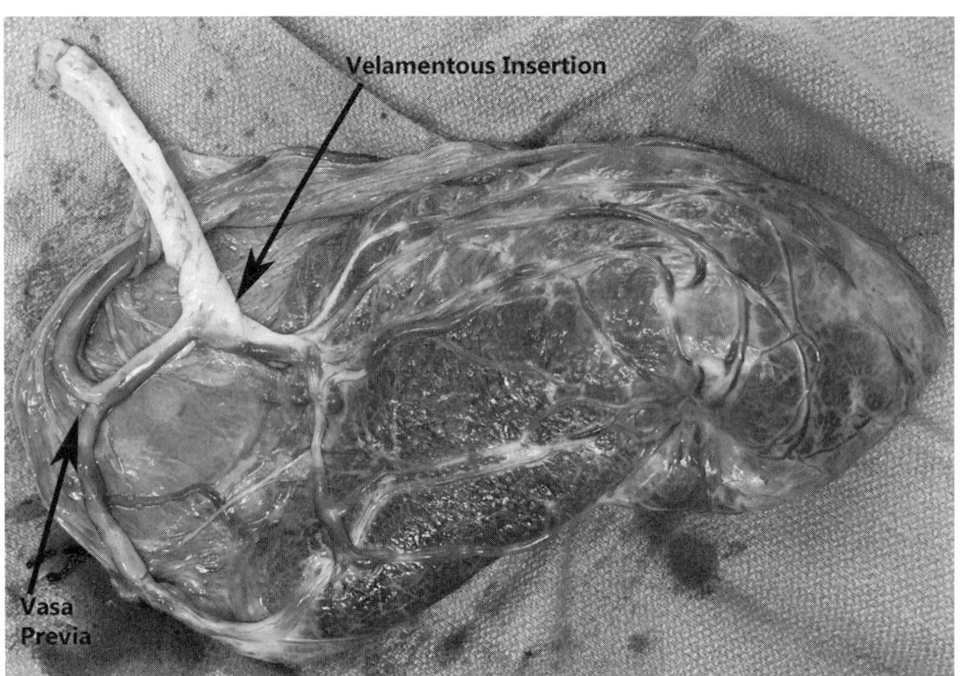

Figure 5.2 Velamentous cord insertion and vasa previa. Courtesy of Elise Hodges and Phillip Bressman, STM, Nashville, TN. 2016.

considerably more frequent in monochorionic twins [23]. A variant of the velamentous cord, known as vasa previa, occurs when unprotected vessels cross the cervical os. Bare vessels running through amniotic membranes are subject to compression, twisting, or rupture and have been associated with fetal growth disorders, anomalies, and stillbirth [23,24]. Variable fetal heart rate decelerations are often seen in labor and third stage complications of premature cord detachment, retained placenta, and postpartum hemorrhage have been reported [25].

When a velamentous insertion is detected by antepartum ultrasound, the fetus should undergo careful scanning for associated disorders and should be managed accordingly. It seems prudent to consider serial growth scans and appropriately timed testing for fetal well-being. Some would suggest scheduled delivery by term induction, although no controlled trials exist to support this [23].

Active management of the third stage of labor in an effort to prevent postpartum hemorrhage is now considered the standard of care [26]. Active management includes uterine massage, controlled cord traction, and prophylactic administration of oxytocin. Velamentous and marginal cord insertions occur in approximately 8% of pregnancies collectively and may complicate the third stage as described previously [25]. In pregnancies with known abnormal cord insertions, aggressive cord traction should be avoided but uterine massage and oxytocin are appropriate. The timing of oxytocin administration before or after placental delivery is often a topic of debate. Data exists, however, that early oxytocin administration does not increase the incidence of retained placenta [27]. Administration before placental delivery to avoid manual extraction may therefore be useful in pregnancies with abnormal cord insertions. Small series have been published describing successful placental delivery after injecting 20 IU of oxytocin diluted in 20–30 mL of saline directly into the umbilical vein [28,29]. This should be contrasted with administration of oxytocin or other pharmacologic agents for a retained placenta (defined as a 30-minute third stage) since no intervention other than manual extraction has been shown to be effective [30].

Vasa previa, with an incidence of 1 in 2,500 pregnancies, is a considerably more serious variant of velamentous cord insertion. Unprotected vessels cross the cervical os and are at risk for hemorrhage with rupture of membranes or labor. Such rupture could lead to sudden and fatal fetal exsanguination. Vasa previa is associated with placenta previa and low-lying placentas, multilobed placentas or accessory lobes,

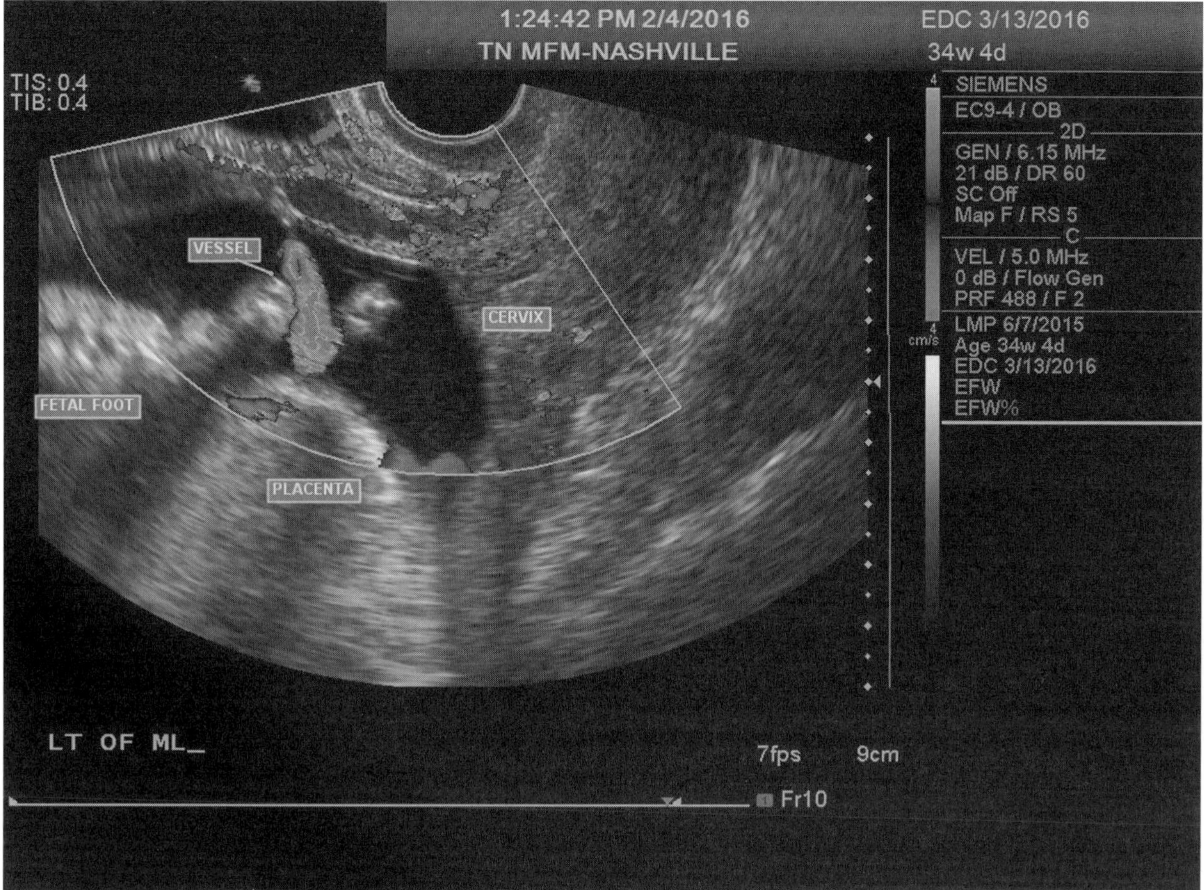

Figure 5.3 Sonogram showing vasa previa-courtesy of Tennessee Maternal Fetal Medicine, Nashville TN, 2016.

and pregnancies resulting from in vitro fertilization. Diagnosis may be made by transvaginal ultrasound as seen in Figure 5.3.

Antenatal hospitalization at 30 weeks, the administration of antenatal steroids, and cesarean delivery at 34 to 37 weeks have been suggested for management [31,32].

Concluding Remarks

Umbilical cords can be evaluated by ultrasound. Conclusions about fetal well-being can be made from fetal heart tracings and umbilical Doppler velocimetry. Amnioinfusion can be used to relieve cord compression and avoid cesarean sections. Nuchal umbilical cords can be fearlessly and expertly managed. Obstetric care providers can do many things, but should not become complacent.

In the past, it has been all too easy to attribute stillbirth to cord complications. Abnormal cord insertions, cord prolapse, cord rupture, and other causes of occlusion account for 3.4–15% of stillbirths. However, cord entanglements, nuchal cords, and true knots should not be considered the cause of stillbirth until other causes have been excluded. Cord occlusion resulting in stillbirth should also leave evidence of constriction of umbilical blood vessels or congestion, edema, or thrombosis in acute cases [24].

It is important to remember that after delivery has been accomplished and attention has been directed to the stabilization of the mother and infant, the placenta and cord should not be automatically relegated to the pan to be later discarded. In cases involving operative vaginal delivery, emergent cesarean section, shoulder dystocia, vaginal breech delivery, thick meconium, suspected maternal infection, recurrent late or variable fetal heart rate decelerations, prolonged fetal heart rate decelerations, Apgar scores of less than 5 at 1 min and/or less than 7 at 5 min, or premature delivery less than 37 weeks, a segment of umbilical cord saved for blood gas evaluation and a section of placenta set aside for pathologic examination may prove invaluable [33].

References

1. Schaffer L, Zimmerman R. Nuchal cords. *UpToDate.* 2015. http://www.uptodate.com/contents/nuchal-cord, accessed 7/2/17.
2. Schaffer L, Burkhardt T, Zimmerman R, Kurmanavicius J. Nuchal cords in term and postterm deliveries – Do we need to know? *Obstetrics and Gynecology* 2005;106:23.
3. Larson J, Rayburn W, Crosby S, Thurnau G. Multiple nuchal cord entanglements and intrapartum complications. *American Journal of Obstetrics and Gynecology* 1995;173:1228.
4. Williams *Obstetrics*, 24th edition, 2014; 538.
5. Henry E, Andres R, Christensen R. Neonatal outcomes following a tight nuchal cord. *Journal of Perinatology* 2013; 33: 231.
6. Schorn M, Blanco J. Management of the nuchal cord. *Journal of Nurse-Midwifery* 1991; 36:131.
7. Flamm B. Tight nuchal cord and shoulder dystocia: A potentially catastrophic combination. *Obstetrics and Gynecology* 1999; 94:853.
8. Mercer J, Skovgaard R, Peareara-Eaves J, Bowman T. Nuchal cord management and nurse-midwifery practice. *Journal of Midwifery and Women's Health* 2005; 50:373.
9. Beall M. Umbilical cord complications. Medscape 2014. http://emedicine.medscape.com/article/262470-overview?pa=%2BXQXD2%2BgrPTTZKBt96Ijymu8o qFarki05%2FE23Wajub85wAcmhHN0EpfY1wq7QYhp jqFQFmc6gRdIHfSEruIFeuN5lPYw%2FtQ7Z8WOOz pssmw%3D, accessed 4/40/17
10. Rossi A, Prefumo F. Impact of cord entanglement on perinatal outcome of monoamniotic twins: A systematic review of the literature. *Ultrasound in Obstetrics and Gynecology* 2013; 41:131.
11. Schultz J. Prolapse of the umbilical cord. *Obstetrics and Gynecology* 1955; 6:657.
12. Savage E, Kohl S, Wynn R. Prolapse of the umbilical cord. *Obstetrics and Gynecology* 1970; 36:502.
13. Levy H, Meier P, Makowski E. Umbilical cord prolapse. *Obstetrics and Gynecology* 1984; 64:499.
14. Lin M. Umbilical cord prolapse. *Obstetrical and Gynecological Survey* 2006; 61:269.
15. Holbrook B, Phelan S. Umbilical cord prolapse. *Obstetric and Gynecological Clinics of North America* 2013; 40:1.
16. Bush M, Eddleman K, Belogolovkin V. Umbilical cord prolapse. UpToDate. 2015.
17. Phelan S, Holbrook B. Umbilical cord prolapse, a plan for an ob emergency. *Contemporary OB/GYN.* September 2013.
18. *Umbilical cord prolapse 2.50. PolicyStat ID 742403. Saint Thomas Midtown Hospital 2014.*
19. Katz Z, Shoham Z, Lancet M, Blickstein I, Mogilner B, Zalel Y. Management of labor with umbilical cord prolapse: a 5-year study. *Obstetrics and Gynecology* 1988; 72:278.
20. Barrett J. Funic reduction for the management of umbilical cord prolapse. *American Journal of Obstetrics and Gynecology* 1991; 165:654.
21. Kinugasa M, Sato T, Tamura M, Suzuki H, Miyazaki Y, Imanaka M. Antepartum detection of cord presentation by transvaginal ultrasonography for term breech presentation: Potential prediction and prevention of cord prolapse. *Journal of Obstetrics and Gynaecology Research* 2007; 33:612.
22. Ezra Y, Strasberg S, Farine D. Does cord presentation on ultrasound predict cord prolapse? *Gynecologic and Obstetric Investigation* 2003; 56:6.
23. Lockwood C, Russo-Stieglitz K. Velamentous umbilical cord insertion and vasa previa. *UpToDate.* 2015. https://www.uptodate.com/contents/velamentous-umbilical-cord-insertion-and-vasa-previa, accessed 7/2/17.
24. Reddy U, Goldenberg R, Silver R, Smith G, Pauli R, Wapner R, Gardosi J, Pinar H, Grafe M, Kupferminc M, Varli I, Erwich J, Fretts R, Willinger M. Stillbirth classification – Developing an international consensus for research. *Obstetrics and Gynecology* 2009; 114:901.
25. Ebbing C, Kiserud T, Johnsen S, Albrechtsen S, Rasmussen S. Third stage of labor risks in velamentous and marginal cord insertion: a population-based study. *ACTA Obstetricia et Gynecologica Scandinavica* 2015; 94:878.
26. Main E, Goffman D, Scavone B, Low L, Bingham D, Fontaine P, Gorlin J, Lagrew D, Levy B. National partnership for maternal safety: Consensus bundle on obstetric hemorrhage. *Obstetrics and Gynecology* 2015; 126:155.
27. Jackson K, Allbert J, Schemmer G, Elliot M, Humphrey A, Taylor, J. A randomized controlled trial comparing oxytocin administration before and after placental delivery in the prevention of postpartum hemorrhage. *American Journal of Obstetrics and Gynecology* 2001; 185:873.
28. Gazvani M, Luckas M, Drakeley A, Emery S, Alfirevic Z, Walkinshaw S. Intraumbilical oxytocin for the

management of retained placenta: a randomized controlled trial. *Obstetrics and Gynecology* 1998; 91:203.

29. Gungorduk K, Asicioglu O, Besimoglu B, Gungorduk O, Yildirm G, Ark C, Tekirdag A. Using intraumbilical vein injection of oxytocin in routine practice with active management of the third stage of labor. *Obstetrics and Gynecology* 2010; 116:619.
30. Duffy J, Mylan S, Showell M, Wilson M, Khan K. Pharmacologic intervention for retained placenta. *Obstetrics and Gynecology* 2015; 125:711.
31. Bronsteen R, Whitten A, Balasubramanian M, Lee W, Lorenz R, Redman M, Goncalves L, Seubert D, Bauer S, Comstock C. Vasa previa. *Obstetrics and Gynecology* 2013; 122:352.
32. Sinkey R, Odibo A, Dashe J. Diagnosis and management of vasa previa. *American Journal of Obstetrics and Gynecology* 2015; 213:615.
33. *Neonatal Encephalopathy and Neurologic Outcome*, 2nd edition. 2014.

Operative Vaginal Delivery

George H. Davis

Introduction

Operative vaginal delivery has been in use for more than two millennia but, until the advent of obstetrical forceps, it was almost exclusively a procedure that involved fetal destruction. The advent of safe cesarean delivery has gradually eroded the need and popularity of operative vaginal delivery, and yet there is still very much a place for obstetrical forceps and vacuum in today's delivery room. The last two decades have seen a resurgence of vacuum-assisted vaginal deliveries.

This chapter deals with the proper use of both forceps and vacuum with an emphasis on the technical aspects. Each is dealt with separately. No attempt is made to compare one approach to the other. While many operative deliveries could be accomplished with either instrument, there are certainly situations where one has an advantage over the other. Any inference that one approach is superior to the other is completely unintentional and no conclusion to that effect should be made.

Scope of the Problem

The opportunity to learn operative vaginal delivery varies greatly across the United States. In an unpublished survey of residency programs, a resident is much more likely to acquire this skill if the program is located in the mid-west, south, or central regions of the country than on either coast.[1] Additionally, the opportunities to learn these skills has diminished. Training experience has changed substantially over the past decade. Accreditation Council of Graduate Medical Education (ACGME) training logs of Ob/Gyn resident experience have demonstrated decreases in both forceps and vacuum-assisted vaginal deliveries with a concomitant increase in cesarean deliveries.[2]

The current ACGME minimum threshold requires at least 15 operative vaginal deliveries during a four-year residency program in obstetrics and gynecology.[3] This can be forceps or vacuum, or both combined. It is hoped, however, that all residents will acquire exposure to both. Despite a growing body of evidence that forceps are more successful than vacuum-assisted deliveries, with a lower incidence of fetal injury, many obstetricians still favor the vacuum for its ease of use, a much shorter learning curve and less risk of maternal trauma.[4]

This chapter follows and adheres to the ACOG clinical management guidelines with an emphasis on proper technique.[5]

Indications

The indications for operative vaginal delivery are essentially the same for both forceps and vacuum. The individual clinical situation and physician preference will dictate which approach is undertaken. While there are numerous clinical indications, they can essentially be placed into the three categories listed in Box 6.1.

The second stage of labor may be prolonged for a number of different reasons. These include an inability of the patient to push effectively, maternal exhaustion, dystocia, and the effects of medications including anesthesia. Classically, failure to progress in the second stage of labor has been an indication of its own and is listed as such in the most recent ACOG practice bulletin. Before choosing an operative intervention, the practitioner should make a reasonable effort to address treatable causes for lack of progression.

Maternal health indications include those situations when the patient should avoid pushing in the second stage. These indications include certain cardiac conditions or intracranial vascular lesions. Other patients may not have the ability to push effectively (such as women with cerebral palsy, spinal bifida, Guillian Barré, etc.) but otherwise have no contraindication to vaginal delivery.

Box 6.1 Indications for operative vaginal delivery

1. Prolonged second stage of labor
2. Maternal health
3. Fetal health

If signs of fetal compromise surface during the second stage of labor, operative vaginal delivery can shorten the second stage. Not all fetal heart rate abnormalities require intervention. Clinical experience and judicious evaluation can discriminate between those indeterminate changes typical of second stage labor and those less common situations where the fetal status is deteriorating. It is frequently the case that a safe operative vaginal delivery can be performed more quickly than a cesarean delivery, thereby shortening the amount of time that the fetus may potentially be compromised.

An unengaged head is an absolute contraindication to operative vaginal delivery. The next section of this chapter will deal with the requirements for a safe operative delivery. Inability to meet these requirements is itself a contraindication. While some of these requirements are soft recommendations, an inability to determine with certainty the position of the fetal head and lack of an experienced operator in attendance should also be considered as absolute contraindications. Some fetal malformations, while amenable to spontaneous vaginal delivery, should also be considered as contraindication. These include hydrocephaly, craniosynostosis, omphalocele, and a distended fetal abdomen from gastrointestinal (GI) obstruction.

Requirements for Safe Operative Vaginal Delivery

A number of excellent texts and atlases are available that discuss and illustrate the techniques for operative vaginal delivery.[6–13] These books include a list of conditions that should met before applying either forceps or vacuum to accomplish the delivery. The list of requirements seen in Box 6.2 generally follows American Congress of Obstetrics and Gynecology (ACOG) recommendations but also combines information from other sources.

Box 6.2 Requirements for safe operative vaginal delivery

1. The cervix must be fully dilated and retracted. Presence of an anterior lip, especially in cases of asynchlitism, may sometimes be permissible.
2. The membranes must be ruptured.
3. The maternal bladder should be empty. An empty rectum is also desirable.
4. The presentation must be cephalic with the fetal head engaged within the maternal pelvis, the exception being the use of Piper forceps for the after-coming head in breech deliveries. Forceps or vacuum should never be applied to the fetal buttocks.
5. The position of the fetal head must be known with certainty.
6. There must be adequate anesthesia. This should be individualized to the patient and the situation. Depending upon circumstances, adequate anesthesia may be general, spinal, epidural, or pudendal. For occasional patients, local anesthesia may be sufficient.
7. Fetal macrosomia is a relative contraindication. The estimated fetal weight should be known and a clinical determination made about whether or not a vaginal delivery should be attempted. A prolonged second stage in the face of known or suspected fetal macrosomia is often an indication that vaginal delivery will be difficult and may predispose to additional complications such as shoulder dystocia.
8. The presence/absence of fetal malformations should be known. Some malformations, such as omphalocele or hydrocephaly, might obstruct vaginal delivery. Others, such as gastroschisis or sirenomelia, may still portend a successful vaginal approach.
9. The maternal pelvis should be adequate for vaginal delivery given the clinic estimation of the fetal size.
10. The patient should be informed of the benefits and risks of operative vaginal delivery and must give consent.
11. An experienced operator must be in attendance.

Types of Forceps Deliveries

The types of forceps deliveries and their criteria go back more than a century. The *American System of Obstetrics* (1889) still referred to those forceps applications that occurred in the superior strait or inferior strait, that is, above or below the ischial spines.[14] By the first edition of *William's Obstetrics* in 1903, high, mid- and low forceps criteria were recognized. The definitions of these criteria were, however, considerably different than those that we use today.[15] From a contemporary standpoint, high forceps should longer be performed and low forceps have been sub-divided to include outlet forceps. The criteria described in Box 6.3 follow the ACOG definitions and apply to vacuum-assisted deliveries as well.

As will be discussed later in this chapter, vacuum-assisted deliveries should meet the aforementioned criteria as well, but are restricted to "outlet vacuum" and "low vacuum." Additionally, rotation should not be attempted with the vacuum.

Box 6.3 Types of operative vaginal deliveries

Outlet The fetal scalp is visible at the introitus without manual separation of the labia. Some authorities describe this observation as being present between contractions. From a more practical standpoint, most practitioners will designate the delivery as "outlet forceps" or "outlet vacuum" if the criteria are met during a contraction.

The fetal skull must have reached the pelvic floor with the head at or on the perineum. The sagittal suture must be in an anteroposterior orientation with no more than 45° of rotation; in other words, between right occiput anterior (ROA) and left occiput anterior (LOA).

Low The leading point of the vertex is at +2 cm or more but the head has not yet reached the pelvic floor. Ideally, this means that the biparietal diameter has reached or exceeded the level of the ischial spines.

Low forceps are subdivided as to "with" or "without" rotation and should be documented as such in the delivery record. Any rotation of no more than 45° is considered to be "without" rotation. If the baby's head requires more than 45° of rotation, it is considered to be "with" rotation.

Mid-Pelvic The station is above +2 cm but the head is engaged.

By the year 2000, most authorities, including the ACOG, had recommended the elimination of high forceps deliveries, as the complication rate clearly outweighed any advantage over cesarean delivery. Lost in this process was a fuller definition of midforceps.

In the third edition of *Dennens's Forceps Deliveries* (1989), the statement is made, "the leading bony point is at the [ischial] spines or below, to +2 station".[16] Technically speaking, the head can be engaged at −3 cm, or even higher. The author agrees with this more complete prior definition and recommends that operative vaginal delivery should not be attempted unless the vertex is at 0 station or lower.

Forceps Deliveries

Anatomy of Obstetrical Forceps

A typical pair of obstetrical forceps consists of the blades, a shank, the lock, and the handle. The blades contain a cephalic curve to accommodate the fetal head and most contain a pelvic curve to align with the maternal pelvis. A few styles contain a perineal curve allowing for simple axis traction. (Figure 6.1).

Blades may be solid, fenestrated, or pseudo-fenestrated. The shanks may be parallel or overlapping. The lock may be English, sliding, or pivot.

Most forceps have a left blade and a right blade. An exception exists for some types of rotating forceps in which the blades are designated as anterior (upper) and posterior (lower). The left blade is the one that goes on the left side of the maternal pelvis. With rare exception, the left blade is the female blade, so called because the lock is designed to receive the right, or male blade. Laufe forceps (see below) are an exception.

The leading edge of the blade is referred to as the tip or the toe and the portion nearest the shank is referred to as the heel.

Choice of Instruments

More than 600 different styles of obstetrical forceps have been described and manufactured. In terms of today's delivery room environment, this chapter will focus on only five modern styles and their variations. If an operative delivery can be safely accomplished, it can be accomplished with one of these five types of forceps. See Box 6.4 for a description of these five major forceps types (Figure 6.2).

In choosing a style of forceps, the first consideration should always be what the individual practitioner has skill and comfort using. The particular advantages of each are listed in Box 6.4. Note that Tucker–McLane forceps are for the unmolded head while Simpson forceps accommodate the molded head (Figure 6.3).

Application of Forceps

Application technique will vary slightly with each practitioner. The description given here is based on the classic textbooks and atlases and confirmed by the

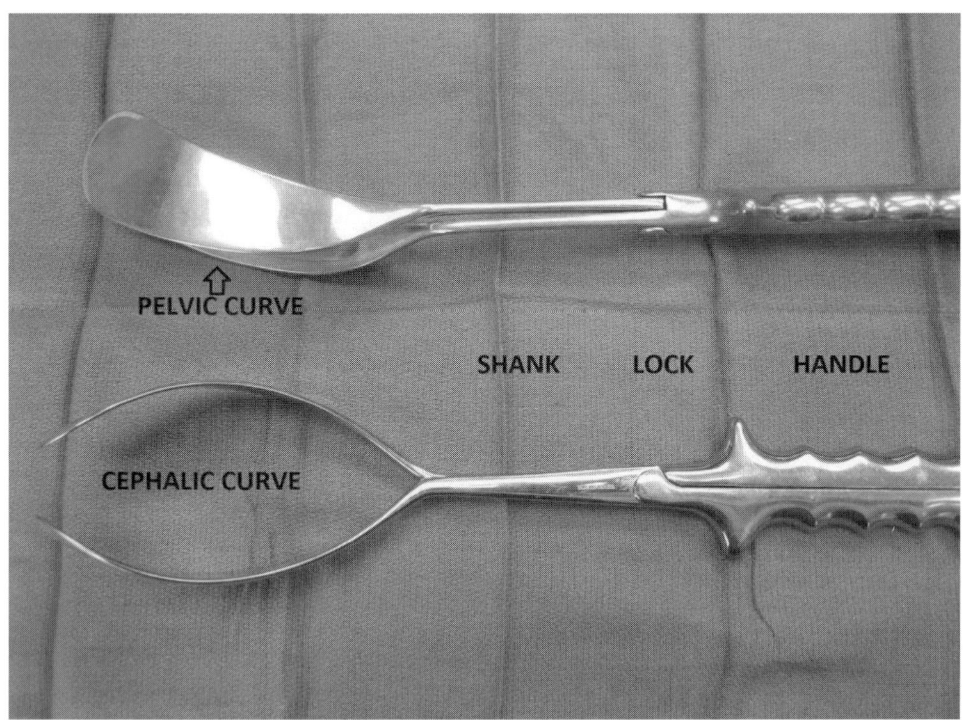

Figure 6.1 Anatomy of the forceps.

author's more than 40 years' experience encompassing more than 1,000 forceps deliveries.

This initial section will assume a vertex presentation to at least +2 cm and with rotation of less than 45°. That is, the position of the fetal head is between ROA and LOA. The patient should be in dorsal lithotomy position with the hips slightly flexed, as in a slight McRoberts position.

The articulated forceps should initially be held near the perineum approximating the way they will fit together when applied to the fetal head, including orientation to the position of the head. This is referred to as a "phantom" application. The left blade is then selected. As a rule, the left blade is held in the operator's left hand and is placed on the left side of the maternal pelvis. The right blade is held in the right hand and is applied to the right side of the maternal pelvis.

The left blade is lightly held near the end of the handle so that it hangs almost vertically with the cephalic curve covering the introitus. It will be noted that the tip of the blade points slightly to the maternal left. It is in this plane that the blade should be inserted. Using the right hand to guide, the blade is gently slid in along the fetal head, avoiding any rotation or twisting of the blade, and keeping the application oriented to about 5 o'clock. To accomplish this, the handle, still vertical will move toward the operator (Figures 6.4a and 6.4b).

Generally speaking, the blade will not be able to advance more than about two-thirds of its length. Properly applied, the heel of the blade will still be slightly outside of the introitus. The end of the handle, still being held lightly in the left hand, should now be swung in a gentle downward arc that courses along the inside of the patient's right thigh. The right hand may be used to guide as needed. This will cause the left blade to easily complete its application to the fetal head. In most cases, this can be accomplished with only fingertip pressure and control (Figure 6.5).

If the position is between occiput anterior (OA) and LOA, nothing more need be done at this point. If the position is ROA, the blade will need to be rotated slightly so that it rests alongside of the left parietal bone of the fetal head (see below).

Attention is then given to the right blade. It is allowed to hang vertically with the cephalic curve against introitus, and it will be noted that the tip of the blade points slightly to the patient's ride side at about 7:00. It is then slid in place using the same technique as for the left blade but swinging the handle in place along the inside of the patient's left thigh. If the position is LOA, this blade will need slight rotation (see below).

Box 6.4 Five major types of obstetric forceps for modern use (Figure 6.2)

Tucker-McLane These forceps typically have solid blades, an overlapping shank, and an English lock. The Luikart modification has pseudo-fenestrated blades while the Elliot and Bailey–Williamson variations have fenestrated blades. The blades have an ample cephalic curve and are ideally suited for low and outlet deliveries of the head with minimal molding (Figure 6.3).

Simpson These forceps typically have fenestrated blades, a parallel shank, and an English lock. The Luikart modification has pseudo-fenestrated blades and the Hawks–Dennen variation includes a perineal curve. The blades are elongated and the cephalic curve is softened. They are ideally suited to low and outlet deliveries where there is more pronounced molding of the fetal head (Figure 6.3). They are also well suited to mid-forceps deliveries when minimal rotation is required.

Laufe These forceps have pseudo-fenestrated blades and a pivot lock that incorporates the handle. There is also a perineal curve. They are commonly referred to as "divergent" forceps. Unlike the other forceps discussed in this chapter, there is no class 1 lever, thereby eliminating any compressive element. They are ideally suited to low and outlet deliveries.

Kielland These forceps have either fenestrated or pseudo-fenestrated blades and a short pelvic curve. The shanks and handle are parallel to the axis of the blades, though slightly offset. There is a sliding lock to accommodate asynchlitism. The Laufe–Kielland–Barton variation incorporates a hinged upper blade and completely eliminates the pelvic curve so that the axis of the blades and the axis of the shanks and handle are in direct alignment. These forceps are ideally suited to mid-forceps deliveries, especially when rotation of more than 45° is required.

Piper These forceps have fenestrated blades, an English lock, and long sweeping parallel shanks to accommodate application to the after coming head in breech deliveries.

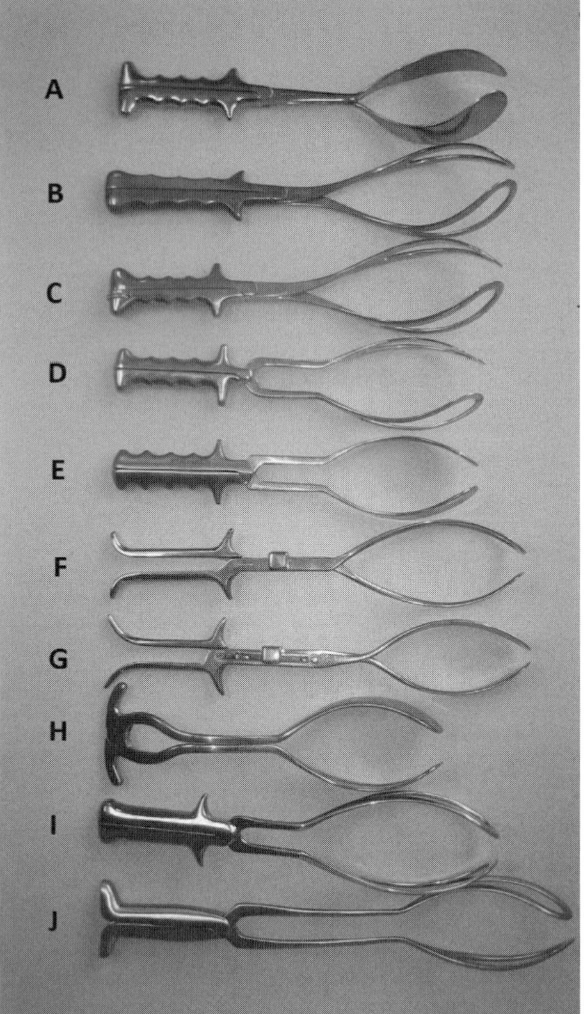

Figure 6.2 Modern types of forceps: (A) Tucker–McLane, (B) Bailey–Williamson, (C) Elliot, (D) Simpson, (E) Luikart–Simpson, (F) Hawk–Dennen, (G) Laufe, (H) Kielland, (I) Laufe–Kielland–Barton, and (J) Piper.

The blades are then locked together. Commonly, the lock will not seem to match up. This is because the natural shape of the maternal pelvis causes the blades to rest slightly too far toward the occiput. The handles must not be twisted to try and get the lock to match up. Rather, the handles should be depressed downward against the perineum. This will accomplish two things simultaneously. First, the handles will orient so that the lock matches up. It may be necessary to move the handles slightly to the right or left to complete the locking. Second, the orientation of the blades to the fetal head should be virtually perfect (Figure 6.6)

With the forceps in place, proper application must be confirmed. The sagittal suture should be aligned with the shanks and the posterior fontanelle should be palpable about 2 cm (one finger breadth) above the shanks. The lambdoid sutures should be equidistant from the right and left blades respectively.

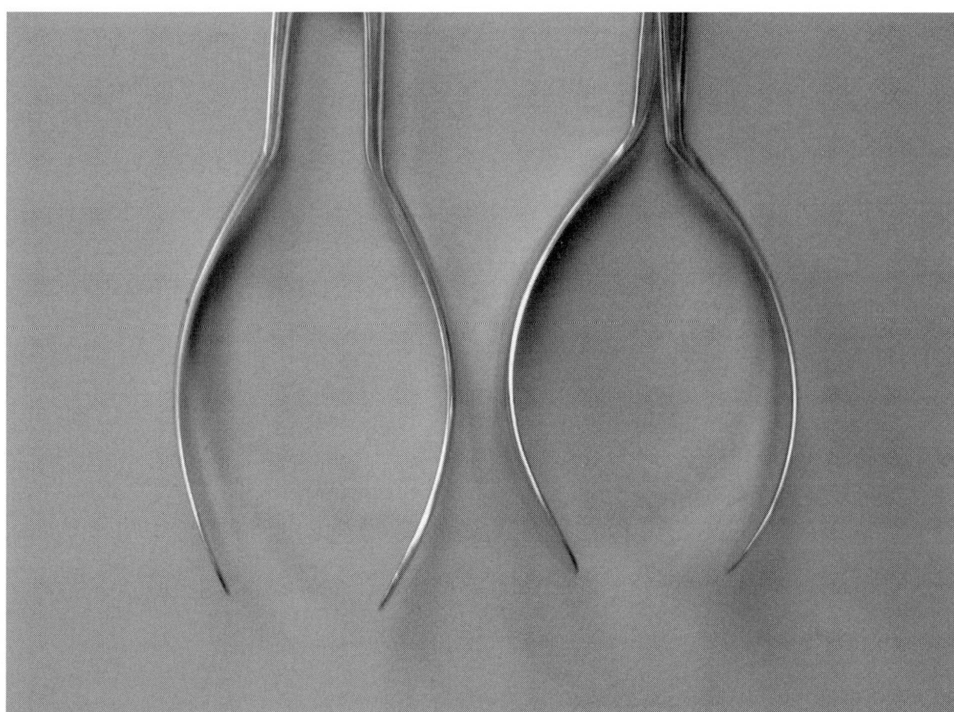

Figure 6.3 Simpson versus Tucker–McLane. Note the elongated cephalic curve for the Simpsons (left) compared to the more rounded cephalic curve for the Tucker McLanes (right).

When applying rotation forceps to a head in a transverse position, between right occiput posterior (ROP) and right occiput anterior (ROA) or between left occiput posterior (LOP) and left occiput anterior (LOA), the anterior blade is inserted first using the above technique. Again, the forceps should first be held in articulated position at the perineum to help visualize what the end orientation will be. Whichever blade will be anterior is then selected for initial application.

Once the blade has been inserted alongside the fetal head in the posterior aspect of the birth canal, it will need to be rotated about the head to reach its anterior resting point. The rotation may proceed in either direction. Some operators prefer to proceed through the shortest arc and some prefer to rotate across the occiput. Experience shows, however, that the easiest course is almost always across the face. The occiput often has molding blocking that pathway and the facial area is flat. The facial features themselves are well protected by the bony features.

The keys to easy and successful rotation of the blade about the head are fairly simple. First, it is important to avoid any twisting of the blade. This will invariably happen if an attempt is made to rotate using the handle. Second, almost all of the rotational force needs to be applied to the inferior edge of the blade, just beyond the heel of the blade. Third, the handle needs to be gently depressed downward as the rotation is progressing.

There are two ways to apply pressure to the edge of the blade. The most common is for the operator to use the hand that is on the same side as the blade. For example, the operator would use the right hand to move the left blade. This is straightforward and simple and easy to learn (Figure 6.7a).

There is another technique that takes a little more practice to learn but is much more effective once learned. The opposite hand is used, that is the left hand for the right blade and the right hand for the left blade. The back of the hand is placed against the outside of the shaft such that the toe of the blade, at its juncture with the shaft, rests in the notch between the index and middle fingers at the back of the hand. The index finger is then curled over the juncture so that the inferior edge of the heel rests alongside the index finger. This aligns all of the forces in the natural axis and the blade can then be rotated by a simple turning of the wrist (Figure 6.7b).

Once the anterior blade has been rotated into position, the posterior blade will be applied in the same manner as the anterior. It can then be rotated slightly,

(a)

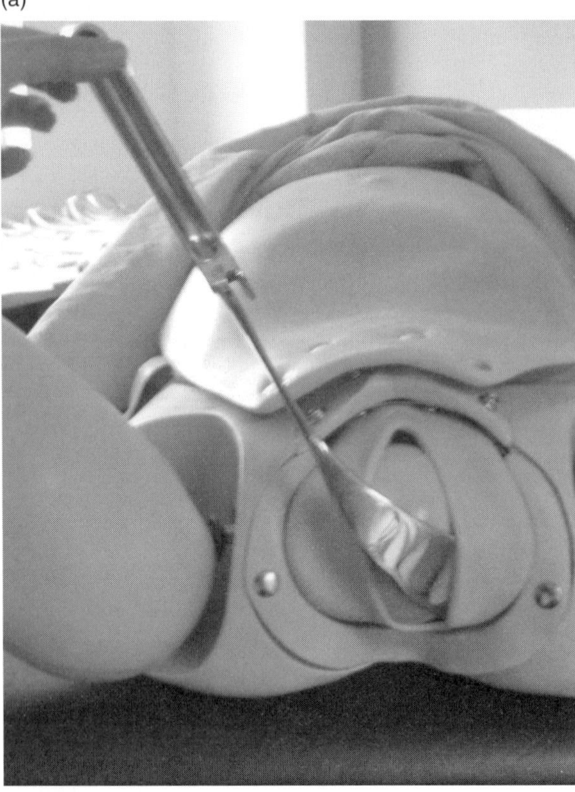

(b)

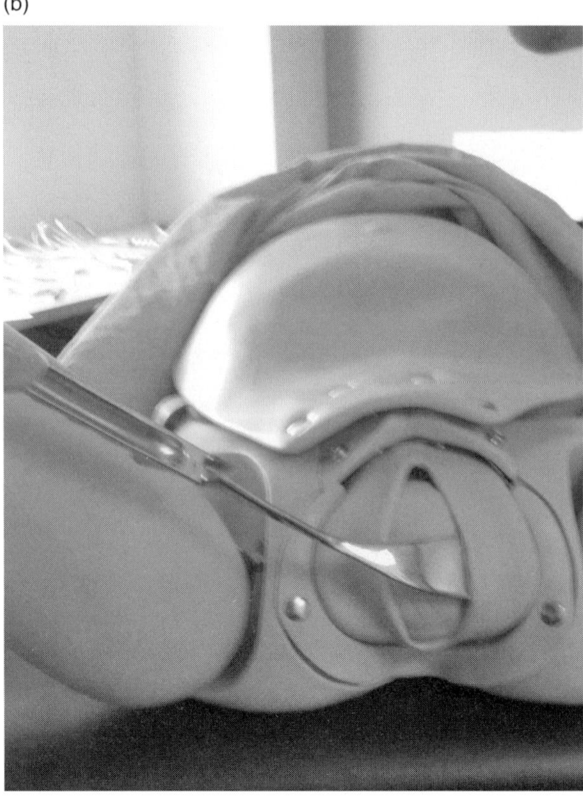

Figure 6.4 Application of outlet forceps: (a) Held upright at perineum and introduced at 5:00; (b) Swung in an arc along the inside of the thigh as blade moves alongside face.

if necessary, and the blades locked. Using Kielland forceps, or a modification of Kiellands, it will be obvious that there is some degree of asynchlitism. If one is attempting to rotate using forceps with a fixed lock, such as Simpsons, the handles will again need to be depressed downward.

Application of Piper forceps to the after coming head may seem challenging, especially since it is seldom used. If one has developed comfort with low and outlet applications, this need not be the case. All of the same principles apply. A vaginal breech delivery should be considered a two-person delivery whenever possible, regardless of whether the forceps are needed. Once the body and extremities are out, the baby is held back up, face down, by one operator. Wrapping the baby in towel or blanket can be helpful. The torso is held with slight elevation of the buttocks.

The left blade is then taken and held vertically by the end of the handle just as with outlet forceps but at the right side of the baby and right side of the maternal pelvis. It will immediately become obvious that the sweeping curve of the shank places the blade directly over the introitus. The blade is then inserted just as with any other forceps, dropping the handle in a gentle sweeping arc along the inside of the right thigh. No rotation should be necessary. The right blade is similarly introduced and the blades locked. Gentle traction is all that is typically needed to deliver the head (Figure 6.8).

Occiput posterior applications can be approached in one of two ways. The easiest is to place the forceps as if it were an occiput anterior position. If this is the case, the anterior fontanelle should be palpable about 2 cm (one finger breadth) above the shanks. The other is to attempt rotation of the head to OA. This should only be attempted by operators skilled in head rotation techniques. See the discussion of head rotation in the next section.

A video instruction of forceps application that incorporates many of these principles can be found at www.youtube.com/watch?v=rloEpKIbnTw

Delivery

First and foremost, it is important to understand that the goal of both forceps and vacuum is to get the

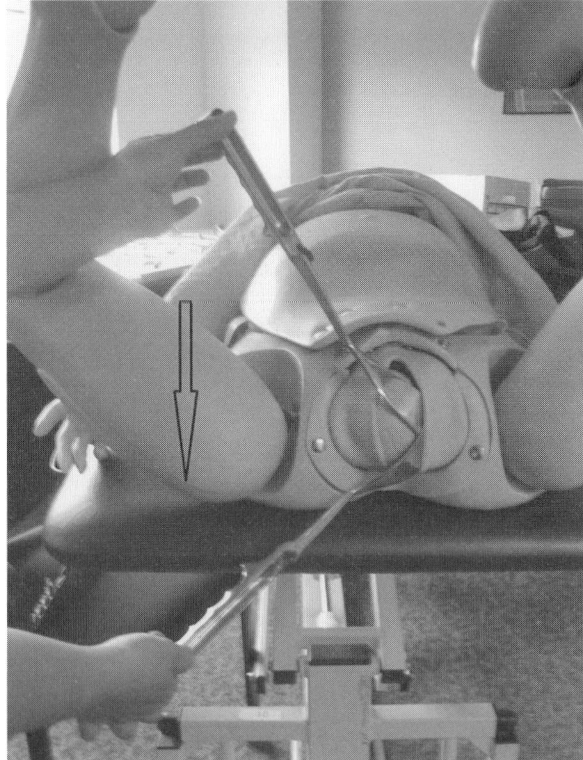

Figure 6.5 Starting and ending points of outlet application.

head under the symphysis pubis. It is *not* the complete delivery of the head. Once the head has cleared the symphysis, the operative instrument(s) should be removed and the delivery should be completed normally. Pipers for the after coming head in a breech delivery are, of course, the exception.

For occiput anterior positions, once the forceps have been applied and checked, the handles are brought into the midline. This will rotate the head minimally, less than 45°, such that the position is now directly OA. This diminishes the outlet marginally but it significantly reduces the risk for vaginal trauma.

Traction should take place with contractions and with whatever additional assistance may be available and safe, such as maternal pushing or fundal pressure. The direction of the traction should be in line with the axis of the blades. For Tucker–McLane, Simpsons and their variations this means that the pull must initially be about 30–45° downward to help get the head under the symphysis. The handles will come upwards as the head clears the symphysis. Frequently, downward pressure on the lock or shanks will help to achieve the proper direction. Forceps with a perineal curve, such

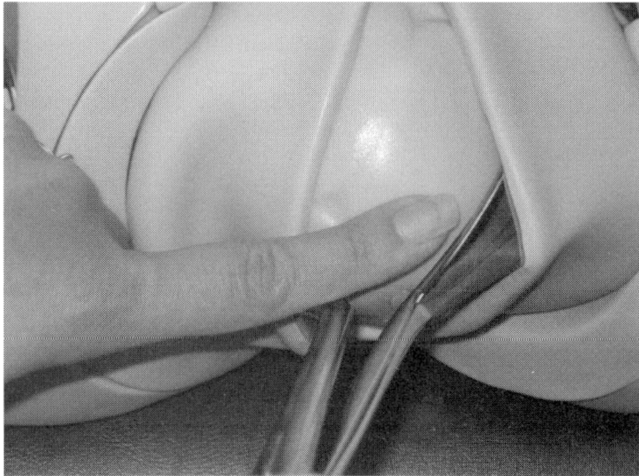

Figure 6.6 Blades in place. Checking for proper alignment.

as Hawk-Dennens or Laufes, automatically create axis traction.

All forceps discussed in this chapter have finger rests at the lock. This is where the hands should be placed. Gripping and or squeezing the handles should be avoided as this can cause undue compression of the head. Every effort should be taken to limit the amount of compression to that naturally created by the maternal pelvis.

The amount of force required will seem considerable to the novice. Nonetheless, it should be limited to what one can apply with upper body strength only. The operator should not have to lean back or place a foot up on the delivery bed. Movement of the head downward should be perceptible with each pull. If complete resistance is noted, the procedure should be stopped and cesarean considered. As the head is coming under the symphysis, the force should be diminished to protect the perineum. Most outlet and low forceps deliveries can be accomplished in one to five contractions. With experience, the operator will gain an appreciation of whether or not to continue beyond that. Each patient and each situation needs to be individualized.

Again, the goal of both forceps and vacuum is to get the head under the symphysis pubis. Once the head has cleared the symphysis, the operative instrument(s) should be removed and the delivery should be completed normally. Typically, torque is created by the blades such that the lock may be tight and the blades difficult to separate. This is especially true of Laufe forceps. Normally, a little slight twisting of the handles will allow the blades to separate. The right blade is removed first, swinging the handle in a gentle arc upward along the inside of the left thigh, reversing

(a)

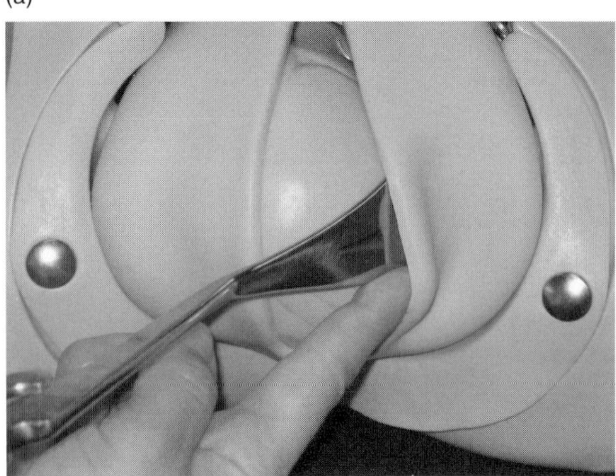

(b)

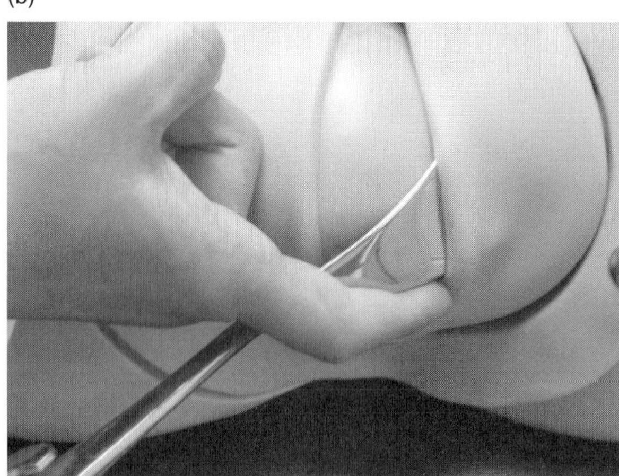

Figure 6.7 Rotation of the blade about the face. (a) Common technique using finger from below to guide blade while depressing the handle with the opposite hand. (b) Alternate technique allowing blade to rotate about the heel of the blade.

the movement of application. The left blade is then removed and the delivery is completed normally.

Rotation of the Head

If the occiput is posterior or transverse, manual rotation should be considered and/or attempted before choosing to apply forceps. It is important to remember the cardinal movements of labor. A failure of internal rotation means that the head is not completely flexed. Virtually without exception, a head in need of rotation is in a deflexion attitude.

Most successful manual rotations can be accomplished by first locating the posterior occiput and the lamdoid sutures. The operator should use whichever hand is on the same side as the occiput, the right for LOP, for example. The hand is inserted such that the edge of the middle finger lies alongside the upper parietal bone. The thumb should lie along the length of the lower parietal bone. With a contraction, flexion of the head is produced by pulling slightly against the fingers and pushing with the thumb. With the patient pushing, this flexion motion is often all that is needed for the head to turn naturally. Once the head has been flexed, the hand can apply a rotational force to the head, primarily through the middle finger.

If rotational forceps are needed, the rotation must be through the axis of the blades. With Kiellands, the handles will circumscribe a small circle as in going around a cyclinder. With Laufe–Kielland–Bartons, the handles are already in the axis of the blades and a simple rotation of the forceps is used. If Simpsons are used, the handles will need to traverse a wide arc, as in going around a cone.

Rotation should first be attempted without disengaging the head. Disengagement, rotation and re-engagement is a more advanced technique requiring a higher level of experience and skill. Once the head is rotated, delivery may continue with the same forceps. Alternatively, some operators prefer to remove the rotation forceps and apply a traditional pair.

Episiotomy

Many of the classic texts on forceps delivery recommend routine episiotomy. To some extent, this is throwback to the day when most deliveries were done under general anesthesia. Once the head comes under the symphysis, and the forceps removed, the decision to perform an episiotomy can be individualized. Occasionally, it will be clear that an episiotomy will aid in the forceps portion of the delivery. No data exist to support its routine use.

There has long been a debate over when to do an episiotomy and what type to perform. That debate is ongoing. The reader is referred to the ACOG bulletin as that discussion is beyond the scope of this chapter.[5] As regards all deliveries, and forceps deliveries in particular, caution should be taken to avoid the early performance of an episiotomy. Waiting until the perineum is well distended will decrease both blood loss and the size of the cut. Ideally, a well-timed episiotomy will take place during the same contraction as the delivery.

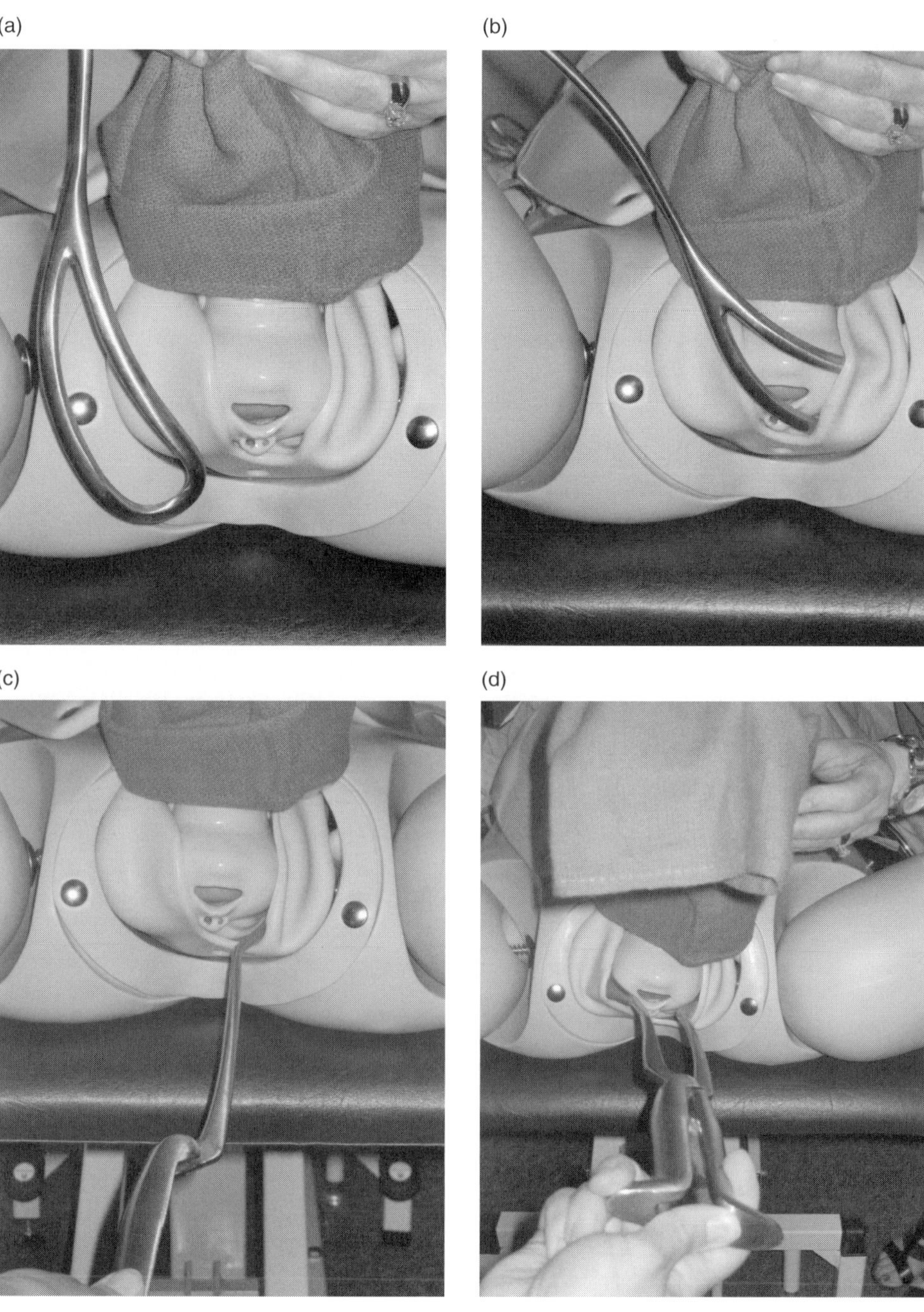

Figure 6.8 Piper forceps. (a) Left blade positioned for introduction. (b) Blade introduced. (c) Blade in place. (d) Both blades in and locked ready for extraction.

Vacuum Deliveries

Contrary to common belief, the vacuum, or ventouse, has been available for hundreds of years. Ambroise Paré (see Chapter 53) is known to have used cupping glasses to elevate depressed skull fractures in the early seventeenth century. In 1706 James Younge reported an unsuccessful use of a cupping glass with a syringe attached.[17] In 1829, Neil Arnott described a theoretical device for obstetrical use including a calculation of the dimensions required and the traction force that could be expected.[18] Twenty years later, following Arnott's descriptions, James Young Simpson (of forceps and chloroform fame) went through a number of designs and trials ultimately coming up with a device that looks eerily similar to the Kabushiki (Dow Corning) silastic cup popular in the 1970s and 1980s (Figure 6.9). Simpson is credited with the first successful vacuum extraction. His fervor for the approach quickly waned and he preferentially returned to his use of the forceps.

Over the next century, more than a dozen different designs appeared but it was not until 1952 when Tage Malmström introduced his rigid metal cup design (in four sizes) that vacuum-assisted deliveries became popular. Concern over complications related to the rigid design led to more flexible models. While effective, these cups were larger and more difficult to apply leading to the smaller, more rigid plastic models favored today.

Several excellent treatises on vacuum extraction are available that go into much more detail than is presented here. Two of the best are by Chalmer[19] and Kuit.[20]

Choice of Instruments

Many different models of vacuum extractor are on the market today (Figure 6.10). The most commonly employed are single-use and disposable. To a large extent, choice will be determined by what is available. Whether a more classic instrument (Malmström, Kabushiki) is used or one of the disposable units, the guidelines which follow apply to all. The Malmström had fallen out of favor because of concerns about neonatal cephalohematomas and consequently relatively few of these units are still in use. This risk is, however, present with all vacuum extractors and experience has shown that proper technique can keep the incidence to a minimum, regardless of which instrument is chosen. Vacuum-assisted delivery should not be used if the gestational age is less than 34 weeks. If the gestational age is uncertain, the physician should err on the side of caution.

Application of Vacuum

Application technique will vary slightly with each practitioner. The description given here is based on the classic textbooks and atlases and confirmed by the author's more than 40 years' experience encompassing more than 100 vacuum-assisted vaginal deliveries.

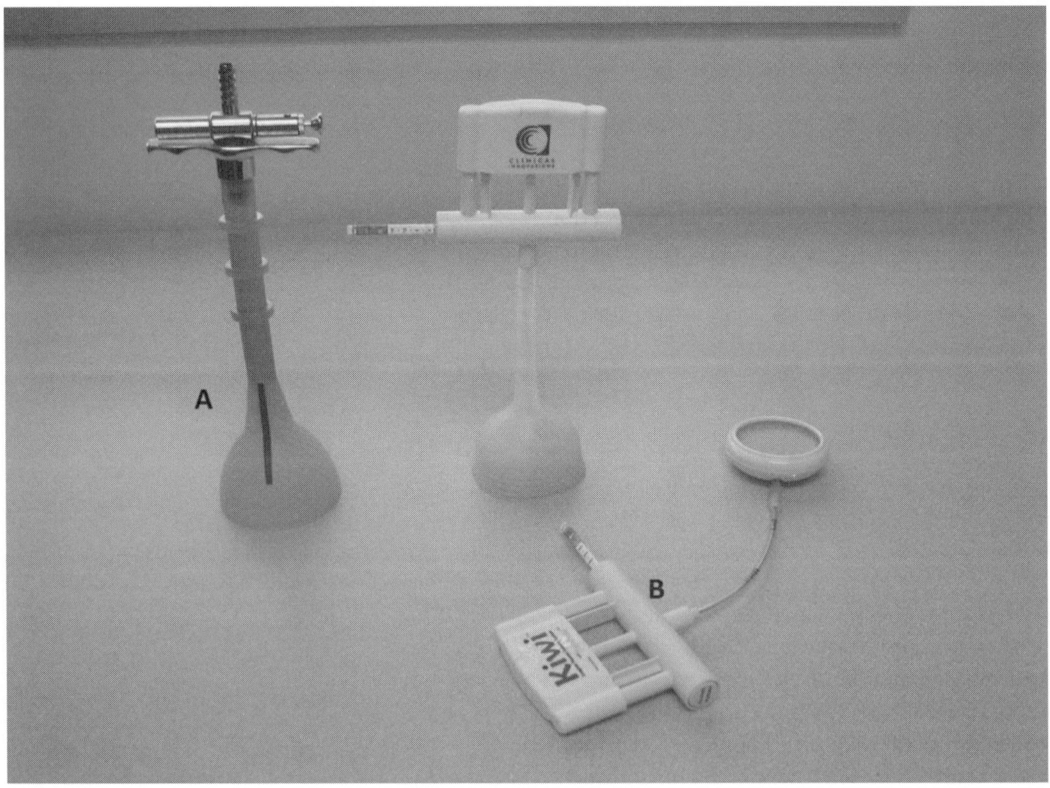

Figure 6.9 Types of vacuum: (A) Kabushiki. (B) Kiwi variations.

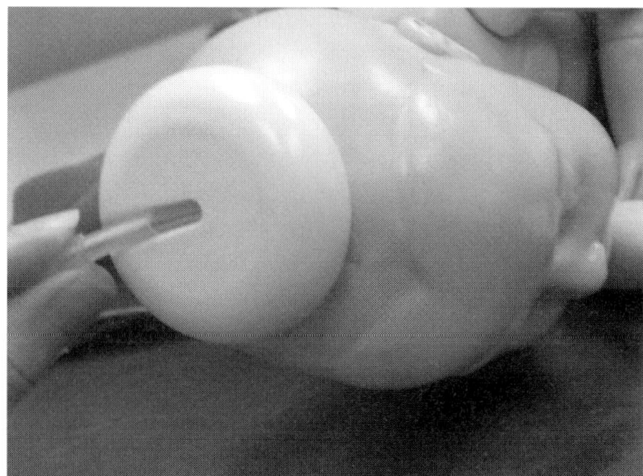

Figure 6.10 Proper placement of vacuum. Note that the cup is behind the anterior fontanelle.

This description will assume a vertex presentation to at least +2 cm and with rotation of less than 45°. That is, the position of the fetal head is between ROA and LOA. Use of the vacuum under other conditions is to be discouraged. The patient should be in dorsal lithotomy position with the hips slightly flexed, as in a slight McRoberts position.

Careful examination should be performed to ascertain position and the location of both the anterior and posterior fontanelles. The cup is then applied to the fetal scalp making sure that no vaginal or cervical tissue is involved. The rim of the cup should rest just anterior to the edge of the posterior fontanelle and at least 2 cm back from the anterior fontanelle. Under no circumstances should the cup lie over any portion of the anterior fontanelle. Some vacuum extractors have a marking that can be aligned with the sagittal suture, allowing the operator to know the position of the fetal head.

Delivery

Suction is then applied. If using wall suction, the goal should be 500–600 mmHg. If using a built-in hand pump, the pressure should rest in the safe operating zone. It had previously been suggested that slowly pumping up the vacuum pressure would result in a more secure application. Subsequent studies have shown that this is not the case and only results in a longer duration of suction. Similarly, there is no evidence that releasing the suction between contractions is of any protective benefit. Some operators will allow the pressure to decrease between contractions but it is advantageous to keep a well applied vacuum in place.

Traction should be coordinated with maternal contractions and aided by maternal efforts. Traction should be directed slightly downward in the midline and rising upward as the head comes under the symphysis. Passive rotation of the head will often occur normally and should be allowed. Under no circumstances should the operator attempt to rotate the head with the vacuum. This creates a high risk for the "cookie-cutter" laceration of the scalp.

The amount of traction should be no more than allowed by the suction application. Too strenuous an effort will result in a "pop-off." Some operators find it useful to pull with one hand while monitoring the application with the other. If the cup shows signs of separation, the amount traction force is reduced.

Many hospitals have protocols that govern the number of pulls (contractions) over which a vacuum may be used. In general, the decision to continue delivery must be re-evaluated continuously. The maximum number of pulls to complete a vacuum extraction and the acceptable number of "pop-offs" (detachments) is unknown. However, in an observational study of 393 singleton term pregnancies, 82% of successful deliveries were achieved within one to three pulls, and more than three pulls was associated with a 45% risk of neonatal trauma.[21] Limiting the effort to no more than three to five pulls and/or two to three "pop-offs" is a sound guideline.

Once the head has cleared the symphysis, the vacuum should be removed, allowing the delivery to be completed normally.

A video instruction of vacuum application that incorporates many of these principles can be found at www.youtube.com/watch?v=eanpNoc0q8U

Use of Forceps, Vectis, or Vacuum at Cesarean

Both forceps and vacuum can be quite useful to assist delivery of the head during cesarean section (CS). Use of the vacuum has the closest correlation with what is done in vaginal delivery. The primary caution is correct placement of the vacuum with avoidance of the anterior fontanelle. When using the vacuum at CS, it is first wise to make sure that the head is disengaged and in flexion. Generally speaking, this application does not need to be rushed. The operator must take the time to ensure a proper application before applying suction and traction.

As in vaginal delivery, forceps are more effective but require a higher level of skill. The type of

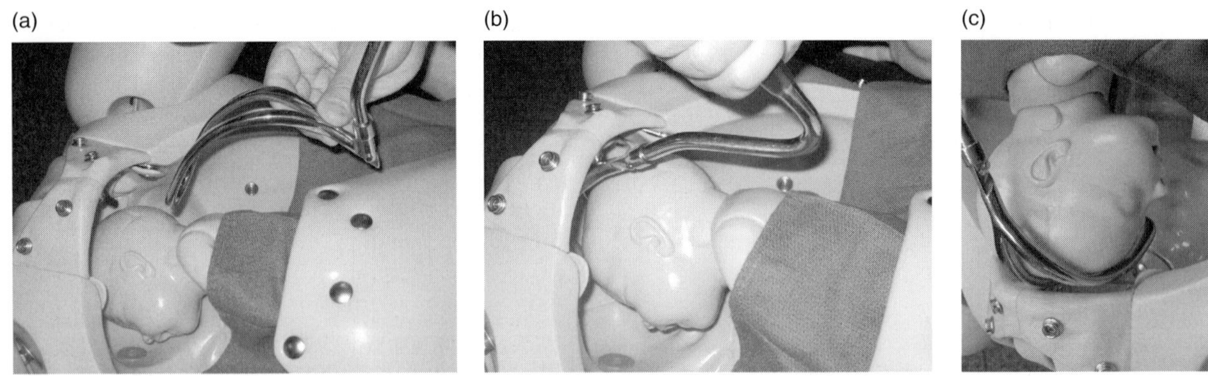

Figure 6.11 Murless vectis. (a) Folded and ready for introduction; (b) applied to side of head; (c) head elevated out of pelvis.

forceps is relatively unimportant. Short-handled forceps, such as Laufe's or short-handled Simpsons, are the most desirable. Negotiation of long handles in the confines of the operative field can be challenging.

Once the head is disengaged, the position must be ascertained. Most commonly in CS, the position will be transverse. A determination should then be made as to whether the occiput is on the maternal left or right. The articulated forceps should then be aligned with the anticipated placement (phantom application), just as in a vaginal application, and whichever blade will be anterior is selected. There is no need to pay attention right or left in this setting. The selected blade is placed along the inferior side of the head and rotated into place anteriorly (see above). The posterior blade is then placed and the handles locked. Straight traction may then be applied. There is no need to attempt any rotation of the head.

Pipers for breech extraction may also be used at cesarean. Short-handled Pipers are available just for this purpose. As with vaginal application, the breech delivery should be accomplished up through the arms and, with an assistant holding the baby (as described earlier), the forceps are applied just as in vaginal application. This is an excellent opportunity for teaching and learning the use of Pipers as it is virtually identical to what is done in the vaginal setting.

The vectis is a single-bladed lever or elevator and is most useful for elevating the head out of the pelvis. The Murless vectis was specifically designed for this purpose and is widely available (Figure 6.11). The hinged handle is opened up to allow the blade to be slid under the impacted head. Placement alongside a parietal bone is preferable but not requisite. With the blade in place, the handle is closed and locked. The handle is then lifted straight upward, disengaging the head.

Concluding Remarks

Sequential use of vacuum and forceps has been associated with increased rates of neonatal complication and should not routinely be performed.[22–24]

Operative vaginal delivery is still, and should remain, an important part of obstetrical care. Although the procedure is safe and effective, risks do exist. In general, a slightly increased risk for maternal trauma is associated with forceps use, whereas newborn trauma is slightly more common with vacuum. For a more detailed discussion of these risks, refer to the ACOG Bulletin.[5]

References

1. Davis GH. "Current Use of Obstetrical Forceps," Presented to 73rd Annual ACOOG Conference, San Antonio, Texas, March 2006.
2. Gupta N, et al. The changing scenario of obstetrics and gynecology residency training. *J Grad Med Educ* 2015 Sep;7(3):401–6.
3. Ciotti M. Minimum Threshold for Obstetrics and Gynecology Procedures. ACGME Memorandum. July 2012.
4. O'Mahony F, Hofmeyr GJ, Menon V. Choice of instruments for assisted vaginal delivery. *Cochrane Database of Syst Rev* 2010; Issue 11. Art. No.: CD005455. DOI: 10.1002/14651858.CD005455.pub2 (meta-analysis).
5. American College of Obstetricians and Gynecologists. Operative Vaginal Delivery. Practice Bulletin 154. November 2015.
6. Hale RW, editor. *Dennen's Forceps Deliveries*. 4th edition. Washington DC: American College of Obstetricians and Gynecologists; 2001.

7. Laufe LE. *Obstetric Forceps*. New York: Harper & Row; 1968.

8. Cunningham FG, Gant NF, Leveno KJ, et al. Forceps delivery and vacuum extraction, in *William's Obstetrics*. 21st edition. New York: McGraw-Hill; 2001.

9. O'Brien WF, Cefalo RC. Forceps delivery and vacuum extraction, in *Obstetrics, Normal and Problem Pregnancies*. Gabbe SG, Niebyl JT, Simpson JL, editors. New York: Churchill Livingstone; 1991.

10. Quilligan EJ, Zuspan F. Forceps, in *Douglas-Stromme Operative Obstetrics*, 4th edition. New York: Appleton-Century-Crofts; 1982.

11. Falls FH, Holt CS. Obstetric forceps delivery in *Atlas of Obstetric Complications*. Philadelphia: Lippincott; 1961.

12. Titus P. *Atlas of Obstetric Technique*. St. Louis: Mosby; 1943.

13. Willson JR. *Atlas of Obstetric Technique*. St. Louis: Mosby; 1961.

14. Hirst BC, editor. *A System of Obstetrics by American Authors, Volume II*. Philadelphia: Lea Brothers; 1889.

15. Williams JW. *Obstetrics, A Text-book for the Use of Students and Practitioners*. New York: Appleton; 1903.

16. Dennen PC. *Dennen's Forceps Deliveries*. 3rd edition. Philadelphia: F. A. Davis; 1989.

17. Hibbard B. *Vacuum Extractors in The Obstetrician's Armamentarium*. San Anselmo: Norman; 2000.

18. Arnott N. *Elements of Physics or Natural Philosophy*. First American Edition. Philadelphia: Carey, Lea & Carey; 1829.

19. Chalmer JA. *The Ventouse*. London: Lloyd-Luke; 1971.

20. Kuit JA. *Clinical and Physical Aspects of Obstetric Vacuum Extraction*. Rotterdam: 1997. file:///C:/Users/George/Downloads/970402%20kuit.pdf. Accessed June 28, 2016.

21. Murphy DJ, Liebling RE, Patel R, et al. Cohort study of operative delivery in the second stage of labour and standard of obstetric care. *BJOG* 2003;110:610–15.

22. Towner D, Castro MA, Eby-Wilkens E, Gilbert WM. Effect of mode of delivery in nulliparous women on neonatal intracranial injury. *N Engl J Med* 1999;341:1709–14.

23. Gardella C, Taylor M, Benedetti T, Hitti J, Critchlow C. The effect of sequential use of vacuum and forceps for assisted vaginal delivery on neonatal and maternal outcomes. *Am J Obstet Gynecol* 2001;185:896–902.

24. Murphy DJ, Macleod M, Bahl R, Strachan B. A cohort study of maternal and neonatal morbidity in relation to use of sequential instruments at operative vaginal delivery. *Eur J Obstet Gynecol Reprod Biol* 2011;156:41–5.

Cesarean Section

Theodore Tsaltas

Introduction

In this chapter the reasons, preparation for, methods, and postoperative care for cesarean section (CS) are discussed.

Statement of the Problem

Cesarean section is the most common major surgical procedure done in the United States. In 2013, the last year for which comprehensive data are available, 1,286,000 cesarean sections (CS) were performed in the United States [1]. The ubiquity of the procedure makes its execution easy to take for granted. CS rates remained at or near 5% as late as 1970, but then began rising as a result of marked improvement in outcomes, introduction of fetal indications, legal concerns, and changing social perceptions of acceptable pregnancy outcomes for both mother and infant. The CS rate in the United States was 32.7% in 2013 [1]. While this number is high, it is by no means the highest in the world. Brazil's rate was 45.9% in 2008, Mexico 37.8%, Argentina 35.2%, and Italy 38.2% [2]. Most frequent indications for CS are currently fetal intolerance to labor and arrest of labor. Other indications include malpresentation, placenta previa, vasa previa, prior vaginal and urethral support procedures, and maternal request. The increased number and proportion of multi-fetal pregnancies has also driven CS rates higher.

History

The lack of anesthesia, antibiotics, and effective suturing made CS extremely dangerous and therefore impracticable throughout most of human history. Records of various quality describe isolated CS performed in the eighteenth and early nineteenth century. The first such case in North America was performed by the patient herself [3]. The first CS by a physician in North America was performed by John Richmond, in 1827 [3]. The patient returned to field work in 24 days. Sutures were not recommended until 1868. It is surprising that the major source of morbidity and mortality was infection, not blood loss, even without sutures [3]. As early as 1878, CS prior to rupture of membranes was recognized as having a lower infectious morbidity.

As late as 1932, maternal mortality remained 4–16% in a review of outcomes from major hospitals [4]. The availability of antibiotics dramatically altered mortality and morbidity, but CS remained very uncommon, with rates of less than 3%. Indications were limited to proven inadequate maternal pelvis (by radiograph), severe pre-eclampsia refractory to induction, and prior CS [5]. There were no fetal indications, as there was no fetal monitoring or ultrasound.

Elective CS

CS on maternal request is an acceptable, although controversial indication. The American College of Obstetricians and Gynecologists (ACOG) admits elective CS from an ethical and patient autonomy point of view [6]. It cautions that the procedure should be done when fulfilling the following criteria in Box 7.1 [7].

Aside from ethical considerations, the debate over elective CS has centered primarily on the relative morbidity of the procedure compared to vaginal delivery or CS in labor for obstetric indications. ACOG has addressed some systemic and coordination of care concerns that must be thoroughly considered when doing purely elective surgery [8]. In some studies on CS safety, data is mixed or obscured by the fact that most severe maternal morbidity occurs in patients with CS.

Geller et al. studied intended planned CS and planned vaginal delivery; there were only 180 elective CS in the study [9]. The vaginal delivery group included labor inductions and CS for obstetric indications. Bleeding and infection were less common among planned CS, while neonatal respiratory

Box 7.1 Criteria for cesarean section for maternal request

- Cesarean delivery on maternal request should not be performed before a gestational age of 39 weeks.
- Cesarean delivery on maternal request should not be motivated by the unavailability of effective pain management.
- Cesarean delivery on maternal request particularly is not recommended for women desiring several children, given that the risks of placenta previa, placenta accreta, and gravid hysterectomy increase with each cesarean delivery

problems were more common. A large 2006 meta-analysis found less bleeding with planned CS, but more neonatal respiratory distress [10]. A 2009 study designed to compare CS in unlabored patients, CS during labor, and vaginal delivery also confirmed less bleeding but more neonatal respiratory problems in the unlabored CS patients [11]. Maternal mortality is increased in CS compared to vaginal delivery (0.013% vs 0.004%) but the absolute risk is extremely low for both [12].

Elective repeat CS also is safer than vaginal birth after cesarean section (VBAC). A large study out of Scotland found neonatal death rates 11-fold higher among VBAC patients compared to repeat CS patients [13]. The risk of uterine rupture in elective repeat CS is also lower; among elective repeat CS patients, it is 1.6/1,000, while in VBAC with spontaneous labor it is 5.2/1000, and in induction VBAC it is 7.7/1,000 [14]. One large review found maternal mortality highest in VBAC as compared to repeat or elective CS (0.13% vs 0.05%), and rates of uterine rupture(0.47% vs 0.03%) were also higher [12]. It is difficult, therefore, on the basis of available data, to limit or condemn elective and repeat CS deliveries.

Prevention of urinary incontinence has been cited as a reason to perform CS. While CS patients have lower rates of stress urinary incontinence at 3 months, there is no difference in rates of incontinence at menopause [15,16]. Concern for urinary tract function is not a reason to perform CS.

Surgical Preparation and Precautions

Many items of surgical preparation and technique deserve reflection and data-based analysis. Various aspects of CS have been addressed in two large review papers [17,18].

Regional anesthesia is the method of choice for CS. Epidural and spinal anesthesia are equally effective but have different advantages. Spinal anesthesia has very rapid onset and is of shorter duration, making it ideal for elective and repeat CS. It has a greater effect on maternal hemodynamics and blood pressure, however. Epidural anesthesia is preferred for labor, and its dose may be readily increased for CS. It has a slower onset of action, less effect on maternal blood pressure, and wears off more slowly. A gradually administered epidural may have advantages in preoperative management of patients with certain forms of heart disease [19].

Patient positioning is an important part of any surgery [8]. Patients for CS should be in the left lateral tilt position to minimize uterine compression of the inferior vena cava. A small amount of Trendelenberg positioning or table flexion can facilitate abdominal exposure. Management of the pannus of an obese patient is an increasingly frequent problem. Taping the pannus up and other methods of increasing exposure can greatly improve ease of surgery.

Deep vein thrombosis (DVT) risk at CS has only been recently addressed in most hospitals. The absolute risk of DVT is low, estimated at 0.23% in one review [20]. A very large review found a much lower incidence, with 0.23% being at the upper end of literature findings [21]. Nonetheless, pregnancy is a hypercoagulable state, as is surgery, and ACOG advises attention to thromboprophylaxis [22]. There is no data to document the superiority of low-molecular-weight heparin, unfractionated heparin or sequential compression devices as the single best modality [23]. This is not surprising considering the low background risk of DVT. The American College of Chest Physicians finds early ambulation to be as effective as other forms of thromboprophylaxis in CS [24]. While data and study quality are mixed, there is good reason to provide some form of thromboprophylaxis during CS. Use of heparin or sequential compression devices has the advantage of not relying upon either patient or staff compliance with early ambulation to achieve prophylaxis.

Urinary catheters are routinely placed for CS; however, despite the broad acceptance of this practice, there is remarkably little data showing any advantage to their use. A large trial found no surgical advantage of placement versus non-placement of a catheter during CS [25]. One potential advantage for placement is ongoing decompression of the bladder in prolonged cases, such as with severe adhesions or those converting to cesarean hysterectomy. Immediate removal of the catheter is not associated with increased urinary retention [26]. It seems a reasonable, low-risk precaution to place a urinary catheter, but to remove it immediately after case completion.

Use of prophylactic antibiotics is essential. As noted earlier, even when suturing was not a part of CS, the major cause of death was infection. Prophylactic antibiotics have dramatically reduced the rate of febrile morbidity. This is true regardless of whether the patient population is high-risk and indigent [27] or privately insured [28]. The choice of antibiotic is equally clearly a first-generation cephalosporin or penicillin [29]. Broader coverage antibiotics do not further reduce the risk of febrile morbidity [30]. Past controversy has occurred over the timing of prophylactic antibiotics, with use after cord clamping recommended at one time. Literature data convincingly show no advantage for this [31]. CS antibiotic prophylaxis should be given immediately prior to skin incision, as for other surgeries [32].

An informal standard exists that CS should be initiated within 30 min of the decision to perform it. In one study this standard was not met in 69% of major perinatal units in the United States [33]. Despite this, decision-to-delivery time did not appear to have a deleterious effect on neonatal outcome in one important study [34]. Caution must be used in interpreting this finding, as many CS are neither urgent or emergent. In emergent and urgent cases, however, decision-to-delivery interval can be a lifesaving difference. Review of severe maternal morbidity shows that delay in management is a major determinant of outcome [35].

Box 7.2 Surgical technique cesarean section

Patient is prepped and draped
Surgical pause
Right handed surgeon is on patient's left
Abdominal incision choice is based on surgical needs.
Skin is cut with scalpel
Subcutaneous tissue is bluntly separated
Fascia is incised with scalpel and scissors
Rectus bellies are bluntly separated
Peritoneal cavity is bluntly entered
Uterine musculature is sharply incised followed by blunt finger entry
Uterine incision is bluntly stretched
Membranes are ruptured if needed
Surgeon's hand is inserted into uterine cavity, fundal pressure is applied by assistant
Fetus is delivered and stimulated if needed
Umbilical cord is cut and clamped
Placenta is removed with traction and inspected
Uterine myometrium is closed with or without exteriorization
Uterine incision is inspected for hemostasis
Fascia is closed with running unlocked suture
Subcutaneous closure is performed if needed
Skin is closed
Final sponge and needle count performed

Surgical Technique

Few factors can have a greater or more immediate impact upon well-being during medical care than poor surgical technique. It is the responsibility of every surgeon to constantly examine, refine, and improve her or his technique in response to his or her own experience, the literature, and the individual patient condition. The development of CS technique fully exemplifies this imperative. A step by step approach to C-section is seen in Box 7.2. A video of a typical cesarean section can be found here: www.learnerstv.com/video/Free-video-Lecture-6923-Medical.htm.

The first descriptions of CS employed the classical incision, a vertical incision made in the upper aspect of the lower uterine segment. A transverse incision was described as early as 1805, although most credit for the first description of the transverse technique is given to Osiander of Oettingen [3]. In an effort to minimize morbidity, a low vertical technique was also introduced, the incision being made vertically in the thinned lower uterine segment. This required the bladder to be displaced and also had the risk of vaginal laceration and limited visualization [3]. Extraperitoneal CS, both by upward and later lateral displacement of the bladder, was developed in a further attempt to minimize infection [36]. Munro Kerr's technique of lower segment transverse incision became the most preferred in the mid-twentieth century [37]. Interestingly, while using a transverse incision, Kerr recommended that the incision be curved downward to minimize vascular injury, in contrast to today's recommendation to curve upward slightly [38]. The ongoing evolution of CS technique is currently best expressed in the Misgav–Ladach technique, as discussed later and fully described in current literature [39].

Operator position should be on the patient's left for a right-handed surgeon. Some right-handed surgeons perform CS from the patient's right in order to use their dominant hand for delivery. This has several important disadvantages. All pelvic surgery is easier when the dominant hand is not limited by motion obstruction from the patient's pubic symphysis. There is also motion confusion between operating from the left and right during training, an important consideration given that CS is the most common laparotomy any obstetrics/gynecologist (OB/Gyn) physician will ever perform. Major text book illustrations show the procedure done from the patient's left side [40].

Choice of abdominal incision must reflect surgical needs, not cosmetics or habit. A transverse incision is adequate for the majority of CS. A vertical incision, however, disturbs fewer vascular and neurologic structures and causes less incisional bleeding. Despite the claims of many individual surgeons, a vertical incision is clearly faster; this is a potentially decisive advantage in cases of maternal hemorrhage or fetal bradycardias [41].

Incisional positioning is in part determined by choice of technique, but also by access to the pelvis and healing considerations. Too low a placement may interfere with both considerations. A Pfannenstiel incision is placed two-finger breadths above the pubic symphysis. This standard is dependent on both the size of the operator's fingers and what is taken as "the pubic symphysis." Incisions are sometimes inappropriately placed almost on the pubic bone. The standard for the Joel–Cohen incision, and related techniques such as the Misgav–Ladach, is 2–3 cm above the upper edge of the symphysis. This is slightly higher and also a clearer standard [42]. The size of the incision should be adequate for delivery. Cosmetic considerations can lead to creation of an incision of inadequate length, resulting in difficulty for exposure and delivery. Spellacy et al. found 15 cm was the minimum length necessary for easy delivery by CS [43].

Multiple studies and reviews have observed that blunt dissection of the subcutaneous tissue is superior to sharp dissection [42,44]. Similarly, blunt or minimal peritoneal entry followed by blunt stretching rather than cutting is also superior [42,44]. The uterine musculature should be superficially incised with a knife sufficiently to allow blunt finger entry. This minimizes risk of fetal knife injury. The uterine incision should then be stretched bluntly rather than cut. Although this is commonly done transversely, superior results are obtained from vertical stretching [45]. A "bladder flap" is commonly made, with inferior displacement of the bladder behind a retractor. This has no advantage, and increases both surgical time and bleeding [46].

It is common to remove the placenta by hand; however, data clearly favors traction removal and use of instruments for extraction of any remaining membranes [47]. After delivery of the infant there has been debate over exteriorization of the uterus. A large meta-analysis found no difference in infection, pain, and bleeding outcomes between exteriorization and repair in situ [48]. It is easier for most surgeons to do the uterine closure with the uterus exteriorized, but all Ob/Gyn surgeons should be comfortable with in situ closure, as adhesions and other conditions can prevent exteriorization.

Extensive debate has occurred over one- versus two-layer closure of the myometrium. The bulk of data demonstrates no advantage for a two-layer closure [49]. Interestingly, this same meta-analysis found a higher rate of uterine dehiscence in locked rather than unlocked closures. A simple running, single-layer uterine closure has the best data support at this time.

Closure of both visceral and parietal peritoneum is not indicated, despite long tradition. Peritoneal healing occurs over an entire surface simultaneously, since the peritoneocytes arise from perivascular, pluripotential stem cells [50]. Destruction of this tissue results in adhesion formation. This has long since been conclusively demonstrated experimentally [51]. There is no indication for peritoneal closure in any circumstance.

Fascial closure is best done by continuous suture, unlocked, although there has been some recent data suggesting interrupted sutures may be of benefit [17,18]. Subcutaneous tissue needs closure only if it exceeds 2 cm in thickness. Closure of subcutaneous tissue is superior to placement of closed suction drains [42,44]. Skin may be closed with either staples or with a subcuticular continuous stitch. There is no advantage for either technique, although the subcuticular stitch avoids the need for staple extraction, minimizing postoperative office visits. it is also popular with patients [52].

Uterotonics are used routinely after CS. Pitocin, in variable concentrations, is most commonly used. Misoprostol has also been used, with the potential disadvantage of fever and chills. Misoprostol may be the preferred agent prior to 36 weeks, since oxytocin receptors are not present on the myometrial cells prior to that time [18].

All these technical details are incorporated into the Misgav–Ladach technique. This method has been shown to have the shortest operating times, lowest blood loss, and lowest febrile morbidity rates [39,42,44]. It is the best technique available for CS at this time.

Intraoperative Complications

Complications of Cesarean section are discussed in Chapter 8.

Special Considerations: The Cesarean Hysterectomy

Cesarean hysterectomy (CH) may be done in emergent and elective conditions. Severe maternal morbidity any occur and is defined by one of five criteria: organ system failure, ICU admission, transfusion of four or more units of packed cells, intubation greater than 12 hours, or any postpartum surgical intervention [53]. CH is included within the definition of severe maternal morbidity, and the other elements of severe morbidity are strongly associated with CH. It is a procedure all Obstetricians will encounter during their careers. Since severe maternal morbidity in the United States is 129 per 1,000 deliveries (1.29%) [54], the practicing obstetrician must be prepared to manage CH and its attendant indications and consequences. A multi-disciplinary team approach, utilizing preplanned protocols and triggers for intervention, has been shown to decrease morbidity in placenta accreta, one of the common reasons for CH [55]. These results are a powerful contrast to the morbidity found in a comprehensive review of CH outcomes and indications [56]. Despite the popular and technically simpler supracervical cesarean hysterectomy, it has no less morbidity than a total cesarean hysterectomy [57].

Postoperative Morbidity

Febrile morbidity remains the major source of postoperative complication. The single greatest source of this is urinary tract infection. Bleeding is greater during CS than vaginal delivery, and hemorrhage more common [17,18,42,44]. As noted previously, bleeding and infection are less when elective CS is performed with the membranes unruptured in a non-laboring patient [9,10,11].

Post-operative Management

Urinary catheters should be removed promptly rather than left in situ until the next morning. Immediate removal is not associated with adverse outcomes [26]. The use of long-acting opioid analgesics has greatly changed and improved CS post-operative care. The addition of ketorolac, given intravenously in the operating room during or immediately after surgery, is extremely effective in reducing pain and subsequent opioid requirements [58].

In the absence of intra-thecal opioid use, other opioids must be given in the immediate post-operative period. Intramuscular (IM) or subcutaneous (SQ) morphine is a preferred choice. Patient-controlled analgesic pumps (PCAs) are much more expensive, deliver three times as much opioids, and have no improvement in effectiveness [59,60]. PCAs also create the impression the patient's pain is so severe that IV medication is required, and they also require IV access. These factors can alter the patient's activity and confidence, further compromising post-operative care beyond the effects of the increased opioid doses of PCAs.

Diet may be advanced as tolerated. The patient may ambulate once regional anesthesia has worn off [17,18]. Depending on the time of the CS, the patient may certainly be discharged the second post-operative day, and even the afternoon of the first post-operative day if in excellent condition.

The first post-operative office visit is ideally at one, not two, weeks. Infection, ileus, bleeding, and other major complications all develop in the first postpartum/post-operative week. If evaluation is delayed until two weeks, the patient either feels well, and questions the purpose for the visit, or has already had her complication, leaving her to wonder why the physician did not see her sooner.

Concluding Remarks

CS is one of the most common major surgeries done in the United States. The details of preparation, execution, and post-operative care make a substantial difference in outcomes. All obstetricians should be prepared to perform CS and should also be confident and prepared for CS complications and cesarean hysterectomies.

References

1. Martin JA, Hamilton BE, Osterman MJK, Curtin SC, Mathews TJ. Births: Final data for 2013. *Mon Vital Stat Rep* 2015 Jan 15;64(1):1–65.

2. Gibbons L, Belizan, JM, Lauer JA, Betran AP, Merialdi M, Althabe F. The Global Numbers and Costs of Additionally Needed and Unnecessary Caesarean Sections Performed per Year: Overuse as a Barrier to Universal Coverage. World Health Report (2010). Background Paper, No 30.

3. Speert, H. *Obstetrics and Gynecology in America – A History*. American College of Obstetricians and Gynecologists, 1980.

4. Plass, ED. Forceps and Cesarean Section, in *White House Conference on Child Health and Protection. Fetal, Newborn, and Maternal Mortality and Morbidity.* Appleton-Century, 1933, pp. 215–247.

5. Smith EF, MacDonald FA. Cesarean section: An evaluation of current practice in the New York Lying-in Hospital. *Obstet Gynecol* 1953;6:593.

6. American College of Obstetricians and Gynecologists. Elective Surgery and Patient Choice. Committee Opinion 578, November 2013.

7. American College of Obstetricians and Gynecologists. Cesarean Delivery on Maternal Request. Committee Opinion 559, April 2013, reaffirmed 2015.

8. American College of Obstetricians and Gynecologists. Patient Safety in the Surgical Environment. Committee Opinion 464. September 2010, reaffirmed 2014.

9. Geller EJ, Wu JM, Jannelli ML, Nguyen TV, Visco AG. Maternal outcomes associated with planned vaginal versus planned primary cesarean delivery. *Am J Perinatol* 2010 Oct;27(9):675–83.

10. Visco AG, Viswanathan M, Lohr KN, Wechter ME, Gartlehner G, Wu JM, et al. Cesarean delivery on maternal request: maternal and neonatal outcomes. *Obstet Gynecol* 2006 Dec;108(6):1517–29.

11. Quiroz LH, Chang H, Blomquist JL, Okoh YK, Handa VL. Scheduled cesarean delivery: Maternal and neonatal risks in primiparous women in a community hospital setting. *Am J Perinatol* 2009 Apr; 26(4): 271–7.

12. Guise JM, Denman MA, Emeis C, Marshall N, Walker M, Fu R, et al. Vaginal birth after cesarean: new insights on maternal and neonatal outcomes. *Obstet Gynecol* 2010 Jun;115(6):1267–78.

13. Smith GC, Pell JP, Cameron AD, Dobbie R. Risk of perinatal death associated with labor after previous cesarean delivery in uncomplicated term pregnancies. *JAMA* 2002 May 22–29;287(20):2684–90.

14. Lydon-Rochelle M, Holt VL, Easterling TR, Martin DP. Risk of uterine rupture during labor among women with a prior cesarean delivery. *N Engl J Med* 2001 Jul 5;345(1):3–8.

15. Hannah ME, Hannah WJ, Hodnett ED, Chalmers B, Kung R, Willan A, et al. Outcomes at 3 months after planned cesarean vs planned vaginal delivery for breech presentation at term: the international randomized Term Breech Trial. *JAMA* 2002 Apr 10;287(14):1822–31.

16. MacLennan AH, Taylor AW, Wilson, DH, Wilson D. The prevalence of pelvic floor disorders and their relationship to gender, age, parity and mode of delivery. *BJOG* 2000 (December) 107 (12):1460–70.

17. Vincenzo B, Baxter JK, Chauhan SP Evidence-based surgery for cesarean delivery. *Am J Obstet Gynecol* 2005;193:1607–17.

18. Dahlke JD, Mendez-Figueroa H, Rouse DJ, Berghella V, Baxter JK, Chauhan SP Evidence-based surgery for cesarean delivery: an updated systematic review. *Am J Obstet Gynecol* 2013 Oct;209(4):294–306.

19. Ng KW, Parsons J, Cyna AM, Middleton P. Spinal versus epidural anaesthesia for caesarean section. *Cochrane Database Syst Rev* 2004; Issue 2. Art. No.: CD003765.

20. Lindqvist P, Dahlback B, Marsal K. Thrombotic risk during pregnancy: A population study. *Obstet Gynecol* 1999;94:595–9.

21. Tooher R, Gates S, Dowswell T, Davis LJ. Prophylaxis for venous thromboembolic disease in pregnancy and the early postnatal period. *Cochrane Database Syst Rev* 2010; Issue 5. Art. No.: CD001689. DOI: 10.1002/14651858.CD001689.pub2.

22. American College of Obstetricians and Gynecologists. Thromboembolism in Pregnancy. August, 2011, reaffirmed 2014.

23. Burrows RF, Gan ET, Gallus AS, Wallace EM, Burrows EA. A randomised double-blind placebo controlled trial of low molecular weight heparin as prophylaxis in preventing venous thrombolic events after caesarean section: a pilot study. *BJOG* 2001;108:835–9.

24. Bates SM, et al, for the American College of Chest Physicians. VTE, thrombophilia, antithrombotic therapy, and pregnancy: Antithrombotic Therapy and Prevention of Thrombosis, 9th ed: American College of Chest Physicians Evidence-Based Clinical Practice Guidelines. *Chest* 2012 Feb;141(2 Suppl):e691S–736S.

25. Nasr AM, El Bigawy AF, Abdelamid AE, Al-Khulaidi S, Al-Inany HG, Sayed EH. Evaluation of the use vs nonuse of urinary catheterization during cesarean delivery: A prospective, multicenter, randomized controlledtrial. *J Perinatol* 2009;29:416–21.

26. Ghoreishi J. Indwelling urinary catheters in cesarean delivery. *Int J Gynaecol Obstet* 2003;83:267–70.

27. Duff, P. Prophylactic antibiotics for cesarean delivery: A simple cost effective strategy for prevention of postoperative morbidity. *Am J Obstet Gynecol.*1987;157:794–8.

28. Watson, WJ, George, RJ, Welter, S, Day, D. High-risk obstetric patients. *J Reprod Med* 1997;42:267–70.

29. Rudge MV, Atallah AN, Peracoli JC, Tristao Ada R, Mendonca Neto M. Randomized controlled trial on prevention of postcesarean infection using penicillin and cephalothin in Brazil. *Acta Obstet Gynecol Scand* 2006;85:945–8.

30. Alekwe LO, Kuti O, Orji EO, Ogunniyi SO. Comparison of ceftriaxone versus triple drug regimen in the prevention of cesarean section infectious morbidities. *J Matern Fetal Neonatal Med* 2008;21:638–42.

31. Sullivan SA, Smith T, Chang E, Hulsey T, Vandorsten JP, Soper D. Administration of cefazolin prior to skin incision is superior to cefazolin at cord clamping in preventing postcesarean infectious morbidity: A randomized, controlled trial. *Am J Obstet Gynecol* 2007;196: 455.e1–5.

32. Costantine MM, Rahman M, Ghulmiyah L, et al. Timing of perioperative antibiotics for cesarean delivery: A metaanalysis. *Am J Obstet Gynecol* 2008;199:301.e1–6.

33. Bloom SL, for the National Institute of Child Health and Human Development Maternal–Fetal Medicine Units Cesarean Registry. Decision to incision times and infant outcome. *Am J Obstet Gynecol.* 2001; 185:S121.

34. Bloom SL, for the National Institute of Child Health and Human Development Maternal-Fetal Medicine Units Network. Decision-to-incision times and maternal and infant outcomes. *Obstet Gynecol* 2006 Jul;108(1):6–11.

35. Onwudiegwu U, Makinde ON, Ezechi OC, Adeyemi A. Decision-caesarean delivery interval in a Nigerian university hospital: implications for maternal morbidity and mortality. *J Obstet Gynecol* 1999 Jan; 19(1):30–3.

36. Water EG, Supravesical extraperitoneal cesarean section: Presentation of a new technique. *Am J Obstet Gynecol* 1940;39:423–32.

37. Powell JL. The Kerr Incision: John Martin Munro Kerr (1868–1960). *J Pelvic Surgery* 2001 May/June; 7(3):177–8.

38. *Williams Obstetrics*, 24th edition. Cunningham FG, Leveno KJ, Bloom SL, Spong CY, et al. McGraw-Hill, 2014, Chapter 30.

39. Holmgren G1, Sjöholm L, Stark M. The Misgav Ladach method for cesarean section: Method description. *Acta Obstet Gynecol Scand* 1999 Aug;78(7):615–21.

40. *Williams Obstetrics*, 24th edition. Cunningham FG, Leveno KJ, Bloom SL, Spong CY, et al. McGraw-Hill, 2014, Chapter 30, figure 6.

41. Wylie BJ, Gilbert S, Landon MB, Spong CY, Rouse DJ, Leveno KJ, et al. and the Eunice Kennedy Shriver National Institute of Child Health and Human Development (NICHD) Maternal-Fetal Medicine Units Network (MFMU). Comparison of transverse and vertical skin incision for emergency cesarean delivery. *Obstet Gynecol* 2010 Jun;115(6):1134–40.

42. Matha M, Hofmeyr GJ. Abdominal surgical incisions for caesarean section. *Cochrane Database Syst Rev* 2007;Issue 1. Art. No.: CD004453.

43. Finan MA, Mastrogiannis DS, Spellacy WN. The "Allis" test for easy cesarean delivery. *Am J Obstet Gynecol* 1991 March; 164(3):772–5.

44. CAESAR study collaborative group. Caesarean section surgical techniques: A randomised factorial trial (CAESAR). *BJOG* 2010 Oct;117(11):1366–76.

45. Cromi A, Ghezzi F, Di Naro E, Siesto G, Loverro G, Bolis P. Blunt expansion of the low transverse uterine incision at cesarean delivery: A randomized comparison of 2 techniques. *Am J Obstet Gynecol* 2008;199:292.e1–292.e6.

46. Hohlagschwandtner M, Ruecklinger E, Husslein P, Joura EA. Is the formation of a bladder flap at cesarean necessary? A randomized trial. *Obstet Gynecol* 2001, December:98 (6)1089–92.

47. Baksu A, Kalan A, Ozkan A, Baksu B, Tekelioğlu M, Goker N. The effect of placental removal method and site of uterine repair on postcesarean endometritis and operative blood loss. *Acta Obstet Gynecol Scand* 2005 Mar;84(3):266–9.

48. Walsh CA, Walsh SR. Extraabdominal vs intraabdominal uterine repairs at cesarean delivery: A metaanalysis. *Am J Obstet Gynecol* 2009;200:625.e1–8 (large meta-analysis showing no difference in outcomes for exteriorization of uterus at repair).

49. Roberge S, Chaillet N, Boutin A, Moore L, Jastrow N, Brassard N, et al. Single- versus double-layer closure of the hysterotomy incision during cesarean delivery and risk of uterine rupture. *Int J Gynaecol Obstet* 2011 Oct;115(1):5–10.

50. Raftery AT. Regeneration of parietal and visceral peritoneum: An electron microscopical study. *J Anat* 1973 115(3):375–92.

51. Connolly WB, Stephens FO. Factors influencing the incidence of intraperitoneal adhesions: An experimental study. *Surgery* 1968 June;63(6):976–9.

52. Mackeen AD, Berghella V, Larsen ML. Techniques and materials for skin closure in caesarean section. *Cochrane Database Syst Rev* 2012;11:CD003577.

53. Geller SE, Rosenberg D, Cox S, Brown M, Simonson L, Kilpatrick S. A scoring system identified near-miss

maternal morbidity during pregnancy. *J Clin Epidemiol* 2004 July;57(7):716–20.

54. Callaghan WM, Creanga AA, Kuklina EV. Severe maternal morbidity among delivery and postpartum hospitalizations in the United States. *Obstet Gynecol* 2012 Nov;120(5):1029–36.

55. Eller AG, Bennett MA, Sharshiner M, Masheter C, Soisson AP, Dodson M, Silver RM. Maternal morbidity in cases of placenta accreta managed by a multidisciplinary care team compared with standard obstetric care. *Obstet Gynecol* 2011 Feb;117(2 Pt 1):331–7.

56. Rossi AC, Lee RH, Chmait RH. Emergency postpartum hysterectomy for uncontrolled postpartum bleeding – A systematic review. *Obstet Gynecol* 2010;115:637–44.

57. Imudia AN, Hobson DT, Awonuga AO, Diamond MP, Bahado-Singh RO, Determinants and complications of emergent cesarean hysterectomy: Supracervical vs total hysterectomy. *Am J Obstet Gynecol* 2010 Sep; 203(3):221.e1–5.

58. Balestrieri P, Simmons G, Hill D, Brown J, Jackson A, Brull SJ, Maneatis TJ, Shefrin A, Bynum L, O'Hara DA. The effect of intravenous ketorolac given intraoperatively versus postoperatively on outcome from gynecologic abdominal surgery. *J Clin Anesth* 1997 Aug;9(5):358–64.

59. Everett B. Salamonson Y. Differences in postoperative opioid consumption in patients prescribed patient-controlled analgesia versus intramuscular injection. *Pain Manag Nurs* 2005 Dec;6(4):137–44.

60. Bayar U. Basaran M. Atasoy N. Ayoglu H. Sade H. Altunkaya H. Comparison of satisfaction and pain relief between patients-controlled analgesia and interval analgesia after laparoscopic ovarian cystectomy. *J Psychosom Obst Gyn* 2008 Jun;29(2):139–45.

Cesarean Delivery Complications and Cesarean Hysterectomy

Melanie D. Altizer

Introduction

Cesarean section is the term used to describe the birth of a fetus through laparotomy and hysterotomy [1]. Cesarean delivery is generally divided into two distinct categories: (1) primary and (2) secondary or repeat. Primary refers to a first-time hysterotomy and secondary is used to describe a uterus that has undergone a prior hysterotomy [1]. Cesarean section is a common procedure performed successfully in the United States for a variety of indications. As with any surgical procedure, complications occur and can range from minor to life-threatening. In order to provide accurate and informed consent, it is imperative that the surgeon be familiar with the risks, benefits, and complications of cesarean section. This chapter will address the most common complications faced by patients and their physicians as a result of cesarean section.

Scope of the Problem

The risks associated with cesarean delivery can be divided into those that are short term, those that are longer term, and those that present risks to future pregnancies. In addition to maternal risk incurred, risks to the newborn also need to be taken into careful consideration. In addition, the clinical situation that prompts the cesarean delivery has relevance in terms of the risk of complications. For example, a primary cesarean section performed for an average-weight woman who is not in labor confers a much lower risk of complications than an emergency cesarean section performed on an obese woman who has chorioamnionitis and has been in labor for hours.

It is important for obstetricians to understand the implications of complications resulting from cesarean section and their impact on the health care system both economically and in lost employee work hours and productivity. Major non-anesthesia-related complications of cesarean section include but are not limited to endometritis, wound infection, dehiscence, and separation, hemorrhage, pelvic organ injury, and thromboembolic events. It is important keep in mind that the risk of complication is greater in patients undergoing an unplanned cesarean delivery during labor than in those cesarean sections that are scheduled [2,3]. Cesarean sections performed during the second stage of labor is usually has a higher association with maternal morbidity than those performed during the first stage of labor [4]. According to the Centers for Disease Control (CDC) in 2014, the cesarean section rate in the United States was 32.2% [5]. The US rate of cesarean hysterectomy is 7.0–8.3 per 1,000 cesarean sections [6]. For purposes of counseling patients regarding risks and benefits, it is helpful to categorize complications of cesarean sections into long term and short term.

Short-term Risks of Cesarean Delivery

Maternal Death. Maternal death is a rare complication of cesarean delivery. Most cases of surgical mortality resulting from cesarean delivery are related to underlying medical comorbidities and obstetrical complications that dictate surgical delivery. It has been estimated that approximately 2 to 6 women die annually in the United States as a result of cesarean delivery (0.2 to 0.6 death/100,000) [7]. The risk of maternal death during childbirth is greater with cesarean delivery compared with vaginal delivery. The overall risk remains still remains low [8–11].

Thromboembolism. A leading cause of maternal mortality related to cesarean delivery is deep vein thrombosis resulting in pulmonary embolism. One study reviewing 1.7 million pregnancies cited a frequency of 246/100,000 cesarean deliveries during the six-week postpartum time span [12].

Other risk factors for thromboembolism are important to consider with cesarean delivery, as they may add to the cumulative risk of a patient including maternal obesity, history of prior thrombotic event, venous stasis resulting from injury, prolonged surgical time, decreased mobility, and genetic and acquired clotting disorders.

Hemorrhage

The average blood loss from a cesarean section is 1,000 mL; however, blood loss estimates are unreliable and underestimated [13,14]. One prospective study quoted a 2% to 4% blood transfusion rate in women who undergo a primary low transverse cesarean section [15]. Cesarean delivery may have a greater blood loss than a vaginal delivery [16,17]. Some studies have suggested a lower risk of hemorrhage in planned cesarean sections as opposed to those that are emergent or unplanned. Planned cesarean sections may also have less risk of severe hemorrhage than operative vaginal deliveries [18]. The most common causes of hemorrhage in this patient population are uterine atony, uterine trauma and injury, extension of hysterotomy incision into the blood vessels supplying the uterus, and abnormal placentation. Extension of the hysterotomy incision may also occur into the vagina resulting in significant bleeding and increased operative time. The risk of hemorrhage requiring blood transfusion increases with increasing number of prior cesarean deliveries [19].

Infection

Infection is one of the most common complications of cesarean delivery [18,20,21]. Infectious complications arising in the setting of a cesarean section can include wound infection, endometritis, or pelvic abscess. Without administration of prophylactic antibiotics, the rates of postpartum endometritis can be as high as 35% to 40% [22]. This rate can vary dramatically based on the specific clinical scenario. Infection rates have been quoted to be as high as 85% for women undergoing cesarean section after prolonged labor and as low as 4% to 5% for those undergoing a planned cesarean delivery without rupture of membranes [22]. Wound infections may occur in 2.5% to 16% of cesareans [23].

Wound complications can include infection, hematoma, seroma, and dehiscence. Wound infection usually develops within 4 to 7 days post cesarean section. A major independent risk factor for development of wound infection is the presence of a subcutaneous hematoma [24]. Infections occurring early in the post-operative course, usually within 24–48 hours, are most often caused by group A or B beta-hemolytic Streptococcus. They typically present with fever and chills; later onset infections, occurring after 48 hours, are more likely caused by the presence of *Staphylococcus epidermidis* or *Staphylococcus aureus*, *Escherichia coli*, *Proteus mirabilis*, or cervicovaginal flora [25,26].

Surgical Injuries

A variety of different soft tissue injuries can occur at the time of cesarean delivery. These injuries can include broad ligament laceration or hematoma, cystotomy, enterotomy, ureteral injury, injury to nerves and blood vessels. One or more of these injuries were found to occur in 0.2 to 0.5% of patients who underwent a primary cesarean delivery [27].

Bladder injuries are the most common injuries to surrounding structures occurring at the time of cesarean delivery [27]. Despite this statistic, they remain rare [27]. One case–control study found the incidence of bladder injury at the time of cesarean delivery to be 0.28% [27]. The risk of bladder injury is higher for cesarean deliveries performed during the second stage of labor or repeat cesarean deliveries [4,27].

Less common injuries are those involving the bowel or ureters. Risk factors for any of these types of injuries are prior pelvic surgery, including prior cesarean delivery, emergency cesarean delivery, and cesarean hysterectomy. Prompt recognition and management of these injuries are crucial to preventing the development of further issues such as sepsis, renal failure, and fistula formation.

Extended Hospitalization. A woman who has had a cesarean delivery typically remains hospitalized longer than one who has had a vaginal delivery; she also has increased risk for readmission [9,15,28]. Patients who deliver abdominally are usually discharged on the third or fourth postpartum day compared with the first or second postpartum day for those who deliver vaginally. The average length of hospitalization may even be longer given the complications that are more common in women who deliver by cesarean section.

Emergency Hysterectomy. The risk of the need for hysterectomy after or during a cesarean delivery is greater than after a vaginal delivery [24,25,29]. An important problem with any study that looks at this issue, however, is that the studies do not control for those women who had a trial of labor before their cesarean delivery. Thus, women undergoing a primary cesarean section who have not labored may have a lower rate of emergent hysterectomy than those who labored before their cesarean delivery.

One study attempted to correct for this issue performed a case–control study of women who had a hysterectomy postpartum (within 14 days of giving birth). Compared with a control group of women who did not have a hysterectomy, those who did have a hysterectomy were 13 times more likely to have been delivered by cesarean section after controlling for prior cesarean delivery, use of prostaglandins or oxytocin, and the use of magnesium sulfate [29].

Pain. Women who undergo cesarean delivery more commonly experience pain after delivery compared with those having vaginal deliveries [30–33]. A study of 242 primiparous women reported that all those who underwent cesarean deliveries (both planned and unplanned) required narcotic pain medications compared with 11% of those who delivered vaginally [15]. Narcotic pain medications can have a significant impact on initial bonding between the mother and the newborn. Narcotics impact breastfeeding success rates and maternal postpartum function. Finally, the risk for postpartum depression may be greater in the presence of narcotic pain medications [15,34,35].

Bowel Dysfunction

A dynamic ileus has been reported to occur as often as 10 to 20% of post-operative cesarean delivery cases [36]. Ileus can be a normal physiologic response to surgery involving the abdomen or pelvis. The exact occurrence of pathologic ileus has been difficult to estimate accurately. Pathologic ileus is the result of multiple factors including infection, operating time, and organ injury. Ogilvie's syndrome (severe post-operative ileus) is characterized by acute pseudo-obstruction and dilation of the cecum and right hemicolon without the presence of an actual anatomic obstruction.

Poor Birth Experience and Psychological Outcome

DiMatteo and colleagues found that women who delivered healthy babies by cesarean section were more likely to report dissatisfaction with their birth experience than those women who delivered vaginally [34]. Women who deliver by cesarean have less initial contact with their newborns and usually have to wait a longer time before first contact with their babies [20,34,35]. This patient population is also less likely to breastfeed than patients who deliver vaginally [37]. In addition, many patients report a feeling of loss, failure, and anger [38]. These feelings are likely the result of many factors, including but not limited to, loss of control, anxiety about undergoing a surgical procedure, stress, pain, fatigue, and the psychological changes that occur in new mothers. Proper establishment of realistic expectations regarding the birthing process is crucial in helping alleviate some of these negative patient experiences.

Septic Pelvic Thrombophlebitis

Patients who undergo cesarean delivery are at an increased risk of septic pelvic thrombophlebitis, which can include both ovarian vein thrombophlebitis and deep septic pelvic thrombophlebitis. The risk is 1–2% with cesarean delivery as opposed to 0.05% with vaginal delivery [39]. These two often occur together. Ovarian vein thrombosis usually presents with fever and abdominal pain within one week of surgery. The pain is usually on the side of the affected ovary. It is possible to see ovarian vein thrombosis on imaging in a small percentage of cases. Deep septic pelvic thrombophlebitis typically presents within a few days of surgery and is associated only with fever and not pain. It is not visualized on imaging studies.

Cesarean Hysterectomy

Cesarean hysterectomy is a term used to describe a hysterectomy that occurs after a cesarean delivery. It can be either planned or unplanned. One of the most common reasons for unplanned, or emergent, cesarean hysterectomy is hemorrhage that can't be controlled by conservative measures. Uterine atony or abnormal placentation account for 30–50% of cesarean hysterectomies [40–43]. Other, less common, contributing factors to cesarean hysterectomy include rupture of the uterus, fibroids, and laceration of uterine vessels [40–43].

One prospective study found the following complication rates: packed red blood cell transfusion (84%), transfusion of other blood products (43%), fever (11%), ileus (5%), bowel injury (1%), cuff abscess (2.7%), and maternal death (1.6%) [43].

The performance of a cesarean hysterectomy can be a stimulating event for the operating room team due to the severe blood loss associated with this procedure. While it is appropriate to initiate conservative measures prior to the decision for cesarean hysterectomy, the patient will continue to lose blood during the efforts for uterine conservation. It is essential to decisively initiate efforts toward conservative management while appropriately recognizing those cases when the efforts have failed to achieve success. Once the surgeon recognizes the situation where conservative management has failed, further delay only increases patient blood loss. Of course, the decision to proceed to cesarean section cannot be made lightly given procedures morbidity and the permanent loss of fertility. A step-by-step description of cesarean hysterectomy is seen in the Box 8.1. A video of a cesarean hysterectomy can be found at www.youtube.com/watch?v=XtPD8atfqzY

Box 8.1 **Steps in the performance of cesarean hysterectomy after delivery of the fetus**

1. Insert a self-retaining retractor such as Bookwalter, Balfour, O'Connor-O'Sullivan, or Alexis-O.
2. Identify, divide and suture ligate the round ligament.
3. The anterior leaf of the broad ligament is opened in a medial fashion toward the vesicouterine fold.
4. The bladder is dissected off of the lower uterine segment. This can be accomplished with a combination of sharp and blunt dissection.
5. The posterior leaf of the broad ligament is then opened parallel to the infundibulopelvic (IP) ligament. Care must be taken to identify and avoid the ureters, which also run parallel to the IP ligament.
6. Identify an avascular area in the posterior leaf of the broad ligament. Create a window in this avascular segment.
7. Advance a Kelly clamp into the hole previously created in the posterior leaf of the broad ligament.
8. Two to three clamps may be utilized: one on the uterine cornu, ligating the uteroovrian ligament, and a second clamp is often placed lateral to the first.
9. The tissue between the medial and lateral clamps is transected and suture ligated with a free tie followed by a transfixaiton suture.
10. Steps 5–9 are repeated on the contralateral side.
11. The bladder is dissected off of the lower uterine segment at the level of the vesicouterine fold. This can be accomplished with a combination of sharp and blunt dissection.
12. Focus at this point shifts to isolating the uterine arteries by skeletonizing away excess connective tissue.
13. Once sufficiently skeletonized, the bilateral uterine arteries are then clamped, transected, and suture ligated. A straight clamp is often utilized to prevent back bleeding from the uterus.
14. The bilateral cardinal and uterosacral ligaments are sequentially clamped, transected, and suture ligated. Care must be taken to hug the uterus in order to avoid clamp placement too laterally, thus risking injury to the ureters.
15. The surgeon can decide to leave or remove the cervix.
16. If the cervix is left in place, as in the case of a supracervical hysterectomy, the cervical stump is sewn closed once the corpus of the uterus has been excised.
17. If the decision is made to remove the cervix, clamps are placed across the cervical vaginal junction and the cervix is removed from the top of the vagina. This can often be difficult to accomplish with a dilated cervix. Some surgeons address this challenge by tagging the cervic with a suture to serve as a landmark to guide excision. Care must be taken to avoid shortening of the vaginal length. The vagina is closed with suture.
18. The pelvis is then irrigated copiously and the abdomen and pelvis are closed once adequate hemostasis is assured.
19. Due to the often emergent nature of the procedure as well as the difficulty level, many surgeons also perform a cystoscopy to visualize efflux from bilateral ureters and insure the bladder is intact.

Fetal and Neonatal Risks Associated with Cesarean Delivery

Cesarean delivery is usually performed for the benefit of the fetus. However, it can also place the fetus at risk for a variety of complications including iatrogenic prematurity, birth trauma, transient tachypnea of the newborn (TTN), respiratory distress (RDS), and death [44].

Respiratory Difficulties

The most well-described respiratory difficulties are those encountered in newborns delivered at term. These respiratory difficulties likely result from a failure of the usual mechanisms to resorb fetal lung fluid that typically occur during vaginal birth. The incidence of TTN is approximately three times more common after elective cesarean delivery than after vaginal delivery [44].

Asthma

Some studies have reported an association between cesarean delivery and the development of asthma. This increased risk of asthma may last into adulthood [45].

Trauma. Babies delivered by cesarean are also at risk of trauma, most commonly mild lacerations that occur during emergency deliveries. The incidence of these lacerations has been reported as 3% [46].

Failure to Breastfeed

Babies delivered by cesarean are less likely to be breastfed compared to those that were delivered vaginally. This is even more likely the case for babies born by unplanned as opposed to planned cesarean [32]. Another study found that mothers who underwent cesarean deliveries of any type are twice as likely to have breastfeeding difficulties compared with those who vaginally [47].

Long-term Risks of Cesarean Delivery

Hospital Readmission

Some studies suggest an increased rate of readmission to the hospital after initial postpartum discharge in patients that had a cesarean delivery as opposed to vaginal delivery [48].

Long-term Pain

Women delivered by cesarean are more likely to report pain in the first two months after delivery than those who deliver vaginally. One survey of more than 1,500 women who had delivered in the previous two years found that those who delivered by cesarean reported incisional pain was a major problem 25% of the time, and a major or minor problem 83% of the time [31]. In the same survey, only 12% of women who delivered vaginally reported perineal pain as a major problem, and a major or minor problem 44% of the time. Some of the patients delivered by cesarean continued to report incisional pain six months out from delivery [31].

Abnormal Placentation

Cesarean delivery increases the risk of abnormal placentation in subsequent pregnancies. The risk of placenta previa, placenta accreta, and placental abruption increases after prior cesarean delivery. These risks increase with increasing number of prior cesarean deliveries [49].

Adhesion Formation

Cesarean delivery is associated with an increased risk of adhesion formation that can be asymptomatic or symptomatic. Symptomatic adhesions can cause a variety of problems including pain, bowel obstruction, infertility, and increased risk of injury to abdominal or pelvic organs in subsequent surgeries. As expected, the incidence of adhesions increases with increasing numbers of repeat cesarean deliveries [4,50,51].

Infertility/Subfertility

No causal relationship between one cesarean delivery and difficulty becoming pregnant in the future has been established although it has been suggested. [51]. No studies examining the effects of multiple cesarean deliveries on future fertility have been conducted.

Stillbirth

Some suggestion of an association between unexplained stillbirth and history of prior cesarean delivery has occurred but more research is needed to confirm or disprove this theory. One theory is that scar tissue formation resulting from a prior cesarean may interfere with placental attachment and function [52].

Uterine Scar Complications

Complications from cesarean delivery can occur in the hysterotomy itself. These include endometriosis, incisional ectopic pregnancy, and postmenstrual spotting. Endometriosis occurring in a hysterotomy incision has been reported in 0.1% patients who have undergone a cesarean delivery [53]. The typical presentation is a tender, palpable mass that increases in size during menstruation and is associated most often with cyclic pain [54,55]. The pain can also be continuous in nature. Spotting after normal menses can occur as a result of a small indentation in the endometrial cavity at the site of the hysterotomy known as a uterine niche. Menstrual fluid can accumulate in this indentation and result in postmenstrual spotting [56]. It is also possible for an embryo to implant into a defect of the hysterotomy scar, resulting in an ectopic pregnancy.

Uterine Rupture

Uterine rupture is a term used to describe the complete disruption of all uterine layers including serosa. Uterine dehiscence is defined by incomplete uterine wall separation where the serosa usually remains intact. Rupture is a life-threatening condition for both mother and fetus whereas dehiscence is not typically associated poor maternal or fetal outcomes. The incidence of uterine rupture in patients who have had one prior cesarean delivery is 0.3–1% [57–59]. The risk of uterine rupture during a trial of labor after cesarean is 0.7% [58]. The type of prior cesarean is an important factor. The risk of uterine rupture after a previous low transverse cesarean delivery is 0.7% versus as high as 12% after a prior classical cesarean delivery [60].

Concluding Remarks

Cesarean section is a common surgery performed in the United States every year usually for fetal indications and less often for maternal indications. It is generally performed without significant risks to the mother and fetus. A number of complications, however, can arise during a cesarean delivery. It is important for the surgeon to be aware of the potential for development of complications and risk factors that predispose patients to a higher chance of suffering one of these complications. It is imperative that complications be recognized and addressed immediately to give patients the best chance of full recovery and function.

References

1. Cunningham, F, et al. *Williams Obstetrics*. 23rd Edition. McGraw Hill Professional. 2009.
2. Armson BA. Is planned cesarean childbirth a safe alternative? *CMAJ*. 2007;176:475.
3. Declercq E, Barger M, Cabral HJ, et al. Maternal outcomes associated with planned primary cesarean births compared with planned vaginal births. *Obstet Gynecol*. 2007;109:669.
4. Alexander JM, Leveno KJ, Rouse DJ, et al. Comparison of maternal and infant outcomes from primary cesarean delivery during the second compared with first stage of labor. *Obstet Gynecol*. 2007;109:917.
5. Martin TA. Hamilton BE. Osterman Michelle. Births in the US, 2014. NCHS Data Brief No. 216 Sept. 2015.
6. Shellhaas CS, Gilbert S, Landon MB, et al. The frequency and complication rates of hysterectomy accompanying cesarean delivery. *Obstet Gynecol*. 2009;114:224.
7. Clark SL, Christmas JT, Frye DR, et al. Maternal mortality in the United States: Predictability and the impact of protocols on fatal postcesarean pulmonary embolism and hypertension-related intracranial hemorrhage. *Am J Obstet Gynecol*. 2014;211:32.e1.
8. Wen SW, Rusen ID, Walker M, et al. Maternal Health Study Group, Canadian Perinatal Surveillance System. Comparison of maternal mortality and morbidity between trial of labor and elective cesarean section among women with previous cesarean delivery. *Am J Obstet Gynecol*. 2004;191:1263–1269.
9. Harper MA, Byington RP, Espeland MA, et al. Pregnancy-related death and health care services. *Obstet Gynecol*. 2003;102:273–278.
10. Lydon-Rochelle M, Holt VL, Easterling TR, Martin DP. Cesarean delivery and postpartum mortality among primiparas in Washington State, 1987–1996. *Obstet Gynecol*. 2001;97:169–174.
11. Schuitemaker N, van Roosmalen J, Dekker G, et al. Maternal mortality after cesarean section in The Netherlands. *Acta Obstet Gynecol Scand*. 1997;76:332–334.
12. Kamel H, Navi BB, Sriram N, et al. Risk of a thrombotic event after the 6-week postpartum period. *N Engl J Med*. 2014;370:1307.
13. Ueland K. Maternal cardiovascular dynamics. VII. Intrapartum blood volume changes. *Am J Obstet Gynecol*. 1976;126:671.
14. Larsson C, Saltvedt S, Wiklund I, et al. Estimation of blood loss after cesarean section and vaginal delivery has low validity with a tendency to exaggeration. *Acta Obstet Gynecol Scand*. 2006;85:1448.
15. Hammad IA, Chauhan SP, Magann EF, Abuhamad AZ. Peripartum complications with cesarean delivery: A review of Maternal-Fetal Medicine Units Network publications. *J Matern Fetal Neonatal Med*. 2014;27:463.
16. Hebert PR, Reed G, Entman SS, Mitchel EF Jr, Berg C, Griffin MR.Serious maternal morbidity after childbirth: Prolonged hospital stays and readmissions. *Obstet Gynecol*. 1999;94:942–947.
17. Sherman SJ, Greenspoon JS, Nelson JM, Paul RH. Obstetric hemorrhage and blood utilization. *J Reprod Med*. 1993;38:929–934.

18. Allen VM, O'Connell CM, Liston RM, Baskett TF. Maternal morbidity associated with cesarean delivery without labor compared with spontaneous onset of labor at term. *Obstet Gynecol.* 2003;102:477–482.
19. Silver, RM, MFMU Network of NICHD. The MFMU cesarean section registry: Maternal morbidity associated with multiple repeat cesarean delivery. *Am J Obstet Gynecol.* 2004;191:s17.
20. Chaim W, Bashiri A, Bar-David J, Shoham-Vardi I, Mazor M. Prevalence and clinical significance of postpartum endometritis and wound infection. *Infect Dis Obstet Gynecol.* 2000;8:77–82.
21. Fisher J, Astbury J, Smith A. Adverse psychological impact of operative obstetric interventions: A prospective longitudinal study. *Aust N Z J Psychiatry.* 1997;31:728–738.
22. Duff P. Pathophysiology and management of postcesarean endomyometritis. *Obstet Gynecol.* 1986;67:269.
23. Owen, J, Andrews, WW. Wound complications after cesarean sections. *Clin Obstet Gynecol.* 1994;37:842.
24. Olsen MA, Butler AM, Willers DM, et al. Risk factors for surgical site infection after low transverse cesarean section. *Infect Control Hosp Epidemiol* 2008;29:477.
25. Selo-Ojeme DO, Bhattacharjee P, Izuwa-Njoku NF, Kadir RA. Emergency peripartum hysterectomy in a tertiary London hospital. *Arch Gynecol Obstet.* 2005;271:154–159. Epub 2005 Feb 3.
26. Figueroa R, Garry D, Maulik D. Emergency peripartum hysterectomy: Experience at a community teaching hospital. *Obstet Gynecol.* 2002;99:971–975.
27. Phipps, MG, Watabe, B, Clemons JL, et al. Risk factors for bladder injury during cesarean delivery. *Obstet Gynecol.* 2005;105:156.
28. Thompson JF, Roberts CL, Currie M, Ellwood DA. Prevalence and persistence of health problems after childbirth: Associations with parity and method of birth. *Birth.* 2002;29:83–94.
29. Kacmar J, Bhimani L, Boyd M, Shah-Hosseini R, Peipert J. Route of delivery as a risk factor for emergent peripartum hysterectomy: A case–control study. *Obstet Gynecol.* 2003;102:141–145.
30. Declercq ER, Sakala C, Corry MP, Applebaum S, Risher P. Listening to Mothers: *Report of the First National U.S. Survey of Women's Childbearing Experiences.* New York: Maternity Center Association, October 2002.
31. Lydon-Rochelle MT, Holt VL, Martin DP. Delivery method and self-reported postpartum general health status among primiparous women. *Paediatr Perinat Epidemiol.* 2001;15:232–240.
32. Almeida EC, Nogueira AA, Candido dos Reis FJ, Rosa e Silva JC. Cesarean section as a cause of chronic pelvic pain. *Int J Gynaecol Obstet.* 2002;79:101–104.
33. DiMatteo MR, Morton SC, Lepper HS, et al. Cesarean childbirth and psychological outcomes: A meta-analysis. *Health Psychol.* 1996;15:303–314.
34. Johnstone SJ, Boyce PM, Hickey AR, Morris-Yatees AD, Harris MG. Obstetric risk factors for postnatal depression in urban and rural community samples. *Aust N Z J Psychiatry.* 2001;35:69–74.
35. LaRosa JA, Saywell RM Jr, Zollinger TW, et al. The incidence of adynamic ileus in postcesarean patients. Patient-controlled analgesia versus intramuscular analgesia. *J Reprod Med.* 1993;38:293.
36. DiMatteo MR, Morton SC, Lepper HS, et al. Cesarean childbirth and psychosocial outcomes: A meta-analysis. *Health Psychol.* 1996;15:303.
37. Clement S. Psychological aspects of caesarean section. *Best Pract Res Clin Obstet Gynaecol.* 2001;15:109.
38. Levine EM, Ghai V, Barton JJ, Strom CM. Mode of delivery and risk of respiratory diseases in newborns. *Obstet Gynecol.* 2001;97:439.
39. Dunnihoo DR, Gallaspy JW, Wise RB, Otterson WN. Postpartum Ovarian Vein Thrombophlebitis: A review. *Obstet Gynecol Surv.* 1991;46:415–427.
40. Bodelon C, Bernabe-Ortiz A, Schiff MA, Reed SD. Factors associated with peripartum hysterectomy. *Obstet Gynecol.* 2009;114:115.
41. Rossi AC, Lee RH, Chmait RH. Emergency postpartum hysterectomy for uncontrolled postpartum bleeding: A systematic review. *Obstet Gynecol.* 2010;115:637.
42. Flood KM, Said S, Geary M, et al. Changing trends in peripartum hysterectomy over the last 4 decades. *Am J Obstet Gynecol.* 2009;200:632.e1.
43. Shellhaas CS, Gilbert S, Landon MB, et al. The frequency and complication rates of hysterectomy accompanying cesarean delivery. *Obstet Gynecol.* 2009;114:224.
44. Bager P, Melbye M, Rostgaard K, Benn CS, Westergaard T. Mode of delivery and risk of allergic rhinitis and asthma. *J Allergy Clin Immunol.* 2003;111:51–56.
45. Alexander JM, Leveno KJ, Hauth J, et al. Fetal injury associated with cesarean delivery. *Obstet Gynecol.* 2006;108:885.
46. Towner D, Castro MA, Eby-Wilkens E, Gilbert WM. Effect of mode of delivery in nulliparous women on neonatal intracranial injury. *N Engl J Med.* 1999;341:1709–1714.

47. Lydon-Rochelle M, Holt VL, Martin DP, Easterling TR. Association between method of delivery and maternal rehospitalization. *JAMA*. 2000;283:2411–2416.
48. Marshall NE, Fu R, Guise JM. Impact of multiple cesarean deliveries on maternal morbidity: A systematic review. *Am J Obstet Gynecol.* 2011;205:262.e1.
49. Tulandi T, Agdi M, Zarei A, et al. Adhesion development and morbidity after repeat cesarean delivery. *Am J Obstet Gynecol.* 2009;201:56.e1.
50. Eijsink JJ, van der Leeuw-Harmsen L, van der Linden PJ. Pregnancy after Caesarean section: Fewer or later? *Hum Reprod.* 2008;23:543.
51. Moraitis AA, Oliver-Williams C, Wood AM, et al. Previous caesarean delivery and the risk of unexplained stillbirth: Retrospective cohort study and meta-analysis. *BJOG.* 2015;122:1467.
52. Andolf E, Thorsell M, Kallen K. Caesarean section and risk for endoemtriosis: A prospective cohort stud of Swedish registries. *BJOG.* 2013;120:1061.
53. Gunes M, Kayikcioglu F, Ozturkoglu E, Haberal A. Incisional endometriosis after cesarean section, episiotomy and other gynecologic procedures. *J Obstet Gynaecol Res.* 2005;31:471.
54. Blanco RG, Parithivel VS, Shah AK, et al. Abdominal wall endometriomas. *Am J Surg.* 2003;185:596.
55. Bij de Vaate AJ, van der Voet LF, Naji O, et al. Prevalence, potential risk factors for development and symptoms related to the presence of uterine niches following Cesarean section: Systematic review. *Ultrasound Obstet Gynecol.* 2014;43:372.
56. National Institutes of Health Consensus Development Conference Panel. National Institutes of Health Consensus Development conference statement: Vaginal birth after cesarean: New insights. March 8–10, 2010. *Obstet Gynecol.* 2010;115:1279.
57. Landon MB, Hauth JC, Leveno KJ, et al. Maternal and perinatal outcomes associated with a trial of labor after prior cesarean delivery. *N Engl J Med.* 2004;351:2581.
58. Guise J-M, Eden K, Emeis C, et al. Vaginal birth after cesarean: New insights. Evidence Report/Technology Assessment No.191. (Prepared by the Oregon Health & Science University Evidence-based Practice Center under Contract No. 290-2007-10057-I). AHRQ Publication No. 10-E003. Agency for Healthcare Research and Quality, Rockville, MD 2010. www.ahrq.gov/clinic/tp/cesarreqtp.htm#Report (Accessed on May 21, 2012).
59. Landon MB, Lynch CD. Optimal timing and mode of delivery after cesarean with previous classical incision or myomectomy: A review of the data. *Semin Perinatol.* 2011;35:257.
60. Glaze S, Ekwalanga P, Roberts G, et al. Peripartum hysterectomy: 1999 to 2006. *Obstet Gynecol.* 2008;111:732.

Vaginal Birth after Cesarean

Sara Petruska

Introduction

Obstetric care providers must facilitate a patient-centered discussion on of the risks and benefits of elective repeat cesarean section (ERCD) and trial of labor after cesarean (TOLAC). It is important to individualize these discussions to include each patient's prior obstetrical history, current pregnancy, postpartum needs, plans for future fertility, and view of her past and future birth experiences. This highly individualized discussion will differ for each patient and is difficult to codify in a decisional model, as different variables are weighed differently by different patients. This chapter will discuss the factors which increase or decrease risks and benefits of repeat cesarean section and TOLAC for obstetrical patients with a prior history of cesarean delivery and review the evidence that guides management of these patients.

Scope of the Problem

Cesarean delivery rates have risen since the 1970s. In the 1990s, efforts to decrease ERCD and increase TOLAC succeeded in reducing the cesarean section rate. The rate of women attempting TOLAC increased, peaking in 1995 when 51.8% of women with a prior cesarean delivery attempted TOLAC.[1] Increased experience with TOLAC revealed an expanded understanding of the risks of TOLAC, most notably uterine rupture. In 1999, the American Congress of Obstetrics and Gynecology (ACOG) issued guidelines that the obstetrician, an anesthesiologist, and/or staff capable of performing an emergency cesarean delivery should be continuously present in the hospital through the active phase of labor for patients undergoing TOLAC.[2] The rate of women attempting TOLAC began to fall, reaching 15.9% in 2008. Since not all TOLACs succeed in vaginal delivery, the successful vaginal birth after cesarean (VBAC) rate was even lower, at about 8% of women with prior cesarean deliveries.[3] In 2010, amid concern about the national cesarean section rate, the Eunice Kennedy Shriver National Institute of Child Health and Human Development (NICHD) and The Office of Medical Applications of Research (OMAR) convened a National Institutes of Health Consensus Development National Institutes of Health (NIH) panel to discuss outcomes of TOLAC. The panel's statement affirmed that TOLAC leads to a successful outcome in a majority of cases and is a reasonable approach for many patients.[4] The panel encouraged organizations and physicians to facilitate the availability of TOLAC for patients.

Risks, Benefits, and Decision Making

Discussion on the route of delivery should begin early in prenatal care to allow time for decision making. The patient should have ample opportunity to change obstetrical provider if necessary for her satisfaction. When weighing the risks and benefits for a particular patient, it is important to begin with the patient's views, obstetric history, and medical history. Her decision on route of delivery for this pregnancy is influenced by her prior birth experience, particularly if she harbors doubts, founded or unfounded, about whether her prior cesarean delivery was truly indicated. Women with a prior history of an unscheduled cesarean section often present with intense feelings about their previous obstetrical experience.[5] Given the degree to which these feelings color the patient's decision making, this should be addressed at the beginning of the discussion.

The obstetrician must identify any contraindications to trial of labor, such as a prior classical incision, prior t-shaped hysterotomy, prior trans-fundal uterine surgery, current placenta previa, or more than two prior cesarean deliveries. A prior low vertical uterine incision has the same risk for uterine rupture as a low segment transverse hysterotomy.[6] The patient's prior operative reports should be requested, but if they are unobtainable, she may still be a candidate for TOLAC as long as the clinical circumstances of her prior cesarean delivery do not suggest that a classical incision may have been used (such as for delivery of a preterm breech infant).[2]

If no contraindications are identified, the risks and benefits of ERCD and TOLAC should be reviewed with the patient. The risks of each route to both patient and fetus are summarized in Table 9.1. The benefits of repeat cesarean delivery include more predictable scheduling, lower chance for uterine rupture and uterine infection, and the ability to complete tubal ligation at the time of delivery if that is desired. The benefits of TOLAC include avoidance of major abdominal surgery, decreased both inpatient and outpatient recovery time, decreased risk for placenta previa and accreta in future pregnancies, less need for narcotics during recovery, and the experience of labor and, if successful, vaginal birth for the patient and potentially her family.

Uterine rupture and its own attendant risks have received the most attention in discussion about risks of TOLAC. Factors that modify a patient's risk for uterine rupture are noted in Table 9.2. Previously, Bujold et al. noted that a single-layer uterine closure was associated with an increased risk for uterine rupture in comparison with a double-layer closure,[7] but in a more recent meta-analysis Bujold and others concluded that, while a double-layer closure may result in a thicker lower uterine segment measured in interpregnancy transvaginal ultrasound, current evidence is insufficient to conclude that this translates into a decreased risk for uterine rupture.[8]

Data on the effect of more than one cesarean scar on the risks of TOLAC have been mixed, but among studies that have noted an increase in uterine rupture, the absolute magnitude of the increased risk was small, from 0.9% with one incision to 1.8% with two incisions.[13] ACOG suggests that it is reasonable to consider TOLAC for patients with two prior cesarean deliveries.[2] The risks of TOLAC in women with more than two cesarean deliveries are not currently well-delineated and in most centers TOLAC for these

Table 9.1 Risks of Trial of Labor after Cesarean Compared with Risks of Elective Repeat Cesarean Section[2,17]

Maternal Risks	**TOLAC**	**ERCD**
Endometritis	**2.9%**	1.5–2.1%
Operative injury	0.4%	**0.42–0.6%**
Blood transfusion	0.7–1.7%	1–1.4%
Hysterectomy	0.2–0.5%	0–0.4%
Uterine rupture	0.7–0.9%	0.4–0.5%
Maternal death	0.02%	0.02–0.04%
Subsequent placenta previa	9 per 1,000 with 1 CS	17 per 1,000 with 2 CS
		30 per 1,000 with 3 CS
Placenta accreta	3.1 per 1,000 with 1 CS	5.7 per 1,000 with 2 CS
		24 per 1,000 with 3 CS
Typical hospital stay	2 days postpartum if VBAC occurs	3–4 days postpartum
Typical analgesia	NSAIDs	NSAIDs and narcotics
Postpartum leave	6 weeks if VBAC	8 weeks
Newborn Complications	**TOLAC**	**ERCD**
HIE	6.7 per 10,000	0
Neonatal death	0.08%	0.05%
Perinatal death	0.13%	0.01%
NICU admission	6.6%	6.0%
Respiratory morbidity	0.1–1.8%	1–5%
Transient tachypnea	3.5%	6.2%
Hyperbilirubinemia	2.2%	5.8%

Table 9.2 Factors That Modify the Risks and Benefits of TOLAC

Factors That Modify Risks of TOLAC	Factors That Modify Benefits of TOLAC	
Increase Risk • Classical incision/myomectomy • More than one prior CD • Less than 18 months between deliveries • Induction of labor, especially with unfavorable cx • No prior vaginal delivery • Birth weight >4,000 g[9] • Infection at prior CD • Thin lower segment on US • Prior preterm CS[10]	Increase Chance of Benefit (successfulVBAC) • Young age • Low BMI • Prior vaginal delivery • Presenting in spontaneous labor • Earlier gestational age • smaller babies • Nonrecurring indication for first section[3]	Increase Value of Benefit • Limited time or assistance for recovery • Plan for several more children (VBAC may avoid several future CD) • Morbid obesity, given increased risks of surgery • Prior addiction, as may avoid narcotics exposure • Personal value patient places on vaginal delivery
Decrease Risk • Two-layer uterine closure • More than 18 months between deliveries • Spontaneous labor • Preterm labor[11] • Prior vaginal delivery[12]	Decrease Chance of Benefit • Preeclampsia • Postdates • Short inter-delivery interval • Macrosomia • Induction of labor • Non-white ethnicity • Advanced maternal age • Gestation over 40 weeks • Pregestational obesity • Increased gestational weight gain • Gestational diabetes • Prior CD for arrest of dilation or descent	Decrease Value of Benefit • Completed childbearing (VBAC will not prevent future CD) • Plan for BTL (will have surgery anyway)

patients would not be encouraged. Patients with twin gestations undergoing TOLAC had similar rates of uterine rupture and maternal and perinatal morbidity to women with singletons attempting TOLAC.[14] Safety of TOLAC for multifetal gestation in patients with more than one prior cesarean delivery has not been evaluated. Inter-delivery interval of less than 18 months was associated with a threefold increased risk for uterine rupture.[15]

When considering the benefits of TOLAC, it is important to address both the likelihood that successful VBAC can occur for this patient and the value that she places on vaginal delivery if it occurs. Since most of the benefits of TOLAC are only realized if the patient has a successful VBAC, it is important to consider her chance for success. The highest rates of morbidity are seen among women who attempt TOLAC but require repeat cesarean delivery in labor. In an important study of over 6,000 women, McMahon et al. demonstrated that the risks for hysterectomy, uterine rupture, and operative injury were increased fivefold among women who delivered by cesarean during failed TOLAC.[16] An important component of the mitigation of risk in TOLAC, therefore, is directive counseling patients toward ERCD when they have a low chance for a successful VBAC. The Maternal Fetal Medicine Units Network have developed calculators to determine a patient's chance for successful VBAC.[17] It can be accessed at https://mfmu.bsc.gwu.edu/PublicBSC/MFMU/VGBirthCalc/vagbirth.html At an obstetrical office visit, the first calculator can be used to assess factors that affect success, such as age, BMI, history of prior vaginal deliveries, and prior history of cesarean for arrest of dilation or descent. If discussion on route of delivery is occurring after a patient has presented in labor, a second calculator at the same site can add additional variables such as estimated gestational age, presence of hypertension, effacement, dilation, and station to refine the calculation.

The American Congress of Obstetrics and Gynecology suggests that, for patients whose calculated success rate is less than 60%, the risk–benefit analysis likely favors delivery by ERCD.[2] It is important to share this information with the patient, and also to understand that the value that she places on vaginal delivery may lead her to choose TOLAC even if her calculated chance for success falls under this recommended threshold. For example, a patient who has 12 weeks paid sick leave, one prior child who is in school, local family support, a partner with a difficult work schedule and a plan for a tubal ligation as her plan for contraception may not place very much value on having a vaginal delivery. On the other hand, a vaginal birth may hold high value to a patient who needs to return to work in 5 weeks, has two small children at home, little family support, a plan for several future pregnancies, and a strong desire for the experience of vaginal delivery.

Through a process of shared decision making, the factors above should be reviewed with the patient. The physician should offer directive counseling toward the route of delivery that his or her experience suggests is most consistent with the patient's goals and safety, but the patient's autonomy should be respected in her decision. The discussion should be fully documented in the prenatal record.

The benefits of TOLAC should be considered separately from the risks. Factors that increase a patient's chance for successful VBAC do not necessarily decrease the risks of TOLAC for her. Some factors, such as morbid obesity, affect the discussion from multiple angles; morbid obesity both increases the value of VBAC by avoiding the increased surgical risks for an obese patient and decreases the likelihood of VBAC by its association with increased need for CD during TOLAC.

For the medically complex patient, the benefit of avoiding the fluid shifts and morbidity of surgery through TOLAC needs to be weighed against the acceptance that for patients such as those with extreme morbid obesity or heart disease, it may not be possible to proceed with the typical pace of a "stat" cesarean delivery in the event that emergent delivery is needed during TOLAC, increasing the risk of morbidity or mortality for the fetus.

Prenatal Care of the Patient with Previous Cesarean Delivery

Decisions on route of delivery should be periodically revisited as the patients may have new questions or new factors may arise which influence the balance of risks and benefits. If breech presentation persists, small, retrospectives studies "suggest that external cephalic version(ECV) is not contraindicated if a woman is at low risk of adverse maternal or neonatal outcomes from ECV and TOLAC."[2] A prospective, observational study of 642 women by Rozenberg et al. found that lower uterine segment thickness under 3.5 mm was associated with increased risk for uterine rupture, but the study was not sufficiently powered to establish a threshold of lower uterine segment thickness that would exclude the possibility of uterine rupture and this cut-off has not been prospectively validated for clinical use in counseling individual patients.[18] In a meta-analysis of the use of ultrasound to predict uterine rupture, Valentin noted that ultrasound techniques to measure the lower uterine segment thickness are variable, and that intra and inter-observer variability are significant.[19] Thus, ultrasound evaluation of the lower uterine segment can be used to add another data point to the discussion, but cannot be used in isolation to plan the route of delivery.

The decision on route of delivery should be revisited if an indication for induction arises. Induction of labor is indeed an option for patients choosing TOLAC. Several studies, however, have shown an increased risk for uterine rupture. This is particularly concerning for patients without a prior history of vaginal delivery, for patients beginning the induction with an unfavorable cervix, or those patients receiving prostaglandins. The risk for uterine rupture increases with higher doses of oxytocin, but a maximum safe level for oxytocin has not been identified.

Studies of mechanical ripening of the cervix have been small and retrospective. The studies only evaluated mechanical dilation in patients with one prior CD, and outcomes have been mixed with some studies showing no increase in risk but another showing an increase in rupture when comparing patients receiving foley bulb ripening with patients in spontaneous labor.[20] Since there is no clear evidence that mechanical ripening strongly modifies the risk for rupture, ACOG suggests that it may be an option when induction is indicated for patients desiring TOLAC who have unfavorable cervices.[2] If the indication for induction is second trimester fetal demise, a small, randomized controlled trial showed that outcomes were similar between patients with and without a prior CD when misoprostol was used for induction.[21]

Management during Trial of Labor after Cesarean

During labor, data on the use of oxytocin for augmentation are mixed. Among studies that suggested an increased risk for uterine rupture the magnitude of the increase was small. Oxytocin augmentation is therefore felt to be acceptable during TOLAC.[2] Cahill reported a dose-related increase in uterine rupture rate with oxytocin administration, particularly above 20 mU/min.[22] Although this study's authors did not conclude that their work was sufficient basis to propose a different oxytocin protocol, consideration should be given to using the lowest effective dose of oxytocin, and obstetricians should be aware that higher doses have been associated with higher risks for uterine rupture. Epidural anesthesia is not associated with failed TOLAC,[23] and as the most common sign of uterine rupture is an abnormal fetal heart rate tracing rather than pain, epidural anesthesia is not believed to mask the presentation of uterine rupture.[24] Retrospective examination of fetal heart rate tracings that preceded uterine rupture showed the most common pattern seen was that of recurrent variable decelerations. Recurrent variable decelerations warrant careful consideration as potential harbingers of uterine rupture when seen in a patient undergoing TOLAC. As changes in the fetal heart tracing are the most common sign of rupture, continuous fetal monitoring should be used for patients undergoing TOLAC. Routine obstetrical indications should be used for placement of internal fetal monitors; these should not be seen as compulsory for TOLAC.[2] Data do not show that intrauterine pressure catheters can be relied upon to help with the diagnosis of uterine rupture.[25]

If VBAC occurs, routine manual exploration of the uterus for has not been shown to improve maternal outcomes,[2] but uterine rupture should be considered for patients with increased vaginal bleeding or unexplained hypovolemia. When these signs exist, evaluation of these patients should include manual exploration and/or ultrasound.

Uterine Rupture during Labor

Uterine rupture includes both complete rupture and incomplete rupture. Incomplete rupture is sometimes called uterine dehiscence; in these cases, the myometrium has separated but the visceral peritoneum over the uterus remains intact.

In addition to abnormal fetal heart rate tracings, other signs and symptoms of uterine rupture include increased vaginal bleeding, acute increase in uterine pain, and loss of fetal station. Perinatal morbidity and mortality are related to the degree to which the placental site remains intact, and risk is greatest in cases when the fetus is extruded from the uterus. In these situations, the chance for permanent neurologic damage to the involved fetus is significant; the chance for perinatal death exceeds 50%.[26] Decision-to-delivery interval is crucial. In Holmgren's series of 35 patients with uterine rupture, no neurologic sequelae were noted among the 17 fetuses delivered in under 18 minutes, but among the 18 neonates delivered more than 18 minutes from the time of decision, three had long-term neurologic deficits. This yields an overall risk of 8.6% for long-term neurologic morbidity following uterine rupture in their study, but the actual risk may be higher as 20% of the children were lost to follow-up.

Maternal mortality with uterine rupture is rare, occurring in 0.2% of 1898 uterine ruptures, which occurred in Canada between 1991 and 2000.[27] McMahon reported that 20% of women with uterine rupture required hysterectomy.[16] When rupture occurs and the uterus is preserved, the risk for recurrent uterine rupture in a subsequent pregnancy is 6–32% depending on the site of rupture. It is therefore recommended that the pregnant patient with previous uterine rupture deliver by ECRD before the onset of labor. Consideration should be given toward late preterm delivery if fetal lung maturity has been demonstrated.[2]

Concluding Remarks

Pregnant patients with histories of previous cesarean deliveries require extensive education on the risks and benefits which are present whether a patient desires to proceed with elective repeat cesarean delivery or trial of labor after cesarean. Obstetricians should carefully consider the factors that are known to modify the risks and benefits of either route and aid the patient in a process of shared decision making. The patient's own experiences and future plans may be very important factors in the process. Support of the option for TOLAC is one way that obstetricians can help to decrease the cesarean section rate, which is an important public health outcome.

References

1. SFG Uddin, AE Simon. Rates and success rates of trial of labor after cesarean delivery in the United States, 1990–2009. *Matern Child Health J* (2013) 17:1309–14.
2. American College of Obstetrics and Gynecology, Practice Bulletin Number 115, 2010.

3. F Cunningham, KJ Leveno, SL Bloom, CY Spong et al. Prior cesarean delivery. *Williams Obstetrics*, Twenty-Fourth Edition. New York: McGraw-Hill; 2013.

4. National Institues of Health Consensus Development Conference Panel: National Institues of Health Consensus Development Conference statement: Vaginal birth after cesarean: New insights. Marcg 8–10, 2010. *Obstet Gynecol* (2010) 115:1279–86.

5. MA Moffat, JS Bell, MA Porter et al. Decision making about mode of delivery among women who have previously had a cesarean section: A qualitative study. *BJOG* (2007) 114:86–93.

6. JN Martin, KG Perry, EE Rogers et al. The care for trial of labor in the patients with a prior low-segment vertical incision. *Am J Obstet Gynecol* (1997) 177:144–8.

7. E Bujold, C Bujold, EF Hamilton et al. The impact of a single-layer or double-layer closure on uterine rupture. *Am J Obstet Gynecol* (2002):186:1326–32.

8. S Roberge, S Demers, V Berghella, N Chaillet, L Moore, E Bujold. Impact of single- vs double-layer closure on adverse outcomes and uterine scar defect: A systematic review and metaanalysis. *Am J Obstet Gynecol* (2014) 211:453–60.

9. MA Elkousy, M Sammel, E Stevens et al. The effect of birth weight on vaginal birth after cesarean delivery success rates. *Am J Obstet Gynecol* (2007) 196:824–30.

10. AC Sciscione, MB Landon, KJ Leveno et al. Previous preterm cesarean delivery and risk of subsequent uterine rupture. *Obstet Gynecol* (2008) 111:648–53.

11. CP Durnwald, DJ Rouse, KJ Leveno et al. The Maternal-Fetal Medicine Units Cesarean Registry: Safety and efficacy of a trial of labor in preterm labor after a prior cesarean delivery. *Am J Obstet Gynecol* (2006) 195:1119–26.

12. CM Zelop, TD Shipp, JT Repke. Effect of previous vaginal delivery on the risk of uterine rupture during a subsequent trial of labor. *Am J Obstet Gynecol* (2000) 183:1184–6.

13. GA Macones, A Cahill, E Pare, DM Stamilio, S Ratcliffe, E Stevens et al. Obstetrics outcomes in women with two prior cesarean deliveries: Is vaginal birth after cesarean delivery an option? *Am J Obstet Gynecol* (2005) 192:1223–8.

14. M.W. Varner, E Thom, CY Spong, MB Landon, KJ Leveno, DJ Rouse et al. Trial of labor after one previous cesarean delivery for multifetal gestation. National Institute of Child Health and Human Development (NICHD) Maternal-Fetal Medicine Units Network (MFMU). *Obstet Gynecol* (2007) 110:814–9.

15. TD Shipp, CM Zelop, JT Repke et al. Interdelivery interval and risk of symptomatic uterine rupture. *Obstet Gynecol* (2001) 97:175–80.

16. MJ McMahon, ER Luther, WA Boews Jr, et al. Comparison of a trial of labor with an elective second cesarean section. *N Engl J Med* (1996) 335:689–95.

17. WA Grobman, Y Lai, MB Landon, CY Spong et al. National Institute of Child Health and Human Development (NICHD) Maternal-Fetal Medicine Units Network (MFMU), "Development of a nomogram for prediction of vaginal birth after cesarean delivery." *Obstet and Gynecol* (2007) 109: 806–12. Calculator at https://mfmunetwork.bsc.gwu.edu/PublicBSC/MFMU/VGBirthCalc/vagbirth.html

18. P Rozenberg, F Goffinet, HJ Philippe, I Nisand. Ultrasonographic measurement of lower uterine segment to assess risk of defects of scarred uterus. *Lancet* (1996) 347: 287–84.

19. L Valentin. Prediction of scar integrity and vaginal birth after cesarean delivery. *Best Pract Res Clin Obstet Gynecol* (2013) 27: 285–95.

20. MK Hoffman, A Sciscione, M Srinivasana, DP Shackleford et al. Uterine rupture in patients with a prior cesarean: The impact of cervical ripening. *Am J Perinatol* (2004) 21:217–22.

21. N Bhattarcharjee, RP Ganguly, SP Saha. Misoprostol for termination of mid-trimester post-cesarean pregnancy. *Aust N Z J Obstet Gynaecol* (2007) 47:23–25.

22. AG Cahill, BM Waterman, DM Stamilio et al. Higher maximum doses of oxytocin are associated with an unacceptably high risk for uterine rupture in patients attempting vaginal birth after cesarean delivery. *Am J Obstet Gynecol* (2008) 199:32–40.

23. MB Landon, S Leidecker, Cy Spog, JC Hauth et al. The MFMU Cesarean Registry: Factors affecting the success of trial of labor after previous cesarean delivery. National Institute of Child Health and Human Development Maternal-Fetal Medicine Units Network. *Am J Obstet Gynecol* (2005) 193: 1016–23.

24. JJ Ridgeway, DL Weyrich, TJ Benedetti. Fetal heart rate changes associated with uterine rupture. *Obstet Gynecol* (2004) 103: 506–12.

25. LD DeVoe, CS Croom, AA Yousef, C Murray. The prediction of "controlled" uterine ruptures by the use of intrauterine pressure catheters. *Obstet Gynecol* (1992) 80:626–9.

26. C Holmgren, JR Scott, TF Porter, MS Esplin, T Bardsley. Uterine rupture with attempted vaginal birth after cesarean delivery, *Obstet and Gynecol* (2012) 119:725–31.

27. S.W Wen, L. Huang, R. Liston et al. Severe maternal morbidity in Canada, 1991–2001. *Canadian Med Assoc J* (2005) 173: 759–61.

Shoulder Dystocia

Christinne Canela

Introduction

Shoulder dystocia is often described as an unpredictable and unpreventable obstetric emergency. Although known risk factors for shoulder dystocia exist, it is known to occur in the absence of these risk factors. Significant risks to the fetus include fracture of the clavicle and/or humerus, temporary or permanent brachial plexus injury, hypoxic ischemic encephalopathy, and potential neonatal death in the most severe cases. Risks to the mother include postpartum hemorrhage, significant obstetric lacerations, and trauma. Recognition is an important first step in its management. Multiple maneuvers have been described to effect delivery of the fetal shoulder once impaction is diagnosed. The goal in shoulder dystocia management is to prevent maternal and neonatal injury but this is, at times, unavoidable. This chapter will provide a review of the management of shoulder dystocia. The maneuvers will be described in detail. Since this is a common cause of litigation in the obstetric field, documentation will also be discussed within the chapter. Appropriate documentation also helps future providers in the management of subsequent pregnancies following shoulder dystocia. Management of subsequent pregnancies is also briefly reviewed.

Scope of the Problem

Shoulder dystocia is most commonly defined as a delivery that requires additional maneuvers to effect delivery of the fetal shoulders after gentle downward traction has failed. Its diagnosis has a subjective component since the provider attending the birth is the one who determines whether additional maneuvers are necessary [1]. Some authors have recommended that the definition should include prolonged head to body delivery time (greater than 60 seconds) as an objective definition, but this has not been widely accepted [2]. Deliveries complicated by shoulder dystocia most commonly involve the anterior shoulder as it gets impacted under the pubic symphysis; less commonly, it involves the posterior shoulder, which may be impacted along the sacral promontory. Reported incidences range from 0.6% to 1.4% [1]. Because of the subjective nature to its definition, concern exists about both under- and overdiagnosis.

The study of shoulder dystocia is important given the associated maternal and fetal complications seen when this event complicates a delivery. It is one of the most common reasons for litigation in the obstetrical field. Even though risk factors are known, shoulder dystocia commonly occurs in the absence of these risk factors and thus remains unpredictable. Any delivering provider should therefore be prepared to manage shoulder dystocia and be proficient in the maneuvers to relieve the impaction. The goals in shoulder dystocia management are to resolve the impaction without causing maternal injury, neonatal injury, or allowing birth asphyxia to occur.

Maternal Complications

The most common maternal complications of shoulder dystocia include postpartum hemorrhage (reported to be 11%) and increased risk of third and fourth degree lacerations (together as high as 7%). Fourth degree lacerations following shoulder dystocia are reported to be 3.8%. In a study involving over 200 shoulder dystocia cases, these complications were found to be equally common in those that resolved with McRoberts' maneuver as opposed to those that resolved with other maneuvers [3.] Maternal morbidity does seem to increase with the number of maneuvers performed to alleviate the shoulder dystocia [4]. In fact, certain "heroic" measures in severe shoulder dystocia cases, such as the Zavanelli maneuver, are associated with significant maternal morbidity [5,6].

Newborn Complications

Brachial plexus injuries, fractures of the clavicle and/or humerus, hypoxic ischemic encephalopathy (HIE), and fetal death are associated with shoulder dystocia.

The reported rates of brachial plexus injuries following shoulder dystocia range from 4% to 40%. Most cases of brachial plexus injuries are temporary and resolve with time. Less than 10% are permanent. The risk of injury to the brachial plexus increases as more maneuvers are performed [7]. It is important to note that many cases of brachial plexus injuries are *not* associated with shoulder dystocia. About 4% of cases reportedly occurred following cesarean delivery. The mechanism of injury to the brachial plexus in these deliveries complicated by shoulder dystocia is thought to be from stretching or compression of the nerves [8]. Stretch injury occurs with hyperextension of one side of the neck, elongating the brachial plexus nerves. Damage to C5–C6 nerve roots leads to Erb-Duschenne's paralysis, which involves the shoulder and elbow only. In these cases, the neonate's upper arm is adducted and internally rotated and the forearm is extended. With increasing stretch, C7 nerve roots may be affected; this can lead to problems with wrist and finger extension. This appearance has been described as "waiter's tip" posture given pronation of the forearm and flexion of the wrist and fingers. With even greater stretch or with twisting of the head to deliver the trunk, the lower roots C8–T1 may become affected, leading to a flail arm. The hands and fingers will be affected along with the other findings noted above. With involvement of T1, Horner syndrome may be seen. Klumpke's palsy is seen when only the C8 and T1 nerve roots are affected and this would be manifested as an isolated hand paralysis and Horner syndrome [8,9].

Delivery of the posterior shoulder by traction techniques increases the risk of fracture of the posterior humerus [10]. Fractures of the clavicle and humerus typically do not lead to long-term sequelae [8].

HIE and even fetal death have occurred following severe cases. HIE occurs secondary to interruption of blood flow within the umbilical cord. Blood flow can be interrupted via external compression from entrapment of a segment of cord between the fetal upper torso or neck and the vagina or via stretching of the cord. It is thought that with prolonged shoulder dystocia, fetal pH decreases by 0.04 per minute [11]. This has been challenged by Leung et al. who found a decline in arterial pH to be only 0.011 per minute [12]. Other studies looking at the head-to-body interval during shoulder dystocia found no clinically significant decrease in cord pH for up to 6 minutes head-to-body delivery interval [8]. Acidosis is reported to occur in 7% of deliveries complicated by shoulder dystocia; 1.5% of neonates experience some hypoxic consequences [13]. Rates of HIE are reported to be 0.3% [11].

Risk Factors for Shoulder Dystocia

Several risk factors for shoulder dystocia have been identified. Fetal macrosomia is the most significant risk factor for shoulder dystocia. Studies have shown that the rates of shoulder dystocia increase with increasing birth weight. Table 10.1 depicts shoulder dystocia rates related to birth weight. One major limiting factor of birth weight is that the actual birth weight is not known to the clinician when clinical decisions are made while caring for the patient. It is well known that estimates of fetal weight are inaccurate whether maternal perception, ultrasound, or Leopold's maneuver are used. Cesarean section rates are higher when the estimated fetal weight is over 4,000 grams, regardless of actual fetal birth weight [14,15].

Gestational and pre-gestational diabetes both increase the risk of shoulder dystocia. Gram for gram, the incidence of shoulder dystocia is increased in diabetic patients compared to those without diabetes. It is thought that this increased risk is related to differences in the growth of infants of diabetic mothers. These infants seem to have higher percentage of body fat, larger shoulder and extremity circumferences, and an asymmetry of somatic growth [15].

A history of previous shoulder dystocia also increases the risk of this event in a future pregnancy. According to the American College of Obstetricians and Gynecology (ACOG), the risk of shoulder dystocia in a subsequent delivery ranges from 1% to

Table 10.1 Birth Weight and Shoulder Dystocia

Birth Weight (g)	Incidence of Shoulder Dystocia (%)
2500–3999	1.5
4000–4499	8.8
4500–4999	17.4
>=5000 gm	17.52

Source: Data from Stotland NE, Caughey AB, Breed EM, Escobar GJ. Risk factors and obstetric complications associated with macrosomia. *Int J Gynecol Obstet.* 2004;87:200–206.

16.7% [1]. It appears that the best predictors of injury include (a) birth weight of the current pregnancy compared to the index pregnancy and (b) severity of prior neonatal injury [1,15]. Operative vaginal delivery is another risk factor. Operative vaginal delivery increases the risk by as much as 35–45% in some studies, especially with the use of a vacuum [14].

Other risk factors identified for shoulder dystocia include maternal obesity/excessive maternal weight gain and labor dysfunction. These risk factors are controversial since studies have had conflicting results. Maternal obesity and excessive weight gain in pregnancy increase the risk of diabetes and fetal macrosomia, two well-known significant risk factors for shoulder dystocia. This makes it difficult to discern which risk factor truly contributed to the shoulder dystocia. It is worth noting that only 5% of obese women experience shoulder dystocia [14].

Attempts to predict the occurrence of shoulder dystocia based on risk factors have poor reliability and poor predictive value. Multiple studies have concluded that shoulder dystocia is an unpredictable event and it is *not* preventable [1,14]. Perhaps, the best use of these risk factors is in the avoidance of performing an operative vaginal delivery when a patient has multiple risk factors for a shoulder dystocia.

Maneuvers to Relieve Shoulder Dystocia

First Line Maneuvers

McRoberts' Maneuver

This is commonly the first maneuver performed by providers. It is performed by hyperflexing the patient's thighs toward the abdomen. This will straighten the maternal sacrum with respect to the lumbar spine, thereby decreasing the angle of inclination of the maternal pelvis [16]. See Figure 10.1.

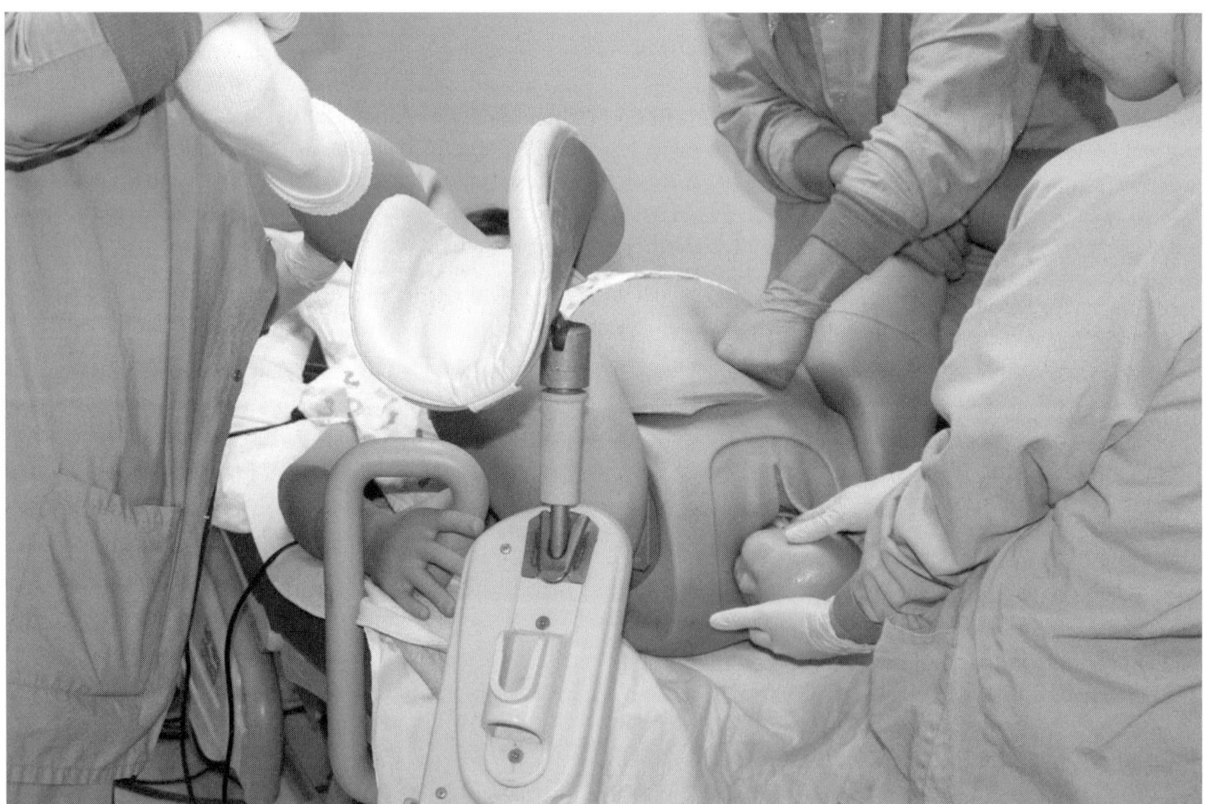

Figure 10.1 McRoberts position and suprapubic pressure. Note hyperflexion and abduction of the mother's hip toward the abdomen. Suprapubic pressure is applied along the area of the fetal back toward the front, leading to adduction of the fetal anterior shoulder, decreasing the bisacromial diameter.

Suprapubic Pressure

This is often performed along with McRoberts' maneuver to alleviate the dystocia. The goal of applying suprapubic pressure is to decrease the fetal bisacromial diameter by adducting the fetal anterior shoulder. Pressure is applied on the suprapubic area in a downward fashion or in a rocking motion from the fetal back toward the front [16,17]. It is important to note that the pressure is applied suprapubically, not on the maternal fundus. Applying fundal pressure only serves to further impact the anterior fetal shoulder into the pubic bone, making the shoulder dystocia worse. See Figure 10.1.

Second Line Maneuvers

Rotational Manuevers

Two rotational maneuvers are described in the literature. As with suprapubic pressure, the aim of these maneuvers is to decrease the fetal bisacromial diameter to allow for delivery of the rest of the fetal body.

Rubin's maneuver is performed by placing a hand into the vagina and applying pressure to the posterior aspect of the most accessible fetal shoulder toward the fetal chest. This will lead to adduction of the fetal shoulder, which would then allow the anterior shoulder to rotate and deliver from behind the pubic bone where is it impacted [16]. See Figure 10.2.

To perform Woods corkscrew maneuver, the delivering provider places a hand on the anterior aspect of the posterior fetal shoulder and rotates the shoulder toward the fetal back. Similar to the motion of unthreading a corkscrew, the goal is to attempt to rotate the fetal shoulder 180°, which allows the fetus to descend while the rotation is occurring [16]. See Figure 10.3.

Delivery of the Posterior Arm

The delivering provider slides a hand along the fetal posterior shoulder and arm. The fetal forearm or wrist is grasped and swept across the anterior fetal chest, thereby delivering the posterior arm. If the fetal forearm is not easily accessible, one can follow the posterior fetal arm and put pressure on the antecubital fossa. This will typically lead to flexion of the fetal arm, allowing access to the fetal forearm. The posterior

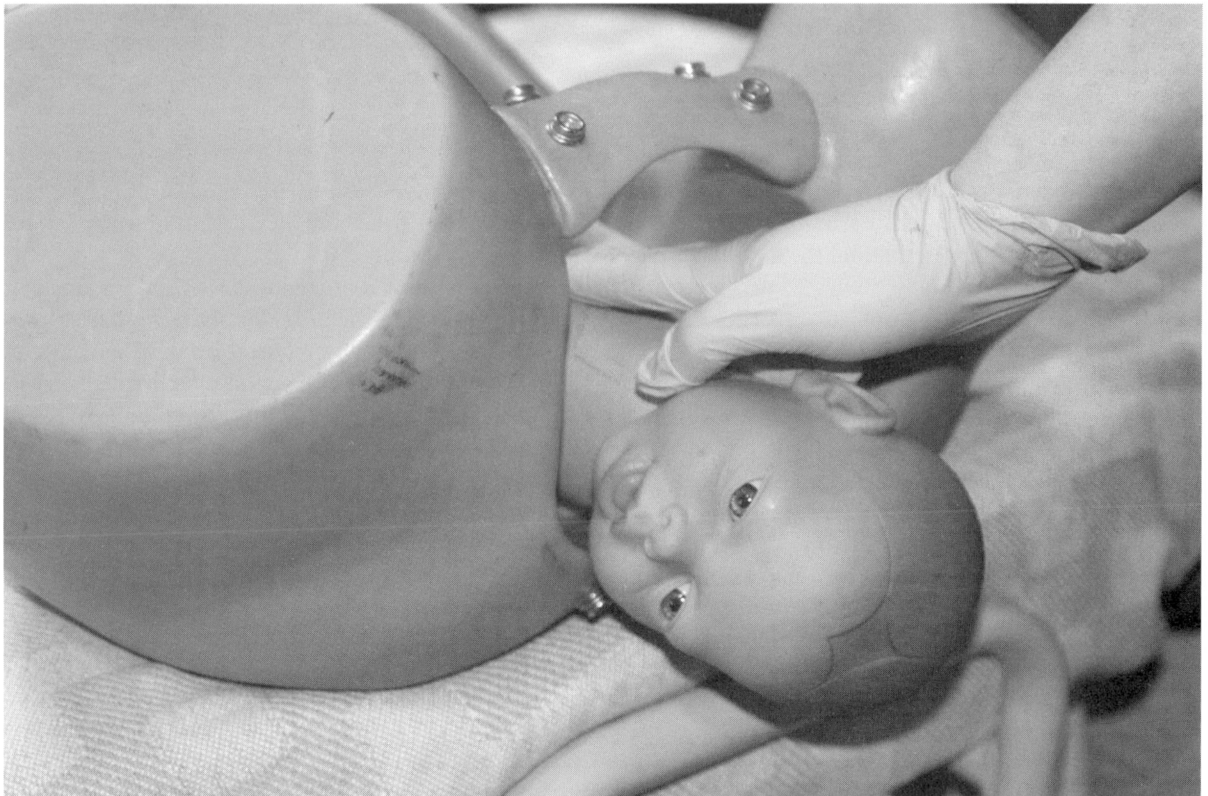

Figure 10.2 Rubin's maneuver. Pressure is applied to the posterior aspect of the most accessible fetal shoulder towards the fetal chest. This results in adduction of the shoulder leading to rotation and delivery of the fetal anterior shoulder.

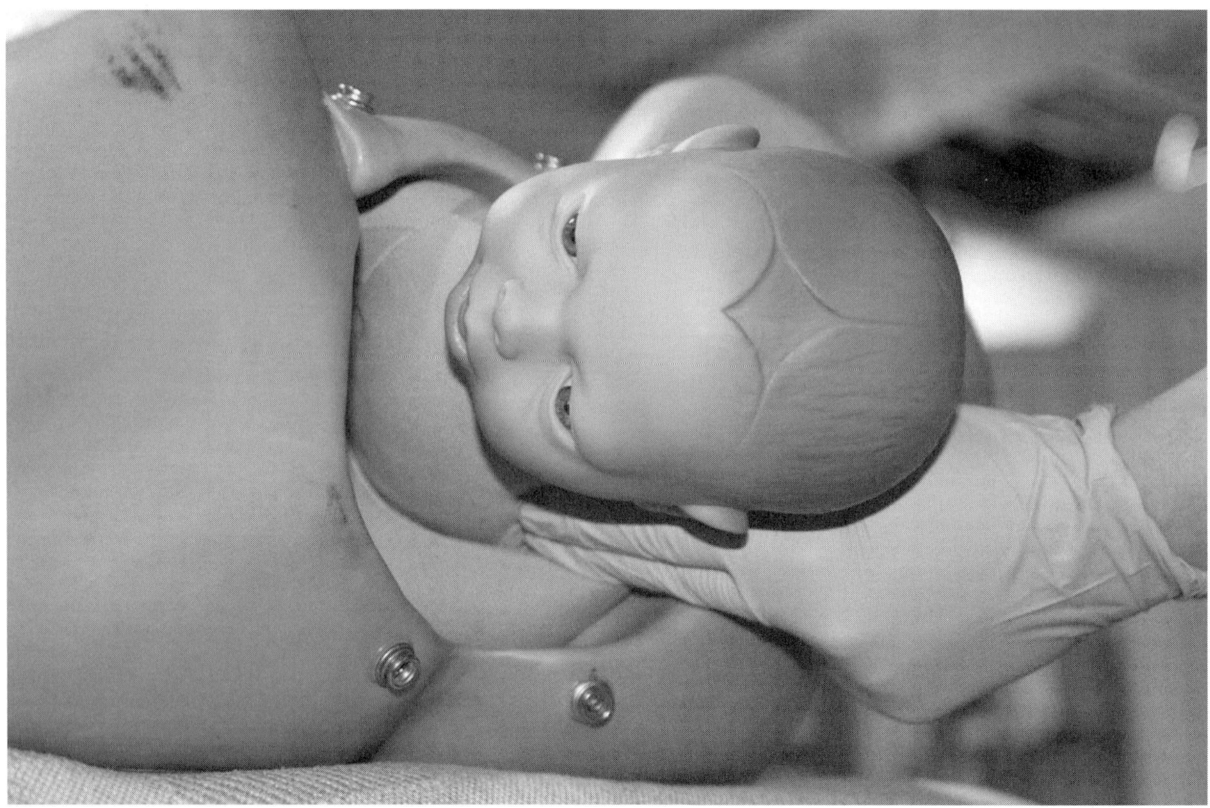

Figure 10.3 Woods Corkscrew manuever. A hand is placed on the anterior aspect of the posterior fetal shoulder to rotate the shoulder toward the fetal back. This will allow the anterior shoulder to descend as the shoulders are rotating.

arm is then delivered as described earlier. With successful delivery of the posterior arm, instead of a fetal bisacromial diameter presentation, the axilloacromial diameter (which is typically about 3 cm shorter) is now the presentation [18]. See Figure 10.4.

Gaskin Manuever

The patient is placed on her hands and knees or in a racing start or "sprinter" position. Gentle downward traction is then applied to the posterior shoulder (the shoulder against the maternal sacrum) or upward traction on the anterior shoulder (the shoulder against the maternal symphysis). This may be a good option for the initial management of a patient without regional anesthesia if McRoberts and suprapubic pressure fail to relieve the shoulder dystocia [19].

Posterior Axillary Traction

Two methods use posterior axillary traction to aid in the delivery of the posterior arm. These maneuvers may be especially helpful in situations in which the fetal arms are extended. With each method, the assistant holds the fetal head and flexes this upward toward the anterior shoulder to make it easier to access the posterior pelvis. Menticoglue describes a maneuver whereby the delivering provider places his or her middle fingers under the fetal posterior axilla and applies downward and outward traction effecting delivery of the posterior shoulder; this is followed by delivery of the posterior arm [10]. With the posterior axilla sling traction procedure, a suction catheter or firm urinary catheter is used as a sling. A loop is created and this loop is threaded under the posterior fetal axilla. Using the other hand, the delivering provider catches this loop and creates a sling around the posterior axilla. Traction is applied to the sling to deliver the posterior shoulder followed by the arm. See Figure 10.5. If this procedure fails to effect delivery, then the sling can be used to rotate the shoulders. With the sling, lateral traction toward the baby's back is applied while the other hand is placed on the anterior shoulder putting pressure toward the fetal chest [20].

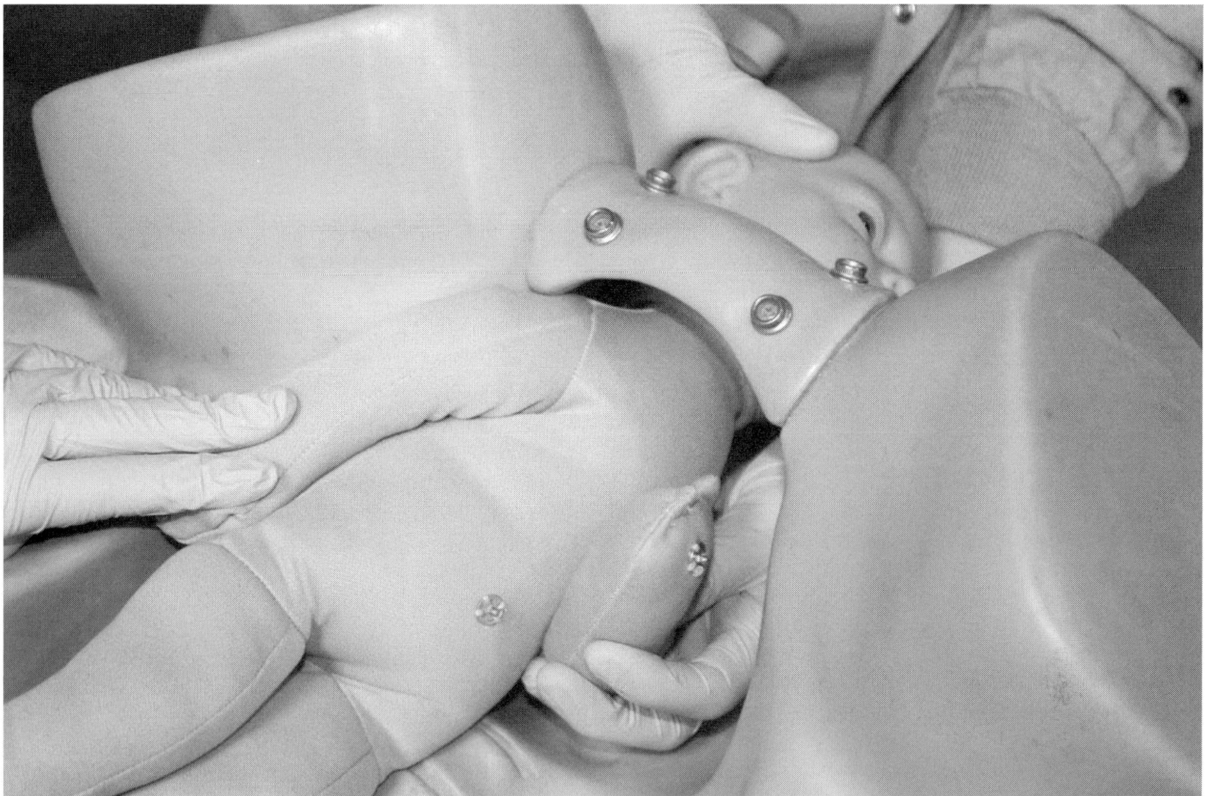

Figure 10.4 Delivery of the posterior arm. The delivering provider is applying pressure on the antecubital fossa, which would result in flexion of the fetal arm. This will allow access to the fetal forearm, which is then swept across the anterior fetal chest leading to delivery of the posterior arm.

Heroic Measures

Intentional Clavicular Fracture

The fetal clavicle can be intentionally fractured by pulling the anterior clavicle outward. This leads to a decrease in the bisacromial diameter. Disadvantages to this method include its difficulty and the possibility of injury to underlying vascular and pulmonary structures.

Zavanelli Maneuver

The fetal head is rotated to its pre-restitution attitude, then flexed and elevated up to the vagina and uterus. Delivery is then accomplished by cesarean section. Tocolytics such as halogenated inhalational anesthetics, Terbutaline, or nitroglycerine may be given to assist with cephalic replacement [16].

Abdominal Rescue

If cephalic replacement or the Zavanelli maneuver is unsuccessful, a low transverse hysterotomy is performed and the fetal shoulders are manually rotated to an oblique diameter through the transabdominal incision. Once the fetal shoulders are rotated, vaginal delivery is then attempted [5,21].

Symphysiotomy

The patient is placed in the lithotomy position and a foley catheter is placed. The urethra is retracted laterally. The skin and subcutaneous tissues are incised with a scalpel to the level of the pubic symphysis. The anterior fibers of the pubic symphysis are also incised. This typically leads to resolution of the dystocia. This is recommended only as a last resort when all the other measures have failed or in cases where immediate access to an operating room facility for Zavenelli or abdominal rescue is not available [16].

Management of Shoulder Dystocia

The providers who attend the birth are responsible for making the diagnosis of shoulder dystocia. Retraction

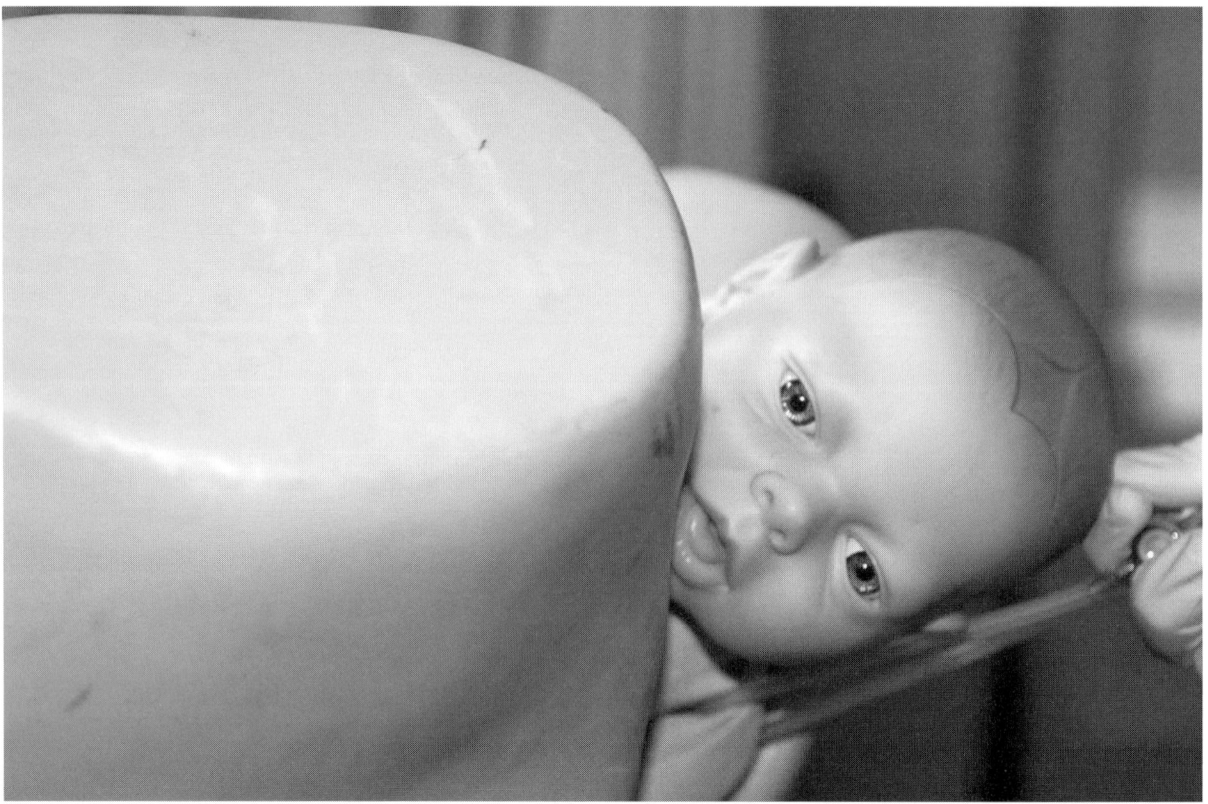

Figure 10.5 Posterior axillary traction. A sling has been created by passing a loop of a suction catheter under the posterior fetal axilla. Downward and outward traction is applied to the sling to deliver the posterior shoulder followed by the posterior arm.

of the fetal head toward the perineum upon delivery of the fetal head, called the "turtle sign" is suggestive of the possibility of shoulder dystocia. If initial attempts to guide the fetal shoulder under the pubic bone fail and the provider deems that additional maneuvers are necessary to effect delivery of the rest of the fetal body, it is important to recognize the situation and inform the other team members about the shoulder dystocia. Grobman emphasized the importance of announcing the shoulder dystocia prior to initiating any other maneuvers. By doing so, the nurses attending the delivery can also call for additional help including additional nursing staff, a second obstetrician, anesthesia personnel and pediatric personnel, if they are needed and readily available [22]. Anesthesia assistance can be helpful if cephalic replacement is necessary. Given the possible risk of fetal injury, pediatric personnel can help with neonatal resuscitation.

It is important to ensure that the delivery bed is in a lowered position or that a stool is available to assist with the performance of some maneuvers. The primary nurse can assist the physician with maneuvers such as McRoberts and suprapubic pressure. A second nurse may also assist with the maneuvers or act as a record keeper. The record keeper should also call out time intervals to help the delivering provider keep track of time. If available, another nurse can help with communication with the family as the delivering provider works to alleviate the dystocia.

Inglis et. al. recommends a "hands off" approach once the shoulder dystocia is diagnosed. This prevents further traction of the fetal head and hopefully will decrease the risk of brachial plexus injury. At this time, the provider can also assess the position of the anterior shoulder as this can help determine the next steps [17]. This time can also be taken to evaluate for the need for an episiotomy. Performing an episiotomy can provide more room to perform additional maneuvers as necessary to relieve shoulder dystocia. The patient is also asked to stop all expulsive efforts.

The American Congress of Obstetricians and Gynecologists (ACOG) recommends using the McRoberts maneuver and suprapubic pressure as the initial steps in the management of shoulder dystocia

[1]. These steps are easy to perform, involve only maternal manipulation, and are known to be effective. Success rates with these maneuvers are reported to be 40–60% [16,22]. If these efforts fail, guidelines are unclear about which maneuver is best performed next. Given that the rates of injury increase with longer interval to resolution of shoulder dystocia and number of maneuvers performed, it makes sense to start with a maneuver that is highly effective and associated with decreased risk of neonatal injury.

A study by Hoffman et al. concluded that delivery of the posterior shoulder should be considered as the next step because of its success rates (as high as 84%) and decreased risk of neonatal injury (12). Rotational maneuvers should then be the next step if delivery of the posterior arm fails [11,17,22]. In this study, Hoffman specifically looked at shoulder dystocia cases where McRoberts' maneuver and suprapubic pressure failed. It was found that delivery of the posterior arm had the highest rate of successful resolution and that the use of the rotational maneuvers were associated with a higher risk of neonatal injury [11]. In this study and others, a strong association was noted between increasing number of maneuvers and the risk of neonatal injury, especially after the fourth maneuver [11]. In a computer model analysis performed by Grimm et al., it was found that delivery of the posterior arm led to a 71% decrease in anterior nerve stretch and an 80% reduction in delivery force. This may explain the lower rates of injury seen with this maneuver [23]. In another study performed by Leung et al., it was found that rotational maneuvers and delivery of the posterior arm were similarly successful in cases of shoulder dystocia where McRoberts maneuver and suprapubic pressure failed (72% vs. 64%). This study, in contrast to Hoffman's study, found that rotational maneuvers were associated with decreased risk of brachial plexus injuries (4.4% vs. 21.4%) and humeral fracture (1.1% vs. 7.1%) [24]. Table 10.2 shows the rates of success of shoulder dystocia maneuvers as seen in these two studies. Table 10.3 describes rates of fetal injury with shoulder dystocia maneuvers according to these two studies. These conflicting results highlight the fact that there is no one "best maneuver" to perform to alleviate shoulder dystocia. It is also important to note that there is no significant loss of efficacy of the different maneuvers for the relief of dystocia regardless of its timing, therefore, at no point in the acute management of shoulder dystocia should any of these maneuvers be abandoned [11].

HIE is a rare complication of shoulder dystocia and seems to be increased after several maneuvers have been performed to relieve the impaction. It is therefore reasonable to consider extraordinary maneuvers to effect delivery once 4–5 min have elapsed since the diagnosis of the dystocia when the fetus remains undelivered [25].

Mnemonics have been developed to help providers and nurses with remembering the management steps when confronted with this event. One such mnemonic is BE CALM, see Box 10.1 for details. Another mnemonic that has been developed is the HELPERR mnemonic and is depicted in Box 10.2 [16,26].

Documentation

Excellent documentation of the shoulder dystocia is very important for multiple reasons. Brachial plexus injuries following this event is the third most common cause of litigation in obstetrics following peripartum HIE which may also follow dystocia [27]. A lack of key information within the records provides opportunities for nonmedical personnel to supply information, which may or may not be accurate. Missing information also opens the case to assumptions and suppositions by expert witnesses. ACOG issued a patient safety checklist for the management of shoulder dystocia and its use may help improve documentation [28]. See Box 10.3 for an example of documentation following shoulder dystocia.

Excellent records on the management of shoulder dystocia are also extremely helpful in the management of subsequent pregnancies. Recurrence rates for shoulder dystocia have been reported to be as high as 16.7% [1,27]. Because of the possibility of recurrence and since the event is traumatic for the patient, it is important that the patient be counseled on the events that occurred during the delivery. Appropriate documentation can assist future obstetricians caring for the patient in making recommendations about future pregnancies.

Management of Subsequent Pregnancies

Given the recurrence rates of 10–16% in pregnancies complicated by shoulder dystocia, it is important to counsel patients immediately after its occurrence, even in mild cases. As mentioned earlier, the most consistent predictors of injury seem to be (a) the birth weight of the infant compared to the index pregnancy,

Table 10.2 Success rates of SD Maneuvers Following Failed McRoberts and Suprapubic Pressure

SD Maneuver	Success Rate (%)				
	First	Second	Third	Fourth	Overall
Hoffman's study results					
Delivery of the posterior arm	87.5	87.5	75.3	88.9	84.4
Rubin maneuver	66.7	80.0	59.3	75	66.0
Woods corkscrew	73.7	79.4	68.4	71.4	72.0
Leung's study results					
Delivery of the posterior arm	77.1	63.6	94.6	No data. Repeated attempts with the previous maneuvers were performed for 11 patients.	
Rotational Manuevers	72	62.5			

Sources: Data from: Hoffman MK, Bailit JL, Ware DW, et al. A comparison of obstetric maneuvers for the acute management of shoulder dystocia. *Obstet Gynecol.* 2011;116(6):1272–78; Leung T, Stuart O, Sahota D, et al. Head-to-body interval and risk off fetal acidosis and hypoxic ischemic encephalopathy in shoulder dystocia: a retrospective review. *BJOG.* 2011;118(4):474–9.

(b) the severity of the dystocia, and (c) presence of neonatal injury [1,15]. These factors should be considered when planning delivery in subsequent pregnancies. Known risk factors for shoulder dystocia include diabetes, obesity, and excessive maternal weight gain during pregnancy. Patients with these findings should be counseled on these risk factors.

In cases of a previous mild shoulder dystocia with no neonatal injury, it is reasonable to obtain a growth sonogram close to term. If estimated fetal weight is less than the index pregnancy with the shoulder dystocia, it is appropriate to allow a trial of labor. The recurrence risk would be expected to be low in this case [29]. If the shoulder dystocia resulted in long-term or permanent injury in a previous pregnancy, then an elective primary cesarean delivery should be offered [29]. The benefit of universal cesarean delivery in patients with a prior shoulder dystocia is questionable since most subsequent deliveries will not be complicated by recurrent shoulder dystocia [1]. Reviewing this information with the patient would be important in the antepartum setting so that the patient and provider can make an appropriate plan of care. ACOG states that following this discussion with the patient, either trial of labor or cesarean delivery is appropriate [1].

Measures to decrease the risk can be instituted prior to subsequent pregnancies in women with previous shoulder dystocia. For example, weight loss may be recommended prior to conception. The patient should also be carefully counseled about appropriate caloric intake and appropriate weight gain during pregnancy. In patients with prior shoulder dystocia, early screening for gestational diabetes is also recommended. If gestational diabetes is diagnosed, attention to careful blood sugar monitoring and control is indicated [29].

Simulation

A discussion of shoulder dystocia would not be complete without discussing simulation. This condition is difficult to manage due to its relatively rare frequency and its unpredictability. Coordination of multiple team members is necessary. Another challenge is that these team members may have not have had the experience of working with each other and some may not have seen a shoulder dystocia previously, yet they are expected to work together well and perform the maneuvers correctly in an emergent setting. This highlights the importance of simulation and training. Simulation and training allows team members to practice the maneuvers, work together, and fine-tune their response to emergencies without exposing patients to harm. Simulation may improve performance of the maneuvers, communication between team members, and documentation. Several studies have found that the institution of standardized shoulder dystocia training protocols decrease rates of fetal brachial plexus injuries in deliveries complicated by shoulder dystocia [22]. This training may be the single most

Table 10.3 Rates of Fetal Injury with SD Maneuvers Following SD Maneuvers

SD Maneuver	Rate of Injury (%)				
	First	Second	Third	Fourth	Overall
Hoffman's Study Results: Percentages reflect total neonatal injuries. The rates of specific neonatal injuries per maneuver were not reported.					
McRoberts maneuver	5.6	8.1	10.5	–	6.1
Suprapubic pressure	5.17	6.1	8.6	12.5	6.4
Delivery of the posterior arm	0	0	2.7	17.78	8.4
Rubin maneuver	0	0	18.5	16.7	14.0
Woods corkscrew	0	0	11.4	14.3	9.5
Leung's Study Results: In this study, suprapubic pressure and McRoberts maneuvers were the first maneuvers initiated, followed by rotational maneuvers or posterior arm delivery.					
Brachial Plexus Injuries					
McRoberts and suprapubic pressure	7.8	–	–		
Posterior arm delivery	–	21.4	3.7		
Rotational maneuvers	–	4.4	0		
Clavicular Injuries					
McRoberts and suprapubic pressure	3.9	–	–		
Posterior arm delivery	–	7.1	0		
Rotational maneuvers	–	5.6	0		
Humeral Fractures					
McRoberts and suprapubic pressure	0	–	–		
Posterior arm delivery	–	7.1	11.1		
Rotational maneuvers	–	1.1	1		

Note A dash (–) was used when data is not available.

Sources: Data from: Hoffman MK, Bailit JL, Ware DW, et al. A comparison of obstetric maneuvers for the acute management of shoulder dystocia. *Obstet Gynecol.* 2011;116(6):1272–8; Leung T, Stuart O, Sahota D, et al. Head-to-body interval and risk off fetal acidosis and hypoxic ischemic encephalopathy in shoulder dystocia: a retrospective review. *BJOG* 2011;118(4):474–9.

Box 10.1 **BE CALM mnemonic**

Breathe. (Do not push, encourage the patient to breathe or pant. Lower the head of the bed)

Elevate the legs (Use McRobert's position)

Call for help. (Additional nursing staff, OB provider able to perform CD, anesthesia provider, pediatric provider, respiratory therapy)

Apply suprapubic pressure (*not* fundal pressure)

En**L**arge the vaginal opening (episiotomy)

Maneuvers – Additional maneuvers may be needed as described earlier.

Source: From ACOG. Managing shoulder dystocia. Optimizing Protocols in Obstetrics. 2013.

Box 10.2 **HELPERR mnemonic**

Help. Call for help.

Evaluate for episiotomy (if necessary)

Legs. Place patient in McRobert's position

Pressure. Apply suprapubic pressure.

Enter maneuvers. Perform the rotational maneuvers as described above.

Remove the posterior arm.

Roll the patient onto all fours (Gaskin maneuver) [27].

Source: From Stitely ML, Gherman RB. Shoulder dystocia: Management and documentation. *Seminars in Perinatology.* 2014;38:194–200.

Box 10.3 Documenting shoulder dystocia

Date
Patient Name/Date of Birth/MRN

Delivering provider:
Timing:
Time shoulder Dystocia was recognized and additional staff called:
Timing of the delivery of the head: fetal head was delivered at ____AM/PM
Timing of the delivery of the posterior shoulder: fetal shoulder was delivered at ____AM/PM.
Head to body interval (seconds): _____

Antepartum documentation:
Assessment of the pelvis for a trial of labor
Estimated fetal weight
Presence of diabetes and degree of control (if present)

Intrapartum documentation:
Mode of delivery of the fetal vertex:
Spontaneous
Operative delivery (Vacuum or Forceps) and indication:
(If it is an operative vaginal delivery, create an additional or supplemental operative note detailing the forceps or vacuum procedure)
Anterior shoulder: Right or Left
Traction on the vertex: None or Standard
Position of the fetal head: ROA, LOA, direct OA, LOP, ROT, direct OP, OT

Upon recognition of a shoulder dystocia, additional staff including Pediatrics and Anesthesia were notified. The patient
was asked to discontinue pushing after delivery of the fetal head.
The McRobert's technique was initiated at ____ AM/PM.
Midline suprapubic pressure was performed by _________ at ______ AM/PM.
The following additional maneuvers were utilized:
Episiotomy _______ (type) at ____ AM/PM
Woods screw maneuver at _____ AM/PM
Attempt at delivery of the posterior arm at ____ AM/PM
Gaskin maneuver at ____ AM/PM
Delivery of the posterior shoulder at ____ AM/PM
Zavanelli at ____ AM/PM

At no time was fundal pressure applied.
At no time was excessive traction on the fetal head applied.
Note which maneuver resulted in delivery of the infant.

Placental delivery: intact/spontaneous/manually extracted

The mother appeared ________________ immediately postpartum.

Condition of the infant at birth:
Birth weight:
Apgar scores:
Neonate moving both arms after delivery: yes or no
Evidence of fetal injury:
Clavicular fracture: yes or no
Humeral fracture: yes or no
Concern for brachia plexus injury: yes or no
Cord Gases sent: yes or no
Cord Gases results:

The following individuals were present at the delivery:
Provider Type and Name:
Nursing Staff:
Anesthesia:
Pediatrics:
Nurse:

Document risk factors for shoulder dystocia
Document any labor abnormality:

Communicate with patient and family about the event as well as recurrence risks
Communicate with Pediatrics if concern for injury or asphyxia exists

effective method of optimizing neonatal outcomes given the unpredictable nature of shoulder dystocia. A video of a simulated shoulder dystocia can be seen at www.youtube.com/watch?v=6s6DwEKc7DA

Concluding Remarks

Shoulder dystocia is an obstetric emergency that requires prompt recognition and management to prevent severe maternal and neonatal consequences. While risk factors for shoulder dystocia are well known, efforts to predict its occurrence have been unsuccessful. Knowledge of the maneuvers to relieve impaction of the fetal shoulders is important. Simulation may help responders to the shoulder dystocia perform the maneuvers correctly and possibly improve outcomes.

References

1. American College of Obstetricians and Gynecologists. Shoulder Dystocia. ACOG Practice Bulletin Number 40. *Obstet Gynecol.* 2002; 100: 1045–50.
2. Spong CY, Beall M, Rodrigues D, et al. An objective definition of shoulder dystocia: Prolonged head-to-body delivery intervals and/or the use of ancillary obstetric maneuvers. *Obstet Gynecol.* 1995; 86: 433–6.
3. Gherman RB, Goodwin TM, Souter I, Neumann K, et al. The McRoberts' maneuver for the alleviation of shoulder dystocia: How successful is it? *Am J Obstet Gynecol.* 1997; 176: 656–61.
4. McFarland MB, Langer O, Piper JM, et al. Perinatal outcome and the type and number of maneuvers in shoulder dystocia. *Int J Gynaecol Obstet.* 1996; 55: 219–24.
5. O'Leary JA. Cephalic replacement for shoulder dystocia: Prevent status and future role of Zavanelli maneuver. *Obstet Gynecol.* 1993; 82: 847–50.
6. Goodwin TM, Banks E, Millar LK, et al. Catastrophic shoulder dystocia and emergency symphysiotomy. *Am J Obstet Gynecol.* 1997; 177 (2): 263–4.
7. Salvatore P, D'Emidio L, Cignini P, et al. Shoulder dystocia: An evidence-based approach. *J Prenat Med.* 2010; 4(3): 35–42.
8. Gurewitsch ED, Allen RH. Reducing the risk of shoulder dystocia and associated brachial plexus injury. *Obstet Gynecol Clin N Am.* 2011;38: 247–69.
9. Roland E, Hill A. Neurological problems of the newborn. In Daroff RB, Jankovic J, Mazziotta JC and

Pomeroy SL (Eds.), *Bradley's Neurology in Clinical Practice*, 7th edition. 2016, pp. 1956–1972. Elsevier.

10. Menticoglou SM. A modified technique to deliver the posterior arm in severe shoulder dystocia. *Obstet Gynecol.* 2006; 108(3 Pt2): 755–7.
11. Hoffman MK, Bailit JL, Ware DW, et al. A comparison of obstetric maneuvers for the acute management of shoulder dystocia. *Obstet Gynecol.* 2011; 117(6): 1272–78.
12. Leung T, Stuart O, Sahota D, et al. Head-to-body interval and risk off fetal acidosis and hypoxic ischemic encephalopathy in shoulder dystocia: A retrospective review. *BJOG.* 2011; 118(4): 474–9.
13. MacKenzie IZ, Shah M, Lean K, et al. Management of shoulder dystocia trends in incidence and maternal and neonatal morbidity. *Obstet Gynecol.* 2007; 110(5): 1059–68.
14. Mehta SH, Sokol RJ. Shoulder dystocia: Risk factors, predictability and preventability. *Semin Perinatol.* 2014; 38: 189–193.
15. American College of Obstetricians and Gynecologists. *Fetal Macrosomia. ACOG Practice Bulletin 22.* Washington, DC; ACOG; 2000.
16. Stitely ML, Gherman RB. Shoulder dystocia: Management and documentation. *Seminars in Perinatology.* 2014; 38: 194–200.
17. Inglis SR, Feier N, Chetiyaar JB et al. Effects of shoulder dystocia training on the incidence of brachial plexus injury. *Am J Obstet Gynecol.* 2011; 204(4):322 e1–e6.
18. Kung J, Swan AV, Arulkumaran S. Delivery of the posterior arm reduces shoulder dystocia dimensions in shoulder dystocia. *Int J Gynecol Obstet.* 2006; 93:233–37.
19. Bruner JP, Drummond SB, Meenan AL, Gaskin IM. All-fours maneuver for reducing shoulder dystocia during labor. *J Reprod Med.* 1998; 43(5):439.
20. Cluver CA, Hofmeyr GJ. Posterior axial sling traction for intractable shoulder dystocia. *BJOG.* 2009;116(13):1818–20.
21. O'Leary JA, Cuva A. Abdominal Rescue after Failed Cephalic Replacement. *Obstet Gynecol.* 1992; 80(3 Pt 2): 514–6.
22. Grobman, W. Shoulder dystocia: Simulation and a team-centered protocol. *Semin Perinatol.* 2014; 38: 205–209.
23. Grimm MJ, Costello RE, Gonik B. Effect of clinician-applied maneuvers on brachial plexus stretch during a shoulder dystocia event: Investigation using a computer simulation model. *Am J Obstet Gynecol.* 2010;203:339.e1–5.
24. Leung TY, Stuart O, Suen SS, et al. Comparison of perinatal outcomes of shoulder dystocia alleviated by different type and sequence of maneuvers: a retrospective review. *BJOG.* 2011; 118: 985–90.
25. Hansen A, Chauhan SP. Shoulder dystocia: Definitions and incidence. *Seminars in Perinatology.* 2014; 38: 184–8.
26. ACOG. Managing Shoulder Dystocia. Optimizing Protocols in Obstetrics. 2013.
27. Gurewitsch ED, Allen RH. Shoulder dystocia. *Clin Perinatol.* 2007; 34: 365–85.
28. Documenting Shoulder Dystocia. Patient Safety Checklist No. 6. American College of Obstetricians and Gynecologists. *Obstet Gynecol.* 2012; 120: 430–1
29. Gurewitsch ED, Johnson TL, Allen RH. After shoulder dystocia: Managing the subsequent pregnancy and delivery. *Semin Perinatol.* 2007; 31(3): 185–95.

Perineal Trauma after Vaginal Delivery: Third and Fourth Degree Lacerations and Hematomas

Anjali Martinez

Introduction

Obstetric perineal trauma is a significant cause of peripartum morbidity with potential significant long-term sequela. Third and fourth degree lacerations, also known as obstetric anal sphincter injury (OASIS), can lead to anal incontinence, pain, and loss of sexual function. Hematomas can lead to life-threatening blood loss. Appropriate identification and treatment of these complications is important to minimize long-term morbidity.

Scope of the Problem

Obstetric anal injury includes both third and fourth degree obstetric lacerations. The incidence of obstetric anal injury has been quoted to be anywhere from 1% to 19% by various sources. A large population based study of over two million deliveries in California estimates the incidence to be 5.8%.[1] Risk factors for obstetric anal injury include nulliparity, operative vaginal delivery, birth weight over 4 kg, prolonged second stage, and shoulder dystocia.

Identification

Identification of an anal sphincter injury is of utmost importance for the proper care and best outcome for the patient. First degree lacerations include the vaginal mucosa and skin over the perineum. Second degree lacerations also include the underlying muscles such as the perineal body and the transverse perineal muscles. A third degree laceration includes the layers of a second degree laceration plus the external anal sphincter but not the anal mucosa. A fourth degree laceration includes all of the above plus the anal mucosa. All patients should have a careful examination including a rectal examination after a vaginal delivery so that occult lacerations are not missed.

Repair

Repair is best done with optimal patient positioning, patient comfort through adequate analgesia, appropriate surgical equipment, and good lighting. Clinicians should therefore consider performing the repair in the operating room rather than the delivery room. If the patient does not already have epidural analgesia, spinal analgesia should be considered. Lithotomy with Allen stirrups or candy cane style stirrups helps with exposure. In addition to the standard instruments used to repair an obstetric laceration, a bulb irrigation syringe and Gelpi retractor are very useful. Allis clamps are often needed to identify and grasp the ends of the torn external anal sphincter. Box 11.1 shows a list of surgical instruments and supplies needed for the repair of third and fourth degree lacerations. Figure 11.1 is a photograph of a Gelpi retractor.

The parts of the anal injury that need to be repaired include the rectal mucosa, the internal anal sphincter, and the external anal sphincter. The rectal mucosa should be reapproximated with a small caliber (3-0 or 4-0) monofilament suture such as polydioxanone (PDS) or braided suture such as polyglactin (vicryl) in a running fashion. It has traditionally been taught that the suture material should not enter the anal canal because of the risk of fistula formation and should be in the submucosal layer. Some newer thoughts exist, however, that entry into the mucosa may not be harmful. Sutures should be close together (less than 0.5 cm apart) to maintain the integrity of the repair.[2] The internal anal sphincter is often overlooked, but is the main contributor toward resting anal tone and therefore continence. It often appears to be a thin, white layer and is sometimes mistaken to be "rectal fascia." The internal anal sphincter is classically repaired with interrupted sutures, but continuous suture may also be employed. 2-0 or 3-0 polyglactin is appropriate for this layer, and sutures should be placed close together

Box 11.1 **Surgical equipment for repair of third and fourth degree obstetric laceration**

Sutures
Needle driver
Smooth forceps
Suture scissors
Allis clamps
Gelpi clamp
Hemostats
Bulb irrigation syringe
Laparotomy sponges
Several pairs of sterile gloves

Box 11.2 **Repair external anal sphincter**

The ends of the external anal sphincter often retract laterally and may not be initially visible. An Allis clamp is very helpful to reach and grasp each of the retracted ends.

2-0 polyglactin or 3-0 polydioxanone suture is used in three or four interrupted sutures to reapproximate the external anal sphincter.

The external sphincter can be repaired in one of two techniques: end-to-end repair or overlapping repair.* See Figure 11.2 to see the difference between these two techniques.

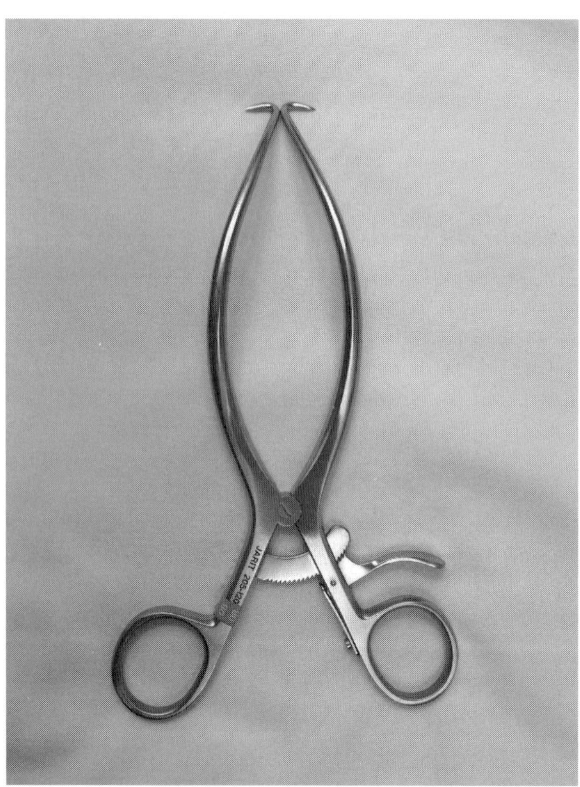

Figure 11.1 Gelpi retractor.

for this layer as well. Irrigation with a bulb irrigation syringe is invaluable during these steps as there is often blood from the rest of laceration obscuring the surgeon's view. If the overlying vaginal tissues obscure the view of the anal mucosa and sphincters, a Gelpi retractor can be very useful. Keeping an examining finger in the rectum during the repair helps delineate the layers and can monitor for inadvertent suture entry into the anal canal. The glove on the examining finger should be changed when moving on to other steps to minimize contamination.

The external anal sphincter can be repaired in one of two ways: an overlapping technique or an end-to-end technique. See Box 11.2 for details of this repair. Figure 11.2 is a schematic of external sphincter repair. A Cochrane review of six randomized trials comparing these two techniques looked at outcomes of anal incontinence (including incontinence of feces and flatus), perineal pain, dyspareunia, and quality of life. The main finding was that the overlapping repair is associated with less risk of fecal urgency and incontinence at 12 months postpartum, but there is no difference between the two techniques at 36 months postpartum. Since this difference at 12 months was based on two of the smaller trials only, the review's conclusion is that either technique is acceptable.[3]

End-to-End Repair

Four interrupted sutures are placed circumferentially around the sphincter end. The superior/cephalad ("3" in the figure) and posterior ("6") are placed first, and the inferior/caudal ("9") and anterior sutures ("12") are placed afterward since they are more proximal to the surgeon.

Overlapping Repair

This method requires 1–2 cm of overlap, so sometimes the inability to mobilize the separated sphincter ends dictates whether an overlapping repair is even feasible.

Three to four interrupted sutures are placed through the overlapping ends from side to side.

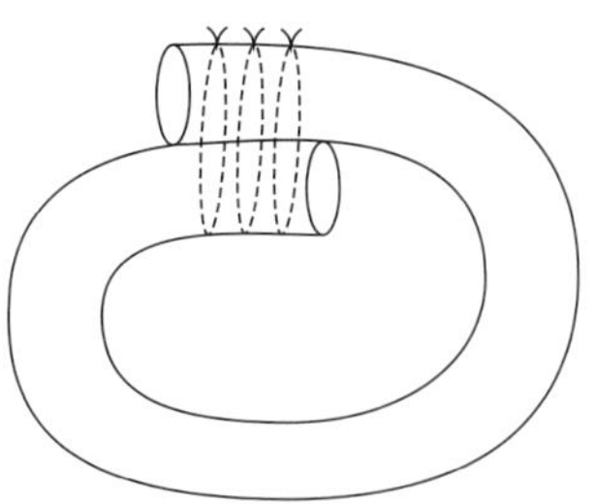

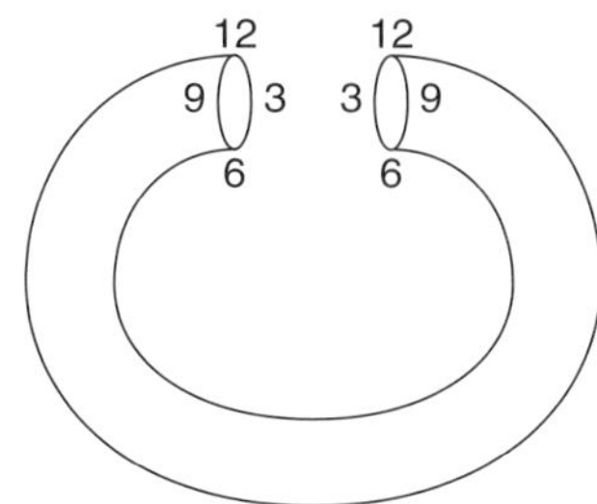

Figure 11.2 Two techniques to repair the external anal sphincter.

For either technique, it is important to incorporate the surrounding fascial sheath and not just the muscle itself to help with the strength of the repair.[2]

Tying one or more of these sutures can distort the tissue relationships and make it difficult to place the additional sutures correctly. As a result, each suture should be held with a clamp until all of the sutures have been placed, then they can be tied.

Although several retrospective studies exist regarding the use prophylactic antibiotics during repair of an obstetric anal sphincter injury, there was only one randomized, placebo-controlled prospective trial that looked at prophylactic antibiotics during repair of an obstetric anal sphincter injury.[4] This trial is the only study that is included in a Cochrane review on the topic. The study showed fewer wound complications (including infection and wound dehiscence) at two weeks postpartum in the group that received antibiotics. The Cochrane review of the study stressed the limitations of a small sample size and large loss to follow-up and does not feel that the evidence is strong enough to recommend for or against prophylactic antibiotics for third and fourth degree laceration repair.[5] Although the data does not unequivocally show an advantage, many providers use that randomized trial as support for using a second generation cephalosporin such as cefotetan or cefoxitin.

The remaining portions of the laceration are repaired as a standard second degree laceration. Some evidence supports particular suturing techniques and suture selection. A meta-analysis of 16 randomized trials looked at if continuous versus interrupted suture technique after repair of second degree lacerations and episiotomies. Effects on postpartum perineal pain and superficial dyspareunia were studied. Continuous suturing caused less short term pain (in the first ten postpartum days). As a secondary factor, this technique offered the economical benefit of requiring less suture.[6] A meta-analysis of 18 studies including data for women with episiotomies and second degree obstetric lacerations looked at short- and long-term pain, superficial dyspareunia, removal of suture material, and wound dehiscence in relation to suture selection. Compared to catgut, meta-analysis shows that synthetic absorbable suture (polyglactin and polyglycolic acid) is associated with less short-term pain (pain in the first 10 postpartum days) and less wound dehiscence but required more suture removal. Rapidly absorbable versus standard synthetic suture was comparable in terms of short-term pain, but the rapidly absorbable version required less suture removal. Long-term pain and dyspareunia were not significantly different among these suture materials.[7]

A video of a perineal laceration repair can be seen at www.youtube.com/watch?v=qARz_we0nSo

Box 11.3 is a summary of which suture material to use during repair of each of the layers of the anal sphincter injury.

Postpartum Care of Third and Fourth Degree Lacerations

Traditional recommendations regarding postpartum care of a repaired obstetric anal sphincter injury are based on expert opinion. Women are encouraged to eat a low fiber and low residue diet for about two weeks. Ample hydration with water and taking a stool softener can also help prevent constipation. Sitz baths are recommended to help with the healing process and can also help with comfort. Of note is the fact that no studies address many of these recommendations.

Complications

Obstetric anal sphincter injury can result in wound complications such as infection or wound breakdown, pain, long-term incontinence of flatus and/or feces, and loss of sexual function. Anal sphincter

Box 11.3 Suture selection for obstetric anal sphincter repair

Layer	Suture
Rectal mucosa	4-0 or 3-0 polyglactin or 4-0 polydioxanone
Internal anal sphincter	3-0 or 2-0 polyglactin or 3-0 polydioxanone
External anal sphincter	2-0 polyglactin or 3-0 polydioxanone

injury increases the risk of early postpartum wound complications. Affected women should have early and frequent follow-up care (within one to two weeks postpartum) to minimize the effect of complications. In a prospective cohort study, the incidence of wound infection was 19.8% and the risk of wound breakdown was 24.6% after obstetric anal sphincter injury.[8] Wound infection can lead to breakdown, but early infection can be treated with oral antibiotics. Infection can be identified based on erythema, edema, and possible purulent drainage. Affected women may have increased perineal pain and/or fever. Wound breakdown can be treated conservatively by debriding any necrotic tissue and keeping the area clean and dry or with early surgical repair if appropriate. Traditionally, wound dehiscence was treated conservatively for months before attempting repair but that method is upsetting to patients because of the fecal incontinence, embarrassment, and loss of sexual function. Early surgical repair may allow for earlier healing and earlier return to sexual activity. For early surgical repair, wound dehiscence is treated with antibiotics and daily debridement until healthy tissue is obtained for repair, ideally within one to two weeks. A Cochrane review looked at two randomized controlled trials and did not find a difference between conservative management and secondary suturing of perineal wounds that have dehisced.[9]

Third and fourth degree lacerations are the most significant risk factor for anal incontinence following delivery. Based on a cohort study, women who have a vaginal delivery without anal sphincter involvement have similar fecal incontinence rates as women who have cesarean deliveries. Operative delivery is a risk for anal incontinence because it is a risk factor for anal injury; it is not an independent risk factor. Similarly, vaginal delivery without anal injury is not an independent risk factor for fecal incontinence.[10] Based on that same study, approximately 10% of women who had obstetric anal injury had anal incontinence 5–10 years later.

Women with pain and/or dyspareunia in the postpartum period should be evaluated for wound infection, breakdown, hematoma, or an abscess. However, some discomfort during healing is normal. Dyspareunia symptoms may be from vaginal atrophy that occurs with postpartum hormonal changes especially with lactation and a decrease in natural lubrication. This temporary atrophy can be treated with local estrogen and will resolve with time and cessation of lactation.

Uncertainty exists concerning advice to women who have had an obstetric anal injury regarding mode of delivery for future pregnancies. Some providers recommend Cesarean delivery to prevent repeat injury or to damage a successful repair; however, Cesarean delivery is associated with other risks. A prospective observational study showed that of 393 women who were continent after a delivery involving anal sphincter repair, only 5.1% of them had a repeat anal sphincter injury in a subsequent vaginal delivery.[11] Several retrospective studies show a risk of a repeat third or fourth degree laceration during a subsequent delivery to be between 2% and 7%.[12–14] There are no consensus guideline about the mode of delivery in a woman with a history of obstetric anal injury, so providers should use a personalized approach.

Pelvic Hematomas

Delivery may be complicated by vulvar, vaginal, or retroperitoneal hematomas. Trauma via operative delivery, rapid descent, and compound neonatal presentation are risk factors for hematoma formation. These occur from disruption of small arteries or veins underlying the soft tissues, even when the overlying tissue remains intact. Vulvar hematomas can be due to branches of the internal pudendal artery or inferior rectal artery, whereas vaginal hematomas are often from vaginal branches of the uterine artery. Retroperitoneal hematomas are often from a vessel originating from the hypogastric artery branches.[15] Although vulvar hematomas are often obvious, vaginal and retroperitoneal hematomas are frequently hidden from view. Women with vaginal hematomas may present with pain or pressure symptoms. Since the vaginal tissues are so distensible, considerable blood loss into the vaginal space may occur. Retroperitoneal hematomas, in particular, are difficult to diagnose because of vague symptoms and a lack of clear physical exam findings. However, retroperitoneal hematomas can lead to massive blood loss and therefore require a high degree of clinical suspicion in a woman who has signs of acute blood loss or hypovolemic shock but no apparent source of bleeding. CT Imaging may be helpful to diagnose a suspected retroperitoneal hematoma, but is only recommended if the patient is hemodynamically stable enough to allow the imaging study. Of note, a retroperitoneal hematoma can occur after either a vaginal or cesarean delivery.

When a hematoma is non-expanding, conservative management such as ice and analgesia with very close observation may be appropriate. The hematoma itself is likely tamponading any further bleeding. A foley catheter should be considered if the size and location of the hematoma or the patient's discomfort will hinder her ability to void.

Vulvar hematomas may require surgical drainage. A large incision is made in the overlying skin to evacuate the blood. If a source vessel is found, it should be ligated. However, bleeding vessels are difficult to isolate because of their small size. The cavity defect should be closed in layers including closing the overlying skin incision.[15]

Vaginal hematomas can also be managed conservatively as described above. Vaginal packing can be used to provide additional tamponade. If the hematoma is expanding, surgical management is required as described above for vulvar hematomas. However, the incision over the vaginal hematoma does not have to be repaired because the vagina can be packed.[15]

Retroperitoneal hematomas often need surgical treatment with evacuation of the clot and ligating the source vessel. Arterial embolization can be used if needed in conjunction with surgical management.

Concluding Remarks

Obstetric anal sphincter injury and hematomas are complications of delivery and providers need to know how to identify and manage them because of the potential for significant morbidity. Of the main risk factors, operative delivery is the main modifiable factor. Appropriate immediate and long-term management can minimize the risk of long-term complications.

References

1. Handa V, Danielsen B, Gilbert W. Obstetric anal sphincter lacerations. *Obstet Gynecol* 2001;98:225–230.
2. Hale R, Ling F. Episiotomy: Procedure and repair techniques. *Am College Obstet Gynecology* 2007. www.scribd.com/doc/285746166/Episiotomy-ACOG (accessed May 15, 2017).
3. Fernando RJ, Sultan AH, Kettle C, Thakar R. Methods of repair for obstetric anal sphincter injury. *Cochrane Database Syst Rev* 2013 Dec 8;12:CD002866.
4. Duggal N, Mercado C, Daniels K, Bujor A, Caughey AB, El-Sayed YY. Antibiotic prophylaxis for prevention of postpartum perineal wound complications: A randomized controlled trial. *Obstet Gynecol* 2008 Jun;111(6):1268–1273.
5. Buppasiri P, Lumbiganon P, Thinkhamrop J, Thinkhamrop B. Antibiotic prophylaxis for third- and fourth-degree perineal tear during vaginal birth. *Cochrane Database Syst Rev* 2014 Oct 7;10:CD005125.
6. Kettle C, Dowswell T, Ismail KM. Continuous and interrupted suturing techniques for repair of episiotomy or second-degree tears. *Cochrane Database Syst Rev* 2012 Nov 14;11:CD000947.
7. Kettle C, Dowswell T, Ismail KM. Absorbable suture materials for primary repair of episiotomy and second degree tears. *Cochrane Database Syst Rev* 2010 Jun 16;(6):CD000006. doi(6):CD000006.
8. Lewicky-Gaupp C, Leader-Cramer A, Johnson LL, Kenton K, Gossett DR. Wound complications after obstetric anal sphincter injuries. *Obstet Gynecol* 2015 May;125(5):1088–1093.
9. Dudley LM, Kettle C, Ismail KM. Secondary suturing compared to non-suturing for broken down perineal wounds following childbirth. *Cochrane Database Syst Rev* 2013 Sep 25;9:CD008977.
10. Evers EC, Blomquist JL, McDermott KC, Handa VL. Obstetrical anal sphincter laceration and anal incontinence 5–10 years after childbirth. *Obstet Gynecol* 2012 11; 207(5):425.e1–425.e6.
11. Fitzpatrick M, Cassidy M, Barassaud ML, Hehir MP, Hanly AM, O'Connell PR, et al. Does anal sphincter injury preclude subsequent vaginal delivery? *Eur J Obstet Gynecol Reprod Biol* 2016 Mar;198:30–34.
12. Boggs EW, Berger H, Urquia M, McDermott CD. Recurrence of obstetric third-degree and fourth-degree anal sphincter injuries. *Obstet Gynecol* 2014 Dec;124(6):1128–1134.

13. Edozien LC, Gurol-Urganci I, Cromwell DA, Adams EJ, Richmond DH, Mahmood TA, et al. Impact of third- and fourth-degree perineal tears at first birth on subsequent pregnancy outcomes: a cohort study. *BJOG* 2014 Dec;121(13):1695–1703.

14. Yogev Y, Hiersch L, Maresky L, Wasserberg N, Wiznitzer A, Melamed N. Third and fourth degree perineal tears – the risk of recurrence in subsequent pregnancy. *J Matern Fetal Neonatal Med* 2014 Jan;27(2):177–181.

15. Francois K, Foley M. Antepartum and postpartum hemorrhage. In: Gabbe S, editor. *Obstetrics: Normal and Problem Pregnancies*. Sixth ed. Chapter 19. Elsevier. 2012. pp. 415−444.

Obstetric Anesthesia

Jeremy P. Campbell and Felicity Plaat

Introduction

This chapter describes the provision of analgesia and anesthesia in obstetric practice. It includes options for non-regional analgesia (pharmacological and non-pharmacological methods) as well as regional analgesia techniques. Anesthesia for obstetric procedures (both regional and general), including the significant complications of these techniques, is described. The importance of informed consent in obstetric anesthesia is discussed.

Scope of the Problem

The safety of obstetric anesthetic techniques has improved over the last thirty years. This is predominantly a consequence of the large increase in the proportion of caesarean sections and other operative procedures during the peripartum period performed under regional rather than general anesthesia. Nevertheless, both regional and general anesthesia are associated with certain risks, which must be discussed with the mother. See Box 12.1 for risks of regional anesthesia and Box 12.2 for risks of general anesthesia. These risks will be and discussed in more detail later in the chapter.

Analgesia for Labor

Labor may well be the most painful experience a woman encounters. The experience is different for each woman and cultural factors, peer group pressures, and personal expectations all influence attitudes toward pain relief in labor. It is essential that women are provided with information and support when considering options for analgesia, and that analgesia be tailored to the individual parturient.

Non-pharmacological Analgesia in Labor

Many non-pharmacological techniques for pain relief in labor have been used over the centuries, including both psychological and physical methods. Unfortunately, there is minimal evidence for the efficacy of any of these methods. Nevertheless, non-pharmacological methods are used by many women in labor and the anesthesiologist must be able to provide unbiased information on all forms of analgesia, including their limitations. Commonly used non-pharmacological techniques include the following.

Transcutaneous Electrical Nerve Stimulation (TENS)

This technique is based on modification of the pain pathway via the "gate theory" of pain transmission. Two pairs of electrodes, placed on either side of the spine, generate electrical impulses that prevent pain signals ascending the spinal cord. The device allows the mother to adjust the level of stimulation, and this enables a degree of self-control, which may increase patient satisfaction. TENS works best for mild pain and it is therefore most useful in early labor when it is often used at home prior to admission to the maternity unit.[1]

Other Techniques

Techniques such as hypnosis and acupuncture require antenatal preparation and a significant investment in terms of time and resources, and evidence for their efficacy is limited. Emotional support, on the other hand, does seem reliably to reduce analgesic requirements during labor, especially when it is provided by trained assistants or doulas.

In the United Kingdom, there is great enthusiasm for immersion (hydrotherapy or water births), with most maternity units having at least one pool. Warm water does seem to reduce the pain of contractions, but cases of fresh water drowning when delivery was managed in water have been reported.

Pharmacological Analgesia in Labor

Inhalational Analgesia (Entonox)

Entonox is a mixture of 50% nitrous oxide in oxygen and is widely used as an analgesic in labor. The

Box 12.1 Risks of regional analgesia/anesthesia

- Hypotension
- Unilateral or partial blockade
- Accidental dural puncture (complicates 0.5–2% of epidurals)
- Total spinal
- Local anesthetic toxicity
- Neurological damage (1 in 80,000 to 1 in 320,000 risk of permanent damage)
- Association with instrumental vaginal delivery

Box 12.2 Risks of general anesthesia

- Failed intubation (1 in 390)
- Aspiration of gastric contents
- Accidental awareness (1 in 670 for cesarean section)
- Increased blood loss
- Increased postoperative pain

woman self-administers the Entonox by producing a small negative pressure via a facemask or mouthpiece attached to the gas source. Entonox needs to be inhaled for about 50 seconds (approximately 10 breaths) before the maximum analgesic effect is produced and therefore the woman should start deep inhalation as soon as the onset of the contraction is felt, and then slow, deep breathing should continue throughout the contraction. Entonox may cause nausea, light-headedness, and drowsiness. Because nitrous oxide inhibits methionine synthase activity, it could theoretically cause bone marrow suppression. Although nitrous oxide is not a potent labor analgesic, studies have suggested that it provides adequate analgesia for many women.[2]

Opioids: Meperidine

Meperidine is the most commonly used opioid used in labor, usually given intramuscularly at a dose of 50–100 mg. It produces predominately sedative and anxiolytic rather than analgesic effects[3] that become apparent after 10–15 minutes and last for around 3 hours. Up to three quarters of parturients require additional analgesia. Meperidine causes nausea and vomiting and can also cause maternal drowsiness and amnesia. It readily crosses the placenta and may cause neonatal respiratory depression if delivery occurs within 1–2 hours of administration, and its use has also been associated with subsequent neonatal behavioral and feeding problems.

Opioids: Patient-Controlled Analgesia

Opioids may be administered intravenously to the parturient via a patient-controlled analgesia (PCA) device, and this provides a useful alternative if regional analgesia is contraindicated or not wanted. Fentanyl and, more recently, remifentanil have been used in PCA regimens for labor analgesia. Remifentanil is particularly suited for use via a PCA because it has a rapid onset of peak effect and a short duration of action. This allows for rapid analgesia during contractions with quick recovery in between contractions and after delivery.[4] The mother requires supplemental oxygen and continuous monitoring of her oxygen saturation during labor and delivery. Because of its rapid metabolism, fetal exposure is low, although there have been case reports of respiratory depression in the mother.

Regional Analgesia

Regional analgesia is without doubt the most effective form of pain relief in labor. This may be provided in two ways: by epidural administration of a mixture of local anesthetic and opioid, or by a combined spinal-epidural (CSE) in which an initial spinal (also called "subarachnoid" or "intrathecal") injection of local anesthetic and opioid is followed by epidural top-ups.

The use of regional analgesia has contributed enormously to improving the safety of maternity care and has greatly facilitated obstetric interventions such as instrumental delivery and cesarean section.

Physiology of Labor Pain

The pain felt during labor and delivery is transmitted via two separate pathways:

First Stage of Labor

The pain of uterine contractions and cervical dilatation is transmitted via visceral afferent fibers through the uterine, cervical and hypogastric plexi to the sympathetic chain, which lies parallel to and either side of the vertebral bodies. From here, the pain fibers enter the white rami communicates to the posterior nerve roots of T11, T12, and L1. Because early labor pain is referred to T11–T12 dermatomes, the pain is felt in the lower abdomen and back. As labor progresses and uterine contractions become more intense, the pain becomes more severe and spreads to the T10 and L1 dermatomes as well.

Second Stage of Labor

The descent of the presenting part into the birth canal causes stretching of the pelvic floor, perineum, and vagina. This produces a second source of pain, which is transmitted by the pudendal nerves and the perineal branches of the posterior cutaneous nerve of the thigh to the S2–S4 nerve roots.

An epidural or CSE placed in the mid to lower lumbar region is therefore ideal to produce a sensory block extending from T10 to S4; this can provide complete analgesia throughout labor and delivery. An added advantage is the ability to extend the block to provide anesthesia for emergency instrumental or operative delivery. Box 12.3 describes indications for regional analgesia and Box 12.4 describes contraindications.

Consent for Regional Anesthesia in Labor

It is essential to seek informed consent from the parturient prior to establishing regional analgesia in labor. Since it is inappropriate to burden women with excessive information when they are in established labor, patients should be provided with antepartum information about epidural analgesia, preferably in the antenatal clinic. Up to half of primigravidas, however, who end up with an epidural did not want one antenatally. It is therefore essential that the anesthesiologist also provide the patient with information at the time of the procedure. The authors' practice is to warn patients of the risk of headache, low blood pressure, partial or complete failure of the block, nerve damage as well as the association with the need for instrumental delivery. The mother is given the opportunity to ask questions and the discussion is documented.[6]

Epidural Insertion

It is mandatory to have large-bore intravenous access prior to establishing regional analgesia for labor. Continuous fetal monitoring should be used throughout insertion of the regional block.

The mother may be positioned in either the sitting or lateral position. Strict aseptic precautions should be used including the use of a hat, mask, sterile gown, gloves, and drape. The skin of the lumbar region should be prepared with a single application of 0.5% chlorhexidine and alcohol and allowed to air dry. The spine is palpated to identify a space at or below Tuffier's line (a horizontal line between the iliac crests that corresponds to the L3/4 intervertebral space). The skin is infiltrated with local anesthetic (usually lidocaine 1–2%). The epidural (Tuohy) needle is advanced into the epidural space using a "loss of resistance" technique with a syringe containing

Box 12.3 Indications for regional analgesia

1. Maternal request
   This is the most common indication for regional analgesia. It should be considered based on the severity of the woman's pain, not cervical dilatation.
2. Maternal cardiovascular and respiratory disease
   Regional analgesia reduces the cardiovascular stress associated with painful uterine contractions, and can facilitate a planned instrumental delivery in order to avoid straining and pushing during the second stage of labor.
3. Obstetric indications
   (i) Pre-eclampsia is the most common obstetric indication for regional analgesia. Effective analgesia helps reduce blood pressure and can also improve renal and placental blood flow.
   (ii) Multiple pregnancy. Epidural analgesia is associated with improved acid–base status of the second twin and facilitates operative delivery if needed.
4. Anesthetic indications
   (i) Obesity
   Early establishment of regional analgesia in the obese parturient can be extended to provide anesthesia should an emergency cesarean section or other operative procedure be required. This may avoid the need for a potentially hazardous general anesthetic.
   (ii) Predicted difficult airway
   Provision of regional analgesia diminishes the need for general anesthesia (and therefore the risk of failed tracheal intubation) should an operative procedure be required.

Box 12.4 Contraindications for regional anesthesia

- Maternal refusal
- Allergy to local anesthetic or opioid drugs
- Lack of resuscitation equipment and trained staff to care for the woman
- Inability to gain large-bore (16G) intravenous access
- Local infection at site of epidural/CSE insertion
- Major coagulopathy or anticoagulation (see later)
- Cardiovascular instability
- Raised intracranial pressure (intrathecal injection or accidental dural puncture with an epidural needle may cause coning)

Special Circumstances

1. Anticoagulants
   (i) Aspirin
   Aspirin therapy is not a contraindication to regional blockade.
   (ii) Low-molecular-weight heparin (LMWH), e.g., enoxaparin, dalteparin
   Following a prophylactic dose of LMWH, a spinal or epidural should not be sited, or an epidural catheter removed, for 12 hours. If a treatment dose of LMWH has been given, it is advised to wait a minimum of 24 hours before siting a regional block or removing a catheter. If LMWH is to be given after administration of a spinal or epidural, the authors recommend waiting a minimum of 4 hours.[5]
2. Thrombocytopenia
   Regional analgesia/anesthesia may be performed in patients with a platelet count above 80×10^9/L. If a patent has thrombocytopenia secondary to pre-eclampsia, the platelet count can fall rapidly. In this situation, it is essential to have a recent (within 6 hours) platelet count before citing a spinal or epidural.
3. Infection
   If a woman is systemically septic, epidural analgesia can exacerbate hypotension due to peripheral vasodilatation, as well as risk introduction of microorganisms into the neuraxial space. Each case needs to be assessed on an individual basis, but in general we avoid regional analgesia/anesthesia in patients who are overtly septic with hypotension. If a patient is pyrexial but has no other signs of infection, we ensure antibiotics are given prior to placing an epidural, and we avoid performing a spinal injection if possible.

saline (as opposed to air, which is associated with a higher incidence of misplacements and complications). Once the epidural space is located, a multi-orifice catheter is passed via the needle into the space and adjusted so that 3–5 cm of catheter is in the space when the needle has been removed. Accidental intravenous or intrathecal placement is excluded by negative aspiration (of blood or cerebrospinal fluid, respectively). The epidural catheter is then secured to the back with a dressing.

Initiation of Epidural Analgesia

A mixture of local anesthetic and opioid is commonly used for regional analgesia in labor. Previously, concentrations of bupivacaine of 0.25–0.5% were used, which provided effective analgesia but left the mother unable to move her legs, feel her contractions, or push effectively. The concentration of local anesthetic used in epidural analgesia regimens has gradually been reduced over the years and today a mixture of 0.1% bupivacaine with 2 mcg/ml fentanyl is widely used. This "low-dose" epidural solution allows a sensory blockade to be established without a significant motor block or hypotension.

The authors recommend administering an initial "test dose" of 10 mL of low-dose mixture, observing the patient for symptoms and signs of accidental intrathecal or intravenous injection. Thereafter, the maintenance dose and method of administration depends on local policy. Many units use intermittent epidural top-ups, but increasingly patient-controlled epidural analgesia (PCEA) regimens are being used in an effort to avoid the risk of accidental intravenous injection of a syringe of low-dose mixture and to reduce staff workload.

After initiation of epidural analgesia, pulse and blood pressure should be checked every 5 minutes for 20 minutes, and thereafter every 30 minutes. Care must be taken to avoid aortocaval compression. It is acceptable for a mother to walk after the epidural has been inserted provided she has adequate motor power, but a companion should be with her at all times.

In the past, initiation of regional analgesia often resulted in maternal hypotension due to sympathetic blockade and therefore standard practice was to administer 500–1,000 ml of intravenous fluid as a preload. With low-dose epidural regimens, hypotension is much less of a problem and fluid preloading is no longer mandatory, although individual maternity units will have their own local policies.

Side Effects and Complications of Regional Analgesia

Hypotension

Administration of local anesthetic into the neuraxial space will result in blockade of nerve conduction in sympathetic fibers, causing vasodilatation. This will cause hypotension due to reduced systemic vascular resistance and venous pooling, which will reduce venous return, cardiac output, and blood pressure. Any degree of aortocaval compression occurring at the same time will further diminish the mother's cardiac output and blood pressure. It is thus essential to avoid reduced cardiac output since the uteroplacental unit does not autoregulate and therefore placental perfusion is proportional to the maternal blood pressure. If hypotension occurs, the mother should be placed in the full lateral position and given high-flow oxygen. A 500 ml bolus of fluid should be administered and, if there is no response to this, ephedrine 3–6 mg and/or phenylephrine 100 mcg boluses should be given intravenously. They may be repeated if necessary. The incidence of hypotension is much lower with today's low-dose epidural mixtures compared with the higher concentrations used in the past.

Unilateral or Partial Blockade

About 80% of epidurals work effectively throughout labor. For those that do not, it is important to review the epidural and identify the problem. An extra top-up to extend a low sensory block may be all that is required. Inadequate analgesia is frequently due to a unilateral block, which may be demonstrated by an unequal sympathetic block in the lower limbs (feet of different temperature). In this situation, the epidural catheter may be withdrawn, leaving 2–3 cm in the epidural space and a top-up administered with the patient lying on the unblocked side. If this fails to achieve adequate analgesia, it is importance to accept early that the catheter is misplaced and to re-site the epidural.

Accidental Dural Puncture

Accidental dural puncture with an epidural needle occurs in approximately 0.5–2% of epidurals. This causes a leak of CSF, which results in a low-pressure post-dural puncture headache (PDPH). Approximately 70% of women who have an accidental dural puncture with a 16–18G epidural needle will develop a PDPH, which usually begins on the first postnatal day and can be very debilitating to a mother caring for a baby. It is classically a frontal and occipital headache, which is postural (worse on sitting or standing and eased by lying down) and is often accompanied by photophobia and neck stiffness. Long-term sequelae include cranial nerve palsies and subdural hematomata.[7]

It is essential that any woman who suffers a dural puncture with an epidural needle is informed about the risk of developing a headache, and she should be actively followed up by an anesthesiologist for several days to assess for headache. Treatment may be conservative, in which the patient is kept well hydrated and given adequate analgesia. However, for those with severe symptoms and a clear diagnosis, an epidural blood patch is needed. This is an injection of up to 20 mL of the patient's own blood into the epidural space and this provides rapid, permanent relief of headache in about 65% of patients; up to one-third will require a second blood patch. Caffeine, sumatriptan, and ACTH have also been used as treatments but are not as effective as a blood patch.[8]

Total Spinal

This occurs when a dose of local anesthetic intended for epidural administration is accidentally given intrathecally due to unrecognized placement of an "epidural" catheter in the subarachnoid space. There is rapid ascent of a sensory, motor, and sympathetic block, resulting in profound hypotension, bradycardia, and, if the mixture reaches the brainstem, apnea, and unconsciousness. Treatment is supportive with intravenous fluids, vasopressors (e.g. phenylephrine), anticholinergics (e.g. atropine) and, if necessary, tracheal intubation and ventilation. There should be a low threshold for emergency delivery of the fetus by cesarean section.

Accidental Intravenous Injection

This occurs as a result of the accidental placement of the epidural catheter in an epidural vein and may result in local anesthetic toxicity. This is a particular concern with epidural mixtures containing bupivacaine, which, when injected intravenously, can cause ventricular arrhythmias that are very resistant to treatment. Symptoms of local anesthetic toxicity include peri-oral tingling and numbness, tinnitus, dizziness, agitation, and confusion progressing to convulsions, unconsciousness, and cardiovascular collapse. Management of these conditions involves stopping administration of the epidural mixture and providing supportive management of the airway, breathing, and circulation. This includes turning the patient into the lateral position, seizure control using a benzodiazepine, and cardiopulmonary resuscitation if cardiac arrest has occurred. Intravenous lipid emulsion (e.g. Intralipid® 20%) can reverse the cardiac and neurological effects of local anesthetics and should be used without delay in patients with suspected local anesthetic toxicity.[9]

Neurological Damage

When neurological problems present in the postnatal period, there may be a tendency to implicate anesthetic interventions, but the majority of reported nerve damage is due to the mechanics of labor or fetal pressure on the nerves. Spinal cord damage should not occur since epidurals for labour analgesia are placed at a vertebral level below the termination of the spinal cord (L1/2). The incidence of permanent neurological damage following neuraxial techniques in obstetrics is very rare, estimated to be between 1 in 80,000 and 1 in 320,000.[10] Any patient with a neurological deficit that is thought to be related to an epidural or spinal needs an urgent magnetic resonance imaging (MRI) scan of the spine to exclude a vertebral canal hematoma or abscess. If present, the patient requires urgent referral to a neurosurgical center for decompression.

Effect on Obstetric Outcomes

Effective regional analgesia can prolong the second stage of labor and there is an association between regional analgesia and instrumental vaginal delivery. There is no evidence that regional analgesia increases the rate of cesarean delivery.[11]

Regional Anesthesia for Cesarean Section

Over the last 30 years, there has been a large increase in the proportion of cesarean sections performed under regional rather than general anesthesia. Regional anesthesia has several important benefits.

Safety

Regional anesthesia for emergency surgery in obstetrics carries a lower risk for the mother than general anesthesia, probably because the dangers of a difficult airway and the risk of aspiration are avoided. This advantage has not been demonstrated in the elective situation. The increasing use of regional anesthesia in obstetrics is likely to have contributed to the large fall in maternal deaths directly attributed to anesthesia over the last few decades.

Blood Loss

There appears to be less bleeding during cesarean section when performed under regional rather than general anesthesia. Regional anesthesia avoids administration of volatile anesthetic agents to the patient, which cause uterine relaxation and exacerbate uterine bleeding.

Postoperative Analgesia and Recovery

In general, the mother who has had a cesarean section under regional anesthesia recovers more quickly than if she has been given a general anesthetic. The ability to administer opioids by the intrathecal or epidural route improves pain relief post-operatively and the patient is more likely to be mobile the following day and also able to eat and drink and care for her baby immediately. Additionally, the ability to be awake during the cesarean section enables the mother to develop early bonding with her baby. This also allows her birthing partner to be present.

Contraindications

The contraindications to regional anesthesia for cesarean section are the same as those for any regional procedure (see Box 12.4).

Pre-operative Preparation

All women undergoing cesarean section under regional anesthesia should undergo a thorough pre-operative anesthetic assessment. This includes assessment of the airway and administration of antacid therapy since a small proportion of regional anesthetics will need to be converted to general anesthesia. Patients undergoing elective cesarean sections should have nothing by mouth (6 hours for food and 2 hours for clear fluids),[12] although all obstetric patients should be considered as being at risk of aspiration. Large-bore intravenous access must be obtained and continuous fetal monitoring should be used while the regional block is being established.

Choice of Technique

Three regional anesthetic techniques are available: spinal, epidural, and combined spinal-epidural anesthesia (CSE).

Spinal Anesthesia

This is popular because it is relatively easy and quick to perform and produces a block that is rapid in onset and reliable.

It is performed with the mother in the sitting or lateral position using the same strict aseptic precautions as for regional analgesia in labor. Following infiltration of the intervertebral space at or below Tuffier's line with local anesthetic, a 25 or 27G needle with a pencil point tip is inserted into the subarachnoid space. Spinal anesthesia should not be inserted above this point because of the risk of damage to the spinal cord. A mixture of 0.5% heavy bupivacaine with an opioid (fentanyl or morphine) is injected intrathecally. The addition of an opioid to the spinal mixture enhances the quality of postoperative analgesia. After the spinal injection has been administered, it is the authors' practice to keep the mother in the full lateral position to avoid aortocaval compression until the height of the block is adequate. The mother is then placed supine with 15° left lateral tilt until delivery of the baby.

Epidural Anesthesia

Epidurals that have been used for labour analgesia may be topped up to provide anesthesia should the mother require an emergency cesarean section or other operative procedure. Epidurals are also occasionally used to provide de novo anesthesia in mothers with certain medical conditions (e.g. pre-existing cardiac disease) because they enable a careful incremental block to be established, which may maintain greater cardiovascular stability than a single-shot spinal.

Various drug regimens may be used to top up an epidural to provide anesthesia for cesarean section. In one regimen, 0.5% bupivacaine is commonly used, although a mixture of 2% lidocaine with epinephrine and bicarbonate ("fast mix") will extend the block more quickly and may be useful in time-critical situations.[13] The volume of these solutions that is required to top up an existing labor epidural is variable and therefore the authors' practice is to give a volume up to 20 ml in divided doses, with serial assessments of the block.

Combined Spinal-Epidural Anesthesia

Combined spinal-epidural anesthesia (CSE) may be used if the duration of surgery is likely to be longer than the anesthetic time provided by a spinal anesthetic (e.g. repeat cesarean section) because the epidural can be used to prolong the block. The epidural may also be used to provide postoperative analgesia.

Fluid and Blood Pressure Management

Hypotension caused by sympathetic blockade with spinal anesthesia can be rapid and profound. For an epidural top-up, the block is slower in onset and hypotension tends to be less pronounced. A balanced crystalloid solution (e.g. Ringer's lactate) is normally administered to the mother during insertion of a spinal anesthetic or administration of an epidural top-up to mitigate against any hypotension. This solution (1 L) may be given to the healthy mother during establishment of the regional block and a further liter during the surgery. Nevertheless, fluid administration does not always eliminate hypotension and treatment with a vasopressor is usually required. Phenylephrine is a pure α-agonist and is the vasopressor of choice. It is the authors' preference to prevent hypotension by giving phenylephrine as a prophylactic infusion as soon as the spinal anesthetic is administered[14] and to measure blood pressure using a non-invasive cuff every minute until delivery of the baby. It should be noted that mothers are often aware of hypotension before it is identified on the monitor: dizziness, nausea, and vomiting are almost always due to hypotension and should be treated with fluids and phenylephrine.

Assessment of the Height of Block

It is essential to assess the height of a regional block before allowing surgery to start and to document this. Several methods can be used to test the level of block including the sensation of cold (using ice or ethyl chloride spray), pinprick sensation, and light touch. Absence of cold sensation has been the most popular method of testing the block but is probably less reliable than testing to light touch. A sensory block extending from T4 to S5 is required bilaterally for a cesarean section. Motor block should also be assessed: the mother should be unable to lift her legs when the block is adequate. In women without a pre-existing epidural, there should be the development of bilateral sympathetic block (as evidenced by warm, dry feet).

Intra-operative Care

Cesarean section carries a risk of endometritis and therefore the mother should receive a prophylactic broad-spectrum antibiotic, administered before surgical incision. Following delivery of the baby, a bolus of intravenous oxytocin is given to assist contraction of the uterus and limit uterine blood loss. Further uterotonics are administered at the request of the obstetrician.

During delivery of the fetus, pressure from the obstetrician on the upper abdomen can often cause the mother to feel uncomfortable; it is important that the anesthesiologist tells her to expect this beforehand. If the obstetrician wishes to exteriorize the uterus to facilitate uterine closure this can also cause some discomfort, although this settles once the uterus is replaced. However, any complaint of pain from the mother must be taken seriously and action taken promptly. If feasible, the surgeons should be asked to stop operating and the anesthesiologist must decide whether the pain can be managed by supplementing regional anesthesia or whether conversion to general anesthesia is required. If she has an epidural this can be topped up with 0.5% bupivacaine, 2% lidocaine and/or fentanyl 50 mcg. Entonox, intravenous opioids (e.g. alfentanil in 10 mcg boluses) and intravenous ketamine have all been used successfully. If these methods are unsuccessful the mother should be given a general anesthetic. Pain during cesarean section under regional anesthesia is the most common cause of successful medicolegal claims against obstetric anesthesiologists and therefore it is essential that its management is clearly documented.

Postoperative Analgesia

The regional anesthetic block will regress after several hours but if intrathecal morphine has been given, it will provide analgesia for up to 24 hours. Its use has been associated with delayed respiratory depression and the mother must therefore be nursed a setting that enables frequent monitoring.

Maternity units will have local protocols for postoperative analgesia. The authors' practice is to prescribe the medications listed in Box 12.5.

> **Box 12.5 Postoperative medications after regional anesthesia for caesarean section**
>
> 1. Regular acetaminophen
> 2. Non-steroidal anti-inflammatory drugs: diclofenac suppository at the end of surgery (with patient consent) followed by regular ibuprofen
> 3. Regular dihydrocodeine
> 4. Oral morphine as required
> 5. If an epidural catheter is in situ, intermittent boluses of low-dose mixture while the patient is in the delivery suite.

General Anesthesia for Cesarean Section

In the past, general anesthesia in obstetrics was an important cause of maternal mortality. This arose principally from hypoxemia as a result of difficulty with intubation of the trachea and/or aspiration of gastric contents. Current practice is therefore to avoid general anesthesia and use regional anesthesia if possible. Nevertheless, general anesthesia must be administered when there are contraindications to regional anesthesia or if there is insufficient time to administer a regional anesthetic.

The Maternal Airway

The incidence of failed tracheal intubation in obstetrics is 1 in 390,[15] nearly 10 times higher than that of the general population. The reasons for this include changes associated with pregnancy such as breast enlargement, weight gain, and pharyngeal wall edema. This may be exacerbated by poor positioning of the mother and overforceful application of cricoid pressure. In addition, general anesthesia in obstetrics is often carried out in stressful, time-critical situations by trainee anesthesiologists during out-of-hours periods with distant consultant supervision, and the anesthesiologist's anxiety may contribute to failure to intubate the trachea.

Aspiration of Gastric Contents

The risk of pulmonary aspiration of gastric contents is increased in obstetrics because of certain physiological changes of pregnancy listed in Box 12.6.

Antacid prophylaxis should be offered to all patients undergoing cesarean section. Various regimens are used but the authors' practice is to administer oral ranitidine and metoclopramide to all patients undergoing elective cesarean section as well as to all at-risk patients in labor. In addition, for women undergoing general anesthesia, 30 ml of 0.3 M sodium citrate is given orally immediately before the anesthetic is administered.

Box 12.6 Physiological changes of pregnancy associated with aspiration

1. Reduced lower esophageal sphincter tone (due to progesterone)
2. Increased intra-abdominal pressure (from the gravid uterus)
3. Increased gastric volumes and reduced gastric pH (due to placental gastrin production)
4. Delayed gastric emptying in labor (exacerbated by the use of opioids)

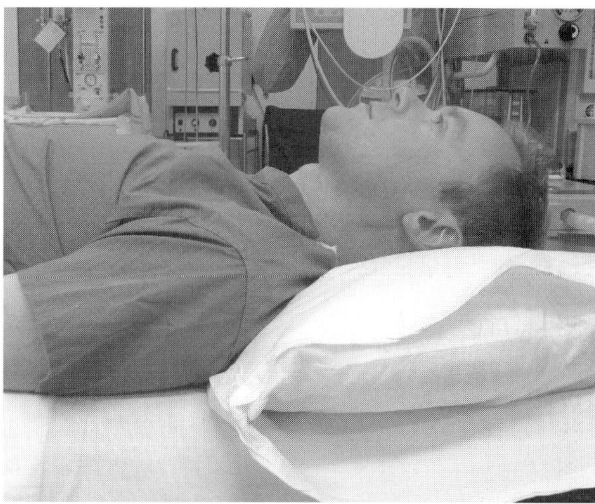

Figure 12.1 A patient in the supine position.

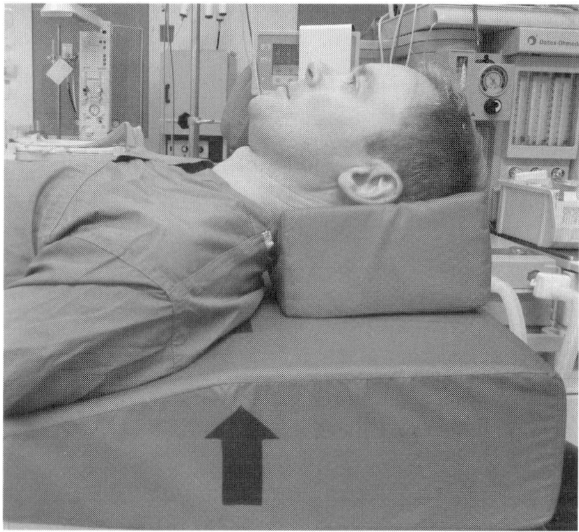

Figure 12.2 A patient in the head elevated (ramped) position – this position may make airway management including intubation easier. Photographs provided by the author.

Conduct of General Anesthesia

It is essential that the patient is in the optimal position prior to induction of general anesthesia. Airway management may be improved when the patient is in the head elevated (ramped) position (in which the external auditory meatus is in the same horizontal line as the suprasternal notch). The ramped position (see Figures 12.1 and 12.2) can be achieved with the use of pillows or specific devices (e.g. Oxford HELP System®). It should also be ensured that the mother is positioned with 15° left lateral tilt to minimize aortocaval compression.

Three minutes of pre-oxygenation should be given using a close-fitting face mask and oropharyngeal suction equipment should be immediately available. Anesthesia is induced with thiopentone or propofol and cricoid pressure applied by a trained assistant. Suxamethonium remains the muscle relaxant of choice for facilitating intubation because it has a rapid onset and offset of action. Once the trachea has been intubated and the correct position confirmed by clinical assessment and with capnography, cricoid pressure may be released. Anesthesia is maintained using a volatile agent (e.g., sevoflurane), often with nitrous oxide. Although volatile agents relax the uterus and may exacerbate uterine bleeding, it is important to use adequate concentrations and to maintain uterine tone using uterotonic agents. Following delivery of the fetus, the patient should be given adequate analgesia (including intravenous morphine) and antiemetics. At the end of the operation the anesthesiologist may administer a transversus abdominis plane (TAP) block to provide additional pain relief. The mother should be extubated when fully awake with intact laryngeal reflexes.

Mothers who have a cesarean section under general anesthesia suffer more pain in the postoperative period compared with those who have had a regional anesthetic. Patients usually require parenteral opioids, and these are often administered via a PCA device.

Problems during General Anesthesia

Failed Intubation

Failed intubation is the dread of the obstetric anesthesiologist. It is important to remember that failure to intubate the mother will not cause harm as long as oxygenation is maintained.

In the United Kingdom, guidelines for the management of difficult and failed tracheal intubation in obstetrics have recently been published.[16] These provide algorithms for the safe provision of general anesthesia in obstetrics, failed tracheal intubation, and the "can't intubate, can't oxygenate" situation. They also include criteria which the anesthesiologist should consider when deciding whether to wake a patient or proceed with surgery following failed tracheal intubation. Because general anesthetics are conducted relatively infrequently in obstetrics, it is essential that all obstetric anesthesiologists maintain their knowledge and skills by regularly practicing drills of these algorithms.

Accidental Awareness

Accidental awareness under general anesthesia (AAGA) is well known to be a particular problem in obstetrics. Concerns about harmful effects of anesthetics on the fetus (both directly, and by the effect on uteroplacental blood flow) have led anesthesiologists in the past to administer "light" anesthesia. A recent national audit in the United Kingdom found that the incidence of AAGA was 1 in 670 for cesarean section (compared to an overall incidence of approximately 1 in 19,000).[17] It is essential that the patient is given an adequate dose of induction agent and volatile agent, and use of a volatile agent monitoring device is mandatory. AAGA causes enormous stress to the mother and often requires a period of counselling.

Concluding Remarks

This chapter has described the provision of analgesia and anesthesia in obstetric practice, including options for non-regional analgesia (pharmacological and non-pharmacological methods) as well as regional analgesia techniques. It has also discussed both regional and general anesthesia for obstetric procedures, including the significant complications of these techniques. Obstetric anesthesia is a safe and reliable benefit to obstetric care for most patients.

References

1. Wee M. Non-regional analgesia 1: Non-pharmacological methods. In: Collis R, Plaat F, Urquhart J, eds. *Textbook of Obstetric Anaesthesia*. London: Greenwich Medical Media, 2002; 47–56.
2. Rosen MA. Nitrous oxide for relief of labor pain: a systematic review. *Am J Obstet Gynecol* 2002; 186: S110–26.
3. Tsui MH, Ngan Kee WD, Ng FF, Lau TK. A double blinded randomised placebo-controlled study of intramuscular pethidine for pain relief in the first stage of labour. *BJOG* 2004; 111: 648–55.
4. Schnabel A, Hahn N, Broscheit J, et al. Remifentanil for labour analgesia: a meta-analysis of randomised controlled trials. *Eur J Anaesthesiol* 2012; 29: 177–85.
5. Association of Anaesthetists of Great Britain and Ireland, Obstetric Anaesthetists' Association and Regional Anaesthesia UK. Regional anaesthesia and patients with abnormalities of coagulation. *Anaesthesia* 2013; 68: 966–72.
6. Campbell JP, Plaat F. Ethical and legal issues in anaesthetics. In: Hakim N, Papalois V, Epstein M, eds. *Ethical and Legal Issues in Modern Surgery*. London: Imperial College Press, 2015; 169–80.
7. MacArthur C, Lewis M, Knox EG. Accidental dural puncture in obstetric patients and long term symptoms. *Br Med J* 1993; 306: 883–5.
8. Fernando R, Price CM. Regional analgesia for labour. In: Collis R, Plaat F, Urquhart J, eds. *Textbook of Obstetric Anaesthesia*. London: Greenwich Medical Media, 2002; 71–97.
9. Neal JM, Mulroy MF, Weinberg GL. American Society of Regional Anesthesia and Pain Medicine checklist for managing local anesthetic systemic toxicity: 2012 version. *Reg Anesth Pain Med* 2012; 37: 16–18.
10. Cook TM, Counsell D, Wildsmith JAW. Major complications of central neuraxial block: Report on the Third National Audit of The Royal College of Anaesthetists. *Br J Anaesth* 2009; 102: 179–90.
11. Cambic CR, Wong CA. Labour analgesia and obstetric outcomes. *Br J Anaesth* 2010; 105 (suppl 1): i50–i60.
12. American Society of Anesthesiologists. Practice guidelines for preoperative fasting and the use of pharmacologic agents to reduce the risk of pulmonary aspiration: Application to healthy patients undergoing elective procedures – an updated report by the American Society of Anesthesiologists Committee on Standards and Practice Parameters. *Anesthesiology* 2011; 114: 495–511.
13. Allam J, Malhotra S, Hemingway C, Yentis SM. Epidural lidocaine-bicarbonate-adrenaline vs levobupivacaine for emergency caesarean section: A randomised controlled trial. *Anaesthesia* 2008; 63: 243–9.
14. Ngan Kee WD, Khaw KS, Ng FF. Prevention of hypotension during spinal anesthesia for cesarean delivery: An effective technique using combination

phenylephrine infusion and crystalloid cohydration. *Anesthesiology* 2005; 103: 744–50.

15. Kinsella SM, Winton AL, Mushambi MC, et al. Failed tracheal intubation during obstetric general anaesthesia: A literature review. *Int J Obstet Anesth* 2015; 24: 356–74.
16. Mushambi MC, Kinsella SM, Popat M, et al. Obstetric Anaesthetists' Association and Difficult Airway Society guidelines for the management of difficult and failed tracheal intubation in obstetrics. *Anaesthesia* 2015; 70: 1286–306.
17. Pandit JJ, Cook TM, the NAP Steering Panel. NAP5. *Accidental Awareness During General Anaesthesia*. London: The Royal College of Anaesthetists and Association of Anaesthetists of Great Britain and Ireland; 2014. ISBN 978-1-900936-11.

Intrapartum Fetal Monitoring

Georgia Ferrell

Introduction

Fetal heart sounds were first detected as early as the 1600s. The first device created for monitoring fetal heart rate was the fetal stethoscope or fetoscope, created in 1917 by David Hollis. Electric-amplified fetoscopes were used as early as the 1940s, and intermittent auscultation of the fetal heart rate was the standard of care well into the 1970s. It wasn't until the 1960s that Doppler technology was used to capture the continuous fetal electrocardiogram (ECG), also known as external fetal monitoring (EFM). It was the 1970s before the fetal scalp electrode (FSE) was introduced as a way to continuously monitor the fetal ECG.[1] In this chapter, intrapartum fetal monitoring will be introduced, and the data for continuous monitoring versus intermittent auscultation will be reviewed. The NICHD classification system will be introduced and defined, and management of intrapartum fetal heart rate tracings will be discussed.

Scope of the Problem

The goal of fetal heart rate monitoring is to identify acidemic or hypoxemic fetuses to ensure timely delivery and prevention of death. The secondary goal is to prevent neurologic injury.[2] The current recommendations of American Congress of Obstetrics and Gynecology (ACOG) and National Institutes of Health (NIH) are that low-risk patients be offered intermittent auscultation (IA) or continuous monitoring in labor. Both organizations recommend that continuous monitoring be performed in high-risk patients: specifically in suspected chorioamnionitis, sepsis, or temperature ≥38°C, severe hypertension (≥160/110 mmHg), oxytocin use, significant meconium, or new vaginal bleeding.[3] When EFM is compared to IA, there is no significant difference noted between low Apgar scores, newborn intensive care unit (NICU) admissions, development of cerebral palsy, or perinatal deaths.[4] The use of continuous EFM did reduce the number of fetal seizures, but these seizures were not associated with long-term neurologic consequences.[5] There is consistent evidence that EFM has a high false positive rate for predicting adverse outcomes; in fact, use of EFM has increased the cesarean section and operative vaginal delivery rate performed for abnormal fetal heart rate tracings. This data is consistent for low-risk and high-risk pregnancies.[4] One meta-analysis in 2013 showed a reduction in perinatal deaths attributed to hypoxia, and one perinatal death prevented per 1,000 births. This study also demonstrated a two- to three-fold increase in the rate of cesarean section.[2] Despite limited data to support improvement in outcomes, EFM continues to be the standard of practice today.

Fetal Monitoring Devices

External fetal monitoring is the most commonly used procedure in obstetrics.[6] It is performed using a Doppler device with computerized logic to interpret and count the Doppler signals. The Doppler captures the fetal cardiac atrial and ventricular contractions and creates a wave form from this data. The computer then uses the wave form to calculate the peak of the wave and determine the interval between fetal cardiac R waves (an R–R interval). Several R–R intervals are calculated and then averaged to reduce artifact. The paper recording speed is 3 cm/minute.

An alternative external form of fetal monitoring is called the Monica. This is a series of electrodes that are placed on the maternal abdomen to detect electrical fetal R–R interval. This device allows maternal ambulation while continuous monitoring is performed. It also has an electrode system that can monitor women with body mass index (BMI) up to 50 using their wireless system.[7]

Internal fetal monitoring is accomplished by using FSE. This bipolar spiral electrode is placed directly on the fetal scalp to monitor the fetal ECG. An additional electrode is placed on the maternal thigh to reduce interference from maternal cardiac activity.

Uterine Contraction Monitoring

External contraction monitoring is performed using tocodynamometry to determine the duration and frequency of maternal contractions. External tocodynamometry is noninvasive and it provides sufficient information for most labors.

Intrauterine pressure catheter (IUPC) can be inserted once fetal membranes are broken and as long as the cervix is dilated 1–2 cm, allowing insertion of the device. IUPCs are useful as they not only measure duration and frequency of contractions, but they also measure strength of contractions in Montevideo units. There is no evidence that using an IUPC improves maternal or fetal outcomes. A systematic review, including three studies and 1,945 women, showed no difference in outcome comparing external or internal monitoring in patients on oxytocin for induction or augmentation of labor.[8] An IUPC is also used for amnioinfusion. This is indicated when a fetal monitoring shows recurrent variable decelerations that do not resolve with maternal repositioning. There is limited evidence that amnioinfusion improved short- or long-term fetal outcomes, but it may reduce the cesarean section rate for "suspected fetal distress."[9] The IUPC is used to infuse sterile normal saline into the uterine cavity. Protocols for amnioinfusion vary from institution to institution. The fetal heart rate (FHR) should be monitored continuously to evaluate for resolution of variable decelerations.

Standardization of EFM Nomenclature

In 2008, after recognition that most women in the United States undergo continuous fetal monitoring, and in an effort to standardize nomenclature and make recommendations based on a universal interpretation system – the American Congress of Obstetricians and Gynecologists, the Eunice Kennedy Shriver National Institute of Child Health and Human Development, and the Society for Maternal-Fetal Medicine sponsored a workshop. This workshop was purposed to focus on updating EFM nomenclature, recommending an interpretative system, and setting research priorities.[10] The outcome from the workshop is the reaffirmation of terms, and the development of a three-tiered classification system for fetal heart rate tracings and management.

NICHD Definitions

Recommendations were made for description and quantification of uterine contractions. Normal uterine activity is defined as five or fewer contractions in 10 minutes, averaged over a 30-minute window. Tachysystole is defined as more than five contractions in 10 minutes averaged over 30 minutes. Tachysystole should be categorized by the presence or absence of FHR decelerations. The terms hyperstimulation and hypercontractility are no longer used.[10]

The NICHD defines variability, baseline, accelerations, and decelerations. These definitions aid in the evaluation of a FHT.

The variability of a fetal heart tracing is defined as absent, minimal, moderate, or marked. Absent variability is defined as no detectable variability, and it is of concern as it represents cerebral hypoxemia and acidosis, signifying failure of compensatory mechanisms to maintain oxygenation to the fetal brain. Minimal variability is defined as an amplitude of 0–5 bpm (Figure 13.1), moderate variability is defined as an amplitude of 6 to 25 bpm (Figure 13.2), and marked variability is defined as amplitude greater than 26 bpm.

A normal baseline is between 110 and 160 bpm. Bradycardia (Figure 13.3) is defined as a baseline lower than 110 bpm, and tachycardia (Figure 13.4) is defined as a baseline greater than 160 bpm. The baseline is determined over a 10-minute window. The baseline must be identifiable 2 minutes out of a 10-minute interval; otherwise the baseline is deemed indeterminate.

Accelerations are classified into two categories: less than 32 weeks and 32 weeks and greater. When a fetus is less than 32 weeks, an acceleration is defined as an abrupt (onset to peak less than or equal to 30 seconds) increase in the fetal baseline by at least 10 bpm for at least 10 seconds. At 32 weeks and greater, an acceleration (Figure 13.5) is defined as an abrupt increase in the fetal baseline by 15 bpm for at least 15 seconds.

Decelerations are classified as early, late, variable, and prolonged. An early deceleration is defined as a gradual (onset to nadir > 30 s) decrease in the fetal baseline that starts at the start of a contraction and ends at the end of a contraction. The peak of the contractions occurs simultaneously with the nadir in the FHR deceleration. Early decelerations are a drop in the FHR in response to vagal stimulation from head compression. They are not concerning.

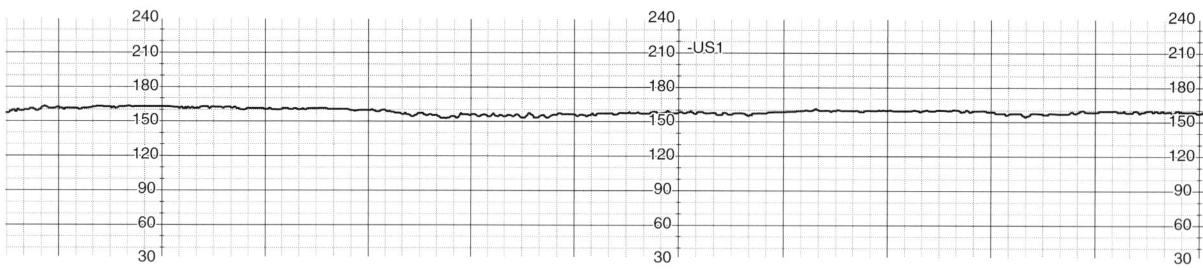

Figure 13.1 This FHR tracing shows minimal variability. New onset of minimal variability may occur for a variety of reasons: fetal sleep cycle, use of narcotics, or CNS depressants including magnesium sulfate, opioids, or fetal acidemia.[10]

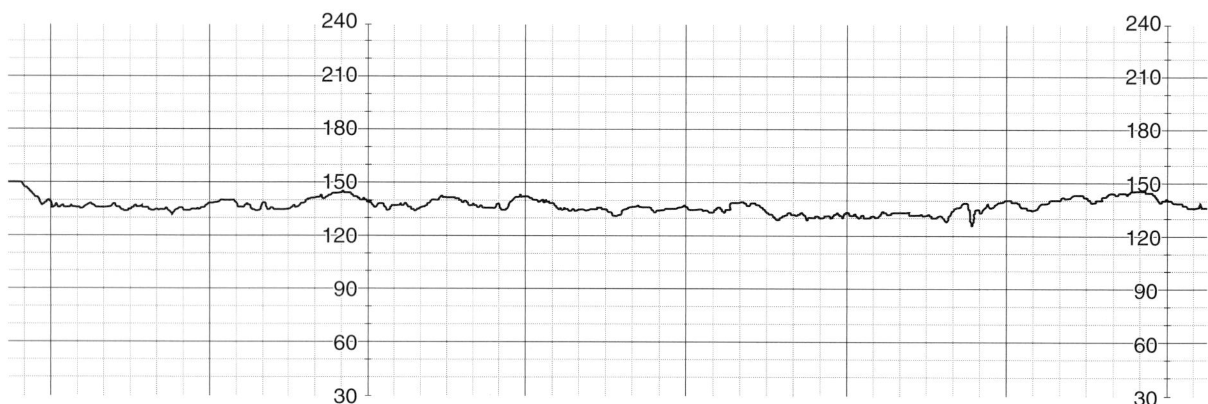

Figure 13.2 This FHR tracing shows moderate variability. This fetus has a normal acid–base status.

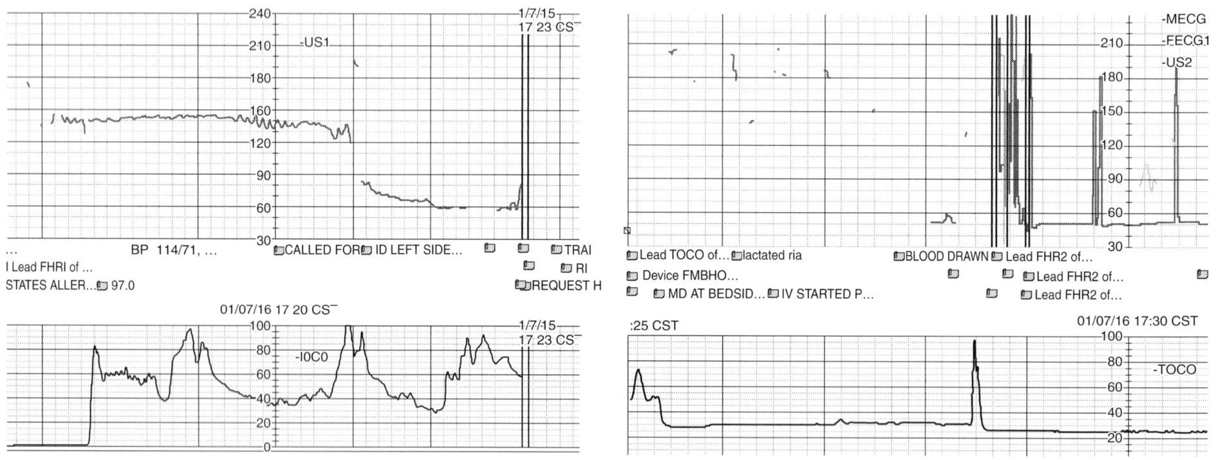

Figure 13.3 This FHT shows a fetal heart rate bradycardia. The baseline drops to 60 bpm; a fetal scalp electrode is then placed and the fetal heart rate a few minutes later is 50 bpm.

A late deceleration (Figure 13.6) is defined as a gradual deceleration in the FHR that starts at the peak of the contraction. The nadir of the late deceleration is after the peak of the contraction. Late decelerations are indicative of placental insufficiency. They are caused by the reflex central nervous system's response to hypoxia and developing acidosis. Late decelerations are also caused by direct myocardial depression.[11]

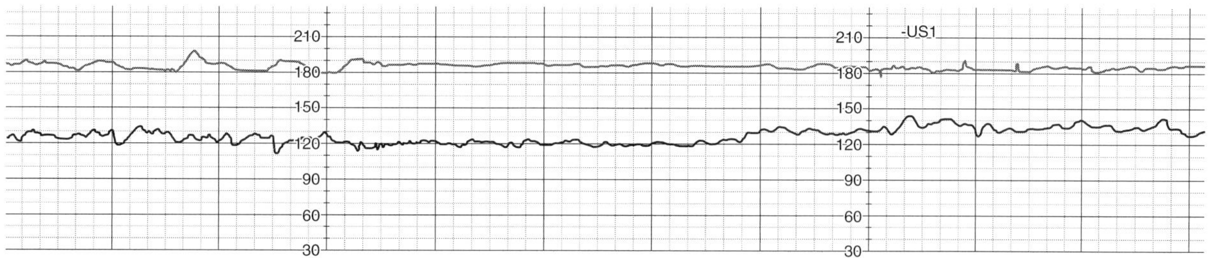

Figure 13.4 This FHT shows a fetal heart rate tachycardia. The lower line is the maternal heart rate. This is the FHT of a patient with chorioamnionitis showing both fetal and maternal tachycardia.

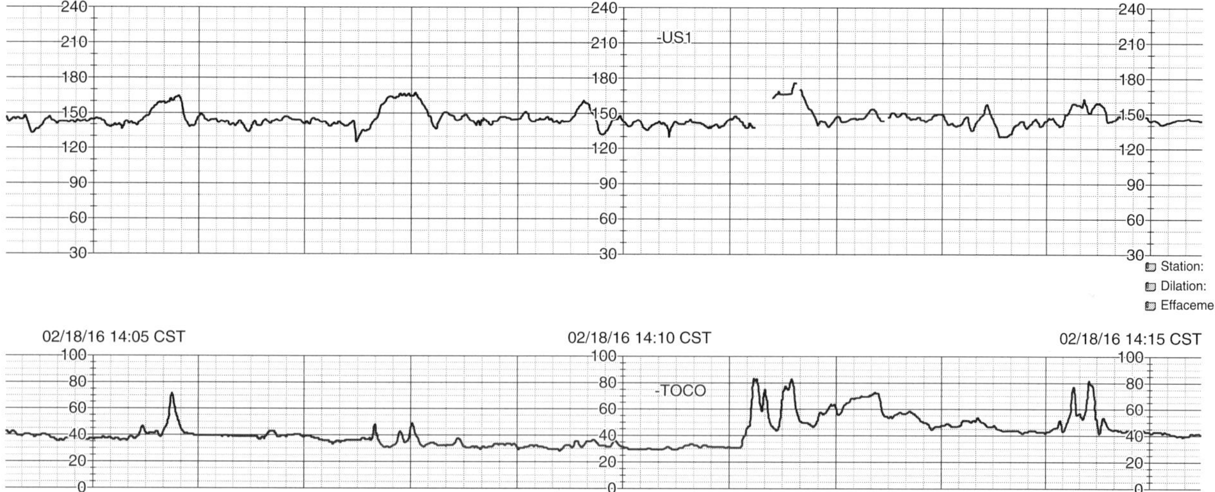

Figure 13.5 This is the FHT of a 39-week fetus. This FHT shows moderate variability with 15 × 15 bpm accelerations.

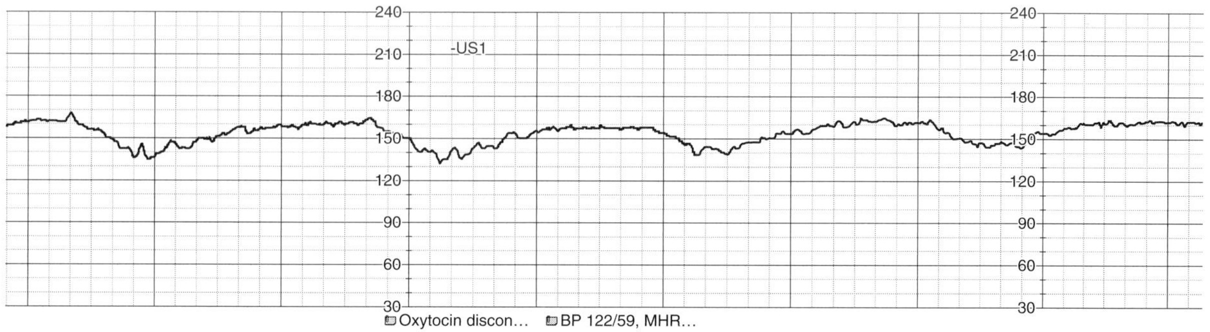

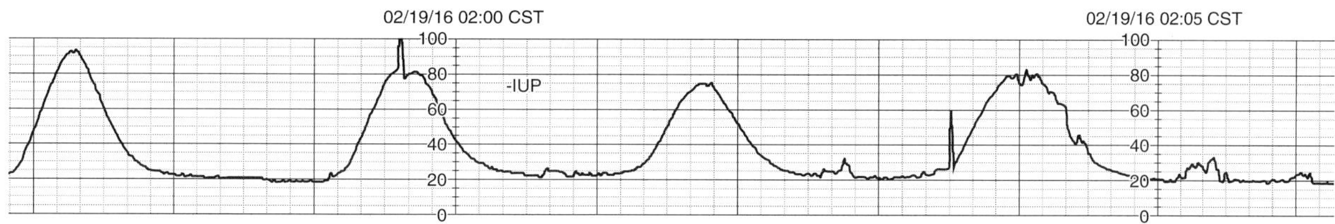

Figure 13.6 This FHT shows recurrent late decelerations with minimal variability in between the decelerations.

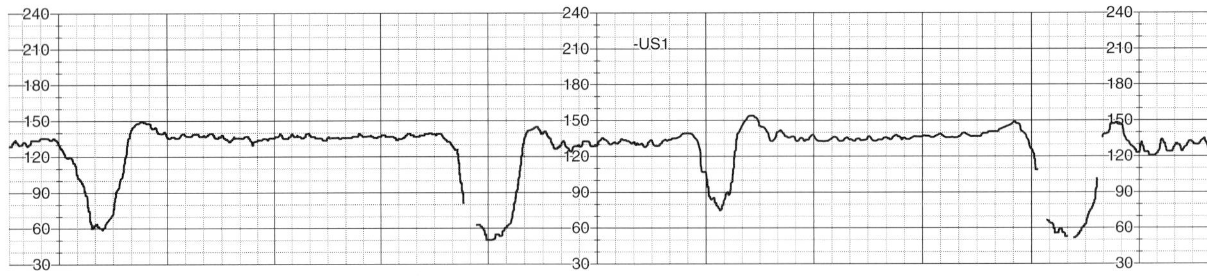

Figure 13.7 This FHR tracing shows recurrent variable decelerations. Notice the "shoulders" on these decelerations.

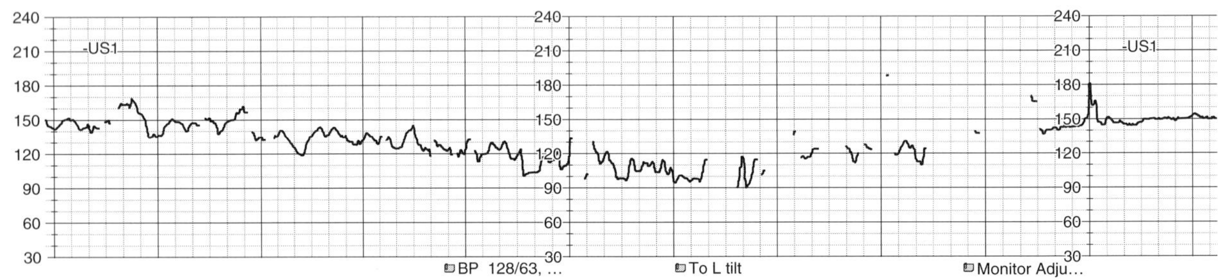

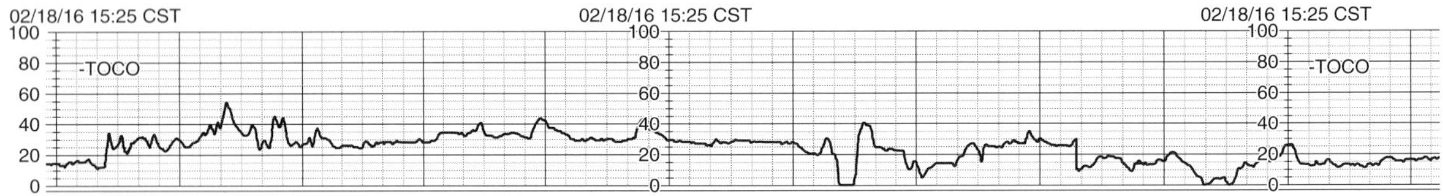

Figure 13.8 This FHT shows a prolonged deceleration. Prior to the start of the deceleration, the baseline shows moderate variability, but as the FHR returns to its baseline of 150, there is minimal variability.

A variable deceleration (Figure 13.7) is defined as an abrupt decline in the FHR of greater than or equal to 15 bpm from the baseline that lasts greater than or equal to 15 seconds and less than 2 minutes from onset to return to baseline. Variable decelerations are caused by cord compression. When the cord is compressed, the thick-walled umbilical arteries remain patent initially allowing deoxygenated blood to return from the baby to the placenta, but the thin-walled vein is compressed occluding oxygenated blood flow to the fetus. This results in a transient tachycardia – the primary shoulder. Eventually the arteries are compressed as well and there is an abrupt drop in the baseline secondary to increase in fetal blood pressure that activates the fetal baroreceptor reflex response. As the compression resolves – the fetal arteries are decompressed primarily, but the thin-walled vein remains occluded – this causes a reflex tachycardia – the posterior shoulder that is often seen at the end of a variable deceleration.[11]

A prolonged deceleration (Figure 13.8) is defined as a decrease in the fetal heart rate of 15 bpm or more that lasts greater than 2 minutes but less than 10 minutes. If a decrease in the baseline persists greater than 10 min, it is defined as a baseline change.

Because the interpretation of fetal monitoring can be subjective, the National Institute of Child Health and Human Development created a standardized three-tiered fetal heart rate interpretation system. ACOG has adopted this system and endorses its use in clinical practice.

Category I

A category I fetal heart rate tracing is an indication of a fetal well-being at the time of the tracing. It is characterized by the following:

A baseline fetal heart rate of 110–160 bpm
Absence of late or variable FHR decelerations
Moderate FHR variability (6–25 bpm)
Early decelerations may be present

Category I FHT are the most common tracings. A study including over 48,000 patients shows that category I patterns were observed at some time during monitoring in over 99% of the tracings.[12]

Category II

A category II FHT is considered an indeterminate finding, meaning that the likelihood of fetal acidosis varies widely across the different category II tracings. Because category II tracings may remain stable for a prolonged period of time, they are the most difficult to evaluate and manage. Category II tracings are also common, and based on a study including 48,000 patients, they are observed at some point in 84% of FHT.[12] A category II FHT is any FHT that is not a category I or category III tracing.

Some category II FHT examples include:

Baseline rate
- Bradycardia not accompanied by absent baseline variability
- Tachycardia

Baseline FHR variability
- Minimal baseline variability
- Absent baseline variability with no recurrent decelerations
- Marked baseline variability

Accelerations

Absence of induced accelerations after fetal stimulation

Periodic or episodic decelerations
- Recurrent variable decelerations accompanied by moderate or minimal variability
- Prolonged deceleration more than 2 minutes but less than 10 minutes
- Recurrent late decelerations with moderate baseline variability
- Variable decelerations with other characteristics such as slow return to baseline, overshoots, or "shoulders" (ACOG Practice Bulletin 116)

Category III

A category III FHT is always abnormal and associated with increased risk of fetal academia, leading to possible cerebral palsy and neonatal hypoxemic ischemic encephalopathy.[13] A category III FHT is characterized by absent FHR variability plus any of the following:

Recurrent late decelerations
Recurrent variable decelerations
Bradycardia
Sinusoidal tracing

Category III tracings require prompt evaluation with in utero resuscitation or delivery to prevent neonatal acidosis and associated morbidity.[10]

Special Fetal Heart Tracings

Sinusoidal FHR

A sinusoidal FHR (Figure 13.9) is characterized by a smooth sine wave with periodicity of three to five cycles per minute, lasting for 20 minutes. This FHR is of concern for fetal hypoxemia typically associated with fetal anemia.[14] Other causes of sinusoidal FHR can be attributed to changes in fetal arterial resistance, fetal sucking movements, and maternal opioid use.[15]

Fetal Arrhythmias

The conduction system of the heart is mature by 16 weeks of gestation. The fetal heart rate should

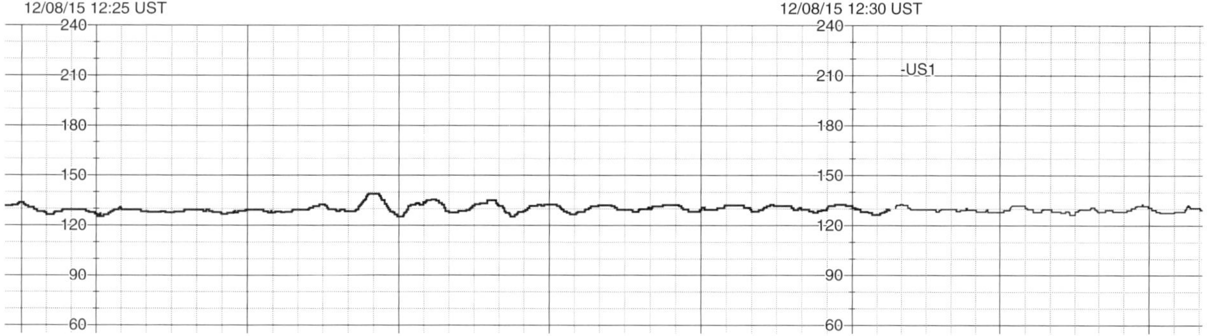

Figure 13.9 This is a FHR tracing showing a sinusoidal pattern. This baby was born with a hematocrit of 26 due to maternal isoimmunization.

be between 110 and 160 bpm by this gestational age.[14] Fetal arrhythmias complicate about 1–2% of pregnancies, and they can compromise fetal well-being.[15] They are typically detected by auscultation at pre-natal visits or by ultrasonography. Two-dimensional ultrasound is used to diagnose the arrhythmia, evaluate cardiac function and anatomy, and evaluate for signs of hydrops fetalis. There is a 10% chance for congenital heart disease associated with a fetal tachycardia, and a 50% chance associated with a fetal bradycardia.

The most common fetal arrhythmia is premature atrial contractions (PACs), causing an irregular rhythm. The main concern with PACs is that they develop into a tachyarrhythmia in 1–3% of fetuses and this can lead to cardiovascular decompensation.[16]

Fetal tachyarrhythmias warrant referral to a fetal cardiology team. The presence of a sustained tachyarrhythmia or an intermittent tachyarrhythmia that is present >50% of the time will ultimately lead to non-immune hydrops fetalis. About 5–10% of fetuses with tachyarrhythmias will have congenital heart disease, with Ebsteins anomaly as the most common abnormality.[17]

Fetal bradyarrhythmias are defined as FHT < 110 bpm, and the most common causes are complete heart block, sinus bradycardia, and blocked atrial bigeminy.[18] In complete heart block, the FHT is usually less than 60 bpm, and complete heart block has a 50% risk for congenital heart disease. Complete heart block can also be caused by exposure to maternal lupus autoantibodies or myocarditis.

Management of Category I FHT

Because category I FHT are considered normal, they are managed expectantly. ACOG recommendations include intermittent monitoring in the first stage of labor every 30 minutes and in the second stage of labor every 15 minutes.[3] In high-risk pregnancies with an increased risk for development of fetal acidosis, the recommendation is for intermittent monitoring every 15 minutes in the first stage of labor and every 5 minutes in the second stage.[19]

Management of Category II FHT

Category II FHT are the most difficult to evaluate and manage, as there is no data to inform on how to manage a FHT that is persistently category II. Intrauterine resuscitative measures can be performed including the following:

Lateral positioning
Administer oxygen
Reduce contraction frequency with by turning off oxytocin or administering terbutaline
Perform amnioinfusion

Frequent reassessment is warranted until the pattern resolves to category I or progresses to category III. Fetal scalp stimulation should be attempted as there is a less than 10% probability of acidosis when fetal scalp stimulation induces FHR acceleration. Positive fetal scalp stimulation indicates normal fetal acid–base status.[20] Similarly, moderate variability is also reassuring with low probability of a fetal acidosis.[21]

ACOG does make recommendations for management of specific category II FHT. Intermittent and recurrent variable decelerations are the most common decelerations in labor.[22] They typically require no intervention, but they do require frequent reevaluation of the frequency, depth, duration, and the FHR variability between variable decelerations. When variable decelerations are recurrent (defined as present with > or equal to 50% of contractions) with increasing depth or duration, they become more indicative of possible developing fetal acidemia.[14] Interventions for relieving cord compression should be implemented. Initially maternal repositioning may relieve a cord compression. If there is no improvement with repositioning, then amnioinfusion can be used.

Recurrent late decelerations, indicative of uteroplacental insufficiency, are commonly caused by maternal hypotension from recent epidural placement, uterine tachysystole, and maternal hypoxia. Frequent monitoring of FHR baseline is warranted, as well as intrauterine resuscitative measures including lateral positioning, maternal oxygen use, IV fluid bolus, and monitoring Pitocin use in an effort to minimize tachysystole.[10] A FHR pattern with recurrent late decelerations, minimal variability, and no response to fetal scalp stimulation is of concern for developing fetal acidemia, prompt interventions should be performed, and need for expedited delivery should be considered.

Fetal tachycardia can be caused by infection as seen earlier in Figure 13.4, certain drugs including terbutaline, cocaine or other stimulants, maternal medical conditions including hyperthyroidism. Obstetric causes such as placental abruption or fetal bleeding should also be considered. Interventions to treat the underlying cause are indicated. Baseline variability

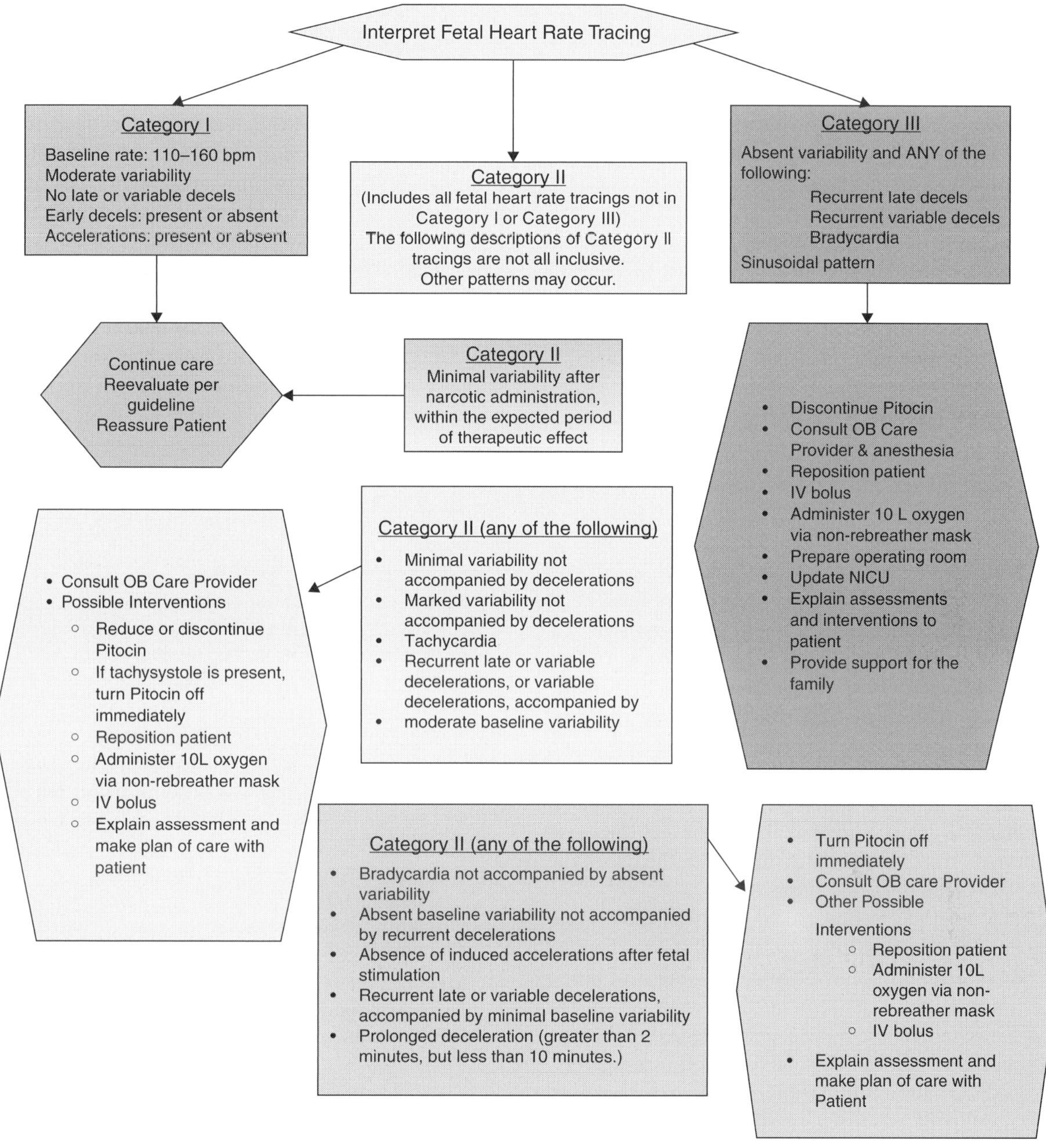

Figure 13.10 Management algorithm of fetal heart rate tracings based on three-tiered category system.[24]

should be evaluated frequently in the setting of fetal tachycardia. Tachycardias alone do not predict fetal hypoxemia or acidemia.[10]

Fetal bradycardia can be caused by maternal hypotension, umbilical cord prolapse or occlusion, rapid fetal descent, tachysystole, placental abruption, or uterine rupture. Interventions to treat the underlying cause are indicated.

Management of Category III FHT

Category III FHT are of concern for fetal acidemia at the time of observation. As a result, the recommendation for intervention is resuscitation measures while preparations for delivery are made such that delivery is expedited if the FHR does not improve.[10] Category III FHT are associated with increased risk for neonatal encephalopathy, cerebral palsy, and neonatal acidosis, but the American Academy of Pediatrics and ACOG have found that Category III tracings do not reliably predict abnormal neurologic outcome.[13] Historically the recommendation for delivery time for Category III FHT has been 30 minutes from the decision to proceed with emergent cesarean section to incision, but there is limited data to support this time frame. Studies have shown that adverse neonatal outcomes have not been established when decision-to-incision interval was over 30 minutes.[23]

The management algorithm (Figure 13.10) outlines management of FHT by category.

Ancillary Intrapartum Testing

Various alternative modes of monitoring fetal status in labor have been introduced, including ST segment analysis (STAN), fetal scalp pH testing, and fetal pulse oximetry. None of these methods have been proven in the literature to improve pregnancy outcomes.

STAN was introduced to monitor the fetal ECG based on the principle that the ST segment will rise or fall with development of fetal hypoxemia. This data is collected via spiral electrode attached to the fetal scalp. Clinicians who use this device must be trained and credentialed. The data has not supported improvements in outcome, specifically there was no decrease in neonatal encephalopathy, cerebral palsy, or perinatal death – overall there was no improvement in maternal or fetal outcomes with the use of the STAN S31 fetal heart monitor.[25]

Fetal scalp pH testing can be useful in the evaluation of a category II or category III FHT. It is performed by visualization of the fetal scalp, cleaning it of blood and amniotic fluid, placement of silicone gel on the fetal scalp, so that when the scalp is pierced, it forms a drop of blood that can then be collected in a heparinized capillary tube for analysis. Its use has decreased for a number of reasons: patient discomfort, physician experience, need for frequently calibrated equipment, and most importantly because similar reassurance can be obtained by fetal scalp stimulation.[26]

Fetal pulse oximetry has not shown improvements in maternal or neonatal outcomes as compared to EFM.[27]

Concluding Remarks

A framework for the evaluation and management of FHT is useful, especially across category II FHT. Management of FHT is directed to identify academic or hypoxemic fetuses using the three-tiered classification system in order to expedite delivery and prevent neurologic injury and death. After delivery, collection of cord pH is useful for determination of fetal acidosis, and the correlation of the FHT with cord pH outcome can be useful. Umbilical artery blood gas should be collected in any fetus with suspected metabolic abnormality, specifically in fetus with 5 or 10 minute Apgar of less than 5, category III FHT, maternal fever, or low birth weight.[28] Although EFM has limitations, there is some data to support reduction in intrapartum fetal death. Continued research is warranted to improve outcomes and reduce long-term neurologic impairment.

References

[1] Dildy GA. Intrapartum assessment of the fetus: Historical and evidence-based practice. *Obstet Gynecol Clin N Am* 2005;32:255–271.

[2] Vintzileos AM, Nochimson DJ, Guzman ER, Knuppel RA, Lake M, Schifrin BS. Intrapartum electronic fetal heart rate monitoring versus intermittent auscultation: A meta-analysis. *SO Obstet Gynecol* 1995 Jan; 85(1):149–55.

[3] American College of Obstetricians and Gynecologists. ACOG Practice Bulletin No. 106: Intrapartum fetal heart rate monitoring: nomenclature, interpretation, and general management principles. *Obstet Gynecol* 2009:114:192.

[4] Alfirevic Z, Devane D, Gyte G. Continuous cardiotocography (CTG) as a form of electronic fetal monitoring (EFM) for fetal assessment during labour. *Cochrane Database Syst Rev* 2006;CD006066.

[5] MacDonald D, Grant A, Sheridan-Pereira M, et al. The Dublin randomized controlled trial of intrapartum fetal heart rate monitoring. *Am J Obstet Gynecol* 1985;152:524.

[6] Martin JA, Hamilton BE, Sutton PD, Ventura SJ, MEnacker F, Munson ML. Births: final data for 2002. *Natl Vital Stat Rep* 2003;52:1–113.

[7] www.monicahealthcare.com. Accessed February 1, 2016.

[8] Bakker JJ, Janssen PF, van Halem K, et al. Internal versus external tocodynamometry during induced or augmented labour. *Cochrane Database Syst Rev* 2013; 8:CD006947.

[9] Hofmeyr GJ. Amnioinfusion for potential or suspected umbilical cord compression in labour. *Cochrane Database Syst Reviews* 1998; Issue 1. Art. No.: CD000013. DOI: 10.1002/14651858.

[10] American College of Obstetricians and Gynecologists. ACOG Practice Bulletin No. 116: Management of intrapartum fetal heart rate tracings. *Obstet Gynecol* 2010 Nov;116(5):1232–40.

[11] Westgate JA, Wibbens B, Bennet L, et al. The intrapartum deceleration in center stage: A physiologic approach to the interpretation of fetal heart rate changes in labor. *Am J Obstet Gynecol* 2007;197:236.

[12] Jackson M, Holmgren CM, Esplin MS, et al. Frequency of fetal heart rate categories and short-term neonatal outcome. *Obstet Gynecol* 2011;118:803.

[13] American Academy of Pediatrics, American College of Obstetricians and Gynecologists. *Neonatal Encephalopathy and Cerebral Palsy: Defining the Pathogenesis and Pathophysiology*. Elk Grove Village, IL: AAP; Washington, DC: ACOG, 2003.

[14] Macones GA, Hankins GD, Spong CY, et al. The 2008 National Institute of Child Health and Human Development workshop report on electronic fetal monitoring: Update on definitions, interpretation, and research guidelines. *Obstet Gynecol* 2008; 112:661.

[15] Johnson TR Jr, Compton AA, Rotmensch J, et al. Significance of the sinusoidal fetal heart rate pattern. *Am J Obstet Gynecol* 1981;139:446.

[16] Copel JA, Liang RI, Demasio K, et al. The clinical significance of the irregular fetal heart rhythm. *Am J Obstet Gynecol* 2000;182:813.

[17] McCurdy CM, Reed KL. Fetal Arrhythmias. In: *Doppler Ultrasound in Obstetrics and Gynecology*, Copel JA, Reed KL (Eds), New York: Raven Press, 1995. p. 253.

[18] Eliasson H, Wahren-Herlenius M, Sonesson SE. Mechanisms in fetal bradyarrhythmia: 65 cases in a single center analyzed by Doppler flow echocardiographic techniques. *Ultrasound Obstet Gynecol* 2011; 37:172.

[19] Liston R, Sawchuck D, Young D, et al. Fetal health surveillance: antepartum and intrapartum consensus guideline. *J Obstet Gynaecol Can* 2007;29:S3.

[20] Skupski DW, Rosenberg CR, Eglinton GS. Intrapartum fetal stimulation tests: A meta-analysis. *Obstet Gynecol* 2002;99:129.

[21] Cahill AG, Roehl KA, Odibo AO, Macones GA. Association and prediction of neonatal acidemia. *Am J Obstet Gynecol* 2012;207:206.e1.

[22] Garite TJ, Dildy GA, McNamara H, Nageotte MP, Boehm FH, Dellinger, EH, et al. A multicenter controlled trialof fetal pulse oximetry in the intrapartum management of nonreassuring fetal heart rate patterns. *Am J Obstet Gynecol* 2000;183:1049–58.

[23] Bloom Sl, Leveno KJ, Spong CY, Gilbert S, Hauth JC, Landon MB, et al. Decision to incision times and maternal and infant outcomes. National Institute of Child Health and Human Development Maternal-Fetal Medicine Units Network. *Obstet Gynecol* 2006;108:6–11.

[24] Guideline for Fetal Monitoring in Labor and Delivery. December 2012. NNEPQIN.

[25] Vayssiere C, Haberstich R, Sebahoun V, et al. Fetal electrocardiogram ST-segment analysis and prediction of neonatal acidosis. *Int J Gynaecol Obstet* 2007;97:110.

[26] Goodwin TM, Milner-Masterson L, Paul RH. Elimination of fetal scalp blood sampling on a large clinical service. *Obstet Gynecol* 1994;83:971–4.

[27] East CE, Begg L, Colditz PB, Lau R. Fetal pulse oximetry for fetal assessment in labour. *Cochrane Database Syst Rev* 2014;10:CD004075.

[28] Page FO, Martin JN, Palmer SM, et al. Correlation of neonatal acid–base status with Apgar scores and fetal heart rate tracings. *Am J Obstet Gynecol* 1986;154:1306.

Obstetric Ultrasound for the Generalist Obstetrician

Stephen Rotholz

Introduction

Routine obstetric ultrasound has become the default standard of care in the United States, and most women will have at least one ultrasound during the course of pregnancy. Thus, routine fetal ultrasound is essentially the United States norm and is expected by both patients and the legal system.

Many textbook chapters go into lengthy and extensive detail about ultrasound technology and abnormal ultrasound findings that may be beyond the need or interest of the generalist obstetrician. The goal for this chapter is to provide a succinct overview of the essential information about obstetric ultrasound needed by generalist providers. Generalist providers should be comfortable with appropriate responsibilities regarding ultrasounds for which they provide interpretation.

Scope of the Problem

What exactly is the responsibility of the generalist obstetrician/gynecologist (Ob/Gyn) regarding the imaging studies performed on their patients? This may depend entirely on who performs and who interprets the images obtained. Acquisition of the obstetric ultrasound images is often performed by a registered diagnostic medical sonographer (RDMS). However, not all ultrasound technicians meet the criteria to be certified as a RDMS as established by the American Registry of Diagnostic Medical Sonographers.

In other words, the generalist obstetrician should be aware that the skill level of the sonographer can vary significantly. After the actual examination is complete, the sonographer typically submits the images and a report to a physician who provides interpretation of the study and who also signs the report. It is not within the scope of practice for the RDMS to provide clinical interpretation. In a radiology center, the interpreting physician would typically be a radiologist with experience in obstetric ultrasound. In a hospital setting, the interpreting physician is usually a radiologist, a generalist obstetrician, or a maternal fetal medicine (MFM) specialist. In a "private office" setting, it is the physicians of the practice who are responsible for the interpretation of the ultrasound examinations they sign off unless it is also formally interpreted by a radiologist or MFM physician. Some family medicine physicians who practice obstetrics will also provide ultrasound interpretation.

It should be stated that the physician who interprets obstetric ultrasound examinations should have adequate training and understanding of the indications for, required content, and potential limitations of obstetric ultrasound. The formal opinion of the American Congress of Obstetrics and Gynecology (ACOG) is that a physician who has completed an Ob/Gyn residency with ultrasound training and is certified by the American Board of Obstetrics and Gynecology meets the criteria for appropriate training.[1]

The responsibility of the generalist to attain and maintain competency in interpretation of obstetric ultrasound may potentially be overlooked as a source of risk. While the generalist is not expected to identify or diagnose ultrasound abnormalities at the level of expertise of the radiologist or MFM, the generalist should be familiar with the published American Institute of Ultrasound in Medicine (AIUM) parameters for obstetric ultrasound and should be able to recognize all the basic anatomy required for the screening exam. The complete AIUM document is available on the AIUM website.[2] The most recent ACOG Practice Bulletin on ultrasound in pregnancy[3] also provides an excellent overview applicable to the generalist obstetrician.

Permanent documentation of the images as well as interpretation should be maintained. The report itself should be part of the patient's permanent medical record. Ideally, images should be stored digitally but hard copy images are still acceptable as long as kept in secure storage for the applicable statute of limitations in your jurisdiction.[4]

This chapter will highlight the basics of what the generalist should understand regarding the AIUM practice parameters and the required elements of ultrasound examinations in all trimesters of pregnancy. The goal is to emphasize familiarity with the relevant normal anatomy, as well as highlight any areas needing further study by the generalist practitioner. This review is directed to the generalist obstetrician and intentionally omits examinations more typically performed by sub-specialists, including but not limited to nuchal translucency as part of the "sequential screen," detailed evaluation of anatomic abnormalities discovered in routine examinations, fetal echocardiography, and "genetic" ultrasounds. There are certainly opportunities for additional training and certification in first trimester screening offered by the Nuchal Translucency Quality Review Program (NTQR) and the Fetal Medicine Foundation. Structural anomalies are also not addressed as these are beyond the scope of our discussion.

Ultrasound Safety

Fetal ultrasound should be performed only when medically indicated and then the lowest possible exposure to the fetus should be emphasized. The energy from sound waves can result in cavitation, which involves the formation of microbubbles. However, cavitation only occurs with high ultrasound power, so it is not of clinical concern in modern obstetric ultrasound. Typical clinical application of this technology is felt to be safe and confers no harm to the developing fetus. Prolonged exposure to ultrasound, however, has been found to alter migration of fetal brain cells in an animal model.[5] While the cited study involved higher energy levels than typically used in clinical practice, this is one basis for the "as low as reasonably achievable" (ALARA) principle as originally promulgated by the AIUM in 2008.[6] The ultimate take-home message from AIUM is "no independently confirmed adverse effects caused by exposure from present diagnostic ultrasound instruments have been reported in human patients in the absence of contrast agents."[7]

Basic Technology and Commonly Used Terms

The ultrasound image displayed on the monitor is generated by software processing of sound waves reflected back from organs, fluids, and tissue interfaces within the uterus and pelvis. Ultrasound coupling gel is used to facilitate sound wave transmission because air is a poor transmitter of these sound waves. Fluids generate few reflected waves and thus appear dark or anechoic. More dense tissues such as bone produce more high velocity reflected waves so they appear more brightly or echogenic on the monitor. Individual two-dimensional images (2D) can be generated at over 200 frames per second so it is thus the software post-processing that allows the appearance of a real-time or moving image.

The higher the frequency of the transducer the better the image resolution, while lower frequency transducers exhibit better tissue penetration. Thus, resolution in obese patients is best with use of lower frequency transducers as the use of high-frequency transducers would not provide the penetration necessary to visualize deep structures.[8] The better the resolution, the more easily the sonographer can distinguish anatomic structures from each other. Many modern ultrasound machines have additional software processing techniques such as tissue harmonic imaging that are designed to assist in improving resolution in the obese patient.

Zoom is a key function of all modern machines. Pushing the zoom knob brings up a "zoom box," which can be adjusted in size and the operator then places over the area of interest. Pushing the zoom knob again then magnifies that specific portion of the image. This is generally preferable to turning the same zoom knob, which magnifies the entire image and may result in the area of interest moving off the screen. More importantly, zooming the entire image does not concentrate the sound waves in the area of interest as it does with the zoom box. Thus, image quality is better when the zoom box is used. Alternatively, some resolution is lost with the use of the zoom function as the pixels themselves are enlarged.

Ultrasound examination in the first trimester can be achieved using either an abdominal transducer or transvaginal (TV) transducer. A transvaginal examination may be preferred when visualization is not optimal with the abdominal probe. This is often the case in early first trimester as well as in obese patients. For most patients, an abdominal transducer with a frequency range of 3–5 MHz should allow adequate tissue penetration while still allowing good resolution, In obese patients, a lower frequency transducer (2.2–2.5 MHz) might be required. TV transducers are typically in the 5–10 MHz range, because less tissue penetration is required due to the proximity of the probe to the uterus and its contents.

Doppler ultrasound is displayed as a shift in wave frequency, reflecting the movement of waves either away from or toward the observer. In today's machines, Doppler generally refers to either pulsed wave (PW) Doppler or color flow Doppler. PW Doppler is often also combined with color flow Doppler. PW Doppler displays blood flowing toward the transducer as red and that away from the transducer as blue; this is typically displayed as a scale in the margin of the monitor screen.

Color flow Doppler is useful in the evaluation of blood flow in fetal vessels as well as maternal vessels. PW Doppler used on vessels will generate a flow velocity waveform with time displayed on the x-axis and the speed of blood on the y-axis in centimeters (cm) per second. From the waveform, one can assess the downstream impedance or resistance to blood flow. This does not measure actual resistance, but rather an index of resistance. For accurate velocity readings, the angle of insonation (angle between the pulsed waves and the vessel) should be zero degrees. This can be achieved either by making the pulsed waves travel directly down the barrel of the vessel or by use of the angle correction knob. The most commonly used PW Doppler index is the systolic/diastolic (S/D) ratio in the fetal umbilical artery. The S/D ratio can be used in evaluating the fetus with intrauterine growth restriction[9] but is not appropriate for screening in low-risk pregnancies.

Measurement of the actual velocity of blood flow is used in determining whether there is moderate to severe anemia in the fetus. This is achieved by measuring the peak systolic flow velocity in the middle cerebral artery (MCA) of the fetus. Anemia is characterized by lower viscosity and thus a higher speed of blood flow. Use of MCA Doppler velocimetry is not performed routinely in low-risk patients.

M-mode is a linear display of cardiac motion with time on the x-axis and motion on the y-axis. It appears as a wavy horizontal line and is commonly used to document fetal cardiac activity prior to 12 weeks of gestation. M-mode can also be used for evaluation of fetal cardiac arrhythmia and as part of fetal echocardiography. To determine the fetal heart rate with M-mode, first push the m-mode button and then use the track ball to move the line in the image through the fetal heart. This will bring up the M-mode display below the fetal image. Once multiple cardiac cycles have been documented, freeze the image and use CALIPER or CALCS setting to select fetal heart rate (FHR). Use the "select bar," which is typically on either side of the track ball to move the caliper lines from either valley to valley or peak to peak. Pressing the "enter" key (generally above the track ball) will then prompt the machine to display the calculated fetal heart rate.

Of note, this same select bar is typically used to "set" the first caliper point when obtaining biometry of fetal structures. After the first caliper is set, the track ball is used to move the second caliper to the desired location for measurement and then the enter key is depressed to allow the software to calculate the distance and the biometric information desired.

Cineloop refers to the ability to scroll backward or forward through the most recently acquired images, which are temporarily stored after the freeze button is pushed. The length of time one can scroll backward or forward varies from machine to machine. Once the desired image is found, it can be saved. It is also possible to save the entire cineloop if desired.

First Trimester

Common indications for first trimester ultrasound examination include but are not limited to confirmation of the number of fetuses, confirmation of cardiac activity, confirmation of gestational age, and estimated date of confinement (EDC), evaluation for possible ectopic pregnancy, and evaluation of possible causes of pelvic pain or bleeding. Box 14.1 describes the current AIUM indications for first trimester ultrasound examination.[2]

In addition to the above-mentioned indications, the common use of first trimester ultrasound has also allowed for the routine early diagnosis of spontaneous abortion, anembryonic pregnancy (e.g. "blighted ovum"), gestational neoplastic neoplasia (molar pregnancy), and ectopic pregnancy.

The presence and location of a gestational sac (GS) and embryo should be noted, and commonly a yolk sac (YS) can be seen. The crown–rump length (CRL) should be documented as it is the most accurate determinant of estimated gestational age (EGA). Ideally images for documentation should utilize zoom or magnification sufficient to have the relevant structure occupy one-third to one-half of the image. The CRL should ideally be measured in the midline sagittal plane taking care not to include the YS.

Box 14.1 AIUM indications for first trimester ultrasound examination

Indications for First Trimester Ultrasound Examination

a. Confirmation of the presence of an intrauterine pregnancy
b. Evaluation of a suspected ectopic pregnancy
c. Defining the cause of vaginal bleeding
d. Evaluation of pelvic pain
e. Estimation of gestational (menstrual) age
f. Diagnosis or evaluation of multiple gestations
g. Confirmation of cardiac activity
h. Imaging as an adjunct to chorionic villus sampling, embryo transfer, and localization and removal of an intrauterine device
i. Assessing for certain fetal anomalies, such as anencephaly, in high-risk patients
j. Evaluation of maternal pelvic masses and / or uterine abnormalities
k. Measuring the nuchal translucency (NT) when part of a screening program for fetal aneuploidy
l. Evaluation of a suspected hydatidiform mole.

Establishment of gestational age is best performed as early in pregnancy as possible. First trimester CRL is the most accurate means of gestational age assessment and is generally felt to have a range of error of ± 5 days. If the ultrasound estimation of gestational age is within 5 days of the menstrual dating, the EDC should be based on dates.

Mean gestational sac diameter can be used when there is no identifiable embryo; however, the CRL is a more accurate measure of gestational age once an embryo is detectable. Cardiac motion should be detectable with an embryo of 5 mm or more, and a follow-up scan to document cardiac activity is indicated when there is an embryo less than 5 mm with no detectable cardiac activity. Figure 14.1 shows the calipers measuring the CRL, and the arrow is on the amniotic membrane.

Cardiac activity should be documented with either a two-dimensional video or M-mode imaging as shown in Figure 14.2. The image demonstrates the measurement from the nadir of one valley to the next. Use of PW Doppler interrogation is not recommended prior to 12 weeks.[10]

Amnionicity and chorionicity should be documented for all multiple gestations. The most accurate time in pregnancy to identify amnionicity/chorionicity is in the first trimester. Figure 14.3 demonstrates a first trimester twin gestation with a "twin peak" or lambda sign documenting dichorionic placentation and two separate sacs. The twin peak sign is formed by the chorion that intervenes between the two amniotic sacs, which also makes the membranes thicker and easier to see with ultrasound.

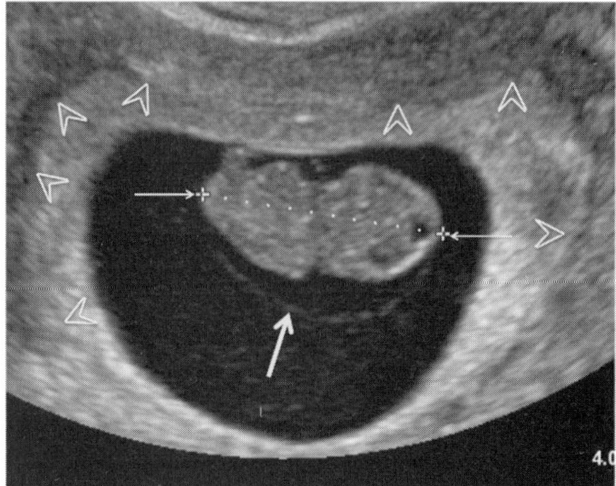

Figure 14.1 Ultrasound image of an early intrauterine pregnancy documenting the presence of the gestational sac and embryo within the uterine wall. Calipers measure crown rump length (CRL). Thick arrow is the amniotic membrane. Thin arrows denote the points of caliper placement for CRL. The arrowheads depict the uterine wall.

The uterus, cervix, adnexae, and cul de sac should be evaluated and documented. The presence of any clinically significant fibroids should be noted, as well as any large ovarian cysts, adnexal masses or significant cul de sac fluid. Figure 14.4 demonstrates a sagittal uterus with caliper measurements in both sagittal and anterior-posterior planes.

Figure 14.5 demonstrates a normal ovary with typical follicular cyst. Each ovary should be documented, but it is common to have difficulty visualizing one or both ovaries in pregnancy. In general, clinically significant cysts can be visualized due to their hypo-echoic appearance.

Second Trimester

The second trimester examination is commonly performed between 18 and 22 weeks gestation as the relevant anatomy is most often visible after 18 weeks. This is also dependent on the quality of the ultrasound machine. ACOG describes three ultrasound

Figure 14.2 M-mode documentation of fetal cardiac activity and fetal heart rate.

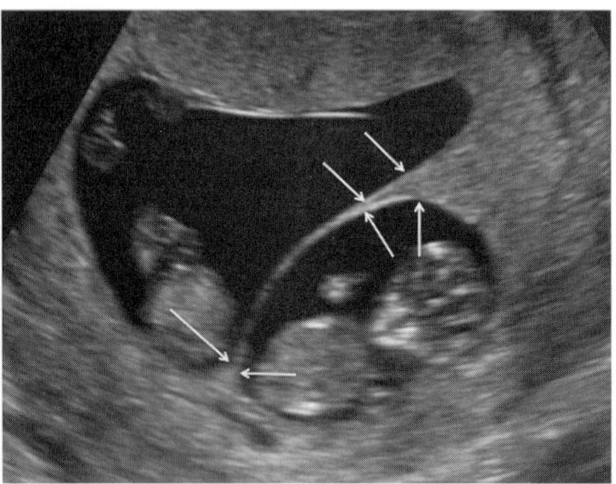

Figure 14.3 First trimester diamniotic, dichorionic twin gestation with the "twin peak" or lambda sign (arrows).

categories used. The terms standard (or basic), limited, and specialized to refer to specific ultrasound examinations in the second and third trimester.[11] The standard or basic examination refers to what could be considered the typical "low-risk" second trimester ultrasound examination used to evaluate fetal number, presentation, cardiac activity, biometry, placentation, as well as an anatomic survey. The limited examination is used to evaluate a specific question such as fetal presentation in labor, evaluation of interval fetal growth, amniotic fluid volume, or cervical length. While cervical length can be a useful measurement in high-risk patients, routine screening of cervical length in low-risk patients is still a matter of debate.[12] Specialized examinations include fetal Doppler interrogation, biophysical profile, assessment of amniotic fluid volume, as well as fetal echocardiography and targeted anatomic evaluation of suspected anomalies. A limited examination does not replace a basic examination, so a patient presenting for examination who has not yet had a basic examination should have an exam including all elements of the basic examination.

Common indications for second trimester ultrasound include but are not limited to evaluation of fetal anatomy to screen for malformation, gestational age, fetal presentation, and placental localization in relation to the cervix. In addition, evaluation of size/dates discrepancy, pelvic mass, suspected fetal

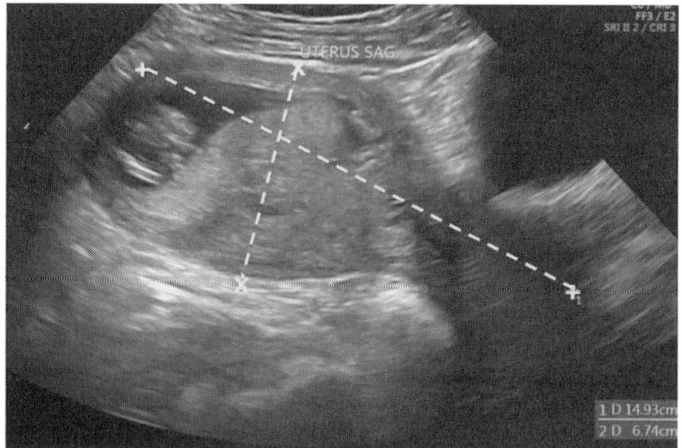

Figure 14.4 Sagittal uterus with caliper measurement of uterine length and the anterior posterior dimensions.

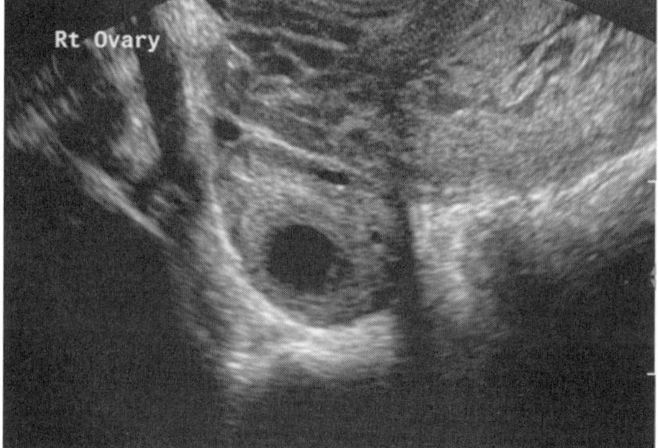

Figure 14.5 Normal ovary with typical follicular cyst.

demise, fetal well-being, amniotic fluid volume, placental abnormalities, and cervical length in high-risk pregnancy is commonly indicated. Ultrasound is also commonly used for guidance of fetal procedures such as amniocentesis or external cephalic version in the third trimester.

Fetal cardiac activity, fetal number, and presentation should all be documented. Figure 14.6 shows a fetus with pulsed-wave Doppler velocimetry to document fetal cardiac activity.

In second trimester multiple gestations, chorionicity should be determined. However, chorionicity is best assessed in the first trimester. The persistence of separate gestational sacs with the intervening membrane and estimate of amniotic fluid in each sac should be documented at any given gestational age (Figure 14.7). In multiple gestation, the most common way to assess the amniotic fluid volume is by measuring the maximal vertical pocket (MVP) in each sac.

Placental location and appearance, as well as relationship to the internal cervical os, are generally easy to determine in second trimester. While the majority of instances of placenta previa and low-lying placenta will resolve with subsequent growth of the uterus, documentation of distance from the lower edge of the placenta to the internal cervical os will help to determine clinical care and direct future follow-up of placental localization to assure that vaginal delivery is safe to pursue. A low-lying placenta is defined as the lower or most inferior leading edge of the placenta within 2 cm of the internal cervical os. Visualization of the lower edge of a posterior placenta may be increasingly difficult as pregnancy progresses due to the acoustic shadowing from the fetus. Figure 14.8 demonstrates a normal posterior placenta with the lower edge several centimeters from the internal os.

Figure 14.9 demonstrates a complete placenta previa with the placenta extending over the internal os.

Figure 14.10 shows a low-lying placenta with the leading edge close to the cervix. If a low-lying placenta is suspected on abdominal ultrasound a transvaginal ultrasound should be considered to definitely rule out a placenta previa.

Figure 14.11 demonstrates the use color Doppler to demonstrate a vasa previa with vessels traversing over the internal cervical os. The vessels of a vasa previa represent a fetal vessel and as such a vaginal delivery is contraindicated.

Documentation of the number of vessels in the umbilical cord as well as placental insertion site of the cord should be attempted. Figure 14.12 provides documentation of a three vessel umbilical cord, and Figure 14.13 reveals a central placental cord insertion site.

The most common biometry used to assess gestational age beyond the first trimester includes measurements of biparietal diameter (BPD), head circumference (HC), abdominal circumference (AC), and femur length. Trans-cerebellar diameter (TCD) is also an accurate measurement. Thus, it is a useful adjunct in dating an intrauterine growth-restricted pregnancy with poor dating as it is typically preserved in intrauterine growth restriction (IUGR). Of particular importance, a given pregnancy should not be re-dated if a good quality first trimester scan is available as the range of error (ROE) increases with advancing gestational age. A good approximation of ROE is plus or minus 10 days at 20 weeks EGA. Estimated

Box 14.2 AIUM indications for second and third trimester ultrasound examination

Indications for Second and Third Trimester Ultrasound Examination

a. Screening for fetal anomalies
b. Evaluation of fetal anatomy
c. Estimation of gestational (menstrual) age
d. Evaluation of fetal growth
e. Evaluation of vaginal bleeding
f. Evaluation of abdominal or pelvic pain
g. Evaluation of cervical insufficiency
h. Determination of fetal presentation
i. Evaluation of suspected multiple gestation
j. Adjunct to amniocentesis or other procedure
k. Evaluation of a significant discrepancy between uterine size and clinical dates
l. Evaluation of a pelvic mass
m. Evaluation of a suspected hydatidiform mole
n. Adjunct to cervical cerclage placement
o. Suspected ectopic pregnancy
p. Suspected fetal death
q. Suspected uterine abnormalities
r. Evaluation of fetal well-being
s. Suspected amniotic fluid abnormalities
t. Suspected placental abruption
u. Adjunct to external cephalic version
v. Evaluation of premature rupture of membranes and / or preterm labor
w. Evaluation of abnormal biochemical markers
x. Follow-up evaluation of a fetal anomaly
y. Follow-up evaluation of placental location for suspected placenta previa
z. History or previous congenital anomaly
aa. Evaluation of the fetal condition in late registrants for prenatal care
bb. Assessment for findings that may increase the risk for aneuploidy.

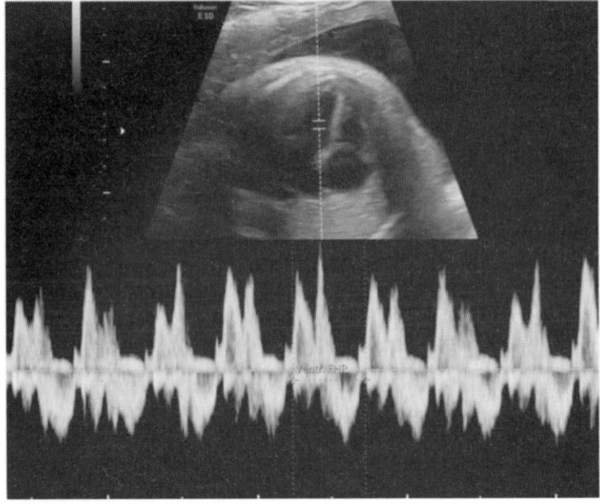

Figure 14.6 Example of the use of pulsed-wave Doppler velocimetry to document fetal cardiac activity.

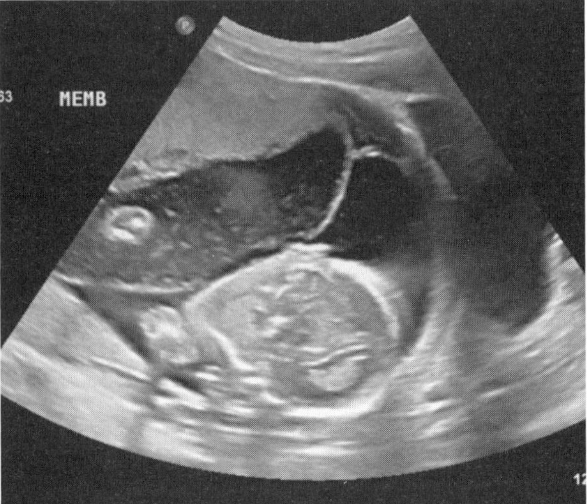

Figure 14.7 Twin gestation documenting intervening membrane.

fetal weight (EFW) is typically calculated based on the above measurements using one of several prediction models, and most modern ultrasound machines have this software included. Of note, interval growth evaluation should not be performed any closer than 2 weeks (preferably every 3–4 weeks), as there may be uncertainty over whether there is actually a growth disturbance or merely a difference in exam technique. Furthermore, fetuses grow in spurts so a short interval ultrasound may not detect growth. Maternal anatomy including uterus, cervix, and adnexal structures should be performed when appropriate. Examples would include large uterine leiomyomas or adnexal masses.

The BPD is measured at the level of the thalami and cavum septum pelucidum (CSP) and is obtained from outer edge of the proximal skull to the inner edge of the distal skull. Figure 14.14 demonstrates measurement of the BPD and HC obtained at this level. The HC is particularly useful when the head is flattened

Figure 14.8 Normal posterior placenta (thick arrows) demonstrating the lower edge (arrowhead) away from the internal cervical os (thin arrow).

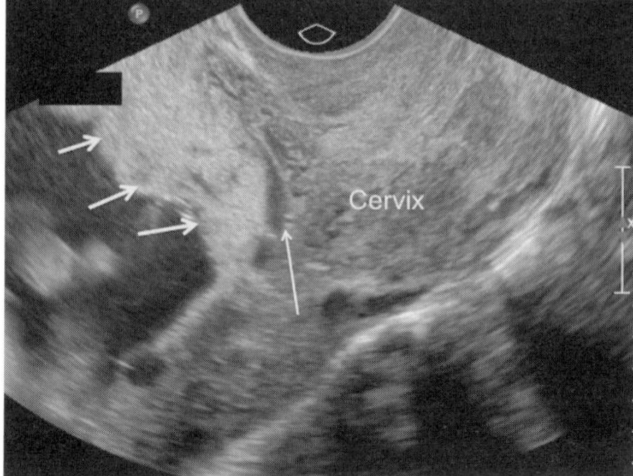

Figure 14.9 Image of a complete placenta previa with lower edge of the placenta (thick arrows) covering the internal cervical os (thin arrow).

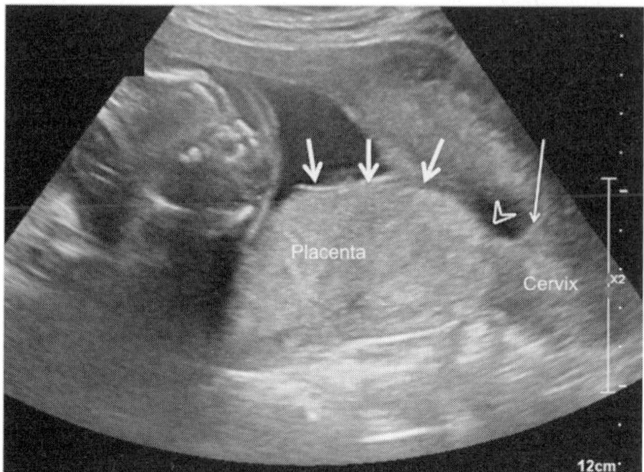

Figure 14.10 Transabdominal ultrasound image of a low-lying posterior placenta (thick arrows) with lower leading edge (arrowhead) less than 1 cm from internal cervical os (thin arrow).

(dolichocephaly) or rounded (brachycephaly) as it is not affected by head shape. The HC is measured around the outer perimeter of the calvarium. Modern machines will typically facilitate obtaining this measurement with the use of an ellipse, rather than measuring the BPD and the occipito-frontal diameter (OFD) separately.

The FL or femoral diaphysis shown in Figure 14.15 is reliable after 14 weeks; care should be taken to not include the distal femoral epiphysis.

The abdominal circumference should be obtained in a transverse view at the skin line at the level of the fetal stomach and is also obtained with use of the ellipse tool as demonstrated in Figure 14.16. Obtaining the proper image of the abdominal circumference can be challenging. Some helpful hints include: (a) obtain a longitudinal view of the fetal spine and rotate the transducer 90 degrees to be perpendicular to the spine (this will help with symmetry), (b) on the axial view, the ribs should be symmetrically imaged, (c) ensure that both the "hockey stick" appearance of the portal vein (actually representing the hepatic portion of the umbilical vein as it curves to become the portal sinus) and the stomach are seen simultaneously, and lastly, (d) that the hepatic vein is not visualized coming from the umbilical ring (would indicate that the image is too low anteriorly on the fetus).

The "fetal anatomic survey" includes a group of anatomic structures that are generally visible after 18 weeks. The documentation of these normal structures can serve to provide reassurance of a normal fetus without major anomaly. However, it must be emphasized that a normal fetal anatomic survey does not "rule out" all potential fetal anomalies, and it does not provide assurance of normal function postnatally.

Excellent obstetrical practice in performance of the ultrasound examination should make the patient aware that a normal anatomic survey does not eliminate the possibility of genetic or anatomic abnormalities. Controversy remains over the sensitivity of fetal anomaly detection and said sensitivity may vary significantly depending on the expertise of the sonographers and physicians interpreting individual examinations. A large review of 36 studies reported an overall sensitivity of 40.4% in anomaly detection with a range of 13.3–82.4%.[13]

Examination of the head, face, and neck should include the lateral ventricles, choroid plexus (CP), midline falx, cavum septum pellucidum, cerebellum,

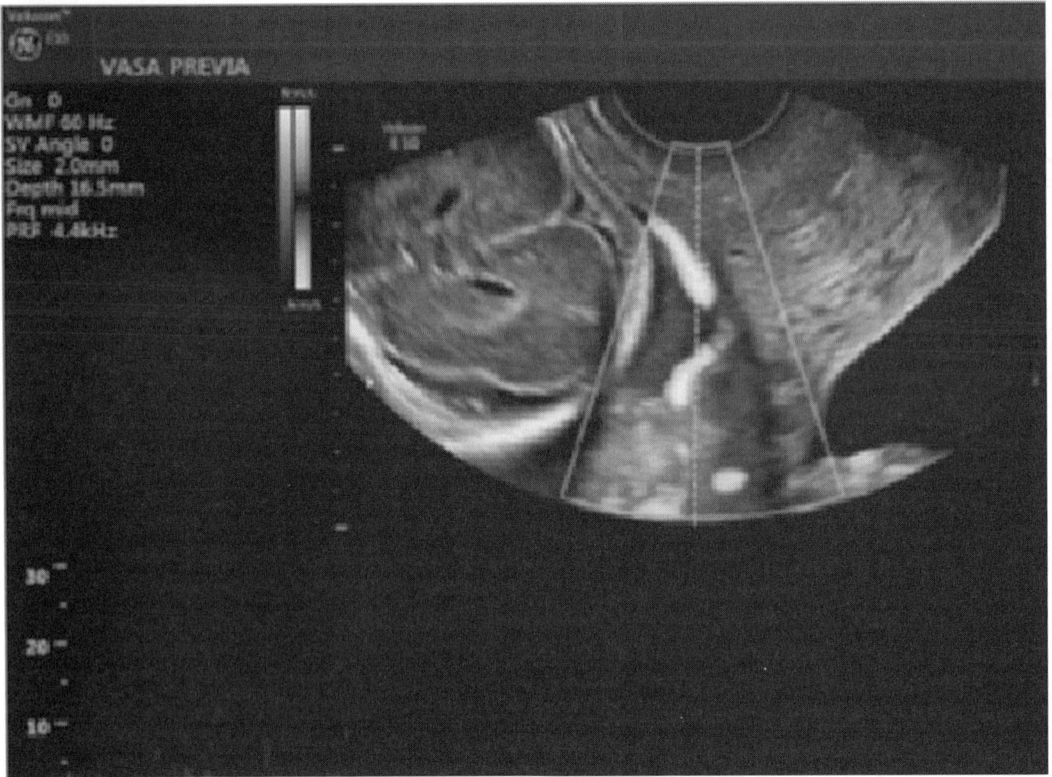

Figure 14.11 Vasa previa with color Doppler demonstrating vessels traversing the internal cervical os.

cisterna magna, and upper lip. In addition, a fetal profile should be obtained. The term "posterior fossa" refers to the occipitobregmatic plane providing an image of the cerebellum and cisterna magna.

Three axial views are required to evaluate the brain. The trans-thalamic view includes the CSP and thalami and is used to measure the BPD and HC, as previously shown in Figure 14.14. The trans-ventricular view includes the lateral ventricles and choroid plexus. The atria of the lateral ventricle should not exceed 10 mm. This measurement is obtained inner edge to inner edge just posterior to the choroid as demonstrated in Figure 14.17.

The trans-cerebellar view includes images of the transverse cerebellum and the cisterna magna as shown in Figure 14.18. The cisterna magna is the hypoechoic fluid filled structure just posterior to the cerebellum. The transverse cerebellar diameter (TCD) is an accurate measure of gestational age and is generally preserved in growth-restricted fetuses.

Figure 14.19 demonstrates a normal fetal profile in second trimester, and Figure 14.20 demonstrates normal fetal lips and nares with an intact upper lip.

Evaluation of the fetal thorax should include a four-chamber heart (4CH), as shown in Figure 14.21. The tricuspid valve attachment is normally lower on the septum than the mitral valve on the left. Also note that the atria should be about equal in size. In a basic examination, an attempt should be made to identify the left and right ventricular outflow tracts (LVOT and RVOT). Observation of the heart should also include the fetal heart rate, as well as its orientation within the chest. Figure 14.22 shows a normal LVOT demonstrating that the anterior wall of the aorta is in continuity with the ventricular septum. In Figure 14.23, the RVOT shows the bifurcation of the pulmonary artery with the ductus arteriosus heading toward the spine and the pulmonary artery wrapping around the aortic root.

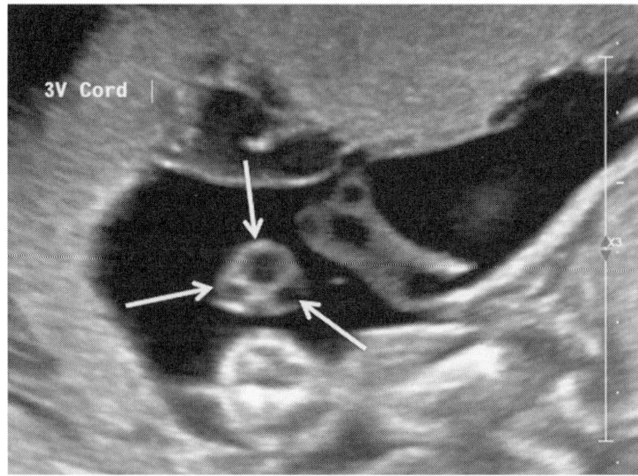

Figure 14.12 Transverse image of an umbilical cord showing that it contains three vessels.

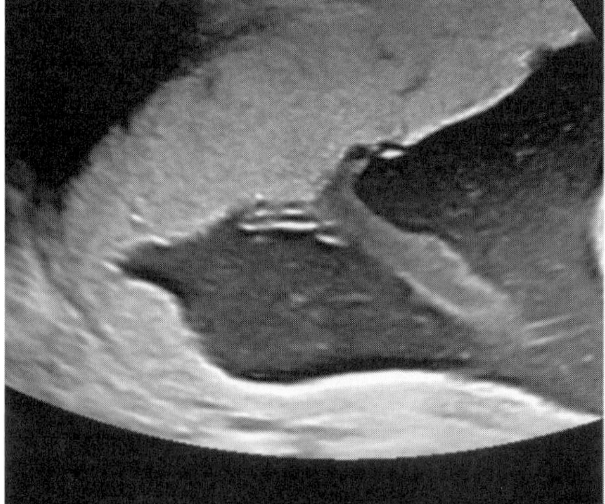

Figure 14.13 Central placental cord insertion in anterior fundal placenta.

Structures that are documented in the fetal abdomen include the stomach (comprising presence or absence as well as situs), kidneys, bladder, fetal umbilical cord insertion site, and umbilical cord vessel number. Figure 14.24 demonstrates presence of both kidneys, and Figure 14.25 demonstrates the umbilical cord insertion site at the fetal abdomen which indicates no evidence of an abdominal wall defect. Figure 14.26 shows a normal fetal bladder, which will typically fill and empty during the course of the examination. An application of color Doppler in this view of the bladder would likely show at least a portion of the two umbilical arteries as they course around the bladder to exit at the umbilical ring.

Evaluation of the fetal spine typically includes a longitudinal mid-sagittal image of the entire spine as well as cross-sectional or axial views of the cervical, thoracic, lumbar, and sacral spine. It is also important to confirm and identify an intact skin line overlying the spine. Of note is that the presence of an open neural tube defect (NTD) in the presence of a documented normal posterior fossa is extremely uncommon, as essentially every fetus with an open NTD will have an abnormal posterior fossa.[14] Figure 14.27 demonstrates a mid-sagittal view of the cervical and upper thoracic spine. The posterior bony elements appear just below the skin with the vertebral body ossification center deep to the hypoechoic spinal canal. The spinal cord itself will be visible later in the pregnancy. In Figure 14.28, an axial view of the lumbar spine shows three ossification centers, which can be visualized by 16–18 weeks.

Interestingly, a screening examination of the fetal extremities only requires documentation that there are four extremities present. While patients commonly assume the examination includes counting "fingers and toes," this is not part of a screening examination. One useful tip is that a view of the lower extremity showing the tibia and fibula in parallel with the foot coming directly toward or away from the viewer (as shown in Figure 14.29) can eliminate the likelihood of a club foot.

Determination of gender is a parental expectation in most cases but is not generally clinically indicated. That being said, determination of gender is typically easily achieved as long as the fetus cooperates in allowing visualization. Figure 14.30 shows male genitalia and Figure 14.31 shows normal female genitalia. It is a good practice to ask the patients whether or not they want to know the gender of their fetus and to document this in the chart.

An objective assessment of amniotic fluid volume can be reasonably achieved with measurement of the maximal vertical pocket (MVP) not containing umbilical cord as shown in Figure 14.32. Use of the MVP compared to the four-quadrant amniotic fluid index (AFI) has been shown in randomized clinical trials to reduce iatrogenic delivery without an increase in adverse pregnancy outcome. A key point in measuring the AFI or the MVP is that the transducer should be perpendicular to the table and not angled, which could create a false impression of a larger pocket.

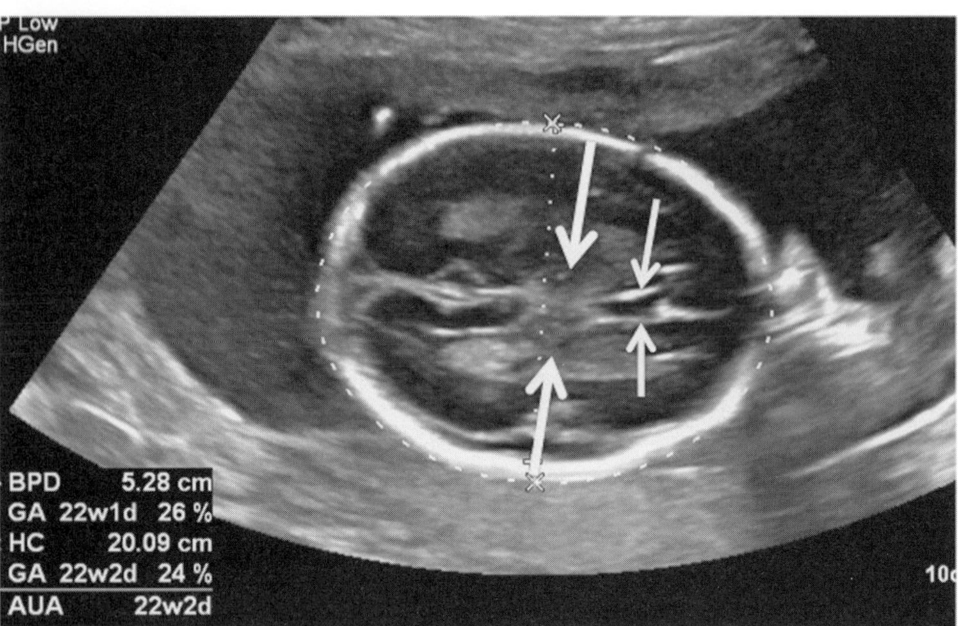

Figure 14.14 Fetal head with biparietal diameter, head circumference, thalami (thick arrows), and cavum septum pellucidum (arrows).

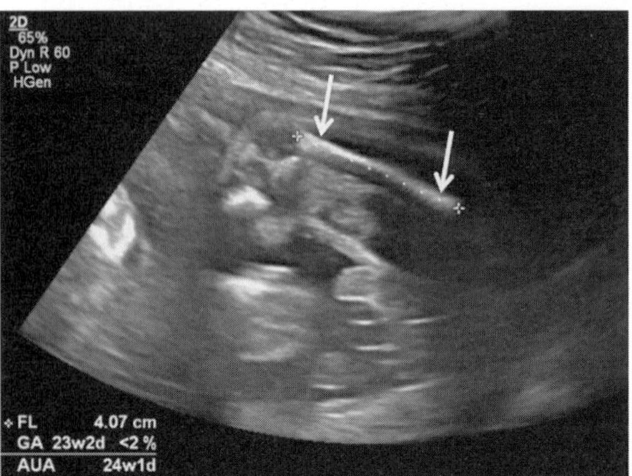

Figure 14.15 Longitudinal image of the femur with caliper placement for the femur length measurement.

Ultrasound in the third trimester is generally indicated for follow-up of fetal growth (assessment of fetal size when there is a size-dates discrepancy or maternal obesity), and assessment of amniotic fluid volume. If a third trimester ultrasound is performed in a patient who has not had a normal fetal anatomic survey, an attempt to evaluate all structures needed for the basic examination should be made.

The fetal biophysical profile (BPP) is a study evaluating fetal well-being in the third trimester, as first described by Manning and Platt in 1980.[15] The ultrasound components include fetal tone, fetal movement, fetal breathing, and an assessment of amniotic fluid volume. Two points are given for each component present, and none are given when absent. The fifth component is a fetal non-stress test (NST). The time allotted for the examination is up to 30 minutes. Two points each are given for a fetus exhibiting at least one 30 second episode of breathing, three trunk movements, and at least one noted limb extension with return to flexion. A MVP equal to 2 cm or greater garners two points as does a reactive NST. A score of 8 or 10 (depending on whether the NST is incorporated) suggests no evidence of fetal academia. While a score of 6 or less may not identify a fetus with academia, it does warrant further and prolonged evaluation.

Three-dimensional (3D) ultrasonography allows the acquisition of a "volume" of an anatomic location that can be viewed in three orthogonal planes corresponding to the sagittal, coronal, and transverse planes. 3D "rendering" creates a topographic or nearly photographic image of the surface of the structure in question such as the fetal face as shown in Figure 14.33.

Potential clinical use of 3D imaging includes evaluation of fetal facial anomalies as well as neural

Figure 14.16 Cross-section image of a fetal abdomen depicting the abdominal circumference with ellipse. Note the labelled portal vein and stomach that should be seen in the proper abdominal circumference view.

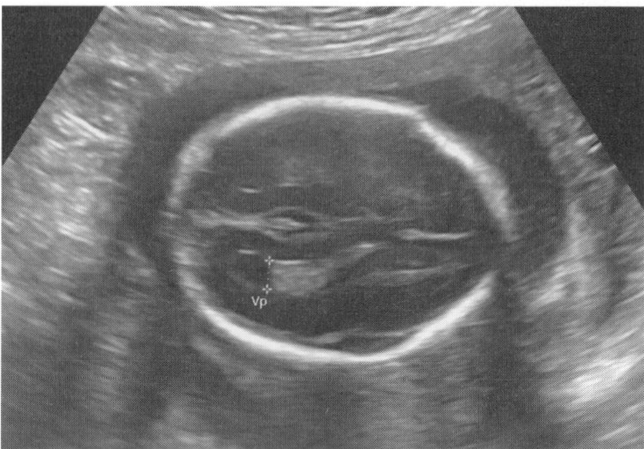

Figure 14.17 Normal lateral ventricle with choroid plexus (thick arrow).

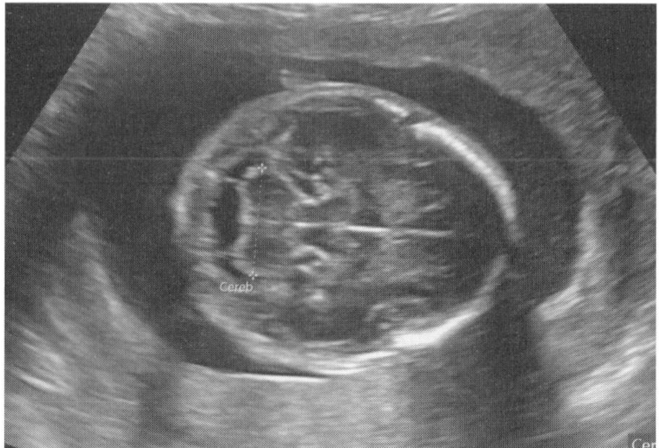

Figure 14.18 Posterior fossa with calipers on measured trans-cerebellar diameter and cisterna magna (arrows).

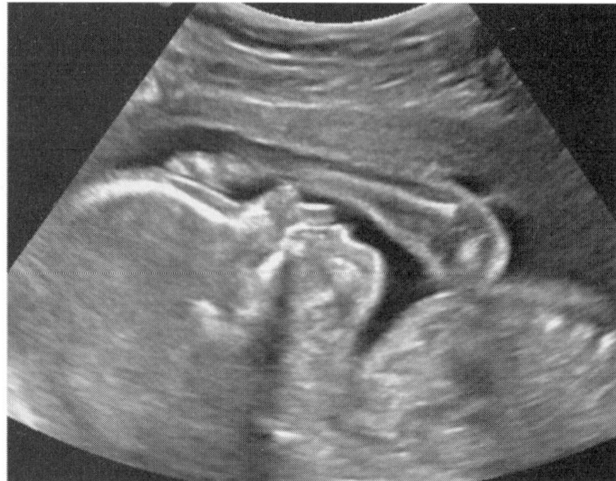

Figure 14.19 Midline sagittal image of the fetal head showing a normal fetal profile.

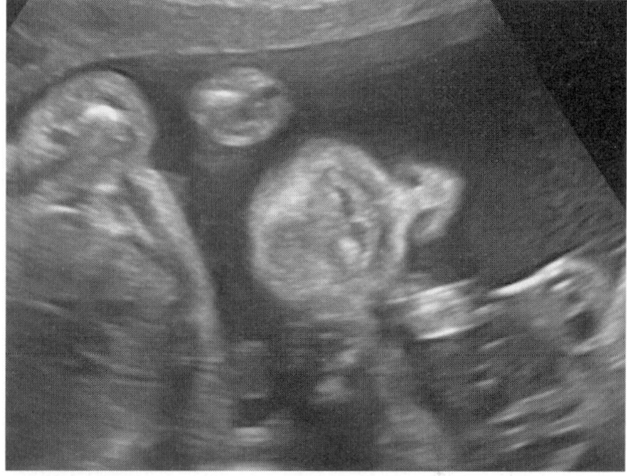

Figure 14.20 Coronal view of the face showing the fetal lips and nares.

tube defects. However, definitive proof any clinical advantage over 2D ultrasound techniques is lacking at this time.

The popularity of "keepsake" ultrasounds has grown significantly along with the availability of 3D imaging transducers and software for generalist obstetric providers. Both ACOG and the AIUM discourage the use of obstetric ultrasound for non-medical purposes. The use of either 2D or 3D ultrasound solely to take photos of the fetus without medical indication is considered to be inappropriate.[16] Nonetheless, many obstetricians have felt this statement applies only to entertainment keepsake video locations that do not

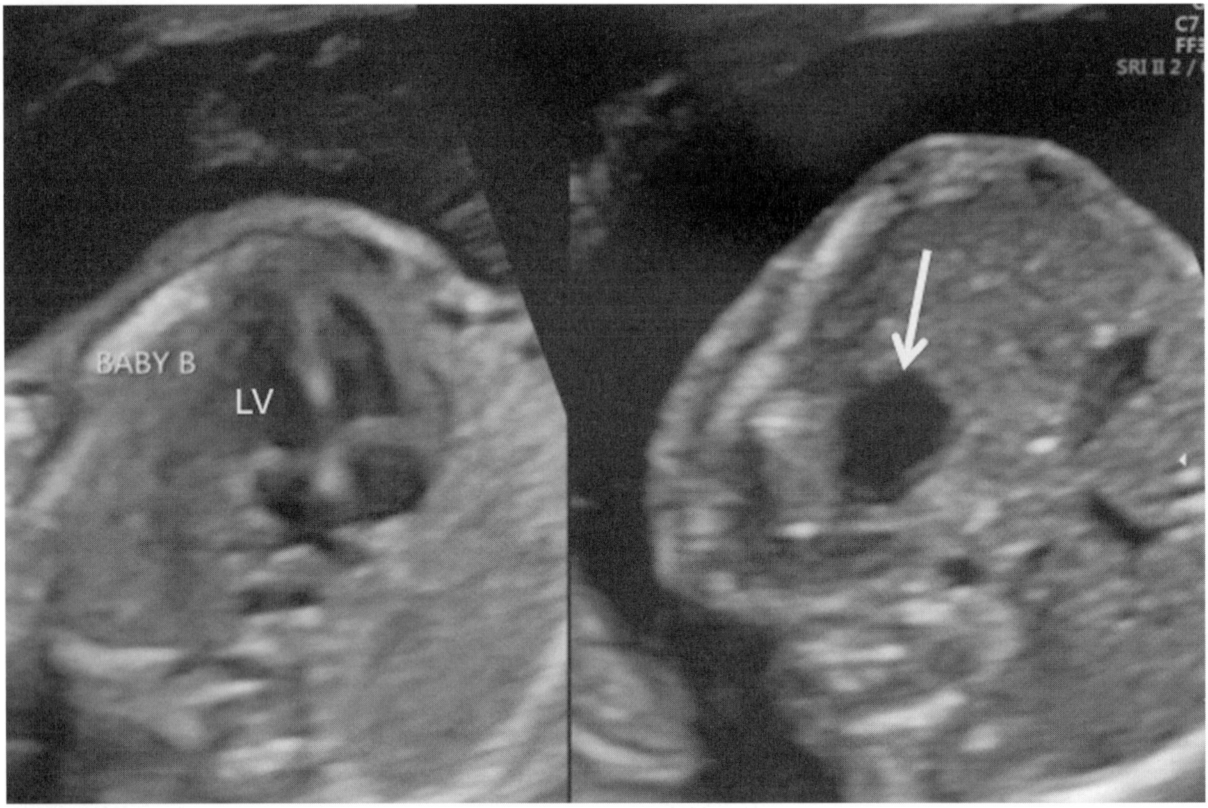

Figure 14.21 Split screen image shows four chamber heart on left image, with correct situs of stomach (arrow) on right image. The stomach is obtained by moving the transducer inferiorly from the same axial plane as the heart. Left ventricle (LV).

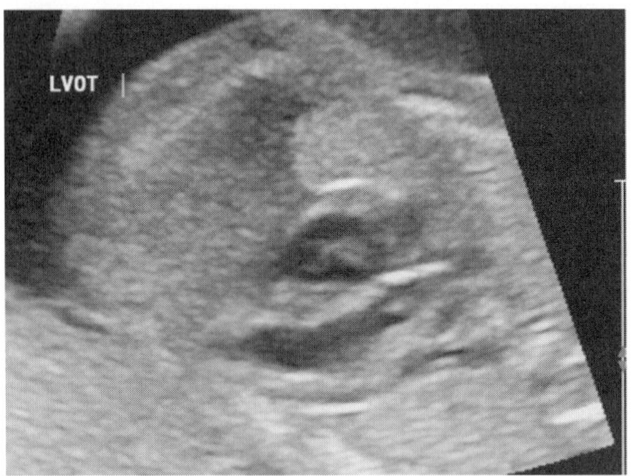

Figure 14.22 Ultrasound image showing the right ventricle (RV) and left ventricle (LV). Image shows the left ventricular outflow tract (LVOT) with arrow on ventricular septum.

provide any medical or obstetric care. Therefore, many obstetric practices now routinely provide images (both 2D and 3D) to their patients as part of their routine obstetric care.

Concluding Remarks

Obstetric ultrasound has clearly become the norm for obstetric care in the United States. The indications for, parameters of, and technological aspects of performing basic obstetric ultrasound are well within the scope of practice for the generalist obstetrician. Each physician who provides interpretation of obstetric ultrasounds should develop and maintain the requisite knowledge required to recognize the anatomy evaluated in the basic ultrasound examination. Furthermore, AIUM accreditation is encouraged.

In addition, although it is beyond the scope of this chapter, a more extensive review of commonly identified normal and abnormal anatomy can help the generalist to recognize that something is abnormal when they are not able to document the normal anatomic structure in question. It is not within the scope of responsibility of the generalist to necessarily be able to identify the anomaly. Rather the generalist needs to be able to recognize that failure to document a normal

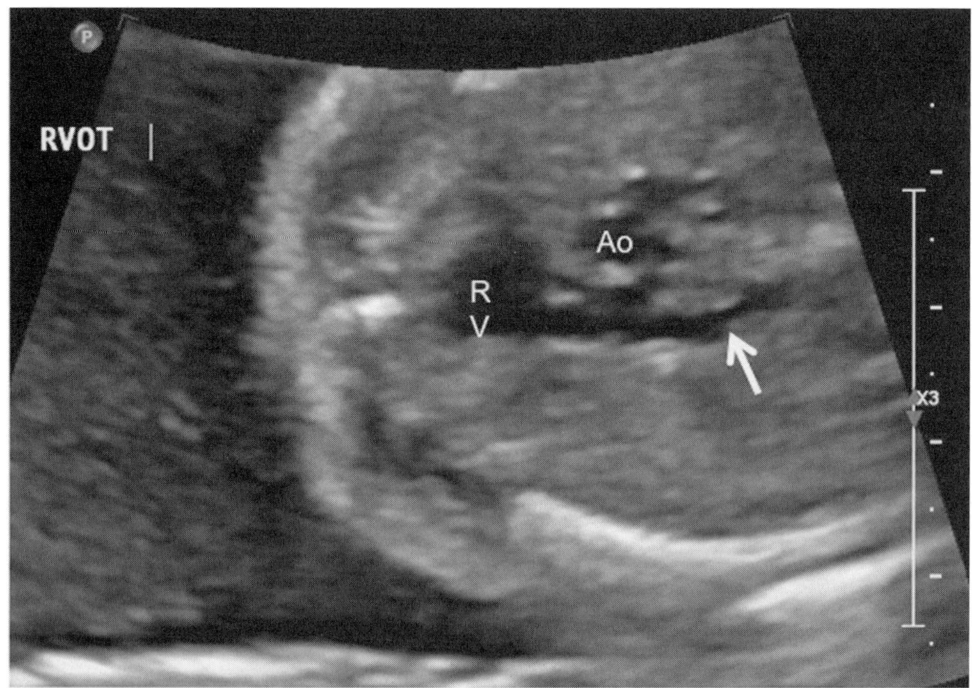

Figure 14.23 Ultrasound image of the right ventricular outflow tract (RVOT) with aortic root (Ao) and ductus arteriosus (arrow). RV = right ventricle.

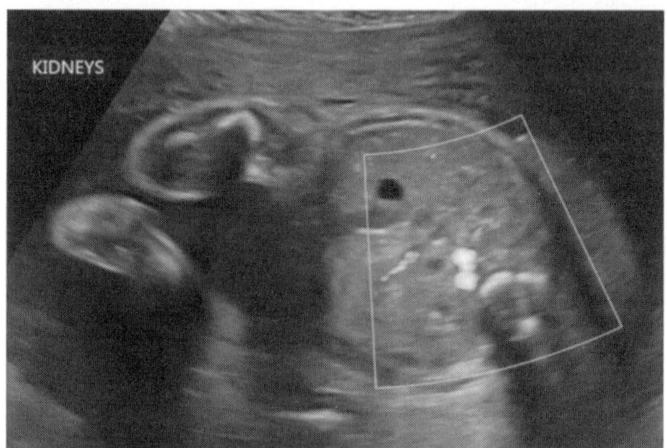

Figure 14.24 Kidneys. Axial view of the fetal abdomen with color Doppler application. The two kidneys are seen cross-sectional view and the color shows the renal arteries.

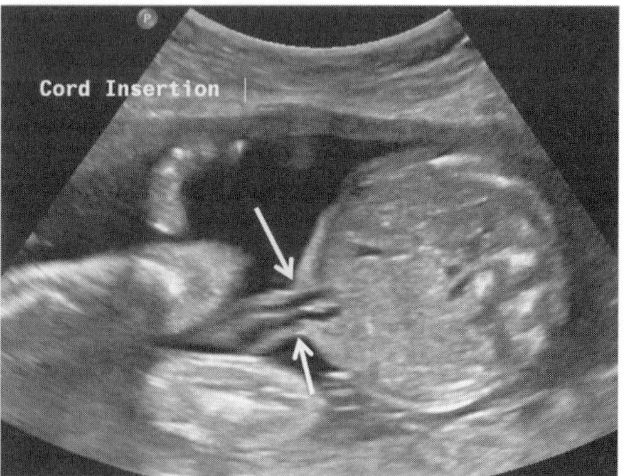

Figure 14.25 Axial view of the fetal abdomen showing the umbilical cord insertion (arrows).

structure should generate a referral to a subspecialist trained to identify and further evaluate the abnormal fetus.

Finally, an oft-ignored aspect of the obstetric ultrasound examination is the patient experience. For many patients, the obstetric ultrasound is one of the best experiences in during pregnancy, and the great majority of patients will be reassured by the results. Therefore, making the experience as comfortable as possible can serve to facilitate a good patient experience and enhance the patient perception of the obstetric practice. While these aspects are not "medically necessary," they contribute to a positive patient experience.

In many ultrasound suites, patients are instructed to fill their bladders by drinking multiple glasses of water in the 1–2 hours prior to their examination and then not to void. This often causes significant patient discomfort, but is also unnecessary in obstetric examinations as the amniotic fluid almost always provides an adequate acoustical window to allow satisfactory

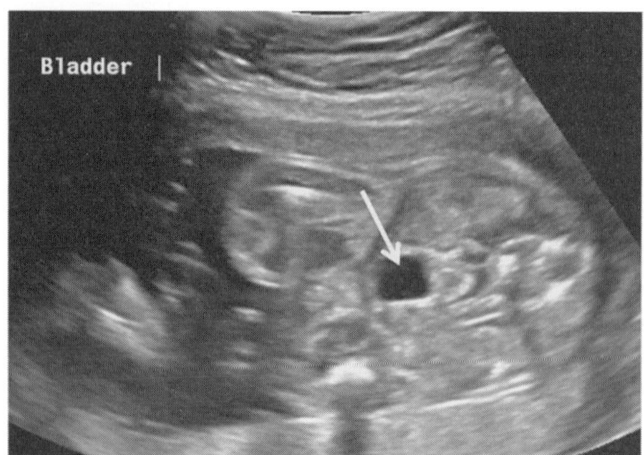

Figure 14.26 Axial view of the fetal abdomen showing the anechoic fetal bladder (arrow).

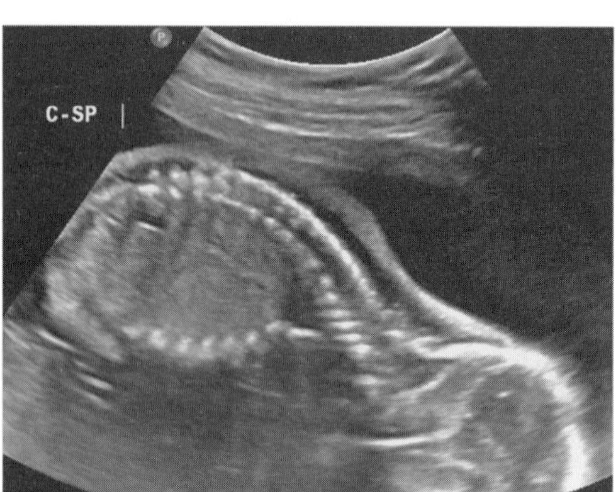

Figure 14.27 Mid-sagittal image of cervical and upper thoracic spine.

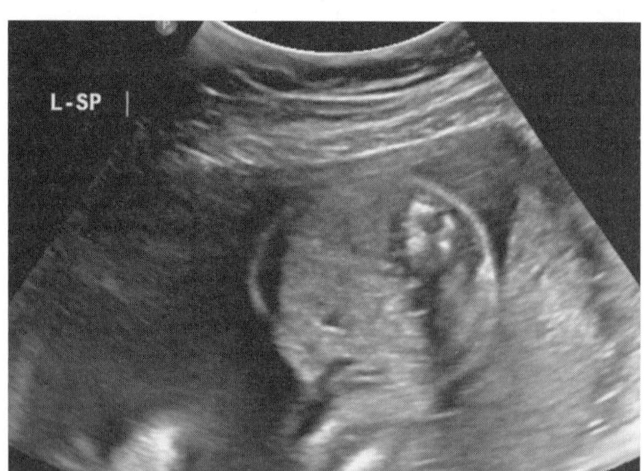

Figure 14.28 Axial image of the lumbar spine.

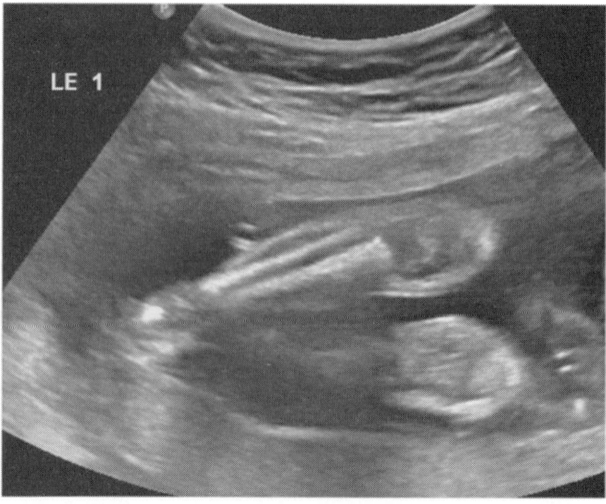

Figure 14.29 Image showing parallel views of tibia and fibula with foot coming toward or away from the sonographer.

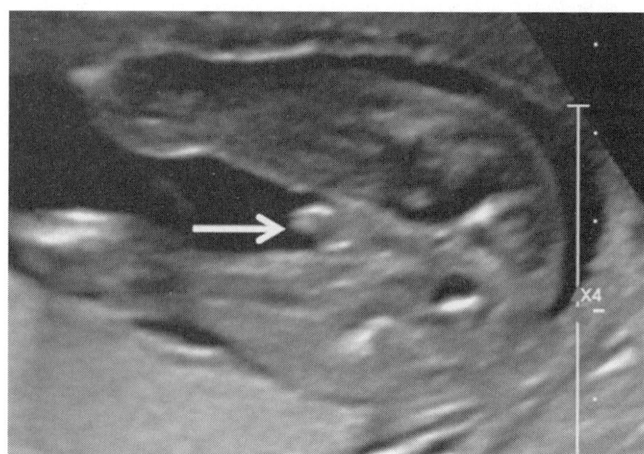

Figure 14.30 Ultrasound image of male genitalia (arrow).

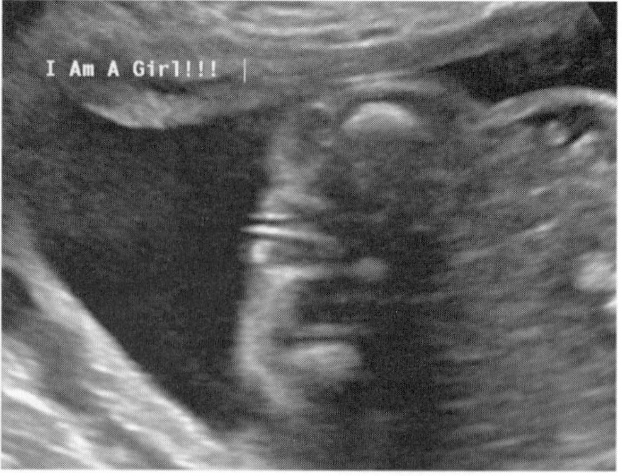

Figure 14.31 Ultrasound image of the female genitalia.

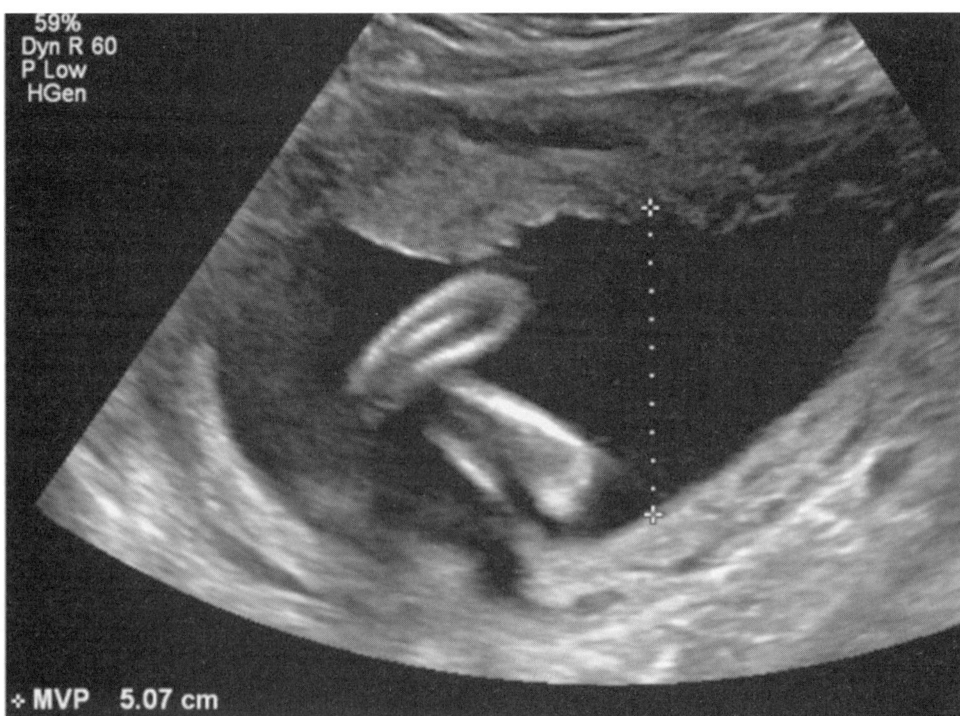

Figure 14.32 Ultrasound image show a measurement of the maximal vertical pocket.

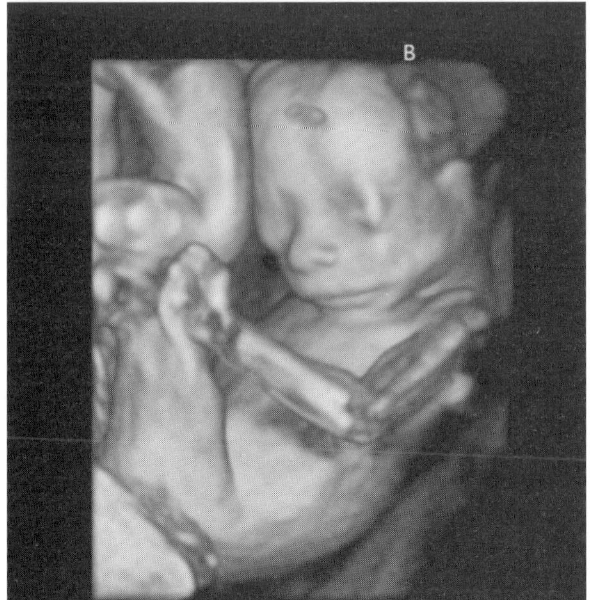

Figure 14.33 3D surface rendering of fetal face and body.

imaging. Allowing the patient to void normally prior to examination is patient friendly and will not tend to have any deleterious effect on the performance of the examination.

Placement of a large TV monitor on the wall in the ultrasound suite can allow the patient to view the examination easily without having to turn her neck sideways to view on the ultrasound monitor; this also allows the examiner to maintain a proper viewing angle for the monitor. Explaining the examination as it progresses can also enhance the patient experience. Simply pointing out the anatomic structures during the exam provides both reassurance and greater patient understanding of the procedure. Finally, providing the patient with a few 2D or 3D photos either in print or on a CD only takes a few minutes and can serve to decrease some patients' perceived need to visit the mall for a "keepsake video."

Acknowledgments

The authors would like to acknowledge Darleen Cioffi-Ragan, BS, RDMS, RDCS, RVT for providing many of the ultrasound images presented herein.

References

1. American College of Obstetricians and Gynecologists. ACOG Practice Bulletin Number 101. Ultrasonography in Pregnancy. February 2009: 5.

2. American Institute of Ultrasound in Medicine. AIUM Practice Parameter for the Performance of Obstetric Ultrasound Examinations. 2013. www.aium.org/resources/guidelines/obstetric.pdf. Accessed May 3, 2016.
3. American College of Obstetricians and Gynecologists. ACOG Practice Bulletin Number 101. Ultrasonography in Pregnancy. February 2009.
4. American Institute of Ultrasound in Medicine. Practice guideline for documentation of an ultrasound examination. *J Ultrasound Med* 2014;33(12):2219–24.
5. Ang ESBC, Gluncic V, Duque A, Schafer ME, Rakic P. Prenatal exposure to ultrasound waves impacts neuronal migration in mice. *Proc Natl Acad Sci* 2006; 103(34): 12903–10.
6. American Institute of Ultrasound in Medicine. Official Statement. As Low as Reasonably Achievable (ALARA) Principle. 2014.
7. American Institute of Ultrasound in Medicine. Official Statement. Prudent Use and Clinical Safety. March 2007.
8. Dasche JS, McIntire DD, Twickler DM. Effect of maternal obesity on the ultrasound detection of anomalous fetuses. *Obstet Gynecol* 2009 May;113(5):1001–7.
9. American College of Obstetricians and Gynecologists. ACOG Practice Bulletin Number 145. Antepartum Fetal Surveillance. July 2014.
10. American Institute of Ultrasound in Medicine. Practice guideline for the performance of obstetric ultrasound examinations. *J Ultrasound Med* 2013:32 (6); 1083–101.
11. American College of Obstetricians and Gynecologists. ACOG Practice Bulletin Number 101. Ultrasonography in Pregnancy. February 2009.
12. American College of Obstetricians and Gynecologists. ACOG Practice Bulletin Number 130. Prediction and Prevention of Preterm Birth. October 2012.
13. Levi S. Ultrasound in prenatal diagnosis: polemics around routine ultrasound screening for second trimester fetal malformations. *Prenat Diagn* 2002;22(4):285–95.
14. Hobbins J. *Obstetric Ultrasound: Artistry in Practice.* Blackwell, 2008, p. 7.
15. Manning FA, Platt LD, Sipos L: Antepartum fetal evaluation: Development of a fetal biophysical profile. *Am J Obstet Gynecol* 1980; 787–95.
16. American College of Obstetricians and Gynecologists. Nonmedical Use of Obstetric Ultrasonography. Committee Opinion Number 297. August 2004.

Prenatal Diagnosis

Heather Anaya and Alexandria Betz

Introduction

Prenatal diagnosis of genetic abnormalities should be offered to all pregnant women. Chromosomal abnormalities will occur in 1 of 160 live births.[1] Biochemical serum screening for Down syndrome (Trisomy 21) was first performed in 1984.[2] Since then, screening techniques have become more accurate and advanced. Most recently, the advent of cell free fetal DNA (cfDNA) aneuploidy screening, which is 99% sensitive for Trisomy 21, has been implemented.[3] Screening tests evaluate for abnormal levels of hormones that suggest an increased risk of Trisomy 21, Trisomy 18, or an open neural tube defect (ONTD). cfDNA screening also detects the fetal sex. The main disadvantage of screening is that not all abnormal fetuses are identified, and false-positive results can occur, leading to additional unnecessary worry and, possibly, invasive procedures. The advantage of serum screening is that it provides a risk assessment for a fetal chromosome abnormality or ONTD without the risk of an invasive procedure.[2] Furthermore, although ultrasound examinations provide information about the fetus, approximately 50% of babies with Trisomy 21 have no abnormalities detectable on ultrasound. Thus, an ultrasound examination cannot be relied upon to effectively screen for Trisomy 21.[4] It is important to understand these screening and diagnostic tests so that appropriate counseling can be provided to the patient. Additionally, some congenital infections are able to be suspected prenatally via ultrasound and confirmed by invasive modalities.

Scope of the Problem

Each year, there are approximately 6,000 babies born with Down syndrome, which is about 1 in every 700 babies born.[5] The incidence of Trisomy 21 increases with advancing maternal age. In 1984, biochemical serum screening for Trisomy 21 in women younger than 35 years was first performed. Low maternal serum alpha-fetoprotein (msAFP) levels were reported to be associated with Trisomy 21. msAFP values are even lower in Trisomy 18. Increasing data has shown the advantages of multiple biochemical markers (particularly msAFP, b-hCG, uE3, PAPP-A, and Inhibin) and biophysical screening (via ultrasound) with substantial improvements in prenatal screening sensitivity. cfDNA provides an excellent screening option for the high-risk population; this option may be extended to the low-risk population in the near future. Chrionic villus sampling (CVS) and amniocentesis are available testing options that have maintained significance in prenatal testing.

Counseling

All pregnant women should be offered aneuploidy screening before 20 weeks of gestation. A woman's provider must be able to discuss strengths, risks, and limitations of all testing. Every screening test has the risk of a false-negative result – where an affected fetus is not detected. Similarly, there is a risk for a false-positive – where an abnormal result is obtained, however there is no abnormality identified. Patients should understand that a "positive screen result" does not mean that the patient's baby has the disease, instead it means that their baby has an increased risk of having a chromosome abnormality beyond the set threshold for that test. When counseling these patients regarding their results, it is important to remember that a risk assessment of 1:200 means that 199 normal fetuses will be require additional testing. An abnormal result on serum screening should prompt a detailed ultrasound examination and discussion of diagnostic options. Similarly, if a woman is a candidate for cfDNA screening and chooses this test, she should be counseled that a positive result should be confirmed with a diagnostic procedure.

Invasive Testing (CVS, Amniocentesis)

CVS and amniocentesis are the two invasive diagnostic options available in pregnancy. CVS is typically offered after 10 weeks of gestation, while an amniocentesis is offered after 15 weeks of gestation. Both tests obtain cells that are sent for fetal karyotyping and are 99.9% accurate in detecting a chromosome abnormality. These tests can also be used in situations where there is a known, identified genetic mutation present in one or both of the parents. The advantage of CVS is that it can be performed earlier in gestation than amniocentesis. These tests can also detect proteins that are elevated with an open neural tube defect. As these are invasive procedures, there is a risk of bleeding, infection, rupture of membranes, and pregnancy loss. The risks associated with CVS and amniocentesis are thought to be similar with regard to pregnancy loss, approximately 1 in 300–500 losses per procedure.[6]

First Trimester Ultrasound: Nuchal Translucency

In the 1990s, the thickness of a fluid collection at the posterior aspect of the fetal neck was noted to be associated with trisomy 21.[7] The thickness of this fluid collection was termed a "nuchal translucency."[2] The nuchal translucency can be measured in fetuses between 11 and 14 weeks gestation.[8] As the normal thickness is dependent upon gestational age and crown–rump length, the nuchal translucency is given a gestational age-specific multiple of the median.[8]

A thickened nuchal translucency (usually defined as greater than 3 mm) is associated with chromosomal abnormalities (such as Trisomy 21 and monosomy X) as well as structural abnormalities (most commonly, heart defects). Other structural abnormalities that are associated with an increased nuchal translucency include a diaphragmatic hernia, severe skeletal defect, and omphalocele.[9] Approximately one-third of fetuses with an increased nuchal translucency will have a chromosome abnormality, with Trisomy 21 representing half of these chromosomal abnormalities.[10] While a thickened nuchal translucency can be a marker for an abnormal fetus, it can also be seen in a normal fetus. In fact, once chromosomal defects are ruled out, in 90% of cases where the nuchal translucency is greater than 3 mm but smaller than 4.5 mm, the fetus can be expected to be healthy. In a fetus with a nuchal translucency between 4.5 and 6.5 mm, 80% of births will result in a healthy neonate. In a fetus with a significantly increased nuchal translucency (greater than 6.5 mm), there is only a 45% chance of a healthy neonate.[11]

Since a thickened nuchal translucency can be associated with significant anatomic abnormalities, all women with this finding should be offered a detailed ultrasound examination and fetal echocardiogram.[12] These pregnancies also remain at an increased risk for miscarriage, fetal demise, low birth weight, and preterm birth.[13]

First Trimester Biochemical Screen

Two maternal serum analytes are utilized in the first trimester screening test: pregnancy-associated plasma protein A (PAPP-A) and the beta subunit of human chorionic gonadotropin (b-hCG). Pregnancies affected by Trisomy 21 typically have a low PAPP-A (0.4 MoM) and an elevated beta-hCG (1.8 MoM).[14] When the PAPP-A and b-hCG results are combined with the nuchal translucency, the Trisomy 21 detection rate is approximately 88% with a 5% screen positive rate.[15] These analytes can also be used to identify pregnancies affected by Trisomy 18 with a detection rate of approximately 90%.[16] In Trisomy 18, the levels of both markers are reduced.[2]

The advantage of the first trimester screen is that women receive results earlier in the pregnancy.[2] These results from the first trimester can be combined with additional analytes collected in the second trimester in a test called the integrated screen. Details of this test can be found in the second trimester biochemical screen section.

Cell-Free Fetal DNA Testing

Cell-free DNA (cfDNA) testing takes advantage of the fact that after 10 weeks of gestation approximately 10–15% of the total cfDNA in the maternal plasma is of placental origin.[17] This provides screening for Trisomy 21, 18, 13, and sex chromosomal abnormalities. The accuracy of the results depends upon the amount of DNA that is present and the chance that an abnormality exists.[18] In some women, the test will be unable to be completed, which is considered a failed result. It is important to remember that this result is still associated with an increased risk and diagnostic testing options should be offered.[18] Unlike the *integrated screen*, cfDNA does not screen for open neural tube defects and so testing for msAFP should be offered to these women if they are interested in this screening.

cfDNA screening is not the appropriate choice for first-line screening for the low-risk population at the present time. For this population, conventional screening methods remain the preferred approach.

Cystic Fibrosis

Cystic fibrosis (CF) is the most common autosomal recessive disease among Caucasian populations with a carrier frequency of 1/25. It is a disease that commonly causes frequent pulmonary infections and pancreatic insufficiency. Life expectancy is reduced with pulmonary complications often leading to death.[19] The gene mutation is on chromosome 7. In the United States, it is reasonable to offer screening for cystic fibrosis to all pregnant women.[19] Screening tests for the most common mutations, however not all of the 1,700 mutations, are tested, making this screening most useful in a high-risk population (such as Ashkenazi Jew and non-Hispanic white).[19] When counseling a patient regarding screening for CF, the clinician must remember that although a negative screen is reassuring, this patient can still have a child affected by cystic fibrosis. If a patient does not opt for screening, cystic fibrosis screening is included in the newborn screening panel; however, this does not give information about the parent's carrier status.[19]

Preconception and Prenatal Carrier Screening for Genetic Diseases in Individuals of Eastern European Jewish Descent

An individual's ancestry is an important component of information to determine additional screening options. There are autosomal recessive conditions that are seen more frequently in certain ethnic populations, in particular Eastern European Jewish (Ashkenazi) descent.[20] The American College of Medical Genetics has recommended additional carrier screening for these women. In particular, these women should be tested for Tay–Sachs disease, Canavan disease, cystic fibrosis, and familial dysautonomia. These carrier tests have a sensitivity of 94–99%. There are additional carrier screening tests that can be offered for more rare diseases. These include Fanconi anemia group C, Niemann–Pick disease type A, Bloom syndrome, mucolipidosis IV, and Gaucher disease.[20]

If these tests are offered, the patient should be counseled that testing is voluntary. In counseling, it is important to remind the patient that if she and her partner screen negative for carrier status, which is reassuring. However, not all carriers can be identified with screening tests, and so the chance remains of the couple having a child that is affected.

Second Trimester Options

Maternal Serum Screen (Quad Marker Screen)

In the second trimester, the levels of msAFP, unconjugated estriol, b-hCG and inhibin A are measured; this is called the *quad marker screen*. The detection rate for Trisomy 21 and 18 is slightly less than the first trimester screen with a Trisomy 21 detection rate of 75% in women younger than 35 years old, and 92% in women older than 35 years with a false-positive rate of 13%.[21] In patients with a fetus affected by Trisomy 21, the average maternal serum AFP is decreased, as is unconjugated estriol; b-hCG and inhibin are increased.[2] In Trisomy 18, the msAFP, b-hCG, and estriol are all reduced.[2]

The integrated screen is a two-part test that combines the results from analytes drawn in the first trimester, the nuchal translucency, and analytes drawn in the second trimester, to assess the risk for certain chromosome abnormalities. Between 10 and 14 weeks, the nuchal translucency is obtained and the first blood draw is performed to evaluate the value of PAPP-A. Then, the patient is instructed to return between 15 and 22 weeks for a second blood draw that measures msAFP, unconjugated estriol, b-hCG, and Inhibin-A. The integrated screen combines these measurements with the nuchal translucency to provide a final risk assessment. This algorithm has a detection rate for Trisomy 21 and 18 of approximately 95% with a 5% false-positive rate. This screening is sensitive and specific, but provides later prenatal diagnosis compared to the first trimester screen.

In contrast to the integrated screen, patients who undergo the sequential screen are notified of the first trimester result.[2]

In the first and second trimester evaluation of risk (FASTER) trial, the detection rate for the integrated screen was 94–96% with a 5% screen positive rate, if using analytes from the first and second trimester, plus the nuchal translucency.[22] The integrated screen can also be performed without incorporating a nuchal measurement and the detection rate is 85–88%.[23]

There is some criticism that this screening test only detects 94–96% of Trisomy 21, compared to the cfDNA screening which detects 99%. In a low-risk population, however, the integrated screen remains the superior test. It is important to remember that serum screening has a high detection rate for abnormal analytes, which can help detect a woman who may have a high risk of adverse pregnancy outcomes. These women may be falsely reassured by a normal cfDNA result, but may still remain at increased risk for other abnormalities, which could have been suspected by an abnormal integrated screen.

Ultrasound Markers for Abnormalities

Trisomy 21

On an ultrasound examination, certain specific findings are associated with Trisomy 21 and, when found, can increase the baseline risk for having an affected pregnancy. These are seen in Box 15.1.[24]

Omphalocele and Gastroschisis

A detailed anatomy ultrasound is performed at 18–20 weeks and can identify a majority of anatomical defects; however, some anomalies can be detected as early as the first trimester. Examples include open neural tube defects, such as anencephaly, and open abdominal wall defects, such as gastroschisis or omphalocele. Open neural tube defects (ONTDs) affect 1–2/1,000 births in the general population. Risk factors for an omphalocele include advanced maternal age and assisted reproductive technology.[25] Low socioeconomic status, tobacco abuse, young maternal age, and vasoactive drug use are risk factors for gastroschisis.[26] Amniocentesis of a patient with gastroschisis will reveal elevated levels of acetylcholinesterase but that may not be the case with omphalocele. This is because nerve endings are open to amniotic fluid only in gastroschisis.

Box 15.1 Abnormal findings on ultrasound associated with Trisomy 21

- Increased nuchal fold > 6 mm (this occurs in only 0.7% of normal fetuses)
- A hypoplastic or absent nasal bone (this occurs in only 1–2% of unaffected pregnancies)
- Short humerus
- Short femur
- Echogenic bowel greater than bone
- Pyelectasis
- Echogenic intracardiac focus as bright as bone (this occurs in 5% of normal pregnancies)

Abnormal Second-Trimester Serum Markers

In Trisomy 21, the PAPP-A, msAFP, and unconjugated estriol tend to be low, while inhibin A and b-HCG are usually elevated.[2]

In Trisomy 18, msAFP, b- hCG, and estriol all tend to be low.

msAFP

An elevated msAFP can be associated with ONTD or abdominal wall defects. This analyte can be affected by an incorrect gestational age, insulin-dependent diabetes mellitus, maternal weight, and ethnicity.[27,28] The msAFP will rise during the screening interval, and so a miscalculated gestational age can result in an inaccurate result. Black women have a 10–15% higher msAFP than non-Blacks. Also, an increased maternal weight will lower the msAFP value as a result of dilution from the larger blood volume.[29] The msAFP cut-off for an abnormal value is 2–2.5 MoM.

If the msAFP is elevated, an ultrasound should be performed to evaluate for an open neural tube defect or abdominal wall defect.[29] Although an ultrasound examination is a highly effective screening tool for open neural tube defects, the patient should be counseled regarding the option of obtaining an amniotic fluid AFP and acetylcholinesterase. The combination of amniotic fluid AFP and acetylcholinesterase has a nearly 100% detection rate for anencephaly and a 96–99% detection rate for spina bifida.[30] If these proteins are elevated but an open neural tube defect or abdominal wall defect is not visualized, other causes should be considered, including exstrophy of the bladder, weeping skin lesions, a sacrococcygeal teratoma, fetal urinary tract obstruction, and congenital Finnish nephrosis.[31]

If the amniotic fluid proteins are normal, then the elevated msAFP is likely due to a problem with the maternal-fetal interface. As a result, these women have an increased risk for intrauterine growth restriction, fetal death, premature delivery, oligohydramnios, placental abruption, and pre-eclampsia.[32] An adverse outcome is highest when the msAFP is greater than 5.0 MoM.[33] Unfortunately, no specific management has been recommended for these women to decrease their risk of poor pregnancy outcomes.

b-hCG

An unexplained elevated b-hCG (greater than 2.0 MoM) is associated with an increased risk of pre-eclampsia, preterm birth, low birth weight, and fetal demise. The risk rises as the level of b-hCG increases. If both the b-hCG and msAFP are elevated, then the risk for adverse pregnancy outcomes is greater than 50%.[34]

Unconjugated Estriol

Low levels of unconjugated estriol (0.01 to 0.15 MoM) are associated with abnormalities including placental steroid sulfatase deficiency and Smith-Lemli-Opitz.[35,36]

Invasive Options

CVS

CVS is a diagnostic, invasive procedure that is usually performed as early as 10 weeks of gestation, which is earlier than the time when an amniocentesis can be offered.[37] A needle is inserted into the placenta to obtain chorionic villi, which are sent for karyotyping. Due to concerns for limb reduction defects, CVS should not be performed before 9 weeks gestation.[38] The placental villi can be accessed from either a transcervical or a transabdominal approach.[39] Vaginal spotting occurs in up to 30% of women after a transcervical CVS.[2] The overall miscarriage rate after CVS is higher than amniocentesis due to the earlier gestational age at which a CVS is performed. The miscarriage rate due to performance of the CVS is thought to be similar to amniocentesis, which is 1 in 300–500.[40]

Amniocentesis

An amniocentesis is a procedure in which a needle is passed through the maternal abdomen into the amniotic fluid. Genetic amniocentesis is typically offered between 15 and 20 weeks of gestation; however, it can be performed at any time during the pregnancy after 15 weeks gestation.[2] It is not offered prior to 15 weeks due to an increased risk of fetal clubfoot.[2] The procedure related loss rate is approximately 1/300–500,[41] with some studies showing no effect of a second trimester amniocentesis on fetal loss.[42] The loss rate does not increase with the number of separate procedures but does increase after three attempts.[43] Complications include vaginal spotting, amniotic fluid leakage (which occurs in 1–2%), and chorioamnionitis (which occurs in less than 1 in 1,000 cases).[2] If there is amniotic fluid leakage, there is a greater than 90% survival rate as resealing of the membranes frequently occurs.[44] Needle injuries to the fetus can occur, however, the procedure is performed under direct ultrasound guidance. The risk of failure of cell culture is rare and occurs in only 0.1% of samples. The diagnostic accuracy is greater than 99%.

FISH and CMA

Fluorescent in situ hybridization (FISH) is performed using labeled DNA sequences that are made for a specific chromosome.[45] FISH is usually performed on chromosomes 13, 18, 21, X, and Y with results available within 48 hours. FISH has a 99.8% concordance rate with standard genetics but allows earlier results for the more common chromosome abnormalities.[46] Chromosomal microarray (CMA) is an emerging technology that is becoming more commonplace as the test of choice for invasive genetic procedures. It has the advantage of providing more detailed information; however, there is a small risk of a result with no known identification in the literature.

Factors Specific for Multiple Gestations

Serum screening in multiple gestations is less accurate than in singletons. This is because an abnormal value from one fetus may be offset by the unaffected fetus.[47] Thus, serum screening tests are not offered to multiple gestations in all institutions. However, an option for prenatal screening is to perform a nuchal translucency measurement on each twin which has a 69% detection rate.[48] With regards to diagnostic chromosome testing in multiple gestations, tissue or fluid should be sampled from both fetuses in a dichorionic diamniotic twin gestation. Monozygotic twins originate from the same gamete, and so both fetuses should possess the same karyotype.[48] However, mitotic nondisjunction, where there are different karyotypes, may rarely occur. Thus, both fetuses in a monochorionic diamniotic gestation should be sampled.

Congenital Infections

Recommendations for Management for Cytomegalovirus (CMV)

See Chapter 46 for more detailed information on congenital infection. One example is the most common cause of viral intrauterine infection, cytomegalovirus (CMV). The rate of transmission from the mother to the fetus is highest in the third trimester, but the disease is more devastating if transmitted in the first trimester,[49] with about 15–20% of infected infants developing complications. The diagnosis can be made from polymerase chain reaction (PCR) on amniotic fluid. Ultrasound findings seen in CMV include: growth restriction, ventriculomegaly, oligohydramnios, echogenic bowel, pleural effusion, brain and liver calcification, and hydrops.[50] These abnormalities may be seen late after the disease is acquired, or may not be seen at all in a fetus that is still affected by CMV. Antenatal treatment options are limited and experimental at this time.

Concluding Remarks

Prenatal screening and diagnostic options should be offered and discussed with all pregnant women. Appropriate counseling takes into account gestational age, patient age, and ethnicity. Prenatal testing encompasses biophysical testing (ultrasound) as well as laboratory evaluation for aneuploidy, anomalies, and congenital infections. Multiple gestation pregnancies have more limited options for prenatal testing.

References

1. Driscoll D, Gross S. Prenatal screening for aneuploidy. *N Engl J Med* 2009;360:2556–2562.
2. American Congress of Obstetricians and Gynecologists: Screening for Fetal Chromosomal Abnormalities, 2007 Jan. Practice Bulletin: 77.
3. Palomaki GE, Kloza EM, Lambert-Messerlian GM, et al. DNA sequencing of maternal plasma to detect Down syndrome: An international clinical validation study. *Genet Med* 2011 Nov;13:913–20.
4. Offerdal K, Blaas H, Eik-Nes S. Prenatal detection of trisomy 21 by second-trimester ultrasound examination and maternal age in a non-selected population of 49 314 births in Norway. *Ultrasound Obstet Gynecol* 2008;32:493–500.
5. Centers for Disease Control and Prevention. *Division of Birth Defects and Developmental Disabilities*; 2016.
6. Caughey AB, Hopkins LM, Norton ME. Chorionic villus sampling compared with amniocentesis and the difference in the rate of pregnancy loss. *Obstet Gynecol* 2006;108: 612–616.
7. Nicolaides KH, Snijders RJ, Gosden CM, Berry C, Campbell S. Ultrasonographically detectable markers of fetal chromosomal abnormalities. *Lancet* 1992;340:704–707.
8. Creasy R, Resnik R, Iams J, Lockwood C, Moore T. *Creasy & Resnik's Maternal-Fetal Medicine Principles and Practice*. 6th rev. ed. Philadelphia: Elsevier Saunders; 2009. p. 227.
9. Souka AP, Snijders RJ, Novakov A, et al. Defects and syndromes in chromosomally normal fetuses with increased nuchal translucency thickness at 10–14 weeks of gestation. *Ultrasound Obstet Gynecol* 1998; 11:391.
10. Snijders RJ, Noble P, Sebire N, Souka A, Nicolaides KH. UK multicentre project on assessment of risk of trisomy 21 by maternal age and fetal nuchal-translucency thickness at 10–14 weeks of gestation. Fetal Medicine Foundation First Trimester Screening Group. *Lancet* 1998;352:343–346.
11. Souka AP, Snijders RJ, Novakov A, et al. Defects and syndromes in chromosomally normal fetuses with increased nuchal translucency thickness at 10–14 weeks of gestation. *Ultrasound Obstet Gynecol* 1998; 11:391.
12. Makrydimas G, Sotiriadis A, Huggon IC, et al. Nuchal translucency and fetal cardiac defects: a pooled analysis of major fetal echocardiography centers. *Am J Obstet Gynecol* 2005;192:89–95.
13. Dugoff L, Hobbins JC, Malone FD, et al. First-trimester maternal serum PAPP-A and free-beta subunit human chorionic gonadotropin concentrations and nuchal translucency are associated with obstetric complications: A population-based screening study (the FASTER Trial). *Am J Obstet Gynecol* 2004;191:1446–1451.
14. Creasy R, Resnik R, Iams J, Lockwood C, Moore T. *Creasy & Resnik's Maternal-Fetal Medicine Principles and Practice*. 6th rev. ed. PA;2009.p. 229.
15. Malone FD, Canick JA, Ball RH, et al. First-trimester or second-trimester screening, or both, for Down's syndrome. *N Engl J Med* 2005;353:2001–2011.
16. Wapner RJ, Thom E, Simpson JL, et al. First-trimester screening for trisomies 21 and 18. *N Engl J Med* 2003; 349:1405–1413.
17. Norton M, Brar H, Weiss J, Karimi A, et al. Non-Invasive Chromosomal Evaluation (NICE) Study: results of a multicenter prospective cohort study for detection of fetal trisomy 21 and trisomy 18. *Am J Obstet Gynecol* 2012;137:1–8.
18. Society for Maternal-Fetal Medicine (SMFM): Prenatal aneuploidy screening using cell-free DNA, 2015 Jun. No. 36.
19. American Congress of Obstetricians and Gynecologists: Update on Carrier Screening for Cystic Fibrosis, 2011 April. No. 486.
20. American Congress of Obstetricians and Gynecologists: Preconception and Prenatal Carrier Screening for Genetic Diseases in Individuals of Eastern European Jewish Descent, 2009 Oct. No. 482.

21. Wapner RJ, Thom E, Simpson JL, et al. First-trimester screening for trisomies 21 and 18. *N Engl J Med* 2003; 349:1405–1413.

22. Cuckle HS, Malone FD, Wright D, et al. Contingent screening for Down syndrome – results from the FaSTER trial. *Prenat Diagn* 2008;28:89–94.

23. Malone F, Canick JA, Ball RH, et al. First-trimester or second-trimester screening, or both, for Down's syndrome. First- and Second-Trimester Evaluation of Risk (FASTER) Research Consortium. *N Engl J Med* 2005;353:2001–2011.

24. Creasy R, Resnik R, Iams J, Lockwood C, Moore T. *Creasy & Resnik's Maternal-Fetal Medicine Principles and Practice*. 6th rev. ed. PA; 2009. p. 225.

25. Creasy R, Resnik R, Iams J, Lockwood C, Moore T. *Creasy & Resnik's Maternal-Fetal Medicine Principles and Practice*. 7th rev. ed. PA; 2014. p. 340.

26. Creasy R, Resnik R, Iams J, Lockwood C, Moore T. *Creasy & Resnik's Maternal-Fetal Medicine Principles and Practice*. 6th rev. ed. PA; 2014.p. 334.

27. O'Brien JE, Dvorin E, Drugan A, et al. Race-ethnicity-specific variation in multiple-marker biochemical screening: alpha-fetoprotein, hCG, and estriol. *Obstet Gynecol* 1997; 89:355.

28. Wald NJ, Cuckle H, Boreham J, et al. Maternal serum alpha-fetoprotein and diabetes mellitus. *Br J Obstet Gynaecol* 1979; 86:101.

29. Creasy R, Resnik R, Iams J, Lockwood C, Moore T. *Creasy & Resnik's Maternal-Fetal Medicine Principles and Practice*. 6th rev. ed. PA; 2009. p. 234.

30. Crandall BF, and Matsumoto M: Routine amniotic fluid alphafetoprotein assay: experience with 40,000 pregnancies. *Am J Med Genet* 1986; 24:143.

31. Creasy R, Resnik R, Iams J, Lockwood C, Moore T. *Creasy & Resnik's Maternal-Fetal Medicine Principles and Practice*. 6th rev. ed. PA; 2009. p. 235.

32. Creasy R, Resnik R, Iams J, Lockwood C, Moore T. *Creasy & Resnik's Maternal-Fetal Medicine Principles and Practice*. 6th rev. ed. PA; 2009. p. 234.

33. Crandall BF, Robinson L, and Grau P. Risks associated with an elevated maternal serum alpha-fetoprotein level. *Am J Obstet Gynecol* 1991;165:581.

34. Kuller JA, Sellati LE, Chescheir NC, et al. Outcome of pregnancies with elevation of both maternal serum alpha-fetoprotein and human chorionic gonadotropin. *Am J Perinatol* 1995; 12:93.

35. Craig W, Palomaki G, Roberson M, Haddow J. Further insights into implications of undetectable or very low unconjugated estriol in maternal serum during the second trimester. *Prenatal Diagnosis* 2011; 31:616–618.

36. Craig WY, Haddow JE, Palomaki GE, et al. Identifying Smith-Lemli-Opitz syndrome in conjunction with prenatal screening for Down syndrome. *Prenat Diagn* 2006;26:842.

37. American Congress of Obstetricians and Gynecologists: Invasive Prenatal Testing for Aneuploidy. 2007 Dec. Practice Bulletin: 88.

38. Chorionic villus sampling and amniocentesis: recommendations for prenatal counseling. Centers for Disease Control and Prevention. MMWR Recomm Rep 1995;44.

39. Jackson LG, Zachary JM, Fowler SE, Desnick RJ, Golbus MS, Ledbetter DH, et al. A randomized comparison of transcervical and transabdominal chorionic-villus sampling. The U.S. National Institute of Child Health and Human Development Chorionic-Villus Sampling and Amniocentesis Study Group. *N Engl J Med* 1992;327:594–598.

40. Caughey AB, Hopkins LM, Norton ME. Chorionic villus sampling compared with amniocentesis and the difference in the rate of pregnancy loss. *Obstet Gynecol* 2006;108:612–616.

41. Eddleman KA, Malone FD, Sullivan L et al. Pregnancy loss rates after midtrimester amniocentesis. *Obstet Gynecol* 2006;108:1067–1072.

42. Mazza V, Pati M, Bertucci E, et al. Age-specific risk of fetal loss post second trimester amniocentesis: analysis of 5,043 cases. *Prenat Diagn* 2007;27:180–183.

43. Marthin T, Liedgren S, Hammar M. Transplacental needle passage and other risk-factors associated with second trimester amniocentesis. *Acta Obstet Gynecol Scand* 1997;76:728–732.

44. Borgida AF, Mills AA, Feldman DM, Rodis JF, Egan JF. Outcome of pregnancies complicated by ruptured membranes after genetic amniocentesis. *Am J Obstet Gynecol* 2000;183:937–939.

45. Creasy R, Resnik R, Iams J, Lockwood C, Moore T. *Creasy & Resnik's Maternal-Fetal Medicine Principles and Practice*. 6th rev. ed. PA; 2009.p. 249.

46. Sawa R, Hayashi Z, Tanaka T, et al. Rapid detection of chromosome aneuploidies by prenatal interphase FISH and its clinical utility in Japan. *J Obstet Gynecol Res* 2001;27:41–47.

47. Creasy R, Resnik R, Iams J, Lockwood C, Moore T. *Creasy & Resnik's Maternal-Fetal Medicine Principles and Practice*. 6th rev. ed. PA; 2009. p. 256.

48. Creasy R, Resnik R, Iams J, Lockwood C, Moore T. *Creasy & Resnik's Maternal-Fetal Medicine Principles and Practice*. 6th rev. ed. PA; 2009. p. 257.

49. Berghella V. *Maternal-Fetal Evidence Based Guidelines*. 2nd ed. UK; 2012. p. 348.

50. Lipitz S, Achiron R, Zalel Y, Mendelson E, Tepperberg M, Gamzu R. Outcome of pregnancies with vertical transmission of primary cytomegalovirus infection. *Obstet Gynecol* 2002;100:428–433.

Genetics

Selman I. Welt

Introduction

All women planning or in a pregnancy should receive genetic counseling. A number of tools for this patient care service are readily available on the Internet and through the medical specialty organizations such as the American Congress of Obstetrics and Gynecology (ACOG), the American College of Osteopathic Obstetrics and Gynecology (ACOOG) and the American Academy of Family Physicians (AAFP). It is estimated that at birth 2–3% of all newborns will have a recognizable structural defect. The number of individuals with defects increases with age, detecting less obvious problems and more subtle, developmental abnormalities with age.[1]

Counseling should include good family and personal genetic and reproductive history. Delineation of the relationships on a pedigree will aid with the relationships and help with the establishment of a genetic pattern.[2] If a genetic disorder is identified in the family, a careful evaluation should be performed to confirm the correct diagnosis of the disorder before additional counseling may proceed. If the disorder follows Mendelian inheritance the advice is fairly straightforward.[3] If it does not, then a more complex analysis is needed and consultation with a geneticist and counselor are needed. Numerous lists of indications for genetic counseling exist; these relate not only to the personal family history but also for populational risks, such as ethnic grouping, maternal age, or maternal medical condition. Examples may be found in text books,[1,4,5] and at several websites. Online Mendelian inheritance in Man,[6] the National Human Genome Research Institute,[7] the NIH Genetic Testing Registry[8] and the Genetic Home reference[9] are all established references.

In a family with a known abnormality and means of transmission, the next step would be to identify how that disorder will affect the index pregnancy and the fetus. Once this is established, a preliminary counseling session is undertaken to determine how far the evaluation will proceed, what the evaluation will mean and what risks and benefits exist for proceeding with additional testing, which may be invasive. A means of confirmation for diagnosis in the mother or baby should be attempted. At this point another decision is made because the means of determining this information may be potentially harmful or the information regarding the fetus may engender a moral dilemma. These daily problems arise in obstetrical care when working in the field of human genetics. Moral dilemmas are beyond the scope of this chapter. Early involvement of an ethicist or genetics counsellor with ethics training is strongly recommended.

Mendelian inheritance deals with the principles of unitary inheritance, allelic segregation and independent assortment.[1] These principles are modified by effects which alter the phenotype of a Mendelian based genotype; such factors as penetrance, expressivity and pleiotropy.[4] Some of these modifications have now been described at a molecular level. Triplet repeats of DNA, increased by chromatid crossing over during meiosis, explains some cases of penetrance and expressivity via anticipation. Imprinting with some of the genetic code in an inactive form explains the Angelman/Prader–Willi complex. Mitochondrial (mtDNA) inheritance may explain some variable expressivity.[5]

Genomics, the study of the genome, its organization and component parts as well as its functional analysis, was first posited in the 1980s with the completion of the Human Genome Project and the compilations and maps subsequently created in the decade of the 2000. Thus there is now extensive source material available for clinical practice.[4–7]

Scope of the Problem

There is a tremendous amount of variation in normal human populations and with this variation we see differences in the indigence and prevalence of disorders related to heredity. This may be secondary to the absence of certain genes in the population but more to the prevalence of such genes. An example is the higher rate of neural tube defects in the British Isles and Ireland than in the United States where many of their descendents are located. It is unclear, even now, how much genetics and how much environment means in this disorder's incidence. In the United States with an estimation of 0.5% chromosomal risk and 0.4% Mendelian inheritance risk plus another 1% compiled multifactorial risk, genetic counseling at the minimum, with a good family pedigree preparation is prudent care.[1]

Chromosomes

Chromosomal disorders work by modified Mendelian principles, unitary inheritance, allelic segregation and independent assortment but in which abnormal numbers of chromosomes, missing and added pieces or DNA and recombination's of DNA create different start and stop functions of DNA. These result in the formation of different protein products.[10] It will be evident below that these recombination's of DNA are extremely important with regard to the effects caused by inversions, translocations, mosaicisms and even chimerism.[11]

Conventional karyology is limited in that G banding is low resolution as are other chromosomal identifying techniques. There is the need for cell culture with specific treatments to arrange for the metaphase plate and proper lysis of cells to see the nuclei clearly. Thus, extended time is required to obtain results and subjective interpretations may occur. Alternatively, automated high throughput analysis is, at present, limited by a likelihood of missing microscopic rearrangements, deletions or duplications in the chromosomes.

Chromosomal terminology has been established by multiple international nomenclature meetings. The important terms to be understood for clinical practice are seen in Box 16.1. Two additional concepts, uniparental disomy and imprinting require specific explanation.

Uniparental disomy is where both members of a chromosome pair are inherited from the same parent. This may have a clinical significance depending upon the chromosomes involved. There are likely several means by which this occurs, one of them being when there is a trisomic conceptus with loss of the extra chromosome.

Box 16.1 Genetic terminology[1]

"P" refers to the short arm of the chromosome (petit) and "Q" to the long arm of the chromosome.

Three individual chromosomes in the complement is trisomy, four could be quadrasomy.

Twenty-three chromosomes to a human complement is a monoploidy (normal for sex cells); a normal complement is a diploidy and three complements is a triploidy.

A slash "/" in the karyology report implies different chromosomal lines as in mosaicism.

"Del" relates to a deletion of a specific chromosomal area.

"Dup" refers to a duplication of a specific chromosomal region.

"Der" refers to a Robertsonian translocation where there is one normal chromosome of each type and one combined chromosome for a total number of 45 instead of 46.

"T" refers to a balanced translocation of a region from one chromosome to another.

"INV" refers to an inversion area of a chromosome.

"R" refers to a ring chromosome with one normal chromosome and one ring with the breakpoints identified.

"I" refers to an isochromosome with one normal chromosome and one isochromosome with the affected area identified.

"Micro" as used for deletions and duplications refers to a very small region of the chromosome as indicated in the karyotype.

Source: From Papaioannou GK, Syngelaki A, Maiz N, Ross JA, Nicolaides KH. *Early Hum Dev*. 2011 Jul;87(7):453–456

Imprinting involves a chromosome inheritance which is silent. The phenotype will depend upon which parent the active chromosome was from as the source. This principle applies to the two conditions Prader–Willi syndrome and Angelman syndrome, which are associated with the same chromosomal region, 15q11.2–q13. The condition depends upon the parental source of the chromosome.[10]

Fluorescence in situ hybridization (FISH) is a technique whereby the fixed metaphase chromosomes are hybridized with a fluorochrome-labeled DNA probe for a specific region of the DNA. This technique allows for specific chromosome identification more rapidly; identification of translocated chromosomal regions; recognition of deletions and additions of specific regions and identification of abnormal chromosomes.

This has been used in the rapid identification of uncultured cells in chorionic villus sampling (CVS) and amniocentesis specimens. Microarray has expanded the identification of chromosomal regions with DNA chips.[11]

Multifactorial Inheritance and Molecular Biology

Diseases with complex inheritance (also called multifactorial inheritance and polygenic inheritance) arise from the interaction of numerous genes with the environment. Some estimates indicate 5% at birth.[4] Through mathematical data of familial aggregation, relative risk ratios, twin studies and concordance, an inference may be made as to the genetic loci and environmental influences which result in the disease manifestation.[12] A number of different conditions fall into these categories but some general rules apply:[12,13] (a) the recurrence risk is higher when more family members are affected; (b) the more serious the defect the higher the recurrence risk; (c) the environment interacts to varying degrees with regard to the final phenotype (e.g. vitamin deficiency, excess hormone production); (d) variations in pharmacogenetics may be in part based upon this form of inheritance.[14] Box 16.2 gives some examples of multifactorial disorders.[13,14]

To establish a better understanding of current developments in prenatal diagnosis, a review of molecular biology is critical. The macromolecule DNA is the basis of the human genome with a large proportion of its constituents being similar in other animals and > 99% similarity among humans. The helical DNA molecule allows for two linear arrays of genetic material.[1] The unwinding of the DNA allows for duplication of the structure and communication to RNA for protein synthesis. It is the precise order of the bases on the DNA that defines the expression of the genetic material. The code is so precise that single base changes create profound effects on the protein product and the starting and stopping points for protein elaboration.

Mutations occur when chemical or physical mutagen agents lead to base modifications.[13] The mechanisms of these changes include: (a) deamination of cytosine, adenine, guanine; (b) methylation of carbon in the nucleic acids; (c) depurination of DNA by thermal fluctuations in the cell; (d) alkylation of the nucleic acids; (e) replacement with nucleic acid analogues; (f) ultraviolet light–induced thymine dimers, alterations in the covalent carbon bonds of adjacent nucleic acids in the DNA. Mechanisms of the DNA mutations are single-nucleotide polymorphisms, missense mutations, nonsense mutations, silence mutations, splice site mutations, frameshift mutations and regulatory polymorphisms.[8,13]

Molecular diagnostic testing of DNA involves restriction endonucleases that cut DNA into specific sequences of nucleotides. There are now hundreds of these enzymes available to cleave DNA at different locations.[8,13,15] Polymerase chain reaction (PCR) is a rapid way of creating multiple copies of DNA when the beginning and ending sequences are known. In multiplex PCR for gene deletion analysis, multiple DNA fragment copies from PCR undergo electrophoresis to determine the presence or absence of the DNA exon. Real-time PCR may amplify and qualify a specific target gene. This is important in discussion of massively parallel genomic or 'shotgun' sequencing.[16] The blot procedures are used to separate fragments of DNA (Southern blot), RNA (Northern blot) and proteins (Western blot).[17]

Microarray technology uses PCR with complementary DNA (cDNA)[18–20] to screen patient DNA for gene mutations or polymorphisms. This is now recommended by the ACOG for every amniotic fluid sample sent for Karyology.[18] An advantage of microarray is the high diagnostic yield, which comes from resolution which may be 50 to 200,000 base pairs compared with banding patterns of 3–10 million bases. Also, cell culture is not always required. The main disadvantages come from the size of the copy

Box 16.2 Multifactorial conditions[11,12]

Birth defects cleft palate/lip, neural tube defects such as spina bifida, pyloric stenosis, congenital dislocation of the hip [1]

Cardiovascular conditions congenital heart disease (esp. Ventricular Septal Defect (VSD)), hypertension, hypercholesterolemia

Neurological/psychiatric conditions Alzheimer disease in later life, schizophrenia, bipolar disorder

Skin conditions psoriasis, moles, eczema

Cancer bowel, breast, ovarian, melanoma, and prostate

Metabolic disease diabetes

Muscular/skeletal disorders arthritis, rheumatic disorders, osteoporosis

Respiratory disorders asthma, allergies, emphysema

number variations, density and genomic distribution of the DNA fragment being assessed.[19,20] Two types of arrays exist with a comparative genomic hybridization for large arrays of microdeletions and microduplications; and the single-nucleotide polymorphisms (SNPs) for smaller arrays which may involve a single nucleotide. The array only assesses those abnormalities of those regions for which the array was created. Because microarray does not require dividing cells, it is useful in the evaluation also of fetal demise or stillbirth where tissue culture is frequently unsuccessful.[19] Single-point mutations and some gain or loss of DNA may not be detected if below the detection boundary; translocations or inversions will only be detected if the oligonucleotide is small and lost in the exchange. Chromosomal mosaicism will not be detected, nor will marker chromosomes, nor triploid status.[1,21,22]

Molecular testing of DNA, although revolutionary, has limitations in accuracy. The test results are heavily dependent upon an accurate clinical diagnosis and the ordering of the most correct test. Testing sensitivity is mathematically restricted by the prevalence of the disease. Some genetic disorders may be caused by different alleles at different loci in different people and families. An abnormal trait may exhibit populational differences in frequency, genetic constitution, and phenotypic expression. Phenotypic penetrance and expressivity may not be determined by the presence or absence of one specific mutation alone but instead may also depend on environmental factors and the presence or activity of other genes.[16]

Genetic Screening and Definitive Testing

Physicians utilize general screening tests and specific diagnostic tests to assess pregnancy risk for genetic disorders in the fetus. Many professionally produced prenatal records for office use contain templates for prenatal screening both by individual and populational criteria.[1] Individual screening parameters include the following:

(a) Maternal age: The risk to the fetus from autosomal aneuploidy increases with maternal age beginning around age 15. By age 35 the risk reaches around 1 in 300. When initial recommendations were made for genetic amniocentesis for maternal age to rule out fetal aneuploidy (primarily trisomy 21), 1:300 was close to the assessed risk to the pregnancy of the amniocentesis procedure and hence became a laboratory standard. This procedural risk has decreased significantly with practitioner experience and the availability of ultrasound direction. The mother can alter her aneuploidy risk by obtaining various tests that are now available and will be discussed further below in populational screening. As maternal age increases, the risks of Trisomy 21, Trisomy 18 and Trisomy 13 continue to rise but risks to the fetus of monosomy X, triploidy and aneuploidies of the sex chromosomes remain stable with maternal age. It also must be noted that as gestational age increases the risk of all the aforementioned chromosomal abnormalities decreases because of the intrinsic biological loss of aneuploidy fetuses through abortion or stillbirth.[21]

(b) Paternal age when the father is greater than 40 years of age or greater than 20 years older than the baby's mother is considered a risk factor for certain autosomal dominant disorders in their children. There is an increased risk in Trisomy 21 and possible mutations in the X chromosomes, which may be carried to future generations. There is no evidence of a detrimental effect on the FGFR2 fibroblast growth factor receptor 2 gene, which may lead to craniosynostosis and to the FGFR3 gene associated with achondroplasia and thanatophoric dysplasia.[23]

(c) Hemoglobinopathies are frequently known to be present in the pregnant woman. If this is not the case, a recommendation for screening in women of African, Southeast Asian, and Mediterranean descent is valuable. A positive finding will establish the basis for genetic counseling and diagnostic testing of the baby's father and perhaps the baby.

(d) Carrier state screenings, as noted in Table 16.1 may be populational or individual. The cystic fibrosis screen is generally recommended to an American patient population and the sickle cell screen is recommended to an African American or African population for genetic reasons but also for maternal pregnancy care reasons.

Table 16.1 Antepartum Record Genetic Screening Form[1,4,21]

Concern	Population	Testing
Aneuploidy and neural tube	AMA advanced maternal age and prior history of aneuploidy or neural tube	NT nuchal translucency
		Quad (sequential) screen
Ventral wall defect	Ventral wall defect	Ultrasound and cell-free DNA
Thalassemia	Italians, Greeks, Mediterranean, Asians	MCV < 80 μm^2
Neural tube defects	Folate deficiency, seizure medications	Maternal serum alpha-fetoprotein (MSAFP) screen, ultrasound
	General populational, screen	
Congenital heart disease	Recurrence population, type 1 diabetes	Ultrasound
	General populational screen	
Sickle cell and other hemoglobinopathies	African and African American	Sickle screen and electrophoresis
	Middle East and Asia	Hemoglobin electrophoresis
Hemophilia A	Family history	Factor VIII carrier screen
Muscular dystrophy	Family history	Dystrophin gene mutation
Huntington's chorea	Family history	Endonuclease and Southern blot
		Looking for a triplet repeat DNA
Fragile X syndrome	Family history	Endonuclease and Southern blot
		Looking for a triplet repeat DNA
Previous stillbirth	Prior history	Ultrasound, metabolic and genetic studies
Phenylketonuria	Caucasian, Native American	Phenylalanine
Tay Sach disease	Ashkenazi Jewish, Cajun French Canadians	Hexoseaminidase A
Canavan disease	Ashkenazi Jewish	Aspartoacylase
Bloom syndrome	Ashkenazi Jewish	The BLM gene
Familial dysautonomia	Ashkenazi Jewish	The IKBKAP gene
Fanconi's anemia	Ashkenazi Jewish	Several genes reported, the FANCC
		The FANCG and the FANCA genes
Gaucher disease	Ashkenazi Jewish	The GBA gene
Mucolipidosis IV	Ashkenazi Jewish	The MCOLN1 gene
Nieman–Pick disease	Ashkenazi Jewish	Several genes reported, the NPC1
		NPC2 and the SMPD1 genes
Cystic fibrosis	Caucasians and Ashkenazi Jewish	The CFTR gene

(E) Ultrasound anatomical survey whether is it performed in midtrimester or increasingly in the late first trimester can be populational but is specifically individual for families with a history of congenital heart disease, dwarfism, Pierre Robin syndrome, facial clefting, ventral wall defects, and some central nervous system (CNS) problems.

Screening Tests in Obstetrics

Population Screening

Population screening may include some of the personal screens as already noted for hemoglobinopathy, by racial background; cystic fibrosis, and in some circumstances phenylketonuria (PKU). Maternal age and reproductive history will overlap with the analyte screens.[21]

Analyte Screening

The best analyte screening example is in the prenatal diagnosis of neural tube defects (NTDs) and open ventral wall defects (OVWDs). These begin by obtaining a sample of maternal blood at a specific gestational and correlating the amount of several chemicals as expressed in multiples of the median (MOM) with a populational graph of groups with neural tube defects, ventral wall defects or chromosomal aneuploidies; a risk factor is then assigned to the correlation. Different practices use different MOMs upon which to take more definitive diagnostic action. The alpha-fetoprotein (AFP) is a product of the fetus with high levels in the fetal serum (FSAFP) and amniotic fluid (AF-AFP). Elevated levels in maternal serum (MSAFP) testify to the fact that AFP has gotten into the maternal serum by a separation in the skin of the fetus or a placental abnormality or connection. Hence this test is helpful in identifying a pregnancy at greater risk for an NTD or a ventral wall defect (VWD). It needs to be clear that there is a range of normal values in pregnancies and the presence of an elevation of the MSAFP may have an explanation other than a NTD. Therefore, when counseling a patient with an elevation in MSAFP value and risk, it is important to explain that screening tests are not diagnostic and that additional testing and evaluation must be performed before establishing a management plan. A decrease in the MSAFP is noted in the population of fetuses with Down syndrome and Trisomy 18, thus in combination with other analytes; Estriol, inhbin A and hCG the quad screen or tetra screen test is valuable in the early part of the second trimester for screening a population for these aneuploidies.[21,24] The point must be made again that this is a screening test and indicates only that additional testing must be performed before any conclusions may be drawn. Factors that may affect interpretation of the analyte results include vegetarian diet, insulin dependence, smoking, race and in vitro conception. The history of the use of the analytes started with the MSAFP and others were added subsequently. Thus we have had the tri of triple screen and now the quad or quadruple screen and other analytes are still under investigation for possible inclusion if mathematic analysis shows benefit. If these additional analytes are able to improve the mathematical calculations, they will be added to future screening.[21]

A second set of analytes is already in use in the first trimester combined with the ultrasound generated nuchal translucency. In the late first trimester, an ultrasound measurement may be made of the nuchal translucency by a certified sonographer and combined with a maternal blood test looking for pregnancy-associated plasma protein A and free beta hCG levels. Again, utilizing populational data bases, a risk figure may be generated for fetal aneuploidy. As an early determinant of risk, a relatively inexpensive study, and a screen with a high sensitivity and specificity, the first trimester testing is currently growing in utilization in obstetrics.[21,25]

There are four major caveats, however, to the use of these screening examinations:

1. The interpretation of the test results must be not be portrayed as a simple yes/no, positive/negative result. Interpretation by trained genetic counselors and physicians are necessary for patient interpretation, and a subsequent plan of additional screening or definitive testing should be outlined for the patient when necessary. When the health care provider's office calls and schedules such counseling, the identification of a positive test is often interpreted by the patient as a definitive abnormality rather than a screening risk figure, which should be further elucidated. This adds great anxiety to the patients' lives and makes them extremely wary of the value of screening tests which are "so frequently wrong."
2. The mathematics of these screening tests are based on populations averages at specific gestational ages in an otherwise normal pregnancy. Thus, multiple gestation, vanished twin, threatened abortion, inappropriate gestational dating, all seriously alter the validation of the screen.
3. Laboratory examinations have standardization procedures and international committees for review. With the exception of certification of the laboratory for ultrasound by national and international bodies, in radiology or obstetrics/gynecology (Ob/Gyn), there is little standardization for physicians' practices. This why the American Institute of Ultrasound Medicine (AIUM) in the United States under the name of Nuchal Translucency Quality Review (NTQR) and the Fetal Medicine Foundation (FMF) in Europe and the Americas have provided a certification process for the combined first trimester screen sonographically with regular follow up of the data

Box 16.3 Conditions associated with elevated MSAFP[24]

Gestational age error	Multifetal gestation	Fetal death
Neural tube defect	Gastroschisis	Omphalocele
Cystic hygroma	Liver necrosis	Cloacal exstrophy
Esophageal or intestinal obstruction		Osteogenesis imperfecta
Renal anomalies – polycytic kidneys, renal agenesis, congenital nephrosis, urinary tract obstruction		
Sacrococcygeal teratoma	Congenital skin abnormality	Pilonidal cyst
Chorioangioma of the placenta		Placental abruption
Placental intervillous thrombosis		Oligohydramnios
Preeclampsia	Fetal growth restriction	
Maternal hepatoma or teratoma		

for each center. When a nuchal thickness (NT) is performed in a laboratory that is not certified for the procedure, the accuracy of the risk value is significantly diminished.

4. When a result of analyte screening is in the high-risk category, the gestational dating is correct, and other confounding factors have been removed, repeating a screen for aneuploidy should not be performed. In some circumstances, repeating a test for MSAFP may be necessary, but in general an elevated value should be investigated sonographically. Box 16.3 enumerates some of the sonographic findings associated with an elevated MSAFP.

Ultrasound Screening

Ultrasound screenings may be used for different purposes and there appears to be ongoing development of greater accuracy and availability. The original ultrasound screen was performed at 18–20 weeks for fetal anatomy, gestational dating, placental location, uterine and adnexal masses or abnormalities, abnormalities of amniotic fluid volume, multiple gestation and hydatidiform mole. Subsequent ultrasound screens have added more and more anatomical findings as imaging has improved.

1. The early first trimester screen is scheduled to establish gestational age, fetal life, assess for multiples and if present establish chronicity. Assessment for uterine and adnexal abnormalities is also indicated. Recent studies show there may be means to determine Trisomy 21 at less than 10 weeks via embryonic measurements.[26]
2. The first trimester genetic screen was established because of the great value which may be placed on a properly imaged and measured fetal nuchal translucency and the associated analyte studies. There continues to be reevaluation of the combined screen with the FMF adding data from the nasal bone, insonation of the fetal ductus venous, fetal tricuspid flow and assessment of the uterine artery blood flow.[25] This data has been taken even further looking at the association with chromosomal defects, other organ system abnormalities (cardiac, bone, eye) unassociated with chromosomal abnormalities, and fetal anatomical surveys in the absence of nuchal translucency abnormalities, which are used to detect unrelated fetal abnormalities.[24,25]
3. The 16–18 weeks ultrasound screen was initially used as an opportunity to detect any major fetal anomalies and the chance to perform genetic amniocentesis. The development of the sonographic markers of aneuploidy have subsequently become widely disseminated.[27] These sonographic markers, called "soft signs" with likelihood ratios of greater than 3 include (a) Nuchal skinfold thickening, (b) echogenic fetal bowel, (c) short humerus and (d) any cardiac defect. There are a number of other markers without a risk ratio of greater than 3. However, if these markers are combined in the same fetus, their combined risk may achieve a risk ratio of 3 or greater and trigger the need for additional testing (Box 16.4).

Box 16.4 Second trimester US markers for aneuploidy[24,27]

Nuchal skin thickening	Renal pelvis dilation	Echogenic intracardiac focus
Echogenic bowel	Short femur	*Short humerus*
Other 'soft signs"		
Brachycephaly or shortened frontal lobe		Flat facies
Clinodactyly (hypoplasia of the fifth digit middle phalanx)		
Nasal bone hypoplasia		Sandal gap of the first and second toes
Shortened ear length		Single transverse palmar crease
Single umbilical artery		Widened iliac angle

Notes: Italics means a relative risk of greater than 3.
Two markers not italicized may achieve a risk greater than 3 when present at the same time.

4. The 18–23 week scan is advocated as providing the most complete assessment of the fetal anatomy for major malformations and for CNS and fetal heart defects.[24,27]
5. Subsequent ultrasound examinations are needed at later gestational ages for several reasons. Follow-up scans on fetal growth patterns, amniotic fluid volume and both CNS and cardiac anatomies add significant clinical information. Aneuploidy risk is increased with selected major fetal anomalies such as cystic hygroma, nonimmune hydrops, ventriculomegaly, holoprosencephaly, Dandy–Walker syndrome, cleft lip and palate, cardiac defects, diaphragmatic hernia, esophageal atresia, omphalocele and clubfoot. When these conditions exist, genetic amniocentesis with microarray is recommended.[24]

Cell-free DNA Testing

Cell-free DNA (cf-DNA) testing is the last of the grouping of non-invasive prenatal testing (NIPT). In a sample of maternal plasma, fetal cf-DNA may be recovered even in a sample with a fetal fraction as low as 3% to 1%. The source of the fetal material is from the apoptotic trophoblast; the sample is therefore subject to inherent errors related to the trophoblast. This fetal fraction is a significant determinant of the success of the study and thus testing is usually not successfully accomplished in samples obtained prior to 10 weeks of gestation. New techniques are now available to clonally amplify the DNA fragments. Using miniaturization and automation, it is now possible to sequence hundreds of millions of DNA fragments using small volumes of reagents. Quantitative PCR may be used to determine Rh genotyping of the fetus, fetal sex determination and perhaps detection of single-gene disorders. In one technique, massively parallel shotgun sequencing (MPSS), and another technique massively parallel genomic sequencing (MPGS), all of the cf-DNA may be sequenced. Laboratories then utilize proprietary mathematical formulas to read the thresholds of samples expected to be of fetal origin. Digital analysis of selected regions (DANSR) is used to identify specific targeted chromosomes and the computers then use a proprietary mathematical model assuming a disomic fetal DNA to assess the risk for a trisomy; this formula is referred to as FORTE. Some laboratories use single-nucleotide polymorphisms (SNP) technology. SNPs are the most common type of genetic variation among people. Each SNP represents a difference in a single DNA building block or nucleotide, which may occur at some specific position in the genome. Next generation aneuploidy testing using SNPs (NATOS) are being used for prenatal diagnosis. Current reliable testing for aneuploidy and chromosomal deletions accrues daily. It is necessary to study the techniques and accuracies of the various commercial laboratories before contracting them for clinical services.[21,24]. Box 16.5 shows the current commercially available tests.[32] Additional research is underway to look at those clinical conditions that may increase the percentage of cf-DNA in the maternal plasma. Already under study are the clinical conditions of preeclampsia, hyperemesis gravidarum, placenta accreta and the hemolysis elevated liver enzymes low platelets (HELLP) syndrome. There is currently an argument in the literature blurring the lines as to whether cf-DNA testing is personal genetic screen or a populational screen. This chapter

Box 16.5 Currently commercially available cf-DNA testing[28]

Trisomy 21 (Down syndrome)	Trisomy 18 (Edwards syndrome)
Trisomy 13 (Patau syndrome)	Fetal gender
45,X (Turner syndrome)	47,XXY(Klinefelter syndrome)
47,XXX (Triple X syndrome)	47,XYY (Jacob's syndrome)
Trisomy 16	Trisomy 22
Del 22q (DiGeorge syndrome)	Del 5p (Cri-du-chat syndrome)
Del 1p36 deletion syndrome	Del 15q (Prader–Willi/ Angelman syndromes)
Del 11q (Jacobsen syndrome	Del 8q (Langer-Giedion syndrome)
Del 4p (Wolf-Hirschhorn syndrome	Trisomy 9

has addressed its utilization as a personal screen but arguments are made that the testing is so safe and the cost is decreasing to potentially make cf-DNA testing a populational, general pregnancy screen.[29–31] The author does not believe the cost or the data yet support this use; the publications of the ACOG agree.[31]

Reports exist that a false-positive cf-DNA may also be the result of an undiagnosed maternal cancer. This occurs at a very low incidence occurrence but must be kept in mind.[32] Box 16.6 enumerates indications and concerns regarding the use of cf-DNA testing. It must be remembered that this is a screening test. There is inherent error in the technique and although very reassuring in many cases, it is not the "gold standard" for an individual's chromosomal complement, which still requires a sample of fetal cells for karyology and microarray.

Invasive Screening

Traditional Invasive screening has not been population based but rather personal and definitive for testing. These techniques have been used to support populational screening in situations such as advanced maternal age or prior simple trisomy fetuses. Now with the progression of the noninvasive diagnostic means, especially ultrasound diagnosis, invasive screening tests are used more exclusively for high-risk personal situations.

Chorionic villus sampling (CVS), transabdominal and transvaginally directed, are generally performed between 10 and 12 weeks of gestation. Early amniocentesis is generally performed between 12 and 15 weeks of gestation. Classical genetic amniocentesis may be performed at any gestational age with greater safety between 16 and 24 weeks gestation. There is also anecdotal evidence that as the pregnancy progresses, material in the amniotic fluid make cell growth and genetic analysis more difficult. Fetal blood sampling, generally through the means of percutaneous umbilical blood sampling (PUBS) may be performed at any time from the second trimester through the end of the pregnancy. The risk of complications to the pregnancy is greater in this procedure so it is generally limited to later in pregnancy or in situations when the amniotic fluid or fluid cells would not be satisfactory for the clinical problem. Placental biopsy may be performed by a technique similar to genetic amniocentesis or PUBS, to obtain a small sample of placental tissue for genetic studies.

Additional new techniques are both invasive and may be personal or populations screening in intent. Preimplantation genetic testing is performed on oocytes or early embryos in the in vitro fertilization (IVF) process. Testing may be accomplished by one of three means: polar body analysis, blastomere biopsy or trophectoderm biopsy. The polar body analysis allows the investigator to take the polar for individual body extruded during meiosis and analyze for maternal Mendelian disorders. The disadvantage is the absence of the paternal component in the study.

Blastomere biopsy is performed at the six-to eight-cell stage or about a 3-day embryo. This is used just prior to implantation by removing a single cell for analysis. Two problems are that (a) the pregnancy rate can be reduced by 10% by obtaining the cell for study and (b) mosaicism in the chromosomal complement is not properly assessed.

In the trophectoderm biopsy, five to seven cells are removed from the 5- to 6-day-old blastocyst. This region gives rise to the trophoblast and thus placenta with no cells removed from the embryonic tissues. This process takes place later in gestation and should be analyzed immediately. If this is not possible, freezing the embryo for later use is possible.

Preimplantation genetic diagnosis (PGD) may be utilized when a couple are using a familial genetic condition rather than infertility as the reason for IVF. PCR for gene disorders and FISH may be used for chromosomal disorders. With only a small number of cells available and a rapid reporting time needed,

Box 16.6 Considering the use of cell-free DNA testing[24,29,30]

When to use cf-DNA testing

Maternal age 35 years or older at delivery

Prenatal ultrasound findings indicating an increased risk of aneuploidy

Prior pregnancy with a simple Trisomy

Screening test result demonstrating an increased risk for aneuploidy including the first trimester, sequential or integrated screen, or a quadruple screen

Parental balanced Robertsonian translocation with an increased risk of fetal trisomy 13 or Trisomy 21

Failure to obtain the first-trimester combined genetic screen or failure of chorionic villus sampling (CVS) or genetic amniocentesis testing for technical reasons.

When not to use cf-DNA testing

Multiple gestation including vanishing twin or triplet

Maternal or placental somatic mosaicism

Maternal obesity (lower fetal cell fractions)[32]

Prior to 10 weeks of gestation

Maternal or paternal chromosomal abnormalities with satellites or unbalanced chromosomes undiagnosed

Maternal organ transplant[32]

Maternal malignancy[32]

Serious consideration must be given to the potential effect on the parents of knowing the fetal gender at an early gestational age.

the procedure is technically challenging. Potential problems in analysis include (a) Failure to amplify the correct gene region of interest, (b) biopsy of a cell without a nucleus and (c) maternal cell contamination. Errors have occurred with this technique so it is not currently recommended by the American Society of Reproductive Medicine (ASRM).[33,34]

Preimplantation genetic screening is used for aneuploidy when an oocyte or embryo is available during IVF. FISH is used in this situation; some labs arrange for microarray. There is a lower successful pregnancy rate after this technique. The ACOG recommends against this form of testing with FISH for advanced maternal age, recurrent pregnancy loss or recurrent implantation failure.[34,35]

Concluding Remarks

As the subject of genomics and the day-to-day clinical dilemmas of genetic counseling become more complex; it is critical that the practicing obstetrician keeps up with the availability of resources in diagnosis and counselling. Two new aids on the horizon have the potentially opposite effect. The use of a computerized decision-making toll should help the clinical with directing the patient and her family to appropriate resources, much as has been outlined in some of the cancer screening genetic testing. The availability of the direct-to-consumer genomewide profiling is potentially dangerous in that a full counseling interpretation is not always provided to the recipient or the family. It has not been shown to alter patient behaviors and is difficult to interpret in varied low-risk populations.[36,37] The future appears to bring more such ethical and cost versus benefit arguments with developments in the field.

References

1. Genetics, in *Williams Obstetrics*, Cunningham, Leveno, Bloom et al. eds. McGraw Hill, New York, 2014, pp. 259–282.
2. www.ndsu.edu/pubweb/~mcclean/plsc431/mendel/mendel9.html. Accessed March 14, 2016.
3. en.wikipedia.org/wiki/Mendelian inheritance. Accessed March 14, 2016.
4. *Thompson & Thompson Genetics in Medicine*, Nussbaum, McInnes, Willard, eds., Saunders, Philadelphia, 2004, pp. 62–65.
5. Welt SI. Genetics, genetic counseling and genetic risk assessment, in *Manual of Obstetrics*, Arthur Evans ed., 8th edn. Wolters Kluwer Health/ Lippincott Williams & Wilkins, 2014, Chapter 29, p. 541.
6. www.omim.org/. Accessed March 14, 2016.
7. www.genome.gov/. Accessed March 14, 2016.
8. www.ncbi.nlm.nih.gov/pmc/articles/PMC3531155/. Accessed March 14, 2016.
9. http://ghr.nlm.nih.gov/. Accessed March 14, 2016.
10. Passarge E. *Color Atlas of Genetics*, Thieme, New York, 2001, pp. 170–349,
11. Welt SI. Genetics, genetic counseling and genetic risk assessment, in *Manual of Obstetrics*, Arthur Evans ed., 8th edn, Wolters Kluwer Health/ Lippincott Williams & Wilkins, 2014, Chapter 29, p. 545.
12. *Thompson & Thompson Genetics in Medicine*, Nussbaum, Mc Innes, Willard, eds., Saunders Philadelphia, 2004, pp. 289–310.
13. Welt SI. Genetics, genetic counseling and genetic risk assessment, in *Manual of Obstetrics*, Arthur Evans, ed., 8th edn, Wolters Kluwer Health/Lippincott Williams & Wilkins, 2014, Chapter 29, pp. 542–524.

14. www.genetics.edu.au/Publications-and-Resources/Genetics-Fact-Sheets. Accessed March 15, 2016.
15. https://en.wikipedia.org/wiki/Restriction_enzyme. Accessed March 15, 2016.
16. Genetics, in *Williams Obstetrics*, Cunningham, Leveno, Bloom et al., eds., McGraw Hill, New York, 2014, p. 277.
17. https://en.wikipedia.org/wiki/Southern_blot. Accessed March 15, 2016.
18. The use of chromosomal microarray analysis in prenatal diagnosis. ACOG Committee Opinion 581, December 2013.
19. www.thefreedictionary.com/complementary+DNA. Accessed March 15, 2016.
20. www.acog.org/-/media/Districts/District-VIII-Junior-Fellows/jfpc.pdf?dmc=1&ts=20160114T1529171067. Accessed March 15, 2016.
21. Welt SI. Genetics, genetic counseling and genetic risk assessment, in *Manual of Obstetrics*, Arthur Evans, ed., 8th edn, Wolters Kluwer Health/Lippincott Williams & Wilkins, 2014, Chapter 29, pp. 551–552.
22. Papaioannou GK, et al. *Early Hum Dev* 2011 Jul;87(7):453–456.
23. www.ncbi.nlm.nih.gov/pmc/articles/PMC3111019/. Accessed March 15, 2016.
24. Genetics, in *Williams Obstetrics*, Cunningham, Leveno, Bloom et al., eds. McGraw Hill, New York, 2014, pp. 287–302.
25. Nicolaides KH, Sebire NJ, Snijders RJM. *The 11–14 Week Scan: The Diagnosis of Fetal Abnormalities*, Parthenon, New York, 1999.
26. Timor-Tritsch, IE, Gupta, SK. Evolving application of first trimester ultrasound. *OBG Management* 2012;24/12; 36–45.
27. Pilu GP, Nicolaides KH, *Diagnosis of Fetal Abnormalities: The 18–23 Weeks Scan*, Parthenon, New York, 1999.
28. info@sequenom.com; www.sequenom.com/laboratories, accessed date March 15, 2016.
29. Welt SI. Genetics, genetic counseling and genetic risk assessment, in *Manual of Obstetrics*, Arthur Evans, eds, 8th edn, Wolters Kluwer Health/Lippincott Williams & Wilkins, 2014, Chapter 29, pp. 556–557.
30. Benn P. Non-invasive prenatal testing using cell free DNA in maternal plasma: Recent developments and future prospects, *J Clin Med* 2014;3:537–565. doi:10.3390/jcm3020537.
31. ACOG Committee Opinion no. 545, 2012.
32. Personal Communication: emechcatie@frontlinemedcom.com.
33. Yaron Y, Jani J, Schmid M, Depker D. Current status for microdeletion syndromes and rare autosomal trisomies using cell-free DNA technology. *OB GYN* 2015;126/5:1095–1099.
34. ACOG committee Opinion 430. March 2009. Preimplantation Genetic screening for aneuploidy. Reaffirmed 2014.
35. Kupperman M, Norton ME, Gates E. computerized prenatal genetic testing decision-assisting toll a randomized controlled trial, *OB GYN* 2009;113(1):53–63.
36. Bloss CS, Schork NS, Topol EJ. Effect of direct-to-consumer genomewide profiling to assess disease risk. *New England J Med* 2011;364:524–534.
37. Berry P, Henneman L, Lakenan PH, et al. Preconception genetic carrier testing and the commercial offer directly-to-consumers. *Hum Reproduc* 2011;26(5):972–977.

Abnormal Fetal Growth

Heidi Leftwich

Introduction

Fetal growth abnormalities continue to be a challenge in obstetric management. Many factors have been implicated in abnormal fetal growth. In early fetal life, it is the genetic predisposition of the infant that accounts for more than environmental, nutritional and hormonal influences. These are more likely to affect fetal growth later in pregnancy. In order to understand abnormal fetal growth, one must first understand normal fetal growth. Fetal growth has been described in three distinct phases, each correlating with gestational ages and with estimations of normal growth velocity. The initial phase is hyperplasia, where there is a rapid increase in the number of cells. This hyperplasia occurs during the first 16 weeks of gestation. Next, a period of both cellular hyperplasia and hypertrophy follows; this lasts until approximately 32 weeks. It is at this time that the cellular hypertrophy takes over, causing the most fetal fat and glycogen deposition and rapid fetal growth.[1] At this time, an average of 30–35 grams/day weight gain is noted versus the 5 grams/day, which occurs at approximately 15 weeks gestation.[2] Insulin and insulin-like growth factor-I (IGF-I) and insulin-like growth factor-II (IGF-II) have been implicated in the regulation of fetal growth and weight gain.[3] A combination of environmental factors, nutritional imbalances, hormonal influences and genetic predisposition can alter the normal fetal growth into a pathologic condition, either fetal growth restriction or macrosomia.

In the past, general classifications were created to define abnormal fetal growth. Fetuses with birth weight less than the 10th percentile were defined as small for gestational age, those between 10th and 90th percentile defined as appropriate for gestational age and those larger than the 90th percentile as large for gestational age.[4] The American Congress of Obstetricians and Gynecologists (ACOG) describes intrauterine growth restriction (IUGR) as an ultrasound estimation of a fetal weight (EFW) below the 10th percentile for gestational age and continues to refer to small for gestational age (SGA) as a measurement to describe neonatal weight after delivery below the 10th percentile.[4] While both pre- and post-delivery thresholds are below the 10th percentile, both values can contain those babies who are merely constitutionally small and those who are truly growth restricted.

Because of lack of uniformity of definition, criteria and management of fetuses with growth restriction has continued to affect physicians caring for these fetuses, both antenatally and post delivery. IUGR is not uncommon; it affects up to 10–15% of pregnancies and has been associated with poor perinatal outcomes including oligohydramnios, stillbirth, cesarean delivery for fetal distress, low Apgar scores at delivery and umbilical artery pH < 7.0.[5,6] While antenatal diagnosis and management of a growth restricted fetus can decrease the risk of these complications, only a startling 25% are diagnosed antenatally.[6,7] with even fewer diagnosed antenatally in the low risk population.[7] The importance of antenatal diagnosis is important. When compared to fetuses diagnosed with IUGR antenatally, those unidentified SGA fetuses showed a found a fourfold increased risk of adverse neonatal outcomes.[8]

No formal consensus has been reached as to a true definition of macrosomia. The term macrosomia is meant to define abnormally large fetal growth. ACOG has defined macrosomia as any weight about 4,500 grams, regardless of gestational age.[9] Other authors have used cutoffs of 4,000, 4,250 and 5,000 grams. Depending on the definition used, the incidence has been noted anywhere from 0.5 to 15%.[9–12] Regardless of the definition, there has been evidence of an increase in perinatal morbidity and mortality with regard to infants with macrosomia compared to their appropriately grown counterparts.[10] Some of these documented risks are an increase in stillbirth, neonatal mortality, birth injury, neonatal asphyxia, meconium aspiration and cesarean delivery.[10] This chapter reviews the various causes of fetal growth abnormalities and discusses the methods of antepartum recognition and diagnosis along with clinical management of pregnancy, labor and delivery.

Scope of the Problem

Fetal growth restriction is associated with an increase in perinatal morbidity and mortality, specifically fetal and neonatal demise, birth asphyxia, meconium aspiration.[13,14] Additionally, neonates are born with a higher incidence of respiratory difficulties, intraventricular hemorrhage and hypothermia.[15] Therefore, infants with fetal growth restriction (FGR) are more likely to require neonatal resuscitation in the delivery room compared to their average for gestational age (AGA) counterparts. They are more likely to experience hypothermia, polycythemia, meconium aspiration, neonatal asphyxia, hypoglycemia and other metabolic abnormalities. Post delivery, the growth restricted infant should be carefully examined for any structural malformations that may not have been detected antenatally; any suspicion for chromosomal abnormalities should be followed with a karyotype of the neonate. Infants born with IUGR also have an increase in neurologic complications, such as cerebral palsy, developmental delay and behavioral dysfunction.[13,14]

After excluding congenital anomalies, more than 50% of stillbirths had preceding IUGR.[7,16] By considering FGR as a cause for the stillbirth in these cases, the rate of what is considered unexplained stillbirth would drop from 65–70% to approximately 15%.[7] Overall, fetuses who do not fulfill their growth potential have a five-to ten-fold increased risk of IUFD.[7,16] In particular, those stillbirths prior to 32 weeks are significantly more likely to be afflicted with fetal growth restriction. Neonates born between 1500 and 2500 grams at term have a 5- to 30-fold elevation in perinatal morbidity and mortality, while those weighing less than 1,500 grams (<3rd percentile) convey a 70- to 100-fold increase.[16] This supports the more recent focus of the IUGR research to those fetuses with EFW less than the 3rd percentile.

According to the National Vital Statistics Report, 7.9% of livebirths in the United States have a birth weight greater than 4,000 grams.[17] Like growth restriction, macrosomia is also associated with poorer perinatal outcomes; many are linked with birth injuries and complications of labor and delivery. Specifically increased rates of brachial plexus injury, skeletal injuries, meconium aspiration, prenatal asphyxia, hypoglycemia and fetal death are seen with macrosomic newborns.[9,10,18] Maternal complications include prolonged labor, increased labor augmentation, cesarean delivery, postpartum hemorrhage, infection, third and fourth degree perineal lacerations, thromboembolic events and anesthesia complications.[9,10,18] It has been shown that long-term complications such as type two diabetes, hypertension and obesity in adulthood are increased in babies born with fetal macrosomia.[18,19]

Prenatal Diagnosis of Abnormal Fetal Growth

Clinical suspicion and assessment for risk factors for abnormal growth patterns needs to be addressed early in the pregnancy and with every prenatal visit to better aid in diagnosis. Unfortunately, methods of detection for abnormal fetal growth have been largely unsuccessful. Compounding the problem, incidence of obesity has increased and the symphysis-fundal height measurements have become even less accurate. Additionally, fetal biometry is more difficult in the obese gravid. A San Francisco, study showed a less than 20% sensitivity for use of the symphysis-fundal height measurement in the detection of both estimated fetal weight less than 10th percentile and greater than the 90th percentile.[20] Therefore, a combination of early establishment of gestational age along with symphysis-fundal height measurements and careful attention to maternal weight gain can be helpful in detecting cases of abnormal fetal growth in low-risk women. While a baseline third trimester sonogram is not recommended in the low-risk population, the at-risk population may benefit from the addition of this modality. It is therefore reasonable to consider obtaining serial growth evaluations in those patients at risk for growth restriction.[21]

Some investigators propose that the difficulty in true detection of abnormal fetal growth comes with the use of a population based growth curve instead of a customized growth curve. These investigators believe a customized growth curve would be more appropriate for the ethnically and culturally diverse population of the United States.[22–24] While fetal growth curves have been published from various populations, one of the earliest used was from Denver, Colorado. A concern with these curves is that they may underestimate SGA in the population living at sea level; given the change in the overall average birth weight, they may also underestimate further the number of FGR cases.[25]

Up to 70% of those diagnosed with SGA are found to be without pathology and considered constitutionally small.[15] A very high head circumference/abdominal circumference ratio is less likely to be associated with a normal fetus and therefore could also be used to aid in identification of true fetal growth restriction.[26] An elevated head circumference/abdominal circumference has been associated with an independent risk for adverse pregnancy outcomes.[26] While some constitutionally small infants are diagnosed falsely as growth restricted, concern also exists for those fetuses in the 10th to 20th percentile as they may experience an increase in poor perinatal outcomes, despite lack of an antenatally diagnosis of IUGR.[27] This is likely due to these specific fetuses not reaching their full growth potential but not measuring small enough to be diagnosed as IUGR.[27] This situation has led many clinicians to adopt the use of a customized versus population-based fetal growth curve. Studies have shown that the customized growth chart may be a better predictor of true growth restriction and therefore adverse outcomes.[22–24] Customized growth curves are not at present the standard of care, but it is important to know of the existence of customized growth curves. Potential exists for specific factors to be present in individual pregnancies that would predict fetal growth potential and therefore help identify deviation from this predicted estimate.

Fetal Growth Restriction

Fetal Growth Restriction Risk Factors

Risk factors for fetal growth restriction can be separated into maternal, fetal and placental. Approximately 40% of fetal growth is attributed to genetic contributions of the mother and fetus and the other 60% can be linked to affects of the fetal environment.[28]

Maternal Risk Factors

Maternal risk factors include chronic conditions such as renal or hypertensive disease, diabetes (especially type 1), antiphospholipid antibody syndrome, hypoxic conditions such as restrictive lung disease or poorly controlled asthma place women at risk for IUGR.[4,29] When uteroplacental perfusion is diminished in pregnancies complicated by maternal hypertensive disorders, there is an increase in the rates of FGR. Similarly, women with vascular disease are more likely to have a decrease in uteroplacental blood flow and therefore increase in FGR.[30] Studies have revealed lower birth weights and higher rates of SGA in those infants born at high altitudes.[31] Oxygen clearly serves an important role in normal fetal growth. Women with chronic pulmonary disease are therefore at risk for FGR. Smoking, alcohol, illicit and prescribed drug use can increase the risk of fetal growth restriction.[32] Maternal smoking status can affect the size of the fetus. For tobacco use, typically the type of fetal growth restriction is symmetric. Interestingly, if smoking cessation occurs prior to the third trimester, the effects of smoking are significantly reduced, making this important in counseling for smoking cessation.[32]

Additionally, poor perinatal history, such as history of IUGR or stillbirth, can increase the likelihood of IUGR.[33] One should be aware that while the risk of developing fetal growth restriction in a subsequent pregnancy is higher if the patient had a prior history of an IUGR pregnancy or stillbirth, these cases may be linked to a chronic maternal disease. Women with low pre-pregnancy body mass index (BMI) and poor gestational weight gain are at an increased risk for having a pregnancy complicated by IUGR.[34]

Fetal Risk Factors

Risk factors pertaining to the fetus such as chromosomal abnormalities, including confined placental mosaicism, are more likely associated with IUGR, as are specific structural malformations. In the placentas of babies with true FGR, confined placental mosaicism is three times more likely than in placentas from appropriately grown infants.[15] Approximately 7% of infants with FGR have a chromosomal abnormality; however, this increases if the diagnosis was made in the first half of pregnancy, especially for trisomy 13 and 18.[35] Multiple gestations are also associated with fetal growth restriction (see Chapter 22). Fetal infections can also be a cause of IUGR and should be assessed for in the prenatal period.[35]

Placental Risk Factors

Adequate uterine blood flow caused by proper trophoblastic invasion of the uterine decidual bed is necessary for supplying adequate nutrients to a growing pregnancy.[36] In many cases of FGR, there is shallow invasion of the cytotrophoblasts in the placental bed.[36] While many cases of IUGR are caused by placental insufficiency, other placental malformations can be associated with an increase in fetal growth restriction including placenta previa, circumvallate placenta, velamentous cord insertion and placental abruption or infarction.[35]

Symmetric versus Asymmetric IUGR

An understanding of the etiology of fetal growth restriction is a key to appropriate management. Long-standing teaching suggests two separate etiologies of IUGR: symmetric and asymmetric. Symmetric growth restriction has been said to be linked to an early insult, presumably viral infections, aneuploidy or chemical exposure.[37] In these cases, there is reduction in both the head and body size, therefore symmetric growth restriction. Asymmetric growth restriction has been described as a result of placental insufficiency, where there is diminished glucose transfer and hepatic storage; therefore, decreasing the size of the abdominal circumference[37] (see Table 17.1). While isolated fetal growth restriction is associated with aneuploidy, karyotypic abnormalities are more common with the addition of soft markers for aneuploidy. Studies have shown that symmetric growth restriction is more likely to be associated with constitutionally small fetuses while the asymmetric fetuses is more likely to be growth restricted and therefore have increased risk of poor perinatal outcomes.[37] While anomalous development, aneuploidy, and infection are causes for increased morbidity and mortality in those infant with symmetric fetal growth restriction, the absence of these factors may reflect a protective effect of the symmetric growth restriction. This may likely represent the cohort of individuals fitting the constitutionally small definition versus true growth restriction. True symmetric IUGR represents approximately 20–30% of those cases of IUGR. This classification may oversimplify growth restriction, as many cases of placental insufficiency show symmetric growth restriction as well as aneuploidy can be seen with a large fetal head and therefore asymmetric growth restriction.[37]

Table 17.1 Etiologies of Symmetric vs Asymmetric IUGR

Symmetric IUGR	Asymmetric IUGR
Chromosomal abnormalities	Placental insufficiency
Congenital malformations	Maternal hypertension
Maternal drug use	Preeclampsia
Congenital infections	Maternal vascular disease
	Chronic pulmonary disease

Management of Fetal Growth Restriction

When suspected, fetal growth restriction should be confirmed by fetal ultrasound. Once confirmed, appropriate evaluation and management are critical. Early onset fetal growth restriction, often symmetric, should prompt evaluation for aneuploidy and infectious etiologies, with early cytomegalovirus infection as the most common of infectious causes.[2] A careful maternal history for cigarette, drug, and alcohol use as well as other toxins known to have an association with fetal growth restriction should be performed. Cutting back and quitting any toxic behaviors would be recommended, should these be a suspected cause. Late onset fetal growth restriction, more likely to be asymmetric in nature, is most probably caused by placental insufficiency and so the focus should remain on identifying maternal vascular disease, rule out preeclampsia workup and monitoring of fetal well-being.[37] Depending on the gestational age, a biophysical profile should be performed to ensure fetal well-being at the time of diagnosis, including amniotic fluid assessment. Additionally, Doppler velocimetry of the umbilical artery should be performed in order to assess for end diastolic flow.[4] Doppler assessment has been a more recent tool used to help predict poor outcomes and therefore appropriate time for delivery.[38–43] Studies have shown that use of umbilical artery Doppler assessment in cases of IUGR has decreased the incidence of perinatal death and therefore should be used in the management of known FGR.[43] This methodology also decreased the rates of unindicated early deliveries. However, it has not been found to be beneficial in the low-risk population.[4,38] A normal umbilical artery Doppler evaluation leads toward a diagnosis of a constitutionally small infant versus a diagnosis of true fetal growth restriction.[38–43] While assessment of the ductus venosus and middle cerebral artery have been used in the assessment of FGR, these are still considered experimental until further randomized controlled trials can be performed and show benefit.[4]

In the early second trimester, forward flow through the cardiac cycle is present due to low impedance in the umbilical artery.[43] An obliteration of the small muscular arteries in the placental villi can cause a decrease in the end-diastolic flow in the umbilical artery.[43] An elevation of the systolic–diastolic ratio, signifying a fall in the end diastolic velocity, starts to occur after an approximately 30% decline in the arteries of the placental tertiary villi.[43] When absent end-diastolic flow is noted, it is associated with a 50% obliteration of these villi.[43] Reversed end-diastolic flow reflects the most severe compromise of placental tertiary villi.[43] This represents an approximately 70% compromise.[43]

Assuming normal end-diastolic flow, follow-up fetal growth ultrasounds should be performed, no sooner than every 2 weeks and no later than every 4 weeks.[4] Continued evaluation of the umbilical artery Doppler velocimetry should be performed to assess for progression to absent or reversed end diastolic flow.[43] Antenatal surveillance should be performed weekly or twice weekly, including at least weekly assessment of the amniotic fluid index.[4] Delivery should be considered in term infants, as there is an increased risk of poor perinatal outcomes including stillbirth.[4] Additionally, those fetuses that are thought to be constitutionally small can benefit from delay of delivery until 38–39 weeks[4]; this would, however, be only for those fetuses with normal umbilical artery Doppler evaluation. Additionally, the likelihood of a constitutionally small infant increases if there has been symmetric IUGR as well as appropriate interval growth, especially when parents themselves are constitutionally small.

While protocols exist on timing of delivery for a term growth restricted fetus,[4] it is ultimately up to the obstetrician to decide on the best management plan for each individual patient. The Disproportionate Intrauterine Growth Intervention Trial at Term (DIGITAT) study randomized women with suspected growth restriction to delivery versus expectant management after 36 weeks and found no difference in their primary composite of adverse neonatal outcome, cesarean deliveries or operative vaginal deliveries.[44] In this study, however, the diagnosis of IUGR was defined as estimated fetal weight or abdominal circumference less than 10th percentile or blunting of the labor curve; the definition was at the discretion of the provider.[44] While this study is promising for those women who desire low intervention related to induction of labor, the study should be reviewed with caution as the primary goal of delivery at term is to prevent stillbirth; stillbirth was not powered for detection in this study and thus cannot be adequately assessed.

Doppler velocimetry of the umbilical artery can be useful in detecting severe growth restriction at gestational age less than 34 weeks.[45] It is less useful in those fetuses over 34 weeks, which adds support toward delivery at term despite normal umbilical artery Doppler assessment.[45] If the etiology of fetal growth restriction, therefore, is unclear, or unlikely to be constitutionally small, or a new diagnosis of IUGR is made at term, delivery is recommended at 37 weeks.[4,45]

When oligohydramnios is present, delivery should be performed prior to full term.[45] Oligohydramnios is defined as a maximum vertical pocket of less than 2 cm or amniotic fluid index less than 5 cm.[46] Oligohydramnios itself has been linked to poor perinatal outcomes, and oligohydramnios in the setting of IUGR significantly increases the risk of perinatal morbidity and mortality.[45] An association with an increase in fetal hypoxia, abnormal antenatal testing and perinatal morbidity and mortality has been documented.[45] Due to these associations, though no randomized controlled trials on timing of delivery have been performed, expert opinion has suggested delivery timing by 34 weeks when oligohydramnios occur in the setting of fetal growth restriction.[45]

In the preterm infant, recommendations are less clear. Typically, delivery would be indicated for worsening maternal hypertension, severe preeclampsia, poor interval growth and reversal of umbilical artery diastolic flow.[46] When planning for delivery at less than 34 weeks gestation, the clinician should administer a course of antenatal corticosteroids for fetal lung maturation.[46] The gestational age at the time of delivery is a significant predictor of neonatal outcome in cases of FGR.[15] It is important to prolong gestational age as much as possible while balancing the risk of stillbirth and hypoxic injury from poor placental perfusion.[45] While the diagnosis of IUGR does not necessitate preterm delivery, absent or reversed end-diastolic flow suggests compromise and increased risk of perinatal morbidity and mortality.[43] Typically delivery would be indicated for absent or reversed end-diastolic flow, however in extreme early gestations, it is reasonable to wait until 32–34 weeks gestation for delivery.[43,45] Risks of intrauterine fetal death need to be addressed and frequent antenatal testing continued should this finding be expectantly managed.[43]

The Growth Intervention Restriction Trial (GRIT) was a randomized controlled trial designed to study whether such expectant management in these compromised infants would be beneficial. GRIT found a higher intrauterine fetal death rate in those fetuses expectantly managed but a higher neonatal death rate in those immediately delivered. No difference in total mortality therefore was discovered.[47]

Concerns for poor antenatal oxygenation in these severely compromised infants may provoke consideration for cesarean delivery in women remote from delivery if there is evidence of fetal deterioration. But when no evidence of acute deterioration was present, cesarean delivery was not associated in improved neonatal outcomes in a study of 2,885 pregnancies between 25 and 34 weeks: cesarean delivery was, in fact, associated with higher rates of respiratory distress syndrome.[48] Therefore, mode of delivery recommendations should be made based on best clinical assessment for the ability to tolerate labor.

Macrosomia

Macrosomia Risk Factors

For macrosomia, known risk factors include gestational and pre-gestational diabetes, although there are many non-glucose-related risk factors.[19] When excluding diabetes, predictive factors in macrosomia included: previous history of macrosomia, increase in maternal weight, non-smoking status, multiparity, male fetus, gestational age over 40 weeks, North American Aboriginal ethnicity, maternal birth weight above 4,000 grams, maternal height and age less than 17 years.[49] This also includes those pregnancies with an abnormal glucola and a negative diagnostic 3-hour glucose tolerance test; however, this was the least predictive of the risk factors.[49] Although shoulder dystocia is an unpredictable event, there is a significant increase in those babies with birth weight above 4,500 grams, from approximately 1.4% to approximately 20%.[50,51]

Diagnosis of Macrosomia

While most discussion regarding fetal growth curves and growth ultrasound evaluation and sensitivity is in the IUGR data, fetal growth measurements can also be inaccurate in the suspected macrosomic infant. Similar to IUGR, the method of diagnosis once fetal macrosomia is suspected, either by history or physical examination, is by fetal biometry. Often, the fetal vertex is too deeply implanted into the pelvis and therefore biometry measurements of the fetal head are inaccurate. An increased abdominal circumference, however, in a LGA infant, specifically greater than 35 cm, has been shown to identify more than 90% of macrosomic infants.[52] If a large fetus is therefore suspected, the clinician can also use the abdominal circumference measurement in the assessment of potential macrosomia.

Management of Fetal Macrosomia

Fetal macrosomia presents challenges with regard to labor and delivery. Unfortunately, due to the imprecise nature of prenatal detection of fetal macrosomia,[9,12] an increase in cesarean delivery and obstetrical interventions due to the suspicion of macrosomia has occurred. Current ACOG guidelines do not support the performance of a primary cesarean birth in the case of suspected macrosomia in a non-diabetic patient, unless the estimated fetal weight is greater than 5,000 grams.[9] Despite this recommendation, providers are still intervening with more frequency when macrosomia is suspected.[12] In fact, a recent study revealed that when clinicians expressed concern for the presence of a large baby (as told to the patients by their provider), there were increases in scheduled cesarean delivery, inductions of labor and labor and delivery interventions.[12] Interestingly, over 30% of the patients sampled stated their provider told them their baby was getting "quite large"; however, only 20% of those patients and 10% of all women studied delivered a baby over 4,000 grams.[12] A protocol at the University of Texas to deliver patients by elective cesarean delivery after estimated fetal weight of greater than or equal to 4,250 grams did show a decrease in shoulder dystocia from 2.4% to 1.1%, with an increase in the overall rate of cesarean rate of 21.7 versus 25.1%.[11] Therefore, options to perform elective primary cesarean delivery for women with diabetes and estimated fetal weight above 4,250 grams or 4,500 grams could be considered.

Concluding Remarks

Abnormal fetal growth is a challenge to practitioners and patients alike. Fetal growth restriction detection rates remain poor and many fetuses with SGA are undiagnosed until delivery. Suspected macrosomia from prenatal diagnosis is often incorrect and leads to increase in interventions and cesarean delivery. When accurately diagnosed, however, clinical management guidelines regarding prenatal care, antenatal surveillance and delivery recommendations have decreased some of the risks associated with these abnormalities in fetal growth. It is important to assess risk factors for abnormal fetal growth in order to help identify and therefore manage these pregnancies accordingly. The best diagnostic tool after history and physical exam is a fetal growth ultrasound evaluation, so suspicion for either fetal growth restriction or macrosomia should be followed up with a prenatal ultrasound for an estimated fetal weight.

References

1. Pollack RN, Divon MY. Intrauterine growth retardation: Definition, classification, and etiology. *Clin Obstet Gynecol* 1992;35:99–107.
2. Resnik R. Intrauterine growth restriction. *Obstet Gynecol* 2002;99(3):490–496.
3. Crossey PA, Pillai CC, Miell JP. Altered placental development and intrauterine growth restriction in IGF binding protein-1 transgenic mice. *J Clin Invest* 2002;110(3):411–418.
4. Fetal Growth Restriction. Practice Bulletin No. 134. American College of Obstetricians and Gynecologists. *Obstet Gynecol* 2013;121:1122–1133.
5. Chauhan SP, Cole J, Sanderson M, Magann EF, Scardo JA. Suspicion of intrauterine growth restriction: Use of abdominal circumference alone or estimated fetal weight below 10%. *J Matern Fetal Neonatal Med* 2006;19(9):557–562.
6. Gardosi J. Clinical strategies for improving the detection of fetal growth restriction. *Clin Perinatol* 2011;38(1):21–31.
7. Figueras F, Gardosi J. Intrauterine growth restriction: New concepts in antenatal surveillance, diagnosis and management. *Am J Obstet Gynecol* 2011;204:288–300.
8. Lindqvist PG, Molin J. Does antenatal identification of small-for-gestational age fetuses significantly improve their outcome? *Ultrasound Obstet Gynecol* 2005;25:258–264.
9. ACOG Practice Bulletin No. 22: Fetal Macrosomia. American College of Obstetricians and Gynecologists, Washington DC; 2000.
10. Zhang X, Decker A, Platt RW, et al. How big is too big? The perinatal consequences of fetal macrosomia. *Am J Obstet Gynecol* 2008;198:517.e1–517.e6.
11. Conway DL, Langer O. Elective delivery of infants with macrosomia in diabetic women: Reduced shoulder dystocia versus increased cesarean deliveries. *Am J Obstet Gynecol* 1998;178:922–925.
12. Cheng EF, et al. Labor and delivery experience of mothers with suspected large babies. *Matern Child Health J* 2015; 19(12):2578–86.
13. Jacobsson B, Ahlin K, Francis A, Hagberg G, Hagberg H, Gardosi J. Cerebral palsy and restricted growth status at birth: Population-based case–control study. *Br J Obstet Gynecol* 2008;115:1250–1255.
14. Jones RAK, Roberton NRC. Small for dates babies: Are they really a problem? *Arch Dis Child* 1986;61:877–880.
15. Rosenberg A. The IUGR Newborn. *Semin Perinatol* 2008;32(3):219–224.
16. Getahun D et al. Risk factors for antepartum and intrapartum stillbirth: A population-based study. *Am J Obstet Gynecol* 2007;196:499–507.
17. Martin JA, Hamilton BE, Ventura SJ, et al. Births: Final data for 2011. National vital statistics reports: From the Centers for Disease Control and Prevention, National Center for Health Statistics, National Vital Statistics System. 2013;62(1):1–69.
18. Weissmann-Brenner A, et al. Maternal and neonatal outcomes of macrosomic pregnancies. *Med Sci Monit* 2012;9:77–81.
19. Mohammadbeigi A, et al. Fetal macrosomia: Risk factors, maternal and perinatal outcome. *Ann Med Health Sci Res* 2013;3(4):546–550.
20. Sparks TN, Cheng YW, Mclaughlin B, Esakoff TF, Caughey AB. Fundal height: A useful screening tool for fetal growth? *J Mat-Fetal Neonat Med* 2011;24(5):708–712.
21. Executive summary: Hypertension in pregnancy: American College of Obstetricians and Gynecologists. *Obstet Gynecol* 2013;122:122–131.
22. Bukowski R, Uchida T, Smith GCS, Malone FD, Ball FH, Nyberg DA, et al. Individualized norms of optimal fetal growth:fetal growth potential. *Obstet Gynecol* 2008;111(5):1065–1076.
23. Clausson B, Gardosi J, Francis A, Cnattingius S. Perinatal outcome in SGA births defined by customised versus population-based birthweight standards. *Br J Obstet Gynecol* 2001;108:830–834.
24. Ego A, et al. Customized versus population-based birth weight standards for identifying growth restricted infants: A French multicenter study. *Am J Obstet Gynecol* 2006;194:1042–1049.
25. Lugo EJ, Tominey TM. The adverse effects of utilizing altitude-inappropriate fetal growth curves. *J Perinatol* 1989;9(2):147–149.
26. David C, Gabrielli S, Pilu G, Boricelli L. The head-to-abdomen circumference ratio: A reappraisal. *Ultrasound Obstet Gynecol* 1995;5(4):256–259.

27. Smith-Bindman R, Chu PW, Ecker J, Feldstein VA, Filly RA, Bacchetti P. Adverse birth outcomes in relation to prenatal sonographic measurements of fetal size. *J Ultrasound Med* 2003;22:347–356.
28. Svensson AC, Pawitan Y, Cnattingius S, Reilly M, Lichtenstein P. Familial aggregation of small-for gestational age births: The importance of fetal genetic effects. *Am J Obstet Gynecol* 2006;194:475–479.
29. McCowan L, Horgan RP. Risk factors for small for gestational age infants. *Best Pract Res Clin Obstet Gynaecol* 2009;23:779–793.
30. Berends AL, de Groot CJM, Sijbrands EJ, Sie MPS, Benneheij SH, Pal R, Heydanus R, Oostra BA, van Duijn CM, Steegers EAP. Shared constitutional risks for maternal vascular-related pregnancy complications and future cardiovascular disease. *Hypertension* 2008;S1:1034–1041.
31. Moore LG, Charles SM, Julian CG. Humans at high altitude: Hypoxia and fetal growth. *Respir Physiol Neurobiol* 2011;178(1):181–190.
32. Shu XO et al. Maternal smoking, alcohol drinking, caffeine consumption, and fetal growth: Results from a prospective study. *Epidemiology* 1995;6:115–120.
33. Ofir K, Kalter A, Moran O, Sivan E, Schiff E, Simchen MJ. Subsequent pregnancy after stillbirth: Obstetrical and medical risks. *J Perinatal Med* 2013;41(5): 543–548.
34. Zeitlin JA, Ancel PY, Saurel-Cubizolles MJ, Papiernik E. Are risk factors the same for small for gestational age versus other preterm births? *Am J Obstet Gynecol* 2001;185(1):208–215.
35. Maulik D. Fetal growth restriction: The etiology. *Clinical Obstet Gynecol* 2006;49(2):228–235.
36. Pardi G, Marconi AM, Cetin I. Placental–fetal interrelationship in IUGR fetuses – A review. *Placenta.* 2002;23:5136–5141.
37. Hadlock FP, Deter RL, Harrist RB. Sonographic detection of abnormal fetal growth patterns. *Clinical Obstet Gynecol* 1984;27:342–351.
38. Alfirevic Z, Stampalija T, Gyte GML. Fetal and umbilical Doppler ultrasound in normal pregnancy. *Cochrane Database Syst Rev* 2010, Issue 8. Art. No.: CD001450. DOI: 10.1002/14651858.CD001450.pub3.
39. Baschat AA. Opinion and review: Doppler application in the delivery timing of the preterm growth-restricted fetus: Another step in the right direction. *Ultrasound Obstet Gynecol* 2004;23:111–118.
40. Hartung J, Kalache KD, Heyna C, Heling KS, et al. Outcome of 60 neonates who had ARED flow prenatally compared with a matched control group of appropriate-for-gestational age preterm neonates. *Ultrasound Obstet Gynecol* 2005;25:566–572.
41. Kaponis A, Harada T, Makrydimas G, Kiyama T, Arata K, Adonakis G, et al. The importance of venous Doppler velocimetry for evaluation of intrauterine growth restriction. *J Ultrasound Med* 2011;30(4):529–545.
42. Kingdom JCP, Burrell SJ, Kaufmann P. Pathology and clinical implications of abnormal umbilical artery Doppler waveform. *Ultrasound Obstet Gynecol* 1997;9:271–286.
43. Berkley E, Chauhan S, Abuhamad A. Doppler assessment of the fetus with intrauterine growth restriction. *Am J Obstet Gynecol* 2012;206(4):300–308.
44. Boers KE, Vijgen SMC, Bijlenga D, van der Post JAM, et al. Induction versus expectant monitoring for intrauterine growth restriction at term: Randomised equivalence trial (DIGITAT). *BMJ* 2010;341:c7087
45. Galan HL. Timing delivery of the growth restricted fetus. *Semin Perinatol* 2011;35:262–269.
46. Spong CY, Mercer BM, D'Alton M, Kilpatrick S, Blackwell S, Saade G. Timing of indicated late-preterm and early-term birth. *Obstet Gynecol* 2011;118:323–333.
47. The GRIT Study Group. A randomised trial of timed delivery for the compromised preterm fetus: Short term outcomes and Bayesian interpretation. *Br J Obstet Gynecol* 2003;110:27–32.
48. Werner EF et al. Mode of delivery and neonatal outcomes in preterm, small-for-gestational-age newborns. *Obstet Gynecol* 2012;120(3):560–564.
49. Okun N, Verma A, Mitchell BF, Flowerdew G. Relative importance of maternal constitutional factors and glucose intolerance of pregnancy in the development of newborn macrosomia. *J Matern Fetal Med* 1997;6:285–290.
50. Nocon JJ, McKenzie DK, Thomas CJ, Hansell RS. Shoulder dystocia: An analysis of risks and obstetric maneuvers. *Am J Obstet Gynecol* 1993;168:1732–1739.
51. Lipscomb KR, Gregory K, Shaw K. The outcome of macrosomic infants weighing at least 4500 grams: Los Angeles and University of Southern California experience. *Obstet Gynecol* 1995;85:558–564.
52. Abdella RMA, Ahmed SAM, Moustata MI. Sonographic evaluation of fetal abdominal circumference and cerebroplacental Doppler indices for the prediction of fetal macrosomia in full term pregnant women. *Middle East Fertility Soc J* 2014;19(1):69–74.

Chapter 18

Alloimmunization and Non-immune Hydrops Fetalis

William Goodnight and Martin Olsen

Introduction

Hydrops fetalis is defined as abnormal fetal fluid collections in at least two fetal compartments, either in soft tissues or serous cavities, which can occur due to diverse etiologies. The most well known is the result of red cell alloimmunization and severe fetal anemia (1). Non-immune hydrops fetalis (NIHF) describes the hydropic fetus in the absence of maternal red cell alloimmunization. NIHF comprises approximately 90% of hydrops fetalis cases affecting 1 in 1,700–3,000 pregnancies and is thus more common than immune hydrops (2,3). Most cases are identified by ultrasound at the time of routine fetal ultrasound examination or in the setting of evaluation for other maternal or fetal indications. Ultrasound examples are seen in Figure 18.1.

Maternal signs and symptoms are few in the majority of cases, but an increased fundal height compared to gestational age may indicate the polyhydramnios that can be present in cases of hydrops. Most diagnoses are made at the time of an obstetric ultrasound for different indications. The diagnosis is made when abnormal fluid is noted in the fetal compartment in more than two locations (Box 18.1).

Scope of the Problem

Given the severity of the majority of the underlying etiologies of non-immune hydrops fetalis, the overall perinatal survival remains poor. Fetal survival ranges from 12% to 24% with some improvement in the prognosis among live born neonates in whom survival may approach 40–50%. Among neonates born with hydrops, most demonstrate ascites and pleural effusions. When live born, the overall survival of neonates with non-immune hydrops fetalis (NIHF) approaches 50% with maximum of 83% among those with lymphatic malformations or isolated chylothorax as the primary etiology. The factors most associated with mortality among live born neonates with hydrops include low serum albumin < 2 g/dl, earlier gestational age at diagnosis, and preterm birth prior to 34 weeks (4). Obstetric complications related to NIHF include symptomatic polyhydramnios, preterm birth (spontaneous and indicated), and increased risk of cesarean delivery.

Alloimmunization in the modern practice of obstetrics is seen significantly less frequently than it was decades ago prior to the routine use of anti-D immunoglobulin in the 1960s. Perinatal mortality for this condition decreased exponentially after this intervention. In the developing world, stillbirth still occurs in 14% of pregnancies and 50% of neonates that survive the pregnancy either die in the neonatal period or develop cerebral injury (5). Alloimmunization management at present more often involves maternal sensitization to atypical antigens such as Kell.

The first section of this chapter will discuss non-immune hydrops. Alloimmunization toward fetal red blood cells will then be discussed followed by a brief discussion of alloimmune thrombocytopenia.

Non-immune Hydrops Fetalis

Pathogenesis and Diagnosis

The pathogenesis of NIHF is dependent on the underlying etiology, but in most cases, it is associated with fetal congestive heart failure with elevated central venous pressure and fetal hypoxia, resulting in increased capillary permeability. Liver congestion results in decreased albumin production and thus a decrease in colloid osmotic pressure. The constellation of low albumin, increased central/lymphatic pressure, and decreased colloid osmotic pressure with capillary damage and increased permeability facilitate formation of serous effusions and skin edema.

NIHF is the fetal expression of a wide variety of etiologies (Table 18.1). While detailed evaluation can

(a)

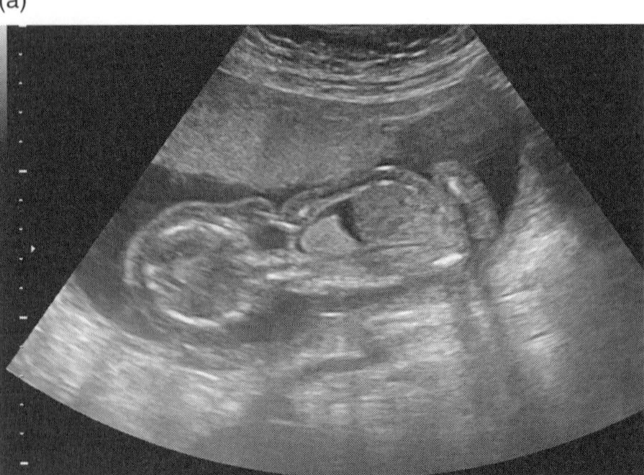

(b)

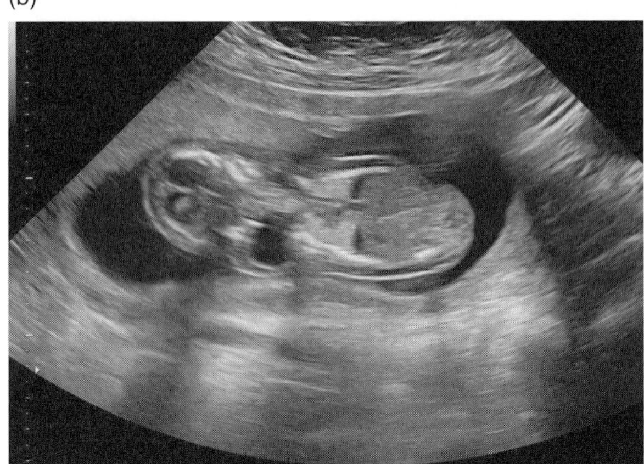

Figures 18.1 (A,B) Edema of fetal soft tissues, ascites and pleural effusions can be seen in these ultrasound images of a 15-week gestation with non-immune hydrops. Figures courtesy Dr. Selman Welt.

Box 18.1 Fetal non-immune hydrops diagnosis

- Abnormal fluid collection in two or more fetal compartments
  - Ascites
  - Pleural effusion
  - Pericardial effusion
  - Skin edema (≥ 5 mm skin thickness)
  - Placental thickness
    - 4 cm (second trimester)
    - 6 cm (third trimester)
  - Polyhydramnios (four-quadrant AFI > 24 cm or maximum vertical pocket of amniotic fluid > 8 cm)
- Absence of maternal red cell alloimmunization (negative maternal antibody screen/negative Comb's test)

reveal the etiology in the majority of cases, up to 20% of cases remain idiopathic in nature. Despite advances in prenatal diagnostic testing, the proportion of idiopathic NIHF remains unchanged over the last three to four decades (2). Determination of the underlying etiology can have direct implications on outcome, recurrence rate in subsequent pregnancies, and potential antenatal interventions.

When fetal hydrops is demonstrated on ultrasound examination, a systematic maternal and fetal evaluation should be undertaken with the goals to (1) determine the underlying etiology and thus provide patient counseling, (2) determine the potential for fetal intervention, and (3) determine recommendations for pregnancy monitoring and delivery planning. Maternal fetal medicine consultation in coordination with reproductive genetic evaluation is recommended. The maternal red cell antibody screen should be confirmed to ensure absence of immune-mediated fetal anemia. A complete detailed anatomic ultrasound including fetal echocardiogram and targeted fetal vascular Doppler evaluation is recommended to determine the presence of other structural anomalies, fetal anemia, or cardiac arrhythmia. The peak systolic velocity of blood flow in the fetal middle cerebral artery will be elevated beyond 1.5 multiples of the median for gestational age in the setting of fetal anemia. Fetal anemia can be present in the setting of congenital infections, most commonly due to parvovirus infection, massive feto-maternal hemorrhage, or in rare cases of fetal hemoglobinopathy such as homozygous alpha-thalassemia (Hemoglobin Bart's). Abnormal middle cerebral artery (MCA) peak systolic Doppler velocity can also identify anemia in the donor twin (PSV > 1.5 multiples of the mean (MoM)) and polycythemia (PSV < 0.8 MoM) in the recipient twin in the setting of twin anemia–polycythemia sequence.

Cardiac Anomalies

The most common fetal cardiac abnormalities noted in NIHF include fetal arrhythmias; in the setting of structural abnormalities, these carry a very poor prognosis. The most common tachyarrhythmias include supraventricular tachycardia, re-entrant tachycardia, and arterial flutter. Maternal administration of antiarrhythmic agents such as a digoxin, sotalol, or flecainide is the primary therapy to correct fetal arrhythmia. In

Table 18.1 Etiologies, Diagnostic Testing, and Potential Interventions for Selected Etiologies of Non-immune Hydrops (2,5)

Etiology	Percentage of NIDF Cases	Diagnosis	Therapy
Cardiovascular	17–35%		
Arrhythmia CHB SVT, flutter		Ultrasound, fetal echo	Maternal/fetal anti-arrhythmia agent for fetal SVT/Flutter (6); trial of dexamethasone, salbuterol for SSA/SSB associated fetal congenital heart block (7)
Structural anomaly (endocardial cushion defect, HLHS), rhabdomyoma		Ultrasound, fetal echo	Rare intracardiac fetal intervention for aortic stenosis (8), rare in utero resection of rhabdomyoma
Thoracic malformation: CPAM/BPS Hydro-/chylothorax	9%	Ultrasound/fetal MRI Diagnostic thoracocentesis	Antenatal corticosteroid course; thoracoamniotic shunting; rare open fetal surgery; needle drainage prior to delivery in large effusion
Hematologic Homozygous α-thalassemia FMH	4–12%	FBS	Intrauterine transfusion
Infection Parvovirus B-19 CMV Adeno/enterovirus	5–7%	Amnio/FBS PCR	IUT for anemia due to parvovirus; possible CMV hyperimmune globulin (9)
Structural anomaly Sacroccoccygeal teratoma AVM Congenital lymphatic dysplasia	1–7%	Ultrasound/MRI	Rare in utero fetal resection
Placenta chorioangioma		Ultrasound	
Chromosomal/Genetic syndrome 45, XO Trisomy 21 Trisomy 18 Noonan syndrome	10–20%	Ultrasound/amnio/FBS	
Inborn errors of metabolism	2–5%	Ultrasound/amnio/FBS	
Monochorionic twin pregnancy complication TTTS/TAPS TRAP	4–8%	Ultrasound/fetal Doppler evaluation	TTTS/TRAP: fetoscopic laser photocoagulation of placental vessels; Selective fetal reduction via RFA/bipolar cord coagulation
Idiopathic	15–25%	Ultrasound/amnio/FBS	

Terminationof pregnancy counseling is appropriate on an individualized basis; Delivery close to term/late preterm period may be preferable.

Abbreviations: FBS – fetal blood sampling; amnio – amniocentesis; PCR – polymerase chain reaction; CPAM – congenital pulmonary adenomatous malformation; BPS – bronchopulmonary sequestration; TTTS – twin–twin transfusion syndrome; TRAP – twin reversed arterial perfusion; TAPS – twin anemia-polycythemia sequence; SVT – supraventricular tachycardia; CMV – cytomegalovirus; AVM – arteriovenous malformation; CHB – congenital heart block.

The majority of therapy beyond IUT for parvovirus and treatment of TTTS/TRAP remains based on case series level evidence and should be undertaken if possible under an investigational protocol or in a fetal therapy center.

some cases, these therapies may reverse fetal hydrops to allow continuation of the pregnancy. Delivery may be indicated in the late preterm or at term with postnatal therapy.

Brady-arrhythmias can be due to malformation of the atrioventricular (AV) conduction pathway due to structural malformations or due to immune-mediated congenital heart block associated with maternal anti-SSA/SSB antibodies commonly associated with lupus or scleroderma. Retrospective studies demonstrated promise in improvement in the long-term outcome when the condition is due to congenital heart block and is treated with dexamethasone. The limited randomized trials have not, however, proven the effectiveness of this therapy.

Other Anomalies

NIHF in the setting of fetal hydrothorax or macrocytic congenital pulmonary adenomatoid malformation can be reversed with thoracentesis or thoraco-amniotic shunting, while reduction in size of large microcystic congenital pulmonary airway malformation (CPAM) has been observed with maternal administration of dexamethasone. Selective laser coagulation of placental vessels is the therapy of choice in the setting of twin–twin transfusion syndrome (TTTS). In cases of hydrops due to fetal twin-reversed arterial perfusion (TRAP), selective reduction of the recipient twin can be effective in increasing the survival of the pump twin. As such, in the setting of NIHF with a fetal structural anomaly, referral to a fetal care center is recommended for possible fetal intervention.

Fetal Anemia

Fetal anemia is a common etiology for NIHF and is potentially amenable to fetal therapy. The most commonly identified infectious etiology for fetal anemia is congenital parvovirus infection. Parvovirus B19 infection in the fetus is associated with infection and suppression of the myeloid precursors resulting in severe anemia and NIHF. In cases of NIHF, elevated peak systolic velocity (PSV) in the middle cerebral artery (MCA) on fetal vascular Doppler assessment is consistent with fetal anemia when PSV > 1.5 multiples of the median (MoM). Fetal blood sampling is then performed to obtain fetal blood for measurement of hematocrit, karyotype, and polymerase chain reaction (PCR) for Toxoplasma gondii, Other, Rubella, Cytomegalovirus and Herpes Simplex (TORCH) infections; intravascular fetal transfusion in then performed.

In addition to Parvovirus B19, fetal infection with cytomegalovirius (CMV), syphilis, and toxoplasmosis may also result in fetal anemia and NIHF, often in association with other fetal findings such as intrauterine growth restriction (IUGR), intracranial calcifications, or other structural anomalies. Non-infectious etiologies associated with fetal anemia include hematologic disorders such as homozygous alpha-thalassemia, red cell aplasia, congenital leukemia, Blackfan Diamond anemia, and Fanconia anemia.

Fetal transfusion (see the following discussion) can result in resolution of the fetal hydrops and may allow the fetus to clear a parvovirus infection. The role of intrauterine transfusion (IUT) for other causes of fetal anemia in NIHF is less clear. CMV hyperimmune globulin has demonstrated some effectiveness in reducing the morbidity due to fetal CMV infection and may be considered. Following an IUT with resolution of anemia/ hydrops in the setting of NIHF due to parvovirus infection, the overall prognosis remains favorable. Based on limited data, the rate of cerebral palsy and neurodevelopmental impairment following IUT for parvovirus infection is estimated to be 2.8 and 5.6% respectively (6).

Management Non-immune Hydrops Fetalis

In the presence of suspected fetal anemia, fetal blood sampling from the umbilical vein can be used as the next diagnostic and potentially therapeutic approach. Fetal blood sampling can confirm anemia, obtain leukocytes for karyotype and genetic assessment including chromosomal microarray, obtain serum for PCR testing for fetal infectious disease, as well as allow therapy with red cell transfusion. Genetic panels for the common genetic etiologies of NIHF are available; these can be obtained if initial evaluation is unclear (7). Fetal blood sampling should be considered as first line management in the setting of suspected fetal anemia and can be considered in the setting of oligohydramnios that prevents ability to perform amniocentesis. In the absence of suspected fetal anemia, genetic and infectious disease testing is recommended; this can be done via amniocentesis. Biochemical assessment of pleural or ascetic fluid may aid in focusing the etiology. The presence of vacuolated cells can be identified in storage metabolic disease. Lymphocytes comprising > 80% of the cell count are associated with chylous ascites.

Low protein is consistent with urinary ascites, and 2 microglobulin is suggestive of infection (8).

Potential interventions for non-immune hydrops are based on the underlying etiology. Given the high risk of fetal death in the setting of NIHF, delivery can be considered in the late preterm or early term setting. The obstetrician must the risks of prematurity with the availability of potential neonatal interventions. In addition, termination of pregnancy can be considered based on the gestational age at the time of the diagnosis.

Antenatal management and assessments will be based on the gestational age and underlying etiology of the disorder. Antenatal management and delivery should be undertaken in a multidisciplinary setting with availability of fetal intervention as indicated by the specific fetal condition. Neonatal subspecialty care including pediatric surgery, cardiology, and pediatric genetics may be needed.

The presence of non-immune hydrops fetalis is a contraindication to expectant management of severe maternal complications in pregnancy such as preeclampsia, preterm labor, or maternal mirror syndrome. The prognosis of non-immune hydrops is especially poor in the setting of prematurity < 34 weeks gestational age (4). The timing of antenatal fetal testing should be individualized to avoid preterm delivery without fetal benefit. Weekly to every other week maternal evaluation to assess for symptoms of mirror syndrome is recommended and assessment of fetal viability can be done at these visits. The initiation of weekly or twice weekly fetal non-stress test or biophysical testing can be initiated after 32–34 weeks or as indicated by the underlying etiology, especially in clinical conditions amenable to prenatal or postnatal treatment such as anemia due to parvovirus infection, TTTS and fetal thoracic malformations. Generally, antenatal corticosteroids have not demonstrated specific improvement or perinatal survival in NIHF, except in hydrops due to fetal thoracic malformations. Antenatal corticosteroids are not contraindicated, however, and should be administered for usual preterm delivery indications.

Delivery

The route of delivery is usually individualized based on the fetal and maternal condition. When palliative care for neonatal management is planned, cesarean delivery is usually reserved for maternal indications with minimal intrapartum fetal heart rate monitoring. The presence of severe fetal malformations or massive ascites or skin edema may result in labor dystocia. Fetal arrhythmia may prevent adequate intrapartum fetal monitoring, thus making cesarean delivery appropriate in individual cases. Intrapartum therapeutic fetal thoracentesis may be indicated in the setting of large effusions to aid in neonatal resuscitation. Fetal paracentesis in the setting of massive ascites may be beneficial to avoid the risk of abdominal dystocia with both cesarean and vaginal delivery and should be individualized based on the specific clinical indication.

Mirror Syndrome

Mirror syndrome, also called Ballantyne's syndrome, is a rare condition in which maternal edema develops when the patient's fetus has hydrops. The maternal symptoms therefore "mirror" the fetal pathology. The condition is felt to be uncommon but also underdiagnosed; incidence of mirror syndrome is thus unclear. Etiology is also unclear, but it has been reported in pregnancies complicated by rhesus isoimmunization, viral infections, fetal and placental tumors, and fetal arrhythmias (9).

In NIHF, expression of fetal placental antigenic factors, such as sFlt1, have been implicated in the development of mirror syndrome, which can have a similar presentation as preeclampsia (17). The most common presentation for mirror syndrome includes maternal peripheral edema, hypertension, and proteinuria (9). Maternal symptoms may also include headache, visual disturbances, and laboratory evaluation may demonstrate anemia, thrombocytopenia, and elevated liver transaminases, creatinine, and uric acid. In the presence of mirror syndrome, expectant treatment of the pregnancy is contraindicated and delivery is the only therapy. In rare circumstances, however, such as anemia due to parvovirus infection or the presence of fetal arrhythmia, prompt correction of the fetal condition may result in improvement in the maternal status. Such correction has allowed continuation of the pregnancy with careful maternal evaluation.

Alloimmunization

Maternal red cell alloimmunization (a synonym is isoimmunization) is caused by the sensitization of a woman's immune system to foreign red-blood-cell-surface antigens. This sensitization leads to maternal production of immunoglobulin G (IgG) antibodies.

Since IgG antibodies can cross the placenta, fetal cells can then be attacked by these antibodies. Severe fetal anemia with the potential for severe hydrops fetalis and fetal death can subsequently occur.

Anti-D, anti-c, anti-E, and anti-Kell antibodies cause the most severe cases of alloimmunization. Generally, anti-D is associated with Rh (–) mothers carrying Rh (+) fetuses, while anti-c, anti-E, and anti-Kell are classified as atypical antibodies Table 18.2 discusses atypical antibody relationships to alloimmunization (10) and the topic is discussed in more detail later.

Pathophysiology of Alloimmunization

In the most well-researched example of alloimmunization, maternal rhesus-D (Rh) alloimmunization, the isoimmunization event is caused by maternal exposure of an Rh (–) woman to Rh (+) blood. Anti-D antibodies are formed in the maternal circulation; these antibodies then can cross the placenta and subsequently sensitize fetal red blood cells for destruction. Macrophages in the reticuloendothelial system then complete the destruction of the fetal red blood cells.

Classic teaching is that alloimmunization can be caused by multiple potential sensitizing events during a pregnancy. The volume of blood available for sensitization is highest at the time of delivery. Concerns about antepartum sensitization also exist. See Box 18.2 for a list of potential antepartum sensitizing events.

Interestingly, the risk of alloimmunization is higher if the fetus has ABO-compatible blood with its mother. The fetus with ABO-incompatible blood has only a 1–2% risk of causing maternal alloimmunization if postpartum anti-D administration is neglected. It is felt that the ABO incompatible fetal blood is destroyed before maternal rhesus sensitization occurs (11). Currently approximately 0.27% of susceptible women become alloimmunized due to failure of medical systems to properly administer Anti-D prophylaxis (12).

Rh (+) women can on rare occasions carry pregnancies at risk for alloimmunization by anti-D. These Rh (+) women are believed to have missing epitopes

Table 18.2 Atypical Red Cell Antibodies and Alloimunization (A1)

Commonly Associated with Alloimunization	Uncommonly Associated with Alloimunization	Rarely Associated with Alloimunization	No Association with Alloimunization
D	Anti-e	Biles	Le(a)
Anti-Kell	C	Co(A)	Le(b)
c	cE	Di(A)	P
E	Ce	Di(b)	
	C (W)	Do(A)	
	Kp(a)	En(A)	
	Kp(b)	Fy(b)	
	K	Good	
	Jk(a)	Heibel	
	S	Jkb	
	Wr(a)	Lu(a)	
	Fy(a)	Lu(b)	
		M	
		Mi(a)	
		Mt(a)	
		N	
		Radin	
		S	
		U	
		Yt(a)	
		Zd	

Box 18.2 Antepartum events postulated to cause maternal sensitization (15)

Spontaneous abortion
Voluntary interruption of pregnancy
Ectopic pregnancy
Amniocentesis
Chorionic villus sampling
Placental abruption
Feto-maternal hemorrhage
Abdominal trauma
External cephalic version
Fetal blood sampling
Evacuation of molar pregnancy
Intrauterine fetal death

on their own D antigens. The Rh (+) mothers then are sensitized to the epitopes present of the fetus which the mothers themselves lack (13). An epitope, also known as an antigenic determinant, is the part of the antigen that is recognized by the immune system.

Initial Care of a Sensitized Woman during Pregnancy

The first step in the care of an alloimmunized patient is to assess the amount of antibody present in the woman's serum. Antibody titers screening tests since they show that the mother is sensitized and the fetus is therefore at risk for severe fetal anemia. The level of antibody titer does not predict disease severity. The indirect anti-globulin (Coomb's) test can detect the degree of alloimmunization (11). The fetal effects of alloimmunization tend to become more severe with each subsequent pregnancy.

A subsequent step is to assess the father of the fetus's genotype. If the father of the fetus is negative for the antigen of concern, then the fetus is not at risk. For example, if the pregnant patient has positive Kell antibodies, but the father of the fetus has no Kell antigens, then the fetus is not at risk. In such a situation, it is obviously important to confirm paternity within the limits available; paternity of the pregnancy is not always definitively known.

Fetal Assessment and Treatment in Anti-D Sensitized Pregnancies

Ultrasonography can be performed to assess the presence or absence of features associated with fetal hydrops. These features include pleural effusions, pericardial effusions, and ascites. These changes are not usually seen until the fetal hemoglobin deficit is at least 7 g/dL below the mean for the fetal gestational age. Other signs of severe feel anemia include polyhydramnios, increased placental thickness over 4 cm, dilation of the cardiac chambers, increase in the umbilical vein diameter, enlargement of the liver, enlargement of the spleen, and visualization of both sides of the fetal bowel wall.

Middle cerebral artery (MCA), peak systolic velocity (PSV), and Doppler assessment are now the standard tools for the prediction of fetal anemia and are used in decision making about which fetuses need intrauterine blood transfusion (14). The middle cerebral artery has been selected for assessment of fetal anemia because it is easily evaluated. The best interval between evaluations has not been determined but every one to two weeks has been recommended (11).

Cordocentesis, also called fetal blood sampling, is performed via ultrasound-guided needle insertion into the fetal umbilical vein. Severe complications for this procedure include fetomaternal hemorrhage, fetal loss, placental abruption, fetal distress, and amnionitis. Cordocentesis is therefore reserved for patients who have ultrasound or MCA evidence of fetal anemia. An intrauterine blood transfusion can be performed immediately after confirmation of severe fetal anemia. Adult donor rhesus-D negative red blood cells are used. Antibody titers are no longer valid or useful after this invasive procedure (11).

Generally speaking, on average three transfusions are required but in very severe cases, even more transfusions are occasionally needed. The risk of intrauterine fetal blood transfusion outweighs the benefits at 34 weeks gestation. These fetuses are therefore delivered early since the risks of late preterm delivery are less than the risk of intrauterine fetal blood transfusion (11).

Care of the Neonate with Severe Anemia Secondary to Alloimmunization

Important preparatory steps to be initiated prior to delivery of a fetus resulting from an alloimunized pregnancy are listed in Box 18.3. Some important components of newborn care for these neonates have not changed for decades. Anemia may require transfusion, sometimes including exchange transfusion. Hyperbilirubinemia can be treated with phototherapy.

Box 18.3 **Planning for delivery of a fetus from an alloimmunized pregnancy (11)**

Obtain consent for exchange transfusion if necessary

Blood for neonatal transfusion must be available. It should be cross-matched with maternal blood

Cord is clamped immediately

Cord should be kept long for possible umbilical vein catheterization

Cord blood is collected for group, bilirubin, and direct agglutinin testing

Calculation of Immunoglobulin Dosage

The standard dose of anti-D immune globulin is insufficient if significant fetal-maternal hemorrhage (FMH) occurs. A 500 IU dose is considered adequate to treat a FMH involving up to 4 mL fetal red cells (15). A Kleihauer–Betke test is used to calculate the volume of fetal red blood cells present in maternal circulation. With a Kleihauer–Betke test, maternal cells are placed in an acid bath, which removes adult hemoglobin but not fetal hemoglobin. After subsequent staining, the adult red blood cells appear washed out, but the fetal cells appear pink. Two thousand cells are counted, the percentage of fetal cells is determined, and a formula using maternal blood volume, maternal hematocrit, percent of fetal cells, and newborn hematocrit is used to determine the volume of fetal red blood cells involved in the fetal-maternal hemorrhage (see Figure 18.2).

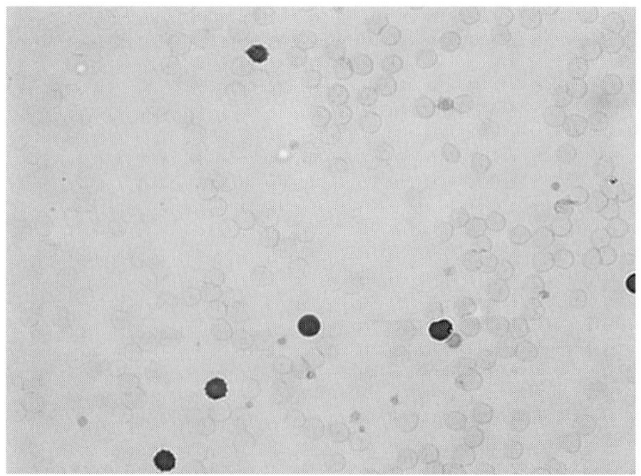

Figure 18.2 Kleihauer–Betke test.

ABO Incompatibility

Incompatibility between maternal ABO blood type and fetal blood type can cause hemolytic disease in the newborn, but the anemia is usually mild. ABO isoimmunization is thus an important concern for pediatricians but it does not commonly affect obstetric management.

Non-rhesus-D Antigens and Atypical Antibodies

Postpartum prophylaxis with anti-D immune globulin has resulted in a dramatic decrease in hemolytic disease of the fetus and newborn. No prophylaxis exists for atypical antigens. Three antibodies are particularly associated with severe disease- anti-D, anti-C, and anti-Kell. A further discussion of atypical antibodies is seen in Table 18.2.

Pregnant patients can be sensitized to these antigens during pregnancy or as result of prior blood transfusion. Two-thirds of women with Kell antibodies, in fact, have a history of a previous blood transfusion (16). Such sensitization could be alleviated with the initiation of policies for a transfusion of Kell negative blood to female children and reproductive age women (17). Such policies are not routine in the United States at the present time.

Treatment of pregnancies complicated by sensitization to atypical antibodies is similar to the management of patient's alloimmunizied to Rh-D (11). As described above, such management may include serial monitoring of maternal antibody titers and feel assessment for anemia including middle cerebral artery peak systolic velocity assessment. Critical maternal titer levels for antibodies to these atypical antigens maybe lower than the recognized critical titer levels for Rhesus D antibodies. It may therefore be appropriate for consultation to occur between the obstetric care providers and the reference laboratory regarding advice for critical titers involving atypical antibodies (11).

Alloimmune Thrombocytopenia

Fetal and neonatal alloimmune thrombocytopenia occurs when maternal alloantibodies are directed against fetal platelets instead of the fetal red cells discussed in the conditions above. The condition can result in fetal or neonatal death or neurologic damage. Intracranial hemorrhage occurs in about 10 to 30% of pregnancies affected by this condition (18). No routine screening program for this condition has currently been implemented. Prenatal diagnosis and treatment are therefore offered to women who have a history of pregnancy with this condition.

Management is controversial. Intravenous immunoglobulins sometimes with and sometimes without corticosteroid have been offered as a noninvasive option (19). Current thinking is that combined therapy with corticosteroids and immunoglobulins is more effective than single agent therapy (20,21). Serial platelet transfusions are an invasive option but carry a significant risk of fetal loss; exsanguination is of course a significant risk in the presence of severe thrombocytopenia (11).

Possible Future Management Changes

Human volunteers are the source for anti-D immune globulin at the present time. Concern exists that transmission of diseases such as Creutzfeldt–Jakob is a potential risk of anti-D immune globulin administration. Fortunately, recombinant Rh immune globulin is undergoing development (14). Cell-free fetal DNA assessment has recently become less expensive. Assessment of cell-free fetal DNA would allow for determination of fetal Rh status; anti-D immune globulin could then be administered only to patients who were carrying Rh (+) fetuses (14,22).

Anti-D prophylaxis for unsensitized Rh (–) women is currently recommended after the sensitizing events listed in Box 18.2. A recent Cochrane review (23) challenged long-standing policies for anti-D immunoglobulin in the antepartum period; anti-D immunoglobulin is commonly given to Rh (–) women at 28 weeks and after miscarriages, ectopic pregnancies, and episodes of vaginal bleeding. The conclusions state: "Existing Studies do not provide conclusive evidence that the use of anti-D during pregnancy benefit either mother or baby in terms of Rhesus alloimmunization during pregnancy...." Perhaps in the future the current standard of practice for administration of antepartum anti-D will be changed. Postpartum administration of anti-D immunoglobulin is of course a well-proven prophylactic medication.

Concluding Remarks

Both NIHF and alloimmunization are conditions that have changed dramatically as the result of modern obstetric care. The routine postpartum administration of anti-D immune globulin has made a common tragedy into a rare event. Other causes of hydrops fetalis can often be managed with resulting neonatal survival.

Prior to efforts to achieve a subsequent pregnancy, preconception consultation is recommended to review underlying etiology if known. The recurrence risk and management of future pregnancies should be discussed at that time.

References

1. Skoll MA, Sharland GK, Allan LD. Is the ultrasound definition of fluid collections in non- immune hydrops fetalis helpful in defining the underlying cause or predicting outcome? *Ultrasound Obstet Gynecol* 1991;1:309–312.
2. Bellini C, Donarini G, Paladini D, Calevo MG, Bellini T, Ramenghi LA., et al. Etiology of non-immune hydorps fetalis: An update. *Am J Med Genet A* 2015 May;167A(5):1082–8.
3. Santolay J, Alley D, Jaffe R, Warsof SL. Antenatal classification of hydrops fetalis. *Obstet Gynecol* 1992;Feb; 79(2):256–9.
4. Huang HR, Tsay PK, Chiang MC, Lien R, Chou YH. Prognostic factors and clinical features in liveborn neonates with hydrops fetalis. *Am J Perinatol* 2007;24(1):33–38.
5. Zipursky A, Paul VK. The global burden of Rh disease. *Arch Dis Child Fetal Neonatal Ed* 2011 Mar;96(2):84–85.
6. van Klink JMM, Koopman HM, Oepkes D, Walther FJ, Lopriore E. Long-term neurodevelopmental outcome after intrauterine transfusion for fetal anemia. *Early Human Develop* 2011;87:589–593.
7. Bahtiyar MO, Emery SP, Dashe JS, WIlkins-Haug LE, Johnson A, Paek BW, et al. The North American fetal therapy network consensus statement. *Obstet Gynec* 2015 Jan; 125(1):118–123.
8. NSG Non-immune hydrops panel. Geenwood Genetics Center. 2016. www.ggc.org/diagnostic/tests-costs/test-finder/ngs-non-immune-hydrops.html. accessed Accessed 9/18/September 18, 2016.
9. Braun T, Brauer M, Fuchs I, Czernik C, Dudenhausen JW, Henrich W, et al. Mirror syndrome: A systematic review of fetal associated conditions, maternal presentation and perinatal outcome. *Fetal Diagn Ther* 2010;27:101–203.
10. Arraut A, Tran SH, Caughey AB. Erthrocyte alloimmunization and pregnancy. *eMedicine J* 2011. http://emedicine.medscape.com/article/273995-overview. Accessed September 18, 2016.
11. Egbor M, Knott P, Bhide A. Red-cell and platelet alloimmunisation in pregnancy. *Best Pract Resear Clin Obstet Gynecol* 2012; 26:119–132.
12. Oepkes D. The modern management of red cell alloimmunisation. *Obstet Gynaecol* 2003;5:15–20.

13. Prasad MR, Krugh D, Rossi KQ, O'Shaughnessy RW. Anti-D in Rh positive pregnancies. *Am J Obstet Gynecol* 2006;195:1158–62.
14. Moise KJ, Argoti PS. Management and prevention of red cell alloimmunization in pregnancy: A systematic review. *Obstet Gynecol* 2012 Nov;120(5):1132–9.
15. The Royal College of Obstetricians and Gynaecologists. The use of anti-D immunoglobulin for rhesus D prophylaxis.*Green-top Guideline* No 22. March 2011. www.rcog.org.uk/en/guidelines-research-services/guidelines/gtg22/ Accessed September 27, 2016.
16. Moise KJ. Fetal anemia due to non-Rhesus-D red-cell alloimmunization. *Semin Fetal Neonatal Med* 2008;13:207–214.
17. Royal College of Obstetricians and Gynaecologist. Guidance on blood transfusion in obstetrics. *Green Top Guideline* No. 47. London: RCOG, 2008. www.rcog.org.uk/files/rcog-corp/uploaded-files/GT47BloodTransfusions1207 amended.pdf. Accessed September 18, 2016.
18. Burrows RF, Kelton JG. Fetal thrombocytopenia and its relation to maternal thrombocytopenia. *Prenat Diagn* 2002;22:96–98.
19. Van den Akker ESA, Oepkes D, Lopriore E, et al. Nonivasive antenatal management of fetal and neonatal alloimmune thrombocytopenia: Safe and effective. *Br J Obstet Gyanecol* 2007;114:469–473.
20. Bertrand G, Drame M, Martageix C, Kaplan C. Prediction of the fetal status in noninvasive management of alloimmune thrombocytopenia. *Blood* 2011 Mar 17;117(11):3209–3213.
21. Berkowitz RL, Kolb EA, McFarland JG, Wissert M, Primani A, Lesser M, et al; Parallel randomized trials of risk-based therapy for fetal alloimmune thrombocytopenia. *Obstet Gynecol* 2006 Jan;107(1):91–96.
22. Kent J, Farrell AM, Soothill P. Routine administration of Anti-D: The ethical case for offering pregnant women fetal RHD genotyping and a review of policy and practice. *BMC Preg Childbirth* 2014;14(87):1–4.
23. McBain RD, Crowther CA, Middleton P. Anti-D administration in pregnancy for preventing Rhesus alloimmunisation (Review) *Cochrane Database Syst Rev* 2015;9:1–31. Art: CD000020.

Chapter 19

Fetal Anomalies

Anitra Beasley

Introduction

Fetal, or congenital, anomalies are important causes of childhood death, chronic illness, and disability. These structural and/or functional anomalies occur during intrauterine life and can be identified prenatally, at birth, or later in life. Although approximately 70% of all congenital anomalies cannot be linked to a specific insult,[1] some known causes and risk factors can be identified. Socioeconomic and demographic factors, genetics, infections, maternal nutrition status, and environmental factors can all contribute to the development of fetal anomalies.

Preconception counseling can be a useful tool for optimization of maternal health and nutrition status. Screening during this period can identify women at risk for specific disorders or at risk for passing a condition onto their children. Prenatal testing can aid in diagnosing abnormalities. This testing enhances maternal informed decision-making; results rarely, however, lead to therapeutic or curative intrauterine interventions.

After delivery, neonatal screening can facilitate life-saving treatments and prevent progression toward some physical, intellectual, visual, or auditory disabilities. Certain neonatal structural anomalies can be ameliorated or surgically corrected and early treatment can be initiated in infants with specific disorders.

Scope of the Problem

Birth defects are common – approximately 3% of liveborn infants have a major congenital anomaly.[2,3] About one half of these anomalies are detected at birth, with the remainder becoming evident during childhood or adult life.[3]

Structural fetal abnormalities are known to develop in at least three ways – malformation, deformation, and disruption. Malformation is the most common mechanism[4] and is defined as an intrinsic abnormality "programmed" into development. The second mechanism, deformation, is when abnormal development is caused by extrinsic mechanical forces. Development of this type of abnormality is especially common during the second trimester when the fetus is constrained within the amniotic sac and uterus.[5] Disruption is a change in form or function that occurs when genetically normal tissue is altered through a specific insult and may be the result of vascular insufficiency, trauma, or teratogens. Abnormalities may also present together as a syndrome, sequence, or association. A syndrome is a cluster of abnormalities that have the same cause while a sequence describes multiple anomalies that developed successively after a single insult. A group of specific abnormalities that occur together but do not seem to be linked in origin defines an association.

Nearly 70% of birth defects do not have an obvious etiology.[1] Although non-genetic factors may cause malformations, genetics are most often responsible.[3]

Chromosomal Abnormalities

The incidence of chromosomal abnormalities is approximately 1 in 155 births.[6] At least 8% of conceptuses are aneuploid, accounting for 50% of first-trimester spontaneous abortions and at least 5% of stillbirths and neonatal deaths.[4] The chromosomal abnormalities that generate the greatest attention are the autosomal trisomies, with the most common found in liveborn infants being trisomy 13, 18, and 21. Down syndrome, or trisomy 21, has a prevalence of approximately 1 in 800 live births[3,6] and is the most common inherited form of intellectual disability.[7] Persons with Down syndrome are distinguished by characteristic craniofacial features, learning disabilities, congenital heart defects, duodenal atresia, childhood leukemia, and early-onset Alzheimer's disease. Trisomy 18 and 13 are less prevalent, being found in 1 in 8,000[6] and 1 in 20,000 livebirths.[3] Both are characterized by growth restriction, distinct facial features, skeletal abnormalities, severe intellectual disability, and are universally lethal within months to years, respectively.

Sex chromosomal abnormalities are less frequently seen. The most common sex chromosome aneuploidy is Klinefelter syndrome (47,XXY) with a prevalence of 1 in 1,000 males. Monosomy X, or is Turner syndrome (45,X), is the only viable momosomy and has an incidence of about 1 in 10,000 liveborn females. It is estimated that 99% of 45,X conceptuses end with spontaneous abortion.[3]

Structural chromosomal abnormalities include deletions, duplications, translocations, isochromosomes, inversions, mosaicism, and ring chromosomes and overall, are present in approximately 1 in 375 newborns.[6] Approximately 1% of liveborn infants are phenotypically abnormal as a result of a single-gene mutation.[3] Common disorders of concern are sickle hemoglobinopathies, thalassemias, cystic fibrosis, and errors of inborn metabolism.

Polygenetic and Multifactorial Disorders

Polygenetic and multifactorial disorders include commonly seen malformations limited to a single organ system, such as, neural tube defects, orofacial clefts, cardiac defects, pyloric stenosis, and omphalocele. Neural tube defects, which include anencephaly, spina bifida, cephalocele, and other rare spinal fusion abnormalities, are the second most common class of major birth defects after structural cardiac anomalies.[2] Isolated neural tube defects are the classic example of multifactorial inheritance, and their development may be influenced by hyperthermia, hyperglycemia, teratogen exposure, ethnicity, family history, fetal gender, and genetic predisposition. After the birth of one child with a multifactorial birth defect, the recurrence risk in subsequent pregnancies is 1–5%.[3,4]

Infections

Infections are a major cause of fetal morbidity and mortality. Common infections that cause mild-to-moderate illness in healthy adults and children can have serious fetal consequences. Cytomegalovirus, human parvovirus B19, toxoplasmosis, and varicella zoster virus can be associated with severe fetal complications when acquired during pregnancy. Epidemic rubella is now less common due to widespread vaccination but when acquired can have similarly devastating consequences. Maternal serologic status, gestational age at the time of infection, and immunologic status can all affect disease outcome.

Teratogenic Disorders

The number of medications and other substances proven or strongly suspected to be human teratogens is small, and, with the exception of alcohol, make minor contributions to the development of fetal anomalies. Alcohol is one of the most frequent non-genetic causes of mental retardation as well as the leading cause of preventable birth defects in the United States.[1] The estimated prevalence of fetal alcohol syndrome is 0.2 to 3 per 1,000 births. Children with fetal alcohol syndrome are characterized by dysmorphic facial features, pre- and/or postnatal growth impairment, and central nervous system neurodevelopmental abnormalities. Alcohol-related cardiac, skeletal, renal, ocular, and auditory birth defects are also seen.[8] Still, the prevalence of fetal alcohol spectrum disorders, which encompass the full range of prenatal alcohol damage, is thought to be even greater and as high as 2–5% in the United States.[9]

Anticonvulsant medications, angiotensin-converting enzyme (ACE) inhibitors and angiotensin-receptor blocking drugs, nonsteroidal anti-inflammatory drugs, radioiodine, heavy metals, retinoids, warfarin, and certain antimicrobial, antiviral, antifungal, antineoplastic, and psychiatric medications have been linked to specific birth defects.

Prevention

Primary prevention of congenital anomalies is ideal and includes strategies such as improving preconception nutrition status, abstention, or restriction of intake of harmful substances during pregnancy, controlling preexisting diabetes, avoiding environmental exposure to hazardous substances, and prepregnancy vaccination from certain diseases.

It is recommended that all low risk women take 400 μg of folic acid daily before conception and through the first trimester of pregnancy to reduce the risk of development of fetal neural tube defects by up to 52%.[10] Women at elevated risk for neural tube defects should take an increased dose of 4 mg of folic acid daily. For a woman with a prior affected child, this decreases the recurrence risk by as much as 72%.[11]

Screening

Genetic screening is used to identify women and their partners who are at increased risk of having a child with an inherited condition, chromosomal abnormality, or birth defect. Some disorders occur with increased frequency in certain ethnic groups, and thus, ethnic background may indicate the need for carrier testing. During pregnancy, biochemical testing and ultrasonography can be used to screen for chromosomal anomalies and severe defects. Newborn screening is mandatory in the United States and designed for the identification of disorders in which early intervention can improve long-term outcomes.

There are many strategies available to screen for structural and chromosomal abnormalities, and currently available noninvasive screening tests have high detection rates. Because technological advances have resulted in improved aneuploidy detection, the American Congress of Obstetricians and Gynecologists (ACOG) now recommends that aneuploidy screening and diagnostic testing be discussed and offered to all women in early pregnancy.[7] Women with positive screening test results should be offered diagnostic testing.

A number of distinct minor abnormalities, or markers, associated with chromosomal aneuploidy are detectable by ultrasound examination. These markers may occur in isolation in a chromosomally normal fetus, but the likelihood of a genetic abnormality increases when multiple markers are present. In contrast, some major abnormalities, such as anencephaly, spina bifida, and abdominal wall defects, are easily detected and rarely missed. Routine inclusion of the four-chamber view of the heart and outflow tracts in screening ultrasounds has resulted in increased in detection of heart defects.[12]

Neural Tube Defects

Anencephaly is easily diagnosed based on the absence of the cranial vault after 10 weeks gestation and is often first suspected when a proper image for measuring the biparietal diameter cannot be obtained. Similarly, characteristic changes in the brain and skull are seen in fetuses with spina bifida, including frontal narrowing of the skull, known as the "lemon sign," and ventriculomegaly (See Figure 19.1). Additionally, the cerebellum is deformed and drawn into posterior fossa, leading to the "banana sign" (see Figure 19.2). Widening of the bony spine is seen on transverse and longitudinal ultrasound views, and in the most severe form of spina bifida, a meningomyelocele sac is seen. Clubfoot and/or lack of movement in the lower extremities is associated with poor prognosis for motor function.[12] Encephalocele is the least common type of neural tube defect and is identified by protrusion of the meninges and possibly brain tissue through a midline cranial defect. Neurologic outcome is poor if brain tissue is contained within the encephalocele

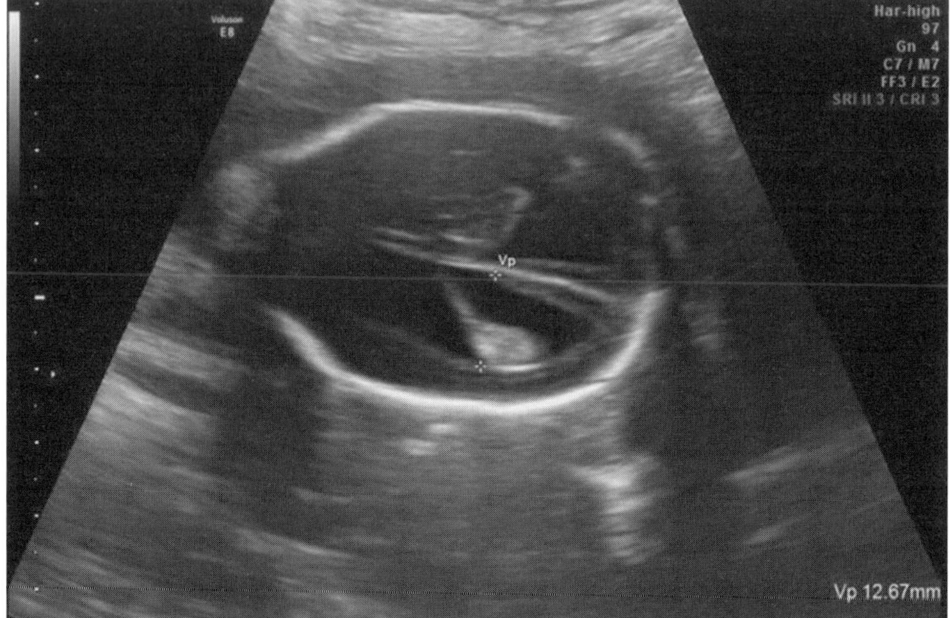

Figure 19.1 Lemon sign.

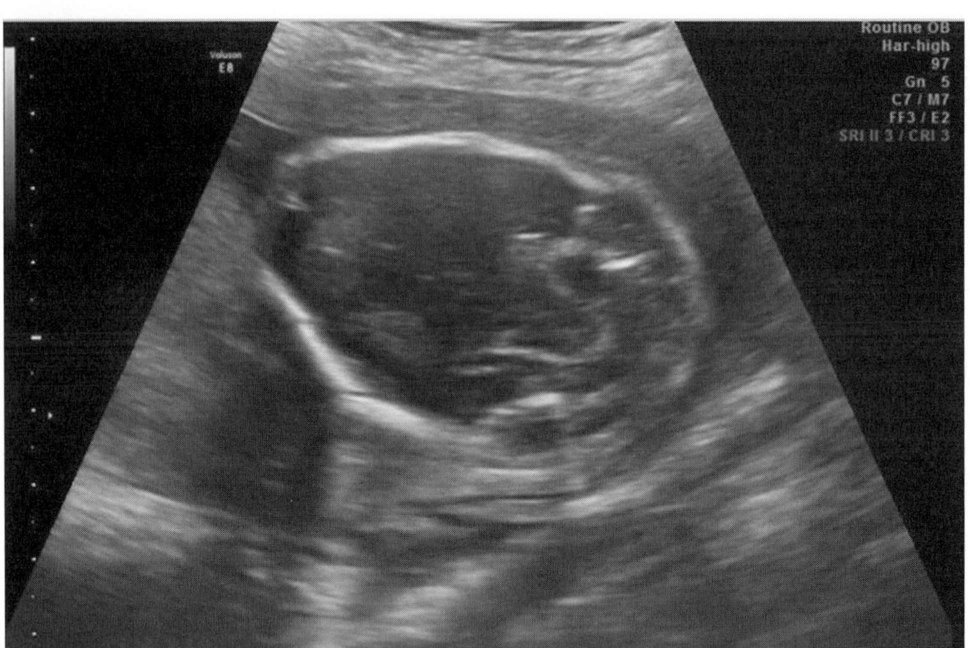

Figure 19.2 Lemon sign with banana sign.

sac; however, in the case of an isolated defect with no brain involvement, neurologic outcome is good.[12]

Orofacial Defects

Isolated orofacial clefts are one of the most common birth defects in the United States,[13] and approximately two-thirds of infants with cleft lip also have cleft palate.[12] Children with a cleft lip and/or palate often have problems with feeding, speech clarity, ear infections, hearing, and dentition.[14] With a screening ultrasound, coronal views of fetal face are usually obtained and can identify a cleft lip. Cleft palate can be seen on oblique views, with a defect in the maxillary ridge. An isolated cleft palate is rarely diagnosed with prenatal ultrasound.[12]

Cardiac Anomalies

The four-chamber view of the heart is part of the standard prenatal screening ultrasound and can be used to identify congenital heart defects, such as septal defects and hypoplastic left heart syndrome. Ventricular septal defects account for approximately a quarter of congenital cardiac anomalies (see Figure 19.3). An atrioventricular canal defect is the most obvious septal defect that can be sonographically seen; it has a strong correlation with Down syndrome, being present in about half of cases. Although large defects can often be detected with standard views, smaller lesions are commonly missed.[12]

Approximately 25% of infants born with a heart defect are considered to have a critical defect[15] and will need surgery or other procedures within the first year of life. These defects include coarctation of the aorta, double-outlet left ventricle, d-transposition of the great arteries, Ebstein anomaly, hypoplastic left heart syndrome, interrupted aortic arch, pulmonary atresia, single ventricle, tetralogy of Fallot, total anomalous pulmonary venous return, tricuspid atresia, and truncus arteriosus.[16] Hypoplastic left heart syndrome is suspected when the left ventricle appears very small and can be better characterized with visualization of the outflow tracts. A fetal echocardiogram may be needed to confirm prenatally suspected congenital heart defects.

Survival of infants with congenital heart defects depends on how severe the defect is, when it is diagnosed, and how it is managed. Approximately 97% of infants born with a noncritical heart defect survive to one year of age and about 95% to 18 years; approximately 75% born with a critical defect survive to one year and about 69% to 18 years. However, those diagnosed with critical defects on or before day of life one have poorer one-year survival compared with those diagnosed after day of life one.[17]

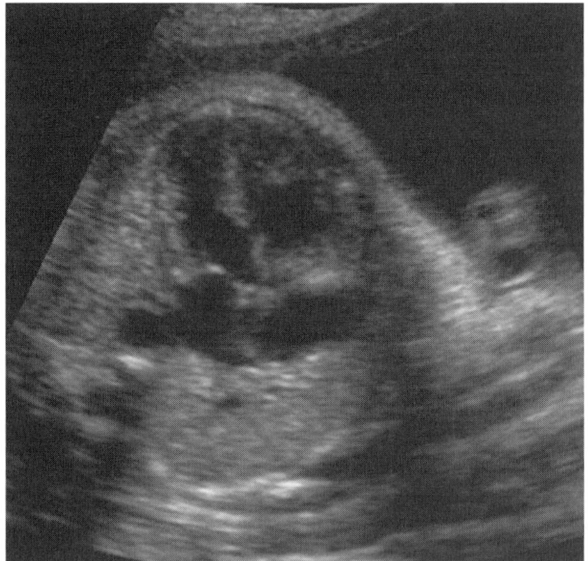

Figure 19.3 Ventricular septal defect (VSD).

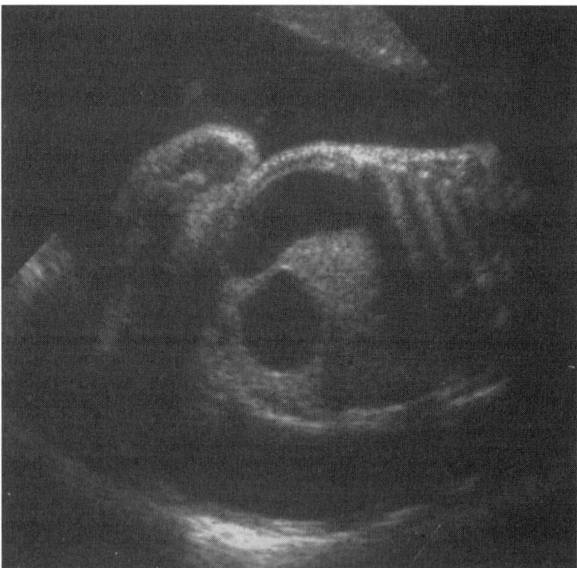

Figure 19.4 Double bubble sign seen with duodenal atresia.

Gastrointestinal Disorders

The fetal stomach can be routinely visualized on ultrasound after the first trimester. If it is small, absent, or does not fill within 60 minutes, esophageal atresia should be suspected. Duodenal atresia, on the other hand, is sonographically diagnosed later and is suspected with visualization of the "double-bubble" sign in which the adjacent fluid-filled dilated stomach and proximal duodenum are seen (Figure 19.4). Polyhydramnios is a common co-finding and trisomy 21 is confirmed in about 30% of cases.[12]

Urologic Anomalies

Sonographically, bladder outlet obstruction is diagnosed when the bladder is abnormally enlarged and emptying is not seen. It occurs almost exclusively in male fetuses and is usually caused by urethral obstruction due to posterior urethral valves. More complex malformations can also cause such obstruction and are more common in female fetuses. With severe obstruction, oligohydramnios, dilated ureters, hydronephrosis, and cystic renal dysplasia can be seen. Longstanding complete obstruction leads to anhydramnios and lethal pulmonary hypoplasia; ureteral reflux results in irreversible renal damage.[12]

Hypospadius is a congenital anomaly of the urethra in male fetuses. This defect is usually isolated and frequently requires surgical repair. Occasionally hypospadias is associated with an undescended testicle; in this case the differential diagnosis includes a disorder of sexual differentiation.

Ambiguous Genitalia

The gender of some neonates cannot be reliably determined at birth. This is extremely distressing to parents and must be addressed as a family emergency. This physician should *not* make a best guess as to the neonate's gender but should allow for appropriate evaluation before assigning gender. A neonate with XX chromosomes who presents with ambiguous genitalia may have congenital adrenal hyperplasia. This salt wasting condition may result in significant morbidity or mortality if undiagnosed.

Abdominal Wall Defects

Omphalocele is a ventral wall defect characterized by protrusion of abdominal contents into the base of the umbilical cord. Intestines, stomach, and liver are the most frequently herniated organs and are covered by a membranous sac. Conversely, gastroschisis is a right paraumbilical herniation of abdominal organs. Most commonly, only bowel is involved but liver, stomach, and bladder can also be present. While there is a 75% likelihood of additional associated birth defects with an omphalocele, gastroschisis is usually isolated and is rarely associated with chromosome abnormalities.[12] These defects are usually surgically managed soon after birth; however, if the defect is large, the repair may need to be staged.

Diagnosis

Whereas genetic screening is used to assess whether an increased risk for a fetal abnormality exists for a particular patient, prenatal diagnosis ascertains whether a specific condition is present. Common indications for genetic testing include advanced maternal age, parental chromosomal rearrangements, heterozygosity for the same single-gene disorder, positive results from aneuploidy screening, previous history of fetal aneulploidy or structural defects, and ultrasonographic detection of structural fetal anomalies. Multiple laboratory techniques can be used to evaluate samples, but testing is most commonly done via karyotype analysis and/or fluorescence in situ hybridization (FISH) with cells obtained through chorionic villus sampling (CVS) or amniocentesis.[18]

Management

After the prenatal diagnosis of a fetal anomaly, the patient should receive detailed information about the natural history of the diagnosed condition. Depending on the anomaly, specialty referral may be indicated as appropriate decision making requires comprehensive and accurate counseling. Effective prenatal therapy is not available for most disorders, and the option of pregnancy termination should be discussed when a genetic disorder or major structural abnormality is detected. If the pregnancy is continued, counseling should include family education and preparation, obstetric management recommendations, and referral to pediatric specialists and tertiary care centers as appropriate. Perinatal palliative care services and comfort care should be discussed in the case of a diagnosis incompatible with long-term survival.[18]

For a limited number of disorders, effective medical and surgical prenatal therapy is available. Fetal pharmacotherapy, defined as medications administered to the mother and delivered transplacentally to the fetus, can be used to treat a small variety of serious conditions. Maternal-fetal surgery is offered for some structural defects that interfere with organ development but could allow for normal fetal development to proceed if corrected. Current fetal conditions for which antenatal surgery may be available include lower urinary tract obstruction, twin-twin transfusion syndrome, myelomeningocele, congenital diaphragmatic hernia, neck masses occluding the trachea, and select tumors associated with developing fetal hydrops. Still, maternal-fetal surgery is a major procedure for the woman and her fetus, with serious implications and complications that can occur acutely, postoperatively, for the duration of the pregnancy, and in subsequent pregnancies. It is highly technical and carries the risk for significant morbidity and mortality. Prenatal surgery should only be offered at facilities with the expertise, multidisciplinary teams, services, and facilities capable of providing the specialized care required. Even though several different procedures have been developed and refined, fetal surgery continues to be plagued by the inability to accurately identify ideal candidates for intervention, determine the optimal timing for surgery, and prevent resultant preterm births.[20]

Myelomeningocele is the most common indication for open fetal surgery[21]; however, prenatal repair can be performed by fetoscopic or open techniques. The Management of Myelomeningocele Study (MOMS) evaluated the outcome of children undergoing open prenatal versus standard postnatal myelomeningocele repair. As compared with postnatal surgery, prenatal procedures decreased the risk of death or need for shunting at 12 months, improved composite mental and motor function scores at 30 months, and improved the degree of hindbrain herniation, motor function, and the likelihood of being able to walk independently. The main complications associated with prenatal surgery were preterm births, intraoperative complications, uterine scar defects, and higher rates of maternal transfusion at delivery. Similar rates of fetal and/or neonatal mortality were found and no maternal deaths occurred.[22] Based on the criteria set from this trial, the ACOG Committee on Obstetric Practice recommends that appropriately qualified women with pregnancies complicated by myelomeningiocele be counseled regarding the option of prenatal maternal-fetal surgery, with the discussion to include the risks and benefits to the woman and her infant and implications for future pregnancies.[19]

Prognosis for fetuses with lower urinary tract obstruction can be poor, and prenatal treatment can be advantageous in cases with preserved renal function. Vesicoamniotic shunting is the main intervention performed; the goal is to maintain amniotic fluid volume to help fetal lung growth, not to preserve renal function. Shunt placement is, however, an invasive procedure that can be complicated by shunt extrusion, retraction, or occlusion, fetal abdominal wall herniation at the site of shunt placement, bladder rupture, intrauterine infection, preterm premature rupture of membranes, preterm labor and fetal death.[21]

Inevitably, some anomalies will not be diagnosed prenatally and will instead be diagnosed at the time of delivery. The birth of an infant with a previously undiagnosed congenital anomaly can be a devastating experience, and many factors can affect how such a birth crisis is handled. Disbelief, denial, and sadness are normal reactions, especially if the problem is unexpected, and feelings of guilt, unfairness, despair, depression, anxiety, anger, failure, and apprehension are common. These feelings may be enhanced when there are preexisting conditions that may have affected the pregnancy or if the mother made lifestyle choices that can be associated with significant disabilities, such as alcohol abuse.[9]

Very little literature is present on the process of delivering the news of a newborn's anomaly to the family at the time of delivery. It seems reasonable to ensure that the mother and family receive the empathy appropriate to the situation. For anomalies with minimal long-term morbidity, it is also sensible to emphasize the positive overall health of the newborn while pointing out the need for further medical attention specific to the treatment of the anomaly.

Management of significant unanticipated infant outcomes must first focus on stabilization of the infant and/or mother. If intensive resuscitation is required, a member of the team should be assigned to provide support and information to the parents. Ideally, the parents should have the opportunity to see and touch their infant before it is moved from the delivery room. The ability to see, touch, and hold the infant with disabilities can decrease fears and misconceptions about the anomalies.[23] Most anomalies can be addressed by the infant's primary caregiver, but a few require the immediate attention of the delivery personnel.

As soon as possible after birth or diagnosis of an infant with an unforeseen anomaly, the infant's primary healthcare provider should meet with the parent(s). It is important to maintain a positive tone that emphasizes the infant's personhood and positive attributes while realistically describing the existing problems. Although it is essential to give complete information about the infant's condition, treatment, and prognosis, parents may not be able to fully retain what is said in the initial meeting.[23]

Meningiomyelocele

Treatment of a myelomeningiocele in the delivery room includes decubitus positioning of the newborn to avoid direct pressure on the lesion and application of a sterile plastic covering or bag, if available, or sterile normal saline soaked gauze to protect the lesion from infection, desiccation, and direct trauma. Any resuscitative measures should be performed with the neonate in the decubitus position. Consultation with a neonatologist and pediatric neurosurgeon should be obtained as soon as possible.[24,25]

Abdominal Wall Defects

In the case of gastroschisis or omphalocele, the defect should be covered immediately after delivery with moist, sterile gauze, and if available, the infant should be placed in a sterile, clear plastic bag that is drawn up over the feet to the chest to essentially cover the defect and limit physical trauma, insensible water losses, and heat loss. The infant should not receive anything by mouth, and an orogastric tube should be placed to minimize gastrointestinal distention. A neonatologist and pediatric surgeon should be consulted for further management.[24,25]

Orofacial Clefts

A cleft lip or palate does not require immediate attention; however, the infant's mother may have many questions and fears. It should be explained that the most important thing to do is to feed the baby to ensure adequate growth until surgery can be performed. If the infant has a cleft lip with an intact palate, feeding, including breastfeeding, may be attempted. If the infant cannot adequately breastfeed because of the cleft, breast milk can be expressed and the infant fed using an alternative feeding method. The infant should be referred to a pediatric surgeon or specialized center for surgical repair. In the interim, close follow-up to check growth and weight gain will be required.[24]

Surgery to repair a cleft lip usually occurs in the first few months of life and should occur within the first year of life. Repair of cleft palate is recommended within the first 18 months of life; however, many children will need additional procedures as they age. Surgical repair can have a cosmetic effect and may improve breathing, hearing, speech, and language development. Other types of treatments and services, such as special dental or orthodontic care or speech therapy may also be needed.[14]

Hypospadias

Hypospadias is usually diagnosed on physical examination after the infant is born. Most newborns with hypospadias will need surgery to correct the defect, but immediate intervention is not required. All patients should have the benefit of urologic consultation, and the infant should not be circumcised as the foreskin will be needed for the future repair.[26]

Concluding Remarks

Birth defects are common – approximately 3% of liveborn infants have a major congenital anomaly.[2,3] When possible, primary prevention is ideal; this includes strategies such as optimizing pre-conception nutrition and medical status, avoidance of harmful substances, and vaccination from certain diseases. Many strategies are available to screen for structural and chromosomal abnormalities, and currently available tests have high detection rates. Patients diagnosed with fetal anomalies require accurate and comprehensive counseling, including the option of pregnancy termination. While fetal therapy is available for some conditions, the vast majority of disorders are not amenable to prenatal management or curative pediatric therapy.

References

1. Teratology, teratogens, and fetotoxic agents. In: F.L.K. Cunningham, S.L. Bloom, C.Y. Spong, J.S. Dashe, B.L. Hoffman, B.M. Casey, J.S. Sheffield, eds. *Williams Obstetrics*. 24th ed. New York: McGraw-Hill; 2013.
2. Centers for Disease Control and Prevention. Update on Overall Prevelance of Major Birth Defects – Atlanta, Georgia, 1978–2005. *Morbidity and Mortality Weekly Report*. 2008;57(1):1–5.
3. Genetic counseling and genetic screening. In: S.G. Gabbe, J.R. Niebyl, J.L. Simpson, et al., editors. *Obstetrics: Normal and Problem Pregnancies*. 6th ed. Philadelphia, PA: Elsevier; 2012.
4. Prenatal Diagnosis. In: F.G. Cunningham, K.J. Leveno, S.L. Bloom, et. al, editors. *Williams Obstetrics*. 24th ed. New York, NY: McGraw Hill; 2013.
5. Developmental Genetics and Birth Defects. In: R.L. Nussbaum, R.R. McInnes, and H.F. Willard, editors. *Thompson & Thompson Genetics in Medicine*. Philadelphia, PA: Elsevier; 2016.
6. Principles of Clinical Cytogenetics and Genome Analysis. In: R.L. Nussbaum, R.R. McInnes, and H.F. Willard, editors. *Thompson & Thompson Genetics in Medicine*. Philidelphia, PA: Elsevier; 2016.
7. Practice Bulletin No. 163: Screening for Fetal Aneuploidy. Obstetrics & Gynecology. Published Ahead of Print.
8. K. Stratton, C. Howe, F. Battaglia, editors. *Fetal Alcohol Syndrome: Diagnosis, Empidemiology, Prevention, and Treatment*. Washington, DC: National Academy Press; 1996.
9. P.A. May, J.P. Gossage, W.O. Kalberg, et al. Prevalence and epidemiologic characteristics of FASD from various research methods with an emphasis on recent in-school studies. *Developmental Disabilities Research Reviews*. 2009;15(3):176–92.
10. N.J. Wald, M.R. Law, J.K. Morris, et al. Quantifying the effect of folic acid. *Lancet*. 2001;358(9298): 2069–73.
11. N Wald, J. Sneddon. Prevention of neural tube defects: Results of the Medical Research Council Vitamin Study. *Lancet*. 1991;338(8760):131.
12. Prenatal Genetic Diagnosis. In: S.G. Gabbe, J.R. Niebyl, J.L. Simpson, et al., editors. *Obstetrics: Normal and Problem Pregnancies*. 6th ed. Philadelphia, PA: Saunders; 2012.
13. S.E. Parker, C.T. Mai, M.A. Canfield, et al. Updated national birth prevalence estimates for selected birth defects in the United States, 2004–2006. *Birth Defects Research Part A: Clinical and Molecular Teratology*. 2010;88(12):1008–16.
14. Centers for Disease Control and Prevention. Birth Defects: Facts About Cleft Lip and Palate. 2015 [May 2016]. Available from: www.cdc.gov/ncbddd/birthdefects/cleftlip.html.
15. M.D. Reller, M.J. Strickland, T. Riehle-Colarusso, et al. Prevalence of congenital heart defects in metropolitan Atlanta, 1998–2005. *J Pediatrics*. 2008; 153(6):807–13.
16. Centers for Disease Control and Prevention. Congenital Heart Defects: Facts About Congenital Heart Defects 2015 [cited 2016 May]. Available from: www.cdc.gov/ncbddd/heartdefects/facts.html.
17. ME Oster, KA Lee, MA Honein, et al. Temporal trends in survival among infants with critical congenital heart defects. *Pediatrics*. 2013; 131(5):e1502–e8.
18. Practice Bulletin No. 162. Prenatal Diagnostic Testing for Genetic Disorders. *Obstetrics & Gynecology*. Published ahead of print.
19. Committee Opinion No. 550. Maternal-fetal surgery for Myelomeningocele. *Obstetrics & Gynecology*. 2013;121(1):218–9.
20. K.D. Wenstrom, S.R. Carr. Fetal surgery: Principles, indications, and evidence. *Obstetrics & Gynecology*. 2014;124(4):817–35.
21. P. Sala, F. Prefumo, D. Pastorino, et al. Fetal surgery: An overview. *Obstetrical & Gynecological Survey*. 2014;69(4):218–28.
22. N.S. Adzick, E.A. Thom, C.Y. Spong, et al. A randomized trial of prenatal versus postnatal repair of myelomeningocele. *New England Journal of Medicine*. 2011;364(11):993–1004.

23. Birth Crisis: Caring for the Family Experiencing Perinatal Death or the Birth of a Child With Medical Complications. In: S.D. Ratcliffe, E.G. Baxley, M.K. Cline, et al, editors. *Family Medicine Obstetrics*. 3rd ed. Philadephia, PA: Elsevier; 2008.

24. *Managing Newborn Problems: A Guide Doctors, Nurses, and Midwives*. Geneva, Switzerland: World Health Organization; 2003.

25. A.K. Rajani, R. Chitkara, L.P. Halamek. Delivery room management of the newborn. *Pediatric Clinics of North America*. 2009;56(3):515–35.

26. Examination of the newborn. In: J.M. Rennie, editor. *Rennie and Robertson's Textbook of Neonatology*. 5th ed. London: Churchill Livingstone Elsevier Limited; 2012.

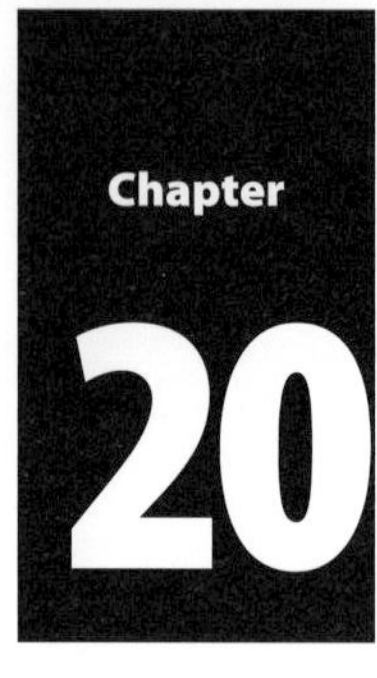

Malpresentation

Martin Olsen

Introduction

Fetal malpresentation is a common obstetric complication. This chapter discusses the diagnosis and management of breech, face, brow, occiput transverse, occiput posterior, transverse lie, and compound presentations.

Scope of the Problem

Abnormal presentation, usually the breech presentation, complicated 3% of total deliveries in a major study.[1] Gardberg et al. described a higher rate of malpresentation. Cephalic malpresentations included persistent occipitoposterior in 5% of overall cases, and face presentation in 1%, brow presentation in 0.14%, breech presentation in 3.1% and a transverse lie in 0.12% of the cases. Primiparity was associated with increased malpresentations.[2]

Approximately 20.6% of deliveries at age 25 to 26 weeks may be complicated by breech presentation; the frequency of breech presentation dropped to 1.7% after 40 weeks gestation in this study.[3] Gestational age is the single greatest influence in the process of fetal malpresentation; other causes include uterine relaxation as a result of parity, hydramnios, uterine anomalies, uterine fibroids, and abdominal placental implantation.[3] One-third of US pregnancies were delivered via cesarean section in 2011; malpresentation was the third leading cause after labor dystocia and fetal heart rate tracing concerns.[4]

Breech Presentation

Risk factors for breech presentation include multiparity, previous breech delivery, polyhydramnios, fetal anomalies, and uterine anomalies.[1]

The American Congress of Obstetricians and Gynecologists' (ACOG) Committee on Obstetric Practice recommended in 2001 that planned vaginal delivery of term singleton breech pregnancies was no longer appropriate,[5] but in 2006 this statement was modified.[6] The 2006 ACOG Committee Opinion stated that the decision regarding mode of delivery can be affected by experience of the health care provider. Cesarean delivery will be the preferred method for most physicians because of the diminished expertise in vaginal breech delivery. Planned vaginal breech delivery of a term singleton breech fetus may be reasonable under hospital-specific protocols and guidelines for both eligibility and labor management. Patients must be informed that the risk of perinatal or neonatal mortality and morbidity may be higher in vaginal breech delivery than in planned cesarean section delivery. The patient's informed consent should be documented.[6] The ACOG's Committee Opinion from 2006 states: "The decision regarding the mode of delivery should depend on the experience of the health care provider. Cesarean delivery will be the preferred mode of delivery for most physicians because of the diminishing expertise in vaginal breech delivery."[6]

Hannah et al. randomized over 2,000 women to planned vaginal birth for breech presentation in one arm and planned cesarean section in the other arm. Fifty-seven percent of the patients in the vaginal delivery arm delivered vaginally. Perinatal mortality, neonatal mortality, and serious neonatal morbidity was higher in planned vaginal delivery group then it was in the planned caesarean group. The authors therefore concluded that planned caesarean section was better than planned vaginal birth for the term fetus.[7]

Further details from the Term Breech trial (done in 2000) by Hannah et al. include requirements for participating institutions in the provision of expertise in vaginal breech delivery; identification of a team of physicians skilled in vaginal delivery was required. Assessment of fetal size in the laboring patient was required.

There were no significant differences in maternal morbidity or mortality between the planned caesarean

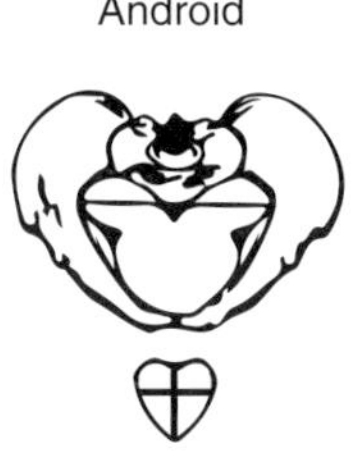

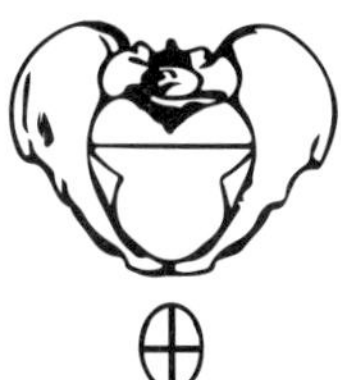

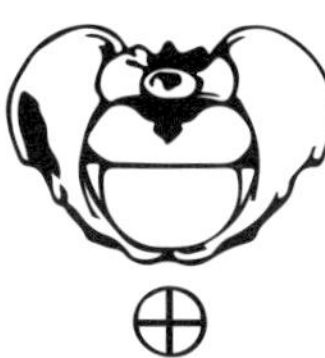

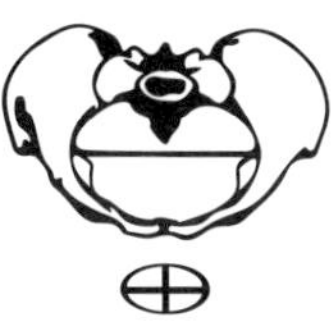

Figure 20.1 Female boney pelvis variations.

section group and the planned vaginal birth group. The authors concluded that a policy of planned cesarean section would result in one baby saved from death or serious morbidity for every 14 additional cesarean sections.[7]

Interestingly, nearly 10% of the patients randomized to caesarean section were delivered vaginally; over half of these patients were delivered vaginally because caesarean section was not possible due to an imminent vaginal delivery. This observation implies to the author that training in vaginal breech delivery remains an essential component of obstetric education.

The Term Breech trial patients were followed after the initial report. At three months, after delivery, the planned cesarean group had more pain on the outside of the abdomen but the planned vaginal delivery group had increased urinary incontinence. The findings otherwise were very similar between the two groups.[8] The Term Breech trial found no differences in breastfeeding, pain, depression, menstrual problems, fatigue, relationship with child, relationship with partners, pain, and subsequent pregnancy, incontinence, urinary problems, sexual problems, fatigue or distressing memories of the birth experience at two years postpartum. A planned cesarean section was associated with higher constipation.[9]

Many authors believe that in selected cases, elective vaginal breech delivery may be appropriate. When specific management protocols are followed in properly selected patients, vaginal delivery of term breech fetus has been safely documented in retrospective studies. Planned vaginal delivery of a term singleton breech fetus may therefore be reasonable under hospital-specific protocol guidelines for eligibility and labor management. Great caution should be exercised in vaginal breech deliveries and detailed patient informed consent should be documented. Patients should be informed that the risk both short-term and long-term perinatal neonatal morbidity and mortality may be higher in vaginal breech deliveries than in planned cesarean deliveries.[6]

Assessment of the maternal pelvis is indicated for additional planning (emergent or otherwise) of potential vaginal delivery of the breech fetus. Female pelvic types are shown in Figure 20.1.

The breech fetus may present in multiple subcategories. Figure 20.2 shows a simulated fetus in the frank breech position. Figure 20.3 shows a complete breech fetus and Figure 20.4 shows an incomplete breech fetus. Figure 20.5 shows an unflexed or hyperextended fetal head. This head position is sometimes called the military position or the sniffing position. If a vaginal breech delivery were to be considered for a fetus with a hyperextended fetal head, the potential for neck injury exists; the military position therefore makes any attempt at vaginal breech delivery contraindicated even in those institutions which perform such planned deliveries.

Criteria and protocols for vaginal breech delivery include the elements provided in Box 20.1. Oxytocin induction or augmentation is not offered. Strict criteria for normal labor progress are followed.[6] Hospitals are, of course, free to add additional criterial such as physical presence of obstetricians and anesthesiologists in the labor and delivery area during the labor of a vaginal breech delivery patient.

The Term Breech trial is controversial especially outside the United States. International variation in the mode of delivery for a singleton breech fetus continues to exist. In 2006 the PREsentation et MODe d'Accouchement (PREMODA) study

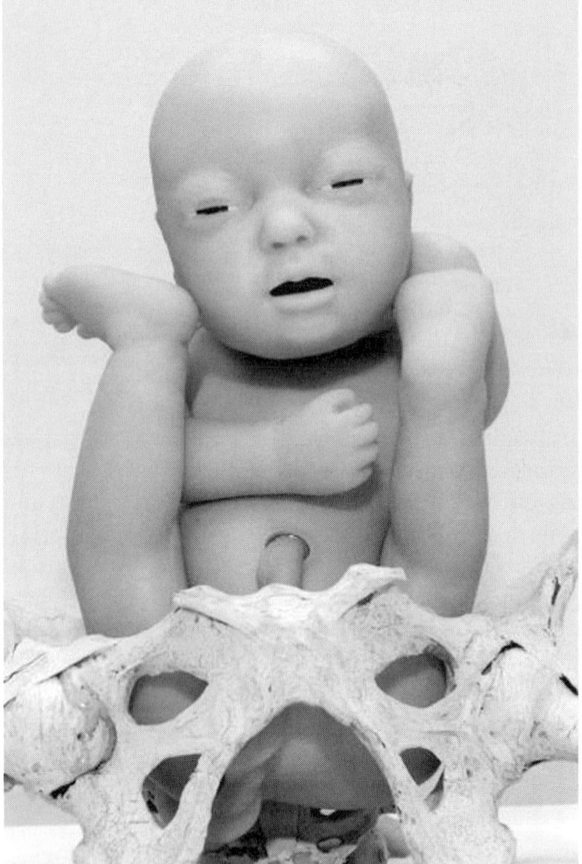

Figure 20.2 Frank breech. Simulated fetus provided by Gaumard Scientific. Photographed by Mr. Jim Sledge, East Tennessee State University.

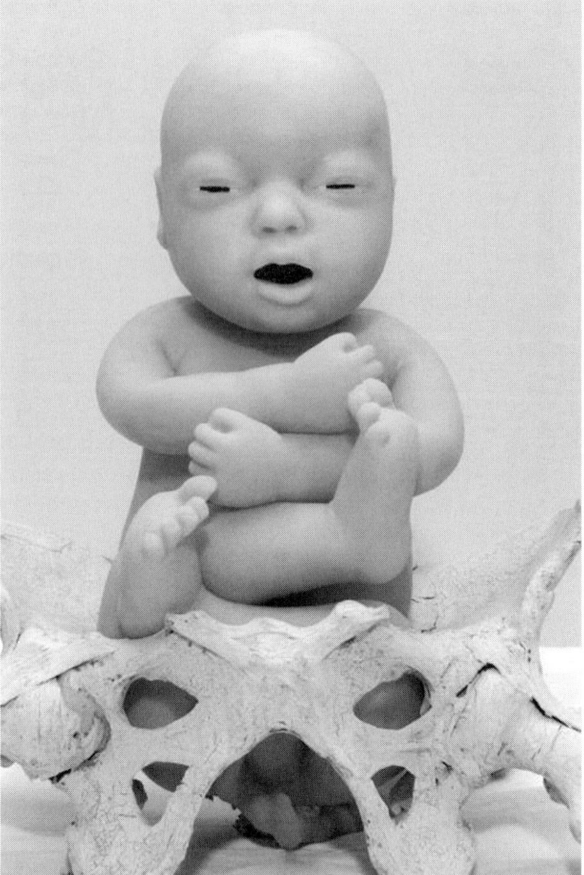

Figure 20.3 Complete breech.

raised questions about the Term Breech trial and concluded that perinatal mortality and serious neonatal morbidity were not as different as previously described for vaginal breech delivery as planned cesarean delivery for term breech fetuses; the study did show an excess of neonates with 5-minute Apgar scores less than 4 and increased risk of intubation in the planned vaginal delivery group. Intensive care admissions and birth trauma were also increased in the planned vaginal delivery group.[10] A national study in the Netherlands[10] showed an increase in the rate of cesarean delivery for breech from 50% to 80% to after the Term Breech trial. Rates of perinatal death, 5-minute Apgar score less than 7 and neonatal trauma declined in the posttrial period. In Denmark, overall rates in cesarean section increased from 80% to 94% in the period immediately after publication of the Term Breech trial; significant declines were observed in intrapartum and neonatal death and in neonatal intensive care admissions. Adverse outcome rates are remained higher in the planned vaginal delivery group.[11]

The author believes that the preponderance of data suggests that planned vaginal breech deliveries should be discouraged in the developed world, but acknowledges that multiple current guidelines suggest that planned vaginal deliveries are a reasonable option.[12] Maternal morbidity was somewhat higher with planned cesarean section in one study.[13] Observational studies have found that delivery by cesarean section increases the risk of placenta previa, placenta accreta, uterine rupture, and the need for a repeat cesarean section in subsequent pregnancies.[14,15]

Joseph et al. argue that specialized clinics and clinicians experienced in vaginal delivery for breech presentation are necessary to support women who choose the vaginal option.[16] All physicians who provide care for women in labor should be familiar with the process of vaginal breech delivery in order to be

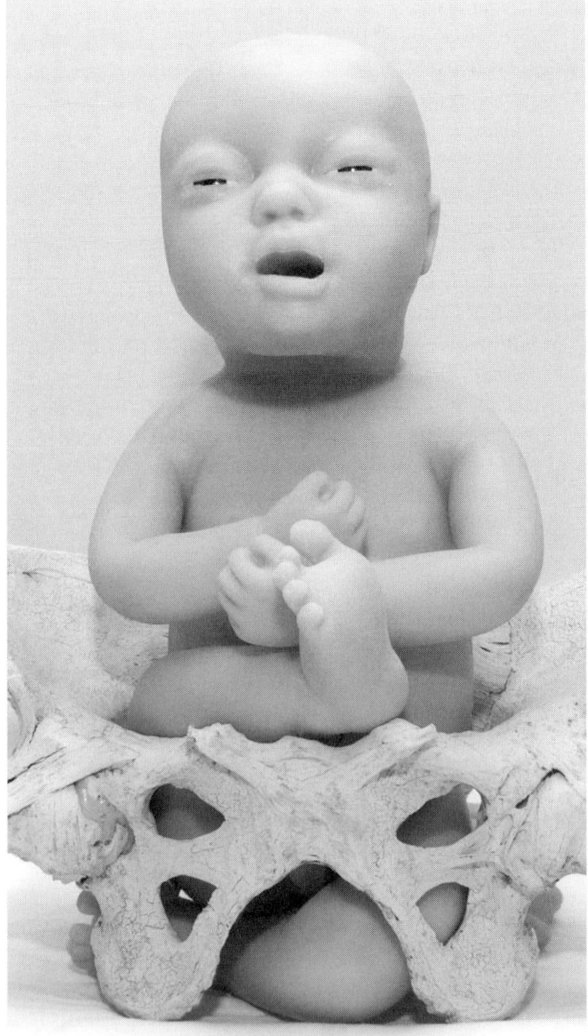

Figure 20.4 Incomplete breech. In labor, this position may be called a footling breech. One leg is up, and the other is presenting part. Risk of cord prolapse is even higher than other forms of breech presentation. Photographed by Mr. Jim Sledge, East Tennessee State University.

prepared for the patient who presents in labor with a breech fetus and will deliver imminent delivery.

The steps in the performance of a vaginal breech delivery are listed in Box 20.2. A very difficult possible issue faced in vaginal breech deliveries is the presence of a fetal nuchal arm. This situation is shown with a simulated fetus in Figure 20.6. A calm approach by the delivering physician is essential to reduce the fetal arm(s) without fracturing the humerus.

American obstetricians have all but abandoned planned singleton breech vaginal deliveries. Planned vaginal delivery of the breech fetus seems limited to breech extraction of the second twin in US training centers[17]; even this is not universally practiced. The level of training in US obstetric residency programs has therefore diminished. The risk to the fetus when an unplanned vaginal breech delivery occurs is unavoidable and may be increased when a physician is inadequately trained.[17]

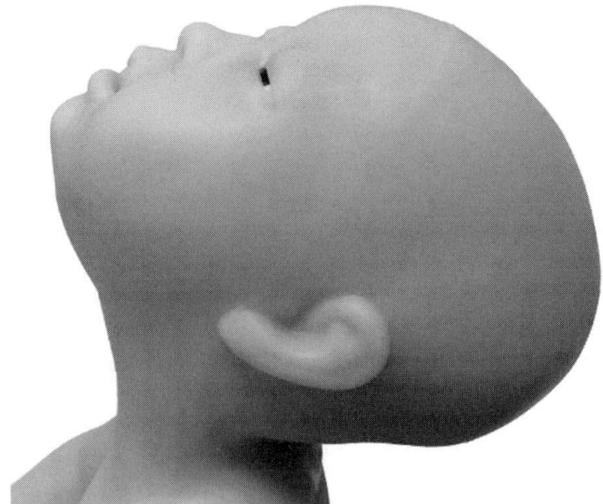

Figure 20.5 Military position.

Box 20.1 Criteria indicated for institutions that deliver breech babies vaginally

(a) Gestational age greater than 37 weeks
(b) Frank or complete breech presentation
(c) No fetal anomalies
(d) Adequate maternal pelvis
(e) Estimated fetal weight between 2,500 and 4,000 g
(f) Documentation of fetal head flexion
(g) Adequate amniotic fluid volume defined as a 3-cm vertical pocket

Simulation training has been shown to improved resident performance in the management of a simulated vaginal breech delivery.[17] Performance of a term breech vaginal delivery is well suited for simulation training. Term breech deliveries are excellent opportunities for simulation training due to the following reasons: (1) the situation is uncommon and so there is little opportunity to practice on real patients; (2) permanent injury may occur if the delivery is performed improperly; (3) additional

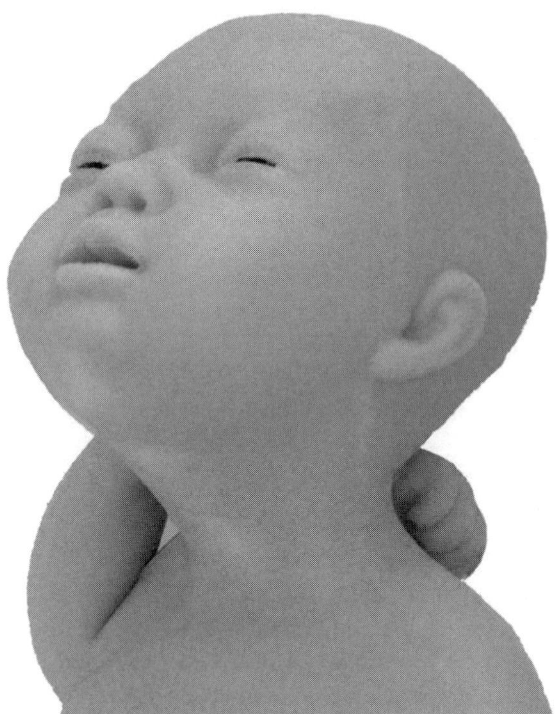

Figure 20.6 Nuchal arm.

emergency complications, such as fetal head entrapment or nuchal arm, may be demonstrated at the time of simulated vaginal breech delivery; and (4) the simulation may be easily accomplished with available birthing models.[17]

When breech presentation is diagnosed prior to the onset of labor, obstetricians should offer and perform external cephalic version. External cephalic version significantly reduces the incidence of noncephalic birth and cesarean delivery without a significant effect on perinatal mortality.[1]

External cephalic version should be performed in a setting in which the fetus can be monitored and an immediate cesarean delivery can be performed if necessary. The procedure can be performed with either one or two operators. Contraindications include third-trimester bleeding, oligohydramnios, ruptured membranes, severe fetal anomalies, and any other contraindications to vaginal birth such as placenta previa, prior classical cesarean section or vasa previa.[1]

A reactive non-stress test should be obtained prior to the procedure. It is thought that administration of beta-mimetic agents may be beneficial.[18] Before the procedure is initiated, the patient should be tilted laterally to prevent supine hypotension. The fetal breech is elevated out of the maternal pelvis with the operator's hand. The version is then performed via the creation of a forward roll of the fetus. If a forward roll is not successful than a backward roll may be attempted. The amount of force exerted is gauged by the patient's pain tolerance. Regional anesthesia is controversial. After the version attempt, the fetus should be monitored for 30 minutes. Rh immunoglobulin should be given to patients who are Rh-negative.

Box 20.2 Vaginal breech delivery technique

Call for help

Notify neonatal care providers that a vaginal breech delivery is imminent; the fetus may require resuscitation

Have a towel ready to support the fetal body and ask for Piper forceps to be available

Allow the fetus to deliver to the umbilicus

Splint the fetal thighs with thumb and index finger to deliver the legs

Wrap towel around the fetal body; assistant will hold fetal body parallel to the floor

Place thumbs on fetal sacrum and index fingers on anterior pelvic girdle. Do not grasp fetal abdomen in order to avoid injury to fetal intra-abdominal contents

Rotate fetus so one scapula is anterior

Squeeze fetal upper arm with index finger and thumb; deliver anterior arm

Rotate fetus so other scapula is anterior; repeat arm delivery on the other side

Instruct assistant to provide pressure on maternal suprapubic area to flex fetal head.

Perform Marceau Smellie Vite maneuver to flex and deliver fetal head; if unsuccessful apply Piper forceps.

Complete delivery and resuscitate fetus

Occiput Posterior

The incidence of persistent occiput posterior ranges from 5 to 12%.[19,20] Occiput posterior has been reported to be increased among African American women; this may be due to deeper anteroposterior outlets in this group of patients.[21] An increased rate of persistent occiput posterior has seen with epidural anesthesia.[22] Occiput posterior is associated with longer first and second stages of labor, prolonged labor, and the need for augmentation.[23] Occiput posterior is associated with a four- to tenfold increase in the risk of cesarean delivery.[20,23] Occiput posterior position doubles the risk of third- or fourth-degree extension.[24] Fitzpatrick et al.[25] found that 78% of patients in the occiput posterior position were able to deliver vaginally and 40% of patients delivered spontaneously. There is a sevenfold increase in anal sphincter disruption, a 5% increase in postpartum infections and an increased duration of labor.[25,26]

The definition of persistent occiput posterior is met when the occiput remains in the posterior quadrant of the pelvis until delivery; this includes deliveries that are spontaneous or those deliveries in which intervention is indicated for non-reassuring fetal status or arrest of descent in the second stage.[27] When occiput posterior presentation is discovered in the active phase or early second stage of labor, the condition usually resolves spontaneously. When spontaneous resolution does not occur, delivery options include cesarean delivery, non-rotational operative vaginal delivery or manual rotation.[27] No evidence exists to support maternal position change as a viable treatment option for rotation of the occiput in the active phase of labor.[28,29]

Prophylactic manual rotation may decrease persistent OP and its associated complications. Nonrotational operative vaginal delivery is appropriate when the maternal pelvis has a narrow anterior segment but ample room posteriorly; this will include patients with an anthropoid type pelvises. Rotation is not recommended if the maternal pelvic has android features or the pregnancy has suspected fetal macrosomia or the biparietal fetal head diameter is above the pelvic inlet.[27]

Numerous variations of manual and digital rotation of fetal occiput exist. Manual rotation of the occiput posterior position is performed by inserting a hand into the vagina with the palm directed upward. The operator's fingers are placed on one side of the fetal head. The direction of rotation is guided toward the side of the fetal back. Once successful rotation to the occiput anterior position is performed maternal expulsive efforts can then expedite a spontaneous delivery or forceps could be used.[30–32]

The relative risks, benefits, and safety of rotational forceps deliveries have been debated and discussed in the literature for decades and are beyond the scope of this discussion. The classic textbooks on forceps delivery include Dennen's forceps and Laufe's forceps. The interested reader is referred to these references. Kielland's forceps are the classic instruments for rotation due to the lack of the pelvic curve but rotations can also be performed with traditional forceps such as Simpson's or Elliott.[27]

Occiput Transverse

With expected management, rotation to occiput anterior position usually occurs in laboring patients diagnosed with occipital transverse. A platypelloid pelvis or android pelvis predisposes the patient to an occiput transverse fetal position. The diagnosis may be difficult do to the edema of the fetal scalp. If significant molding has occurred, the obstetrician may need to palpate the helix of the fetal ear to confirm the presentation. Occiput transverse position may rotate spontaneously but digital rotation may be considered. For the left occiput transverse position, the index and middle fingers of the operator's right hand are placed along the lambdoidal suture. The thumb is placed along the parietal bone. Counterclockwise rotation is then preformed. The technique is similar for the right occiput transverse position. In these cases, the operator uses the left hand and rotation is performed in the clockwise direction.

After a successful rotation, the operator should leave fingers in place to hold the fetal head in the occiput anterior position while maternal expulsive efforts are used to promote the descent of the fetal head or conversely forceps may be applied.[30,31]

Instrumental rotation of the occiput transverse position can be accomplished with either classical forceps, such as Elliot or Simpson forceps, or Kielland forceps. The Barton forceps were designed specifically to deliver a transverse fetal head in a patient with a platypelloid pelvis. Discussion of these forceps in rotational maneuvers is beyond the scope of this chapter.

Face Presentation

Hyperextension of the fetal head may result in face presentation. Contraction of the pelvic inlet, anencephalic, fetus, fetal macrosomia or high parity are associated with face presentation.[1] The fetal chin replaces the occiput as the landmark for the fetus with a face presentation; These pregnancies are therefore described as mentum anterior, mentum posterior or mentum transverse. Figure 20.7 shows a simulated fetus with a face presentation, mentum anterior.

Vaginal manipulation is associated with fetal morbidity and is contraindicated.[33] The mentum transverse fetus may rotate spontaneously to a mentum anterior position with the potential for vaginal delivery. The

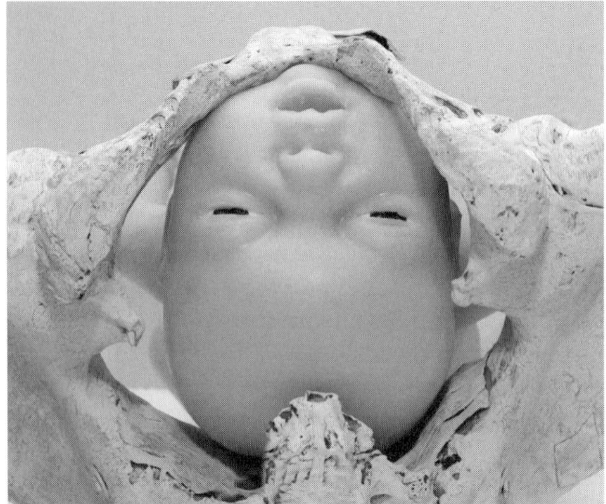

Figure 20.7 Face presentation mentum anterior. Photographed by Mr. Jim Sledge, East Tennessee State University.

fetus in mentum anterior deliveries may have significant bruising of the face. The persistent mentum posterior fetus cannot deliver vaginally. The patient with a mentum posterior fetus can be managed expectantly in the earlier phases of labor in hopes that spontaneous rotation to a mentum anterior position will occur.

Forceps can be considered for the mentum anterior fetus. Either Kielland forceps or classical forceps such as Simpsons or Elliots may be used for the intramentum delivery of the face presentation.[1]

Brow Presentation

Brow presentation occurs because of partial deflexion of the fetal head. Incidence is approximately 0.07%.[33]

More than 50% of pregnancies with brow presentations convert to vertex presentation or a face presentation. The fetus should not be manipulated vaginally to attempt conversion to a face or vertex presentation because such attempts are dangerous and are therefore contraindicated. In the absence of spontaneous conversion to a mentum anterior or vertex presentation, the delivery must be via cesarean section.

Transverse Lie

Transverse lie occurs in approximately 0.3% of pregnancies.[34] A simulated transverse lie is seen in Figure 20.8. Phelan et al.[35] point out that 83% of patients at 37 weeks' gestation or later with transverse lie will convert to a longitudinal lie if expectant management is under taken. Expectant management may, however, result in neonatal and maternal morbidity

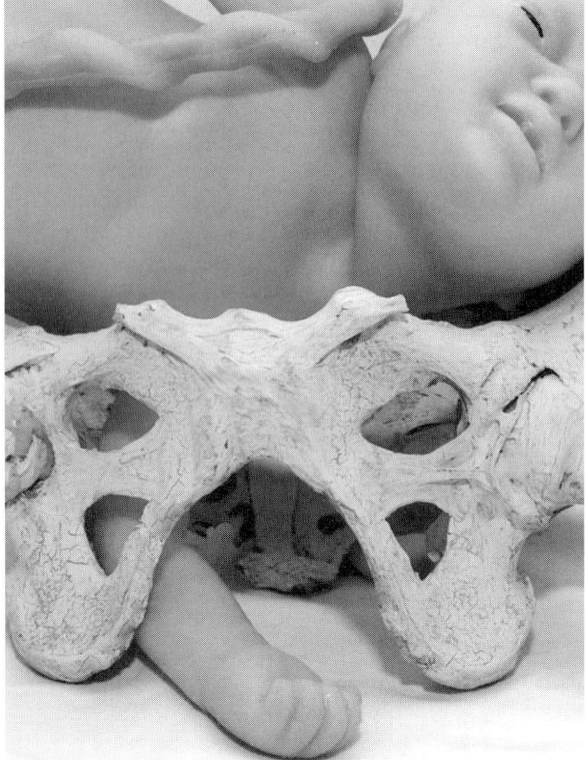

Figure 20.8 Transverse lie.

since the patients are at risk of cord prolapse and uterine rupture. The authors of this paper recommend that external cephalic version beyond 37 weeks gestation be considered; cesarean delivery for patients with failed version or persistent transverse lie would then be performed. When performing a cesarean section, a classical uterine incision should be considered to allow for an atraumatic delivery of the fetus. At the time of cesarean section, consideration should also be given to the performance of an intra-abdominal version to convert the fetus to a longitudinal lie-either cephalic or breech.[36]

Compound Presentation

Compound presentation involves the prolapse of an extremity alongside the presenting fetal head or the presenting fetal breech. Compound presentations are found more in preterm deliveries. Three forms of compound presentation exist – hand head, hand breech, and foot head. A simulated hand head compound presentation is shown in Figure 20.9. Management is expectant and often the prolapsed arm retracts and

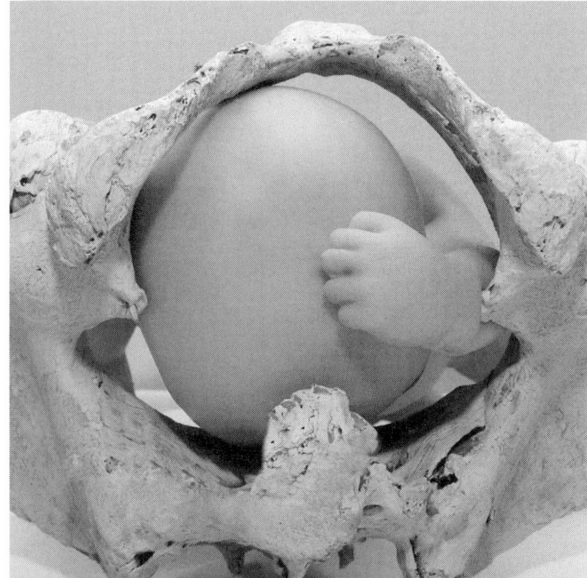

Figure 20.9 Compound presentation: hand-head. Photographed by Mr. Jim Sledge, East Tennessee State University.

allows descent of the fetal head or breech. The risk of cord prolapse is increased in cases with compound presentation and upper extremity injuries have been reported in newborns who experienced hand-head compound presentations during labor.[37,38]

Concluding Remarks

Fetal malpresentations are commonly encountered in obstetric practice. Obstetric providers must be able to calmly and decisively diagnose and manage breech, occiput transverse, occiput posterior, transverse lie, face, brow, and compound presentations. Breech presentations in particular may present emergently; the clinician must be able to perform a vaginal breech delivery in patients whose delivery is imminent even in facilities that usually perform cesarean section for breech presentation

References

1. Stitely, M. L., & Gherman, R. B. (2005). Labor with abnormal presentation and position. *Obstet Gynecol Clin North Am,* 32(2), 165–179. doi:10.1016/j.ogc.2004.12.005
2. Gardberg, M., Leonova, Y., & Laakkonen, E. (2011). Malpresentations – impact on mode of delivery. *Acta Obstet Gynecol Scand,* 90(5), 540–542. doi:10.1111/j.1600-0412.2011.01105.x
3. Hickok, D. E., Gordon, D. C., Milberg, J. A., Williams, M. A., & Daling, J. R. (1992). The frequency of breech presentation by gestational age at birth: A large population-based study. *Am J Obstet Gynecol,* 166(3), 851–852.
4. Caughey, A.B., Cahill, A.G., Guise, J.M., & Rouse, D.J. (2014) Safe prevention of the primary cesarean delivery. *Am J Obstet Gynecol,* 210;(3) 179–193.
5. Practice, A. C. o. O. (2006). ACOG Committee Opinion No. 340. Mode of term singleton breech delivery. *Obstet Gynecol,* 108(1), 235–237.
6. Practice, C. o. O. (2002). ACOG committee opinion. Mode of term singleton breech delivery. Number 265, December 2001. American College of Obstetricians and Gynecologists. *Int J Gynaecol Obstet,* 77(1), 65–66.
7. Hannah, M. E., Hannah, W. J., Hewson, S. A., Hodnett, E. D., Saigal, S., & Willan, A. R. (2000). Planned caesarean section versus planned vaginal birth for breech presentation at term: a randomised multicentre trial. Term Breech Trial Collaborative Group. *Lancet,* 356(9239), 1375–1383.
8. Hannah, M. E., Hannah, W. J., Hodnett, E. D., Chalmers, B., Kung, R., Willan, A., … TermBreech Trial 3-Month Follow-up Collaborative Group. (2002). Outcomes at 3 months after planned cesarean vs planned vaginal delivery for breech presentation at term: the international randomized Term Breech Trial. *JAMA,* 287(14), 1822–1831.
9. Hannah, M. E., Whyte, H., Hannah, W. J., Hewson, S., Amankwah, K., Cheng, M., … Term Breech Trial Collaborative Group. (2004). Maternal outcomes at 2 years after planned cesarean section versus planned vaginal birth for breech presentation at term: the international randomized Term Breech Trial. *Am J Obstet Gynecol,* 191(3), 917–927. doi:10.1016/j.ajog.2004.08.004
10. Rietberg, C. C., Elferink-Stinkens, P. M., & Visser, G. H. (2005). The effect of the Term Breech Trial on medical intervention behaviour and neonatal outcome in The Netherlands: an analysis of 35,453 term breech infants. *Br J Obstet Gynaecol,* 112(2), 205–209. doi:10.1111/j.1471-0528.2004.00317.x
11. Hartnack Tharin, J. E., Rasmussen, S., & Krebs, L. (2011). Consequences of the Term Breech Trial in Denmark. *Acta Obstet Gynecol Scand,* 90(7), 767–771. doi:10.1111/j.1600-0412.2011.01143.x
12. Royal College of Obstetricians and Gynaecologists. (April 2001). The management of breech presentation. Guideline No. 20. London: RCOG.
13. Hofmeyr, G. J., Hannah, M. E., & Lawrie, T. A. (2003). Planned caesarean section for term breech delivery. *Cochrane Database Syst Rev*(3), CD000166. doi:10.1002/14651858.CD000166

14. Mozurkewich, E. L., & Hutton, E. K. (2000). Elective repeat cesarean delivery versus trial of labor: a meta-analysis of the literature from 1989 to 1999. *Am J Obstet Gynecol,* 183(5), 1187–1197. doi:10.1067/mob.2000.108890

15. Lydon-Rochelle, M., Holt, V.L., Easterling, T. R., & Martin D. P. (2001). First-birth cesarean and placental abruption or previa at second birth(1). *Obstet Gynecol,* 97(5 Pt 1), 765–769.

16. Joseph, K. S., Pressey, T., Lyons, J., Bartholomew, S., Liu, S., Muraca, G., & Liston, R. M. (2015). Once more unto the breech: Planned vaginal delivery compared with planned cesarean delivery. *Obstet Gynecol,* 125(5), 1162–1167. doi:10.1097/AOG.0000000000000824

17. Deering, S., Brown, J., Hodor, J., & Satin, A. J. (2006). Simulation training and resident performance of singleton vaginal breech delivery. *Obstet Gynecol,* 107(1), 86–89. doi:10.1097/01.AOG.0000192168.48738.77

18. Hofmeyr, G. J. (2004). Interventions to help external cephalic version for breech presentation at term. *Cochrane Database Syst Rev*(1), CD000184. doi:10.1002/14651858.CD000184.pub2

19. Gardberg, M., & Tuppurainen, M. (1994). Persistent occiput posterior presentation – A clinical problem. *Act Obstet Gynecol Scand* Jan;73(1):45–7.

20. Lieberman, E., Davidson, K., Lee-Parritz, A., & Shearer, E. (2005). Changes in fetal position during labor and their association with epidural analgesia. *Obstet Gynecol,* 105(5 Pt 1), 974–982. doi:10.1097/01.AOG.0000158861.43593.49

21. Kotaska, A., Menticoglou, S., Gagnon, R., Farine, D., Basso, M., Bos, H., ... Society of Obstetricians and Gynaecologists of Canada. (2009). SOGC clinical practice guideline: Vaginal delivery of breech presentation: no. 226, June 2009. *Int J Gynaecol Obstet,* 107(2), 169–176.

22. Sizer, A. R., & Nirmal, D. M. (2000). Occipitoposterior position: Associated factors and obstetric outcome in nulliparas. *Obstet Gynecol,* 96(5 Pt 1), 749–752.

23. Ponkey, S. E., Cohen, A. P., Heffner, L. J., & Lieberman, E. (2003). Persistent fetal occiput posterior position: obstetric outcomes. *Obstet Gynecol,* 101(5 Pt 1), 915–920.

24. Cheng, Y. W., Shaffer, B. L., & Caughey, A. B. (2006). Associated factors and outcomes of persistent occiput posterior position: A retrospective cohort study from 1976 to 2001. *J Matern Fetal Neonatal Med,* 19(9), 563–568. doi:10.1080/14767050600682487

25. Fitzpatrick, M., McQuillan, K., & O'Herlihy, C. (2001) Influence of persistent occiput posterior position on delivery outcome. *Obstet Gynecol.* 98(6), 1027–1031.

26. Phillips R. D., & Freeman, M. (1974) The management of the persistent occiput posterior position. *Obstet Gynecol,* 43(2), 171–177.

27. Barth, W. H. (2015). Persistent occiput posterior. *Obstet Gynecol,* 125(3), 695–709. doi:10.1097/AOG.0000000000000647

28. Hunter, S., Hofmeyr, G. J., & Kulier, R. (2007). Hands and knees posture in late pregnancy or labour for fetal malposition (lateral or posterior). *Cochrane Database Syst Rev*(4), CD001063. doi:10.1002/14651858.CD001063.pub3

29. Stremler, R., Hodnett, E., Petryshen, P., Stevens, B., Weston, J., & Willan, A. R. (2005). Randomized controlled trial of hands-and-knees positioning for occipitoposterior position in labor. *Birth,* 32(4), 243–251. doi:10.1111/j.0730-7659.2005.00382.x

30. Walkowiak, R. G. (1971). Manual rotation of the transverse posterior occiput. *Obstet Gynecol,* 37(3), 464–467.

31. Lowenstein, A., & Zevin, R. (1971). Digital rotation of the vertex. *Obstet Gynecol,* 37(5), 790–791.

32. Cargill, Y. M., MacKinnon, C. J., Arsenault, M. Y., Bartellas, E., Daniels, S., Gleason, T., ... Clinical Practice Obstetrics Committee. (2004). Guidelines for operative vaginal birth. *J Obstet Gynaecol Can,* 26(8), 747–761.

33. Cruikshank, D. P., & Cruikshank, J. E. (1981). Face and brow presentation: A review. *Clin Obstet Gynecol,* 24(2), 333–351.

34. Cruikshank, D. P., & White, C. A. (1973). Obstetric malpresentations: Twenty years' experience. *Am J Obstet Gynecol,* 116(8), 1097–1104.

35. Phelan, J. P., Boucher, M., Mueller, E., McCart, D., Horenstein, J., & Clark, S. L. (1986). The nonlaboring transverse lie. A management dilemma. *J Reprod Med,* 31(3), 184–186.

36. Pelosi, M. A., Apuzzio, J., Fricchione, D., & Gowda, V. V. (1979). The "intra-abdominal version technique" for delivery of transverse lie by low-segment cesarean section. *Am J Obstet Gynecol,* 135(8), 1009–1011.

37. Buchanan, E. P., Richardson, R., & Tse, R. (2013) Isolated lower brachial plexus (Klumpe) palsy with compound arm presentations: Case report. *J Hand Surg,* 38A Aug. 1567–1570.

38. Tebes, C. C., Mehta, P., Calhoun, D. A., & Richards, D. S. (1999) Congenital ischemic forearm necrosis associated with a compound presentation. *J Mat Fet Med,* 8:231–233.

Intraamniotic Infection

Ann E. Williford

Introduction

Intraamniotic infection, often called chorioamnionitis or amniotic fluid infection, is an infection of the placenta, membranes, decidua or amniotic fluid. Chorioamnionitis is most commonly caused by an ascending infection from the lower genital tract. Infection is polymicrobial and the most frequently isolated bacteria include ureaplasma, mycoplasma, anaerobes, enteric gram-negative bacilli and group beta streptococcus. See Box 21.1.

A closed internal cervical os along with cervical mucus typically prevents ascension of vaginal bacteria to the upper reproductive tract. Uncommonly, chorioamnionitis is caused by inoculation of bacteria during an invasive process such as an amniocentesis or from bacteremia, as in the case of a *Listeria monocytogenes* infection.

Clinical chorioamnionitis is a common source of maternal febrile morbidity and results in 20–40% of early onset neonatal sepsis and pneumonia. It has also been associated with fetal white matter brain injury from a fetal immune response as well as cerebral palsy [2].

Scope of the Problem

The incidence of chorioamnionitis decreases as gestational age increases and is lowest at term and highest in preterm deliveries. In one study by Newton, chorioamnionitis was diagnosed in 41% of women with premature rupture of membranes (PROM) < 27 weeks gestation, 15% of PROM diagnosed at 28–36 weeks and in 2% of PROM diagnosed at term [3]. Similarly, chorioamnionitis is diagnosed in 75% of patients who developed labor after being admitted for preterm PROM as well as in one-third of cases of preterm labor with in tact membranes [4]. A 33% risk of preexisting intraamniotic infection exists in cases of cervical insufficiency [5].

Risk factors for chorioamnionitis include prolonged rupture of membranes, nulliparity, multiple vaginal exams, prolonged labor, and internal monitoring. Meconium-stained fluid, the presence of genital pathogens including group beta streptococcus or sexually transmitted infections, a history of intraamniotic infection, and diminished host immune response due to smoking, drug use, immunodeficiency and obesity also increase the risk of an intraamniotic infection [6,7].

Chorioamnionitis is considered treated once the infected products of conception are delivered, but management with broad spectrum antibiotics are used to control the infection and decrease maternal and neonatal sequela [8]. Unfortunately, the severity of maternal or fetal illness is not conveyed simply by the diagnosis of chorioamnionitis. Additionally, there is no unanimous approach to diagnosis. Further investigation is needed to refine the definition of an intraamniotic infection and improve cost-effective management for this condition.

Approach to Diagnosis

There is no consensus to the work-up and diagnosis of chorioamnionitis. Currently, to make a clinical diagnosis of chorioamnionitis, the patient must have a fever characterized by a maternal temperature of ≥ 38°C or 100.4°F with no other obvious source of infection. The presumed diagnosis is strengthened by the presence of risk factors and other signs and symptoms of infection. Maternal and fetal tachycardia (>100 beats per minute and >160 beats per minute, respectively) are present in 50–80% of cases of chorioamnionitis [9], maternal leukocytosis (white blood cell count >15,000/mm^3) is reported in 70–90% of cases, and uterine tenderness and or a foul odor to the amniotic fluid are reported in 4–25% of cases [10]. Of note, white blood cell count is often elevated in labor,

Box 21.1 Common organisms identified in amniotic fluid in patients with intraamniotic infection [1]

Ureaplasma urealyticum
Gram-negative anaerobes
Mycoplasma hominis
Bacteroids bivius
Gardnerella vaginalis
Group B *Streptococcus*

Box 21.2 Clinical signs and symptoms of chorioamnionitis

Maternal fever ≥ 38°C
Maternal leukocytosis (greater than 15,000 cells/mm^3)
Maternal tachycardia (greater than 100 beats/minute)
Fetal tachycardia (greater than 160 beats/minute)
Uterine tenderness
Foul odor of the amniotic fluid

often between 10,000 and 16,000/mm^3, and increases linearly with the duration of labor [11]. Therefore leukocytosis accompanied by a left shift is more supportive of an infectious process.

Fever is caused by pyrogens produced by the patient in response to infection, injury, or inflammation. These pyrogens include IL-1 alpha, IL-1 beta, IL-6, TNF-alpha, TNF-beta, and interferon alpha. The pyrogens reset the hypothalamic thermoregulatory center to a higher temperature. The measurement of maternal temperature during labor is important. Oral, tympanic or axillary temperature measuring devices are all available with oral temperature correlating best with core temperature [12]. It is also important to remember that axillary temperature is 1–2°C lower than oral temperature. Maternal fever should be confirmed with an oral temperature (see Box 21.2).

Differential Diagnosis

Intrapartum fever can also be secondary to a non-infectious cause. Most women who develop a fever during labor are often presumed to have an intraamniotic infection and are treated with broad spectrum antibiotics since fever is the most objective sign of chorioamnionitis and no clinical or laboratory findings reliably distinguish between infectious and non-infectious causes. Non-infectious causes are common, however, and should be considered including hyperthyroidism, elevated ambient temperature, the use of prostaglandin in the induction of labor, dehydration or an epidural fever.

The etiology of an epidural fever is unknown, but historical studies comparing maternal temperature before and after the availability of epidural anesthesia suggest that the epidural itself is the cause of increased temperature [13]. Most women do not experience increase in temperature after an epidural is placed, but for those women who do, temperature increases an average of 0.33°F per hour and increases with increasing duration of epidural anesthesia exposure [14,15]. There is no safe or proven way to decrease the risk of epidural-related temperature elevation.

Other common infectious causes of maternal febrile morbidity in the peripartum period include pyelonephritis, appendicitis, cholecystitis, pneumonia, influenza or infection of any other organ system. If the diagnosis is uncertain, ancillary testing including diagnostic imaging, urine microscopy, urine culture, chest X-ray or rapid influenza testing may help to support a diagnosis.

Amniocentesis can be used for the purpose of diagnosing chorioamnionitis. It is typically used in the setting of refractory preterm labor to determine if continued tocolysis is appropriate or to distinguish an intraamniotic infection from other causes of maternal fever and abdominal pain especially if treatment would result in delivery of an immature fetus. An amniotic fluid culture is the gold standard in determining an infection. It takes several days for results and therefore its usefulness is limited. Gram stain, glucose concentration, white blood cell concentration and leukocyte esterase level can be used for a more rapid diagnosis. Caution is advised before action is initiated prior to obtaining culture results [7]. If amniotic fluid has a positive gram stain (the presence of any bacteria and at least six leukocytes per high-power field), elevated white blood cell concentration, low glucose concentration and positive leukocyte esterase level, there is a 90% sensitivity and 80% specificity for predicting a positive amniotic fluid culture in patients with preterm labor [16].

For patients with cervical insufficiency, routine performance of an amniocentesis is not recommended to diagnose a subclinical intraamniotic infection before attempting to prolong pregnancy. The reason for this is the 48-hour delay in results; additionally rapid testing of the amniotic fluid has a poor predictive value. Lack of data supports contentions that routine amniocentesis decreases maternal and fetal morbidity [7].

Management

Management of chorioamnionitis includes prompt initiation of antibiotics, antipyretics, hydration and induction or augmentation of labor. The cure is delivery of the infected placenta and membranes. Broad spectrum antibiotics that cover beta-lactamase-producing aerobes and anaerobes will control infection and minimize maternal and fetal morbidity and should be started promptly after diagnosis. No randomized controlled trials have compared different antibiotic regimens [8]. The standard treatment includes ampicillin 2 grams IV every 6 hours until delivery plus gentamicin 1.5 mg/kg IV every 8 hours. Gentamicin can also be given in a single daily dose of 5 mg/kg; this is a more convenient dosing and does not result in toxic maternal levels in women with normal renal function. Daily dosing also leads to appropriate fetal serum levels as opposed to the standard dosing, which results in lower fetal drug concentration [17]. For women with normal kidney function, there is no indication for monitoring gentamicin levels. For those women with renal insufficiency, the gentamicin dose should be adjusted with the help of a pharmacist based on creatinine clearance and serial serum gentamicin levels. Other antibiotic regimen options for chorioamnionitis include ampicillin-sulbactam 3 grams IV every six hours or cefoxitin 2 grams IV every six hours.

For patients who were receiving penicillin for group beta streptococcus prophylaxis, it is advised to discontinue the penicillin and start ampicillin and gentamicin for broader coverage. For penicillin-allergic patients, vancomycin 1 gram IV every 12 hours can be substituted for the ampicillin. If mode of delivery includes a cesarean section, adding clindamycin 900 mg IV or metronidazole 500 mg IV to cover for anaerobic bacteria 30 to 60 minutes prior to incision reduces the rate of post-cesarean endometritis.

The duration of antibiotic therapy is controversial, as only small randomized control trials or observational studies have compared outcomes. Most suggest no additional doses of antibiotic therapy after delivery, especially if the patient delivered vaginally or has no other risk factors for postpartum endometritis [18–20]. An alternative is to continue antibiotics for one additional postpartum dose or until the patient is asymptomatic and afebrile for at least 24 hours. Patients most likely to benefit from this regimen include those patients delivered by cesarean section (C/S). This is seen because the prevalence of persistent postpartum fever is 15% in C/S patients compared to 1% after a vaginal delivery. Additionally, the incidence of postpartum endometritis is higher following a cesarean section [21].

In chorioamnionitis, an antipyretic can be administered to reduce fever as maternal fever and fetal acidosis are associated with a 12.5% risk of neonatal encephalopathy [22]. It may also reduce fetal tachycardia, which is common in an intraamniotic infection and is not predictive of a fetal academia. This strategy may decrease the incidence of cesarean delivery for non-reassuring fetal status. Acetaminophen is often the drug of choice to reduce maternal fever.

After an intraamniotic infection is diagnosed, the fetus should be continuously monitored for the development of fetal compromise. A fetal infection does not have a specific fetal heart rate pattern, but a category III tracing is predictive of fetal acidosis and delivery should be expedited. Cesarean sections are reserved for standard obstetrical indications as there is no evidence that duration of infection coincides with adverse fetal outcomes [23].

Fetal management after the diagnosis of chorioamnionitis is also controversial. Current guidelines from the American Academy of Pediatrics for neonates at risk for sepsis, which includes the maternal diagnosis of chorioamnionitis, consists of observation, a blood culture at birth, white blood cell count with differential plus C-reactive protein (CRP) collected at 6–12 hours of life and broad spectrum antibiotics. It is also recommended that broad spectrum antibiotics be continued even if the blood culture is negative if the mother received antibiotics during labor and delivery [24]. Some authors disagree with these guidelines, believing that following these guidelines results in treatment of well-appearing neonates delivered by patients who received antibiotics after the diagnosis of chorioamnionitis was made by an isolated maternal fever during labor and delivery and no other signs or symptoms of infection. These neonates have a low likelihood of infection and over treatment can have possible deleterious effects on the neonate including exposure to antimicrobial therapy, alterations to neonatal gut flora, admission to the neonatal intensive care unit plus its inherent risks, separation of the neonate from their families and increased healthcare cost [25].

Maternal Outcome

In patients diagnosed with chorioamnionitis, there is an increase in labor abnormalities, cesarean section, uterine atony and postpartum hemorrhage [26]. This suggests a deleterious effect of chorioamnionitis on uterine function. In a study by Satin et al., chorioamnionitis diagnosed late in labor was associated with a marked increase in cesarean section rate for labor dystocia compared to controls, 40% versus 10% [27]. There is also an increased risk of wound infection after a cesarean section, development of pelvic abscess, ovarian vein thrombosis, septic pelvic thrombophlebitis and postpartum endometritis in patients diagnosed with chorioamnionitis [7].

Bacteremia occurs in 5–10% of cases of chorioamnionitis, which may lead to sepsis and a worse maternal outcome. If treatment with broad spectrum antibiotics is initiated promptly, life-threatening maternal conditions including sepsis, acute respiratory distress syndrome and coagulopathy are rare. Maternal sepsis following an intraamniotic infection is 1.4% [28]. Blood cultures should not be sent routinely, but are useful in those patients who do not respond to empiric therapy or those women who appear critically ill. Assessment of Lactate level is also helpful in patients when sepsis is considered. If serum lactate is elevated, rapid resuscitation and treatment improves outcomes.

Fetal Outcome

Fetal infection may result from aspiration or swallowing of infected fluid or from hematogenous spread. Overall, chorioamnionitis is associated with 20–40% of early neonatal sepsis and pneumonia. Other adverse outcomes from intraamniotic infection include perinatal death, asphyxia, meningitis and intraventricular hemorrhage. Preterm infants have a higher rate of complications from chorioamnionitis compared to term infants, in particular, perinatal death (25% versus 6% in preterm and term infants, respectively), grades 3 and 4 intraventricular hemorrhage (24% versus 8%), neonatal sepsis (28% versus 6%), pneumonia (20% compared to 6%) and respiratory distress (62% compared to 35%) [29].

Preterm premature rupture of membranes plus the diagnosis of an intrauterine infection is associated with an increased risk of neurodevelopmental impairment [30,31]. Similarly, a meta-analysis by Wu et al. showed potential long-term disabilities resulting from intraamniotic infection at or near term including neurodevelopmental delay, cerebral white matter changes and potential long-term disabilities including cerebral palsy [32]. It is thought that with chorioamnionitis, a fetal immune response is activated and high levels of cytokines and chemokines like tumor necrosis factor can cause cerebral ischemia, damage and ultimately neonatal brain injury [33]. Fetal involvement is a more important predictor of neonatal outcome than isolated maternal inflammation [34]. Funisitis and chorionic vasculitis on placental pathology are histological manifestations of the fetal inflammatory response syndrome, therefore, it is important to send the placenta to pathology when a diagnosis of chorioamnionitis is made [35].

Prevention

To decrease the incidence of chorioamnionitis, it is recommended that, in patients who present with premature rupture of membranes at 37 0/7 weeks gestation and the onset of labor is not spontaneous at the time of presentation, labor should be induced. There is a higher rate of chorioamnionitis in those induced with prostaglandins compared to oxytocin [36]. Therefore, oxytocin is generally used for induction of labor in patients admitted with premature rupture of membranes. Mechanical dilation with a Foley balloon has a theoretical risk for infection, but there is insufficient data at this time to recommend against mechanical dilation of the cervix [37]. In patients who are diagnosed with preterm premature rupture of membranes, clinical chorioamnionitis is a clear indication for delivery. Induction of labor did significantly reduce the risk of chorioamnionitis in patients between 34 and 37 weeks gestation when compared to expectant management (1.6% at 34 weeks versus 5.3% at 37 weeks), however, the optimal gestational age for delivery remains controversial [38,39]. Currently, delivery is recommended for all women with ruptured membranes at 34 0/7 weeks. Prior to 34 weeks and after viability, antibiotics reduce the risk of intraamniotic infection, improve neonatal outcomes and prolong latency.

Group B *Streptococcus*

Group B *Streptococcus* (GBS) is an encapsulated gram-positive coccus that can colonize the genital and gastrointestinal tract. Colonization occurs in 10–40%

of pregnant women [40]. Vertical transmission can lead to early-onset GBS infection in neonates less than 7 days of age and it is also a cause of an intraamniotic infection. Several randomized controlled trials in the 1980s demonstrated a reduction in early-onset GBS infection with intrapartum administration of intravenous penicillin or ampicillin to women who carry GBS [41–43].

The Centers for Disease Control (CDC) has recommended guidelines for universal screening of all pregnant women to identify those at risk for having a newborn with early-onset GBS [44]. A GBS culture should be obtained at 35–37 weeks gestation and the culture is reasonably predictive of a patient's GBS status for roughly five weeks. A culture can be obtained by a health care provider or by the patient herself. A swab should culture the lower vagina and the rectum with insertion of the swab through the anal sphincter. The swab should then be placed into a nonnutrient transport medium and transported at room temperature. In the lab, the swab is then placed into a selective enrichment broth, incubated overnight at 37°C and subcultured onto a blood agar plate. It takes 48 hours to definitively exclude GBS in culture. Rapid diagnostic testing is available, however, the CDC does not support their use to replace routine antepartum culture at 35–37 weeks.

Intrapartum antibiotic prophylaxis at the onset of labor until delivery should be administered to those patients at risk for newborns developing early-onset GBS after delivery. This includes women who have a positive GBS culture and women with unknown GBS status and when the gestational age is less than 37 weeks, duration of ruptured membranes is ≥ 18 hours or an intrapartum maternal temperature ≥ 100°F. Chemoprophylaxis should be administered to those patients in labor who have a history of a neonate who was diagnosed with early-onset GBS disease after birth or if the patient had GBS bacteria during the current pregnancy. In those cases, a culture does not need to be obtained at 35–37 weeks gestation [44].

The recommended therapy for GBS prophylaxis is penicillin G 5 million units IV initially and then 2.5–3 million units IV every 4 hours until delivery. Ampicillin 2 grams IV initially and then 1 gram every 4 hours until delivery is also an acceptable regimen. Thus far, there are no consistent trends in development of antibiotic resistance to this regimen. For patients with a low-risk penicillin allergy (patients who develop a maculopapular rash without uricaria or pruritus), cefazolin 2 grams IV initially and then 1 gram IV every 8 hours until delivery is regimen of choice. If a patient has a high risk of anaphylaxis due to penicillin, then sensitivities should be sent at the time of culture. If the cultured GBS is sensitive to clindamycin and erythromycin, then the patient should receive clindamycin 900 mg IV every 8 hours until delivery. If the GBS isolate is resistant to clindamycin or the susceptibility results are not available, the patient should receive vancomycin 1 gram IV every 12 hours until delivery for prophylaxis [45]. For penicillin, ampicillin and cefazolin, prophylaxis is most effective if administered at least four hours before delivery [46]. Since timing of delivery cannot be predicted, chemoprophylaxis should be started at the onset of labor or rupture of membranes and continued until delivery.

Concluding Remarks

Chorioamnionitis can cause adverse neonatal outcomes and significant maternal and neonatal morbidity, therefore, it should be diagnosed and treated promptly. However, diagnosis is problematic and health care providers often err of the side of treatment when an intraamniotic infection is suspected. Treatment includes antibiotic therapy to control the intrauterine infection and antipyretics. Cure for chorioamnionitis is delivery of the infected products of conception. Overtreatment can have deleterious effects on both the mother and the neonate. Recently, an expert panel has recommended new terminology and restricted the term "chorioamnionitis" to pathologic diagnosis. The new terminology includes isolated maternal fever as well as intrauterine inflammation, infection, or both, in which the author coined the term "TRIPLE I." This expert panel has also identified multiple areas of research gaps and opportunities for the future [25].

References

1. Sperling RS, Newton E, Gibbs RS. Intraamniotic infection in low-birth-weight infants. *J Infect Dis* 1988; 157:113.
2. Cornette L. Fetal and neonatal inflammatory response and adverse outcome. *Semin Fetal Neonatal Med* 2004; 9:459.
3. Newton ER. Chorioamnionitis and intraamniotic infection. *Clin Obstet Gynecol* 1993; 36:795.
4. Yoon BH, Romero R, Moon JB, et al. Clinical significance of intra-amniotic inflammation in patients

with preterm labor and intact membranes. *Am J Obstet Gynecol* 2001; 185:1130.

5. Harger JH. Cerclage and cervical insufficiency: An evidence-based analysis [published erratum appears in *Obstet Gynecol* 2003;101:205]. *Obstet Gynecol* 2002;100:1313–27.
6. Soper DE, Mayhall CG, Dalton HP. Risk factors for intraamniotic infection: A prospective epidemiologic study. *Am J Obstet Gynecol* 1989;161;562–6.
7. Tita AT, Ramin SM, Barss VA. Intraamniotic infection (chorioamnionitis). In: *UpToDate, Post*, TW (Ed), UpToDate, Waltham, MA, 2016.
8. Chapman E, Reveiz L, Illanes E, Bonfill Cosp X. Antibiotic regimens for management of intra-amniotic infection. *Cochrane Database Syst Rev* 2014; 12:CD010976.
9. Tita AT, Andrews WW. Diagnosis and management of clinical chorioamnionitis. *Clin Preinatol* 2010; 37:339.
10. Newton ER. Chorioamnionitis and intraamniotic infection. *Clin Obstet Gynecol* 1993; 36:795.
11. Acker DB, Johnson MP, Sachs BP, Friedman EA. The leukocyte count in labor. *Am J Obstet Gynecol* 1985; 153:737.
12. Banerjee S, Cashman P, Yentis SM, Steer PJ. Maternal temperature monitoring during labor: Concordance and variability among monitoring sites. *Obstet Gynecol* 2004; 103:287.
13. Yancey MK, Zhang J, Schwarz J, et al. Labor epidural analgesia and intrapartum maternal hyperthermia. *Obstet Gynecol* 2001; 98:763.
14. Lieberman E, Lang JM, Frigoletto F Jr, et al. Epidural analgesia, intrapartum fever, and neonatal sepsis evaluation. *Pediatrics* 1997; 99:415.
15. Goetzl L, Rivers J, Zighelboim I, et al. Intrapartum epidural analgesia and maternal temperature regulation. *Obstet Gynecol* 2007; 109:687.
16. Abdel-Razeq SS, Buhimschi IA, Bahtiyar MO, et al. Interpretation of amniotic fluid white blood cell count in "bloody tap" amniocenteses in women with symptoms of preterm labor. *Obstet Gynecol* 2010; 116:344.
17. Locksmith GJ, Chin A, Vu T, et al. High compared with standard gentamicin dosing for chorioamnionitis: A comparison of maternal and fetal serum drug levels. *Obstet Gynecol* 2005; 105:473.
18. Turnquest MA, How HY, Cook CR, et al. Chorioamnionitis: Is continuation of antibiotic therapy necessary after cesarean section? *Am J Obstet Gynecol* 1998; 179:1261.
19. Edwards RK, Duff P. Single additional dose postpartum therapy for women with chorioamnionitis. *Obstet Gynecol* 2003; 102:957.
20. Chapman SJ, Oven J. Randomized trial of single-dose versus multiple-dose cefotetan for the postpartum treatment of intrapartum chorioamnionitis. *Am J Obstet Gynecol* 1997; 177:831.
21. Black LP, Hinson L, Duff P. Limited course of antibiotic treatment for chorioamnionitis. *Obstet Gynecol* 2012; 119:1102.
22. Impey LW, Greenwood CE, Black RS, et al. The relationship between intrapartum maternal fever and neonatal acidosis as risk factors for neonatal encephalopathy. *Am J Obstet Gynecol* 2008; 1998:49.e1.
23. Rouse DJ, Landon M, Leveno KJ, et al. The maternal-fetal medicine units cesarean registry: Chorioamnionitis at term and its duration-relationship to outcomes. *Am J Obstet Gynecol* 2004; 191:211.
24. Polin RA, the committee on fetus and newborn. Management of neonates with suspected or proven early-onset bacterial sepsis. *Pediatrics* 2012; 129:1006.
25. Higgins RD, Saade G, Polin RA, Grobman WA, Buhimischi IA, Watterberg K, Silver RM, Raju TNK. Evaluation and management of women and newborns with a maternal diagnosis of chorioamnionitis. *Obstet Gynecol* 2016; 127:426.
26. Mark SP, Croughan-Minihane MS, Kilpatrick SJ. Chorioamnionitis and uterine function. *Obstet Gyncol* 2000; 95:909.
27. Satin AJ, Maberry MC, Leveno KJ, et al. Chorioamnionitis: A harbinger of dystocia. *Obstet Gynecol* 1992; 79:913.
28. Edwards SE, Grobman WA, Lappen JR, et al. Modified obstetric early warning scoring systems (MOEWS): Validating the diagnostic performance for severe sepsis in women with chorioamnionitis. *Am J Obstet Gynecol* 2015; 212:536.e1.
29. Morales WJ, Washington SR 3rd, Lazar AJ. The effect of chorioamnionitis on perinatal outcome in preterm gestation. *J Perinatol* 1987; 7:105.
30. Spinillo A, Capuzzo E, Satronati M, Ometto A, Orcesi S, Fazzi E. Effect of preterm premature rupture of membranes on neurodevelopmental outcome: Follow up at two years of age. *Br J Obstet Gynaecol* 1995; 102:882.
31. Yoon BH, Romero R, Park JS, Kim CJ, Kim SH, Choi JH, et al. Fetal exposure to an intra-amniotic inflammation and the development of cerebral palsy at the age of three years. *Am J Obstet Gynecol* 2000; 182:675.
32. Wu YW, Escobar GJ, Grether JK, et al. Chorioamnionitis and cerebral palsy in term and near-term infants. *JAMA* 2003; 290:2677.
33. Kadhim H, Tabarki B, Verellen G, et al. Inflammatory cytokines in the pathogenesis of the periventricular leukomalacia. *Neurology* 2001; 56:1278.

34. Pappas A, Kendrick DE, Shankaran S, et al. Chorioamnionitis and early childhood outcomes among extremely low-gestational-age neonates. *JAMA Pediatr* 2014; 168:137

35. Pacora P, Chaiworapongsa T, Maymon E, et al. Funisitis and chorionic vasculitis: The histological counterpart of the fetal inflammatory response syndrome. *J Matern Fetal Neonatal Med* 2002; 11:18.

36. Hannah ME, Ohlsson A, Farine D, Hewson SA, Hodnett ED, Myhr TL, et al. Induction of labor compared with expectant management for prelabor rupture of membranes at term. TERMPROM Study Group. *N Engl J Med* 1996; 334:1005.

37. Premature rupture of membranes. Practice Bulletin No. 160. American College of Obstetricians and Gynecologists. *Obstet Gynecol* 2016; 127:e39–51.

38. van der Ham DP, van der Heyden JL, Opmeer BC, Mulder AL, Moonen RM, van Beek JH, et al. Management of late-preterm premature rupture of membranes: The PPROMEXIL-2 trial. *Am J Obstet Gynecol* 2012; 207(276):e1–10.

39. van der Ham DP, Vijgen SM, Nijhuis JG, van Beek JJ, Opmeer BC, Mulder AL, et al. Induction of labor versus expectant management in women with preterm prelabor rupture of membranes between 34 and 37 weeks: A randomized controlled trial. PPROMEXIL trial group. *PLoS Med* 2012; 9:e1001208.

40. Regen JA, Klebanoff MA, Nugent RP. The epidemiology of group B streptococcal colonization in pregnancy. Vaginal Infection and Prematurity Study Group. *Obstet Gynecol* 1991; 77:604.

41. Boyer KM, Gotoff SP. Prevention of early-onset neonatal group B streptococcal disease with selective intrapartum chemoprophylaxis. *N Engl J Med* 1986; 314:1665.

42. Easmon CS, Hastings MJ, Deeley J, et al. The effect of intrapartum chemprophylaxis on the vertical transmission of group B streptococci. *Br J Obstet Gynaecol* 1983; 90:633.

43. Boyer KM, Gadzala CA, Kelly PD, Gotoff SP. Selective intrapartum chemoprophylaxis of neonatal group B streptococcal early-onset disease. III. Interruptio of mother-to-infant transmission. *J Infect Dis* 1983; 148:810.

44. Verani JR, McGee L, Schrag SJ, Division of Bacterial Diseases, National Center for Immunization and Respiratory Diseases Control and Prevention (CDC). Prevention of perinatal group B streptococcal disease – Revised guidelines from CDC, 2010. *MMWR Recomm Rep* 2010; 59:1.

45. Baker CJ, Ramin SM, Sexton DJ, Barss VA. Neonatal group B streptococcal disease: Prevention. In: *UpToDate, Post*, TW (Ed), UpToDate, Waltham, MA, 2016.

46. Edwards MS, Nizet V, Baker CJ. Group B streptococcal infections. In: *Infectious Diseases of the Fetus and Newborn Infant*, 7th ed, Remington JS, Klein JO, Wilson CB, et al. (Eds), Elsevier Sauders, Philadelphia 2011. p. 419.

Multifetal Pregnancy

Fidelma B. Rigby

Introduction

Over the past three decades, the incidence of twin births in the United States has increased by 76% [1]. Higher order gestations (triplets and above) increased by 400% [1] for a portion of this timeframe [2]. Given the increased maternal and perinatal mortality associated with multiple gestations, this increase has had significant effects in maternal and fetal welfare (see Box 22.1 for a discussion on the abbreviations used in this chapter).

Scope of the Problem

Although multifetal pregnancies account for 3% of births in the United States, they constitute 15% of preterm births in less than 37 weeks and 25% of very low birthweight infants who are less than 2,500 grams. The neonatal death rate (from birth to day 28) is 7.8/1,000 pregnancies in singletons. This increases by a multiple of seven in twins and by 22 times in triplets. The infant death rate from birth to one year is 11.2/1,000 births in singletons and rises by a factor of six in twins and by a factor of 17 in triplets. The prevalence of cerebral palsy is 2 per 1,000 live birth in singletons and rises by a factor of nine, 31 and 100 and 11 in twin, triplet and quadruplet pregnancies. Prematurity is the major risk factor for this rise [3].

In natural conceptions, dizygotic (DZ) twins occur in approximately 1–1.5% of all pregnancies and monozygotic (MZ) twins occur in 1/250 pregnancies. It is the DZ twinning rate that varies the most. Maternal history of twins, increased maternal age, African heritage, and assisted reproductive techniques (ART) all increase the DZ twinning rate. Increasing maternal age and the use of ART in the United States are thought to be the driver behind the increasing multiple gestation rate over the past three decades [1]. Certain ethnicities such as Asian descent can decrease DZ twinning rates. ART has also been suggested to increase even the MZ twinning rate [4] by two-five times, although some authors suggest this is most common in higher order ART pregnancies [5] Increased maternal risks associated with multiple gestations are seen in Table 22.4.

Zygosity/Chorionicity/Epidemiology

The specific type of multifetal gestation plays a large role in the possibility of adverse outcomes. Twins are either monozygotic (MZ) (coming from a single egg that divides) or dizygotic (DZ) coming from two separate fertilized eggs). MZ is also referred to as identical twins. DZ twins are always dichorionic/ diamniotic (DC/DA). MZ twins, on the other hand, can be either dichorionic/ diamniotic (DC/DA), monochorionic/ diamniotic (MC/DA) or monochorionic/ monoamniotic (MC/MA). A rare subset of monochorionic twins would be conjoined twins. It is the timing of fertilized egg division that determines chorionicity (see Table 22.1).

Accurate diagnosis of chorionicity is very important as it determines many risk factors for the pregnancy. This can be most easily accomplished by first trimester sonography. By five weeks, it is often possible to see separate gestational sacs and yolk sacs while the crown–rump length and heart tones are visible as early as six weeks. Between 11 and 14 weeks, the thickness of the dividing membrane and presence of T sign or lambda sign (thickness as the membranes insert into the placenta) helps determine chorionicity [6]. The lambda sign is also called the twin peak sign.

Discordance for gender (with rare exceptions) would suggest diamniotic dichorionic- (DI/DI) gestation. Determining zygosity can be more difficult: if anything is shared (i.e. diamniotic-monochorionic (DI/Mono)) then the twins should be MZ. However, if everything is separate (Di/DI) and the sexes are concordant, MZ is still possible if the egg divided before

Box 22.1 Abbreviations used in this chapter

ART	assisted reproductive technology
DC	dichorionic
DZ	dizygotic
EGA	estimated gestational age
EFW	estimated fetal weight
FFN	fetal fibronectin
IUFD	intrauterine fetal demise
IUGR	intrauterine growth restriction
IVF	in vitro fertilization
MC	monochorionic
MA	monoamniotic
NEC	necrotizing enterocolitis
PTB	preterm birth
RDS	respiratory distress syndrome
TTTS	twin–twin transfusion syndrome
TRAP	twin reversed arterial perfusion

three days. Further genetic testing (i.e., blood typing or human leukocyte antigen (HLA) typing) would be needed to determine zygosity in these cases [6].

Fetal Risks with Multiple Gestations

Multifetal gestations have significantly increased morbidity and mortality, which increases with each fetal number (see Table 22.2).

Low birthweights, prematurity, cerebral palsy and infant mortality are among the most significant issues [7–10]. As compared to singletons, twins have a fivefold increased risk of stillbirth. They have a sevenfold increased risk of neonatal death and fourfold increased risk of cerebral palsy, much of this related to prematurity. The increased cerebral palsy risk is associated with threefold increase in high-grade intraventricular hemorrhage [10].

Fetal Anomalies

Multifetal pregnancies also carry an increased risk for congenital anomalies. A recent study from England notes a 1.7 relative risk for twins (vs singletons) and the risk for MC gestation is 1.8 that of DC gestations. This study noted an increased risk for all major anomalies except for chromosomal changes [11].

Monochorionic Gestations

The chorionicity of the gestation plays a major role in the frequency of twin-specific risks. The more membranes the fetuses share, the higher risk the gestation becomes due to vascular components in the placentas.

Twin–Twin Transfusion Syndrome (TTTS)

The most frequent risk with a monochorionic (MC) gestation is the twin–twin transfusion syndrome (TTTS), which complicates up to 10% of these gestations and is the main cause of morbidity and mortality in a MC/DA gestation. Connecting vessels in the donor twin's placenta move blood into the recipient twin [12]. The donor twin becomes much smaller with very low fluid (sometimes referred to as a "stuck twin") while the recipient twin develops polyhydramnios and eventually fluid collections leading to hydrops. Management for this is based on gestational age and severity of syndrome at the time of diagnosis (see Table 22.3) [13].

Ultrasound parameters such as the presence of oligohydramnios in the donor sac and polyhydramnios in the recipient sac are used to stage the severity of the syndrome. The treatment of choice, especially for early and severe cases, would be fetoscopic laser photocoagulation. This coagulates the connecting blood vessels. This would be considered for Quintero Stages II–IV between 16 and 26 weeks. There can be significant complications (1% abruption to 30% PPROM) so many centers reserve this for early and severe disease. This often requires travel to a center that specializes in this disorder, which further limits its availability. Serial amnio reduction (removing amniotic fluid from the larger twin's sac) can be done by local maternal fetal medicine providers. This can be effective in lower risk TTTS but for the more severe cases, it is not as effective and can sometimes need to be done as frequently as every other day [12,14].

Twin Anemia Polycythemia Arterial Sequence (TAPS)

A more recently described complication has been anemia of the donor twin and polycythemia of the recipient twin without the typical polyhydramnios and oligohydramnios. This can complicate 3–5% of MC gestations and up to 13% of the gestations treated with laser for TTTS. Diagnosis is made with middle cerebral artery (MCA) discrepancies (> 1.5 MOM for donor and <1.1 MOM for recipient twin). It is due to very small vessel connections causing slow unbalanced transfusions. Treatment for this condition remains unclear with fetoscopic laser or intrauterine transfusion reserved for very select cases [15].

Table 22.1 Gestational Timing and Split of Monozygotic Twins

Twin Zygosity	Day Eggs Divide	Placentation	Amniotic Sacs	Yolk Sacs	Dividing Membrane	Sex
DZ	N/A (separate from beginning)	DC/DA Separate or fused	2	2	Thick (lambda sign)	Concordant or discordant
MZ	Day 0–3 (29%)	DC/DA Separate or fused	2	2	Thick (lambda sign)	Concordant
	Day 4–7 (70%)	MC/DA One placenta	2	2	Thin (T sign)	Concordant
	Day 8–12 (1%)	MC/MA One placenta	1	1	Absent	Concordant
	After day 12 (Rare)	MC/MA One placenta Conjoined Always same position	1	1	Absent	Concordant

Table 22.2 Fetal Risks and Multiple Gestations

Gestation Type	Birthweight	EGA	<37 Weeks (%)	<32 Weeks (%)	LBW (%)	VLBW (%)	CP Per 1,000 Live Births	Infant Mortality Per 1,000 Live Births
Singleton	3296	38.1	10.4	1.6	6.5	1.1	1.6	5.4
Twin	2336	35.3	58.8	11.4	57.2	10.2	7	23.6
Triplet	1660	31.9	94.4	36.8	95.4	34.8	28	52.5
Quad	1291	29.5	98.3	64.5	98	73.4	–	96.3

Abbreviations: LBW, low birth weight; VLBW, very low birthweight; CP, cerebral palsy.

Sources: Data obtained from:

Peterson B, Nelson KB, Watson L, Stanley F. Twins, triplets, and cerebral palsy in births in Western Australia in the 1980s. *BMJ* 1993;307:1239–43.

Multifetal gestations: twin, triplet, and higher order multi-fetal pregnancies. Practice Bulletin No.144. American College of Obstetricians and Gynecologists. ***Obstet Gynecol*** 2014;123: 1118–32.

Luke **B**, Brown MB. The changing risk of infant mortality by gestation, plurality, and race: 1989–1991 versus 1999–2001. ***Pediatrics*** 2006;118 (6):2488–97.

Martin JA, Hamilton BE, Sutton, PD et al. Births: Final data for 2006. National Vital Statistics Reports, Volume 57, Number 7.

Monoamniotic Twin Gestation

This subset of twins is of the highest risk for perinatal mortality, ranging from 10% to 40%. This increased mortality arises from prematurity, congenital anomalies, placental vascular anastomoses and cord entanglement [12,16]. Optimal management for this very high risk subset of twin gestations (1/10,000 pregnancies) is limited by a lack of randomized controlled studies. A recent Cochrane Database review came to no definitive conclusions [17]. A recent retrospective review [15] recommended close fetal surveillance after 26–28 weeks with delivery by 33 weeks due to the prospective risk for nonrespiratory neonatal complications being lower than the prospective risk for neonatal death at that EGA. Current consensus would be intensive fetal surveillance after 26–28 weeks with strong consideration for delivery at approximately 33 weeks [12,17].

Twin Reversed Arterial Perfusion (TRAP)

Twin reversed arterial perfusion syndrome (TRAP) occurs when a normal twin (the pump twin) perfuses

Table 22.3 Quintero Staging of Twin–Twin Transfusion

Stage	Poly/Oligo Hydramnios	Absent bladder donor	Doppler Flow Changes	Hydrops	Demise
I	✓	–	–	–	–
II	✓	✓	–	–	–
III	✓	✓	✓	–	–
IV	✓	✓	✓	✓	–
V	✓	✓	✓	✓	✓

Notes: Polyhydramnios: greater than 8 cm maximum vertical pocket. Oligohydramnios: less than 2 cm maximum vertical pocket.

Source: From Quintero RA, Morales WJ, Allen MH, et al. Staging for twin–twin transfusion system. *J. Perinatol.* 1999;19 (8) Part 1: 550–5.

a nonviable co-twin (the cardiac twin) through placental channels. The pump twin experiences high output failure and has up to 50% mortality. Interruption of the anastomoses can be accomplished via bipolar or laser cord coagulation. Recent studies recommend a proactive approach with definitive treatment once continued growth of the acardiac twin is documented (without waiting for compromise of the pump twin) [12].

Conjoined Twins

These should be suspected when monoamniotic twins remain in the same relative positions to each other on subsequent scans. Mortality is high with only 18% of prenatally diagnosed conjoined twins surviving. Long-term outcomes will be predicted by the degree of sharing vital organs and treatment options will be individualized [12].

Demise of Co-Twin in Monochorionic Gestation

In monochorionic gestations, demise of a co-twin may have dire consequences for the surviving twin based on the degree of vascular anastomoses. Vascular damage to multiple organs, especially the central nervous system (CNS), can occur. Originally these vascular events were thought to result through emboli from the demised twin's circulation and these occurred over days to weeks. Recent studies suggest these adverse outcomes are the result of acute events from sudden and profound hypotension and anemia immediately following the demise. This results in very poor tissue perfusion. Thus the subsequent damage is from a very acute event so early delivery of the remaining twin is no longer recommended and expectant management can be done [18].

Maternal Risks

Multifetal gestations have a significantly increased risk of pregnancy complications, which increase with increasing fetal number. These include anemia, urinary tract infection, hyperemesis, pre-eclampsia, eclampsia, preterm labor, gestational diabetes, cesarean section, third trimester bleeding, postpartum hemorrhage, puerperal endometritis and maternal death. The incidence of these risks is directly proportional to the fetal number. For example, hypertensive complications have been found to occur in 6.5% of singletons, 12.7% of twins and 20% of triplets [19,20] Preterm birth is also significantly higher with deliveries less than 32 weeks occurring in 1.6% of singletons, 11.4% of twins, 36.8% of triplets and 64.% 5 of quads (see Table 22.4) [7–9,21].

One of the main drivers of prematurity is pre-eclampsia, which occurs in 10% of multiple gestations vs. 4.4% of singletons [17]. Hypertension can also increase the risk of abruption: triplets have a 1.3 adjusted odds ratio for this (vs. twins) while quads have a 1.34 adjusted odds ratio [22]. Indeed multiple gestations are at risk for other hemorrhagic complications of pregnancy including third trimester bleeding (1.3% singleton vs 1.6% multiple gestation) and postpartum hemorrhage (4.7% singleton vs 9.1% multiple gestation) [22].

Assisted Reproductive Technology (ART) and Maternal Fetal Risks

ART has played a significant role in the increasing rate of multifetal gestations, with a recent small downtrend. The most recent available data suggest that in cycles completed in 2010, 26% of pregnancies after in

Table 22.4 Maternal Complications in Twin Pregnancies (%)

	Singleton	Twin	RR
Hyperemesis	1.7	5.1	3.0
Threatened Ab	18.6	26.5	1.4
Anemia	16.2	27.5	1.7
Abruption	0.5	0.9	2.0
Gest. HTN	17.8	23.8	1.3
Pre-eclampsia	3.4	12.5	3.7
Eclampsia	0.1	0.2	3.4
Antenatal thromboembolism	0.1	0.5	3.3
Primary PPH	0.9	3.1	3.4
Secondary PPH	0.6	1.7	2.9
Post-partum thromboembolism	0.2	0.6	2.6

PPH: post-partum hemorrhage.

Source: Data from Campbell DM, Templeton A. Maternal complications of twin pregnancy. *Int J Gynecol Obstet* 2004;84:71–3.

vitro fertilization (IVF) are twins while 1.3% are higher order multiples [19]. Some research suggests that multiple gestations conceived by IVF may pose additional risks over those conceived spontaneously. The risks of preterm birth (PTB) between 32 and 36 weeks has an odds ratio of 1.48 [21] and pre-eclampsia may show a 2.1-fold increase [23,24]. Other concerns for ART conceived pregnancies (independent of multiple gestation) include chromosomal anomalies (if intracytoplasmic sperm injection (ICSI) is used) and possible genomic imprinting concerns (such as Beckwith–Wiedermann and Angelman's syndromes) [24].

Antenatal Care

Maternal Nutrition and Weight Gain

Maternal Physiology

Significant physiologic changes occur in multiple gestations out of proportion to those of singleton gestations. These include increased plasma volume, a higher basal metabolic rate and resistance to carbohydrate metabolism. By 20 weeks gestation, the blood volume increases by 50–70% with a smaller 25% increase in erythrocytes. Maternal energy expenditure increases more with each trimester and overall is increased 10% over a singleton pregnancy. Overall this can necessitate a 40% increase in caloric requirements with twins [25].

Maternal Weight Gain

Overall weight gain and its timing in gestation can influence the overall health of the twin pregnancy. In twins, it is particularly important to have the majority of the weight gain by 20 weeks. Optimal outcomes are typically associated with 24 pounds by 24 weeks. New body mass index (BMI) based weight gains for twin pregnancies are 37–54 pounds for normal weight, 31–50 pounds for overweight and 24–42 pounds for obese women. These ideal weight gain would optimize twin birthweights and help decrease premature birth. To help accomplish micronutrient goals, a multivitamin with 30 mg of elemental iron and 1 mg of folic acid is recommended. Fe, folate, vitamin D and B12 levels should be checked in the first trimester to see if additional supplementation may be required [25]. Of course, it is also important for the patient to avoid gaining more than the recommended weight: the goal should be to stay within the recommended guidelines.

Antepartum Management

Preterm Birth Risk Prediction

As preterm birth is a major concern with multifetal gestations, much has been studied in this arena. The first question is whether testing can be used to predict asymptomatic women at risk. Methods considered have included transvaginal sonography, fetal fibronectin (FFN) screening and home uterine monitoring. None of these have proved successful. The use of FFN as a predictor of PTB in twins may help triage symptomatic patients, although more study in this area is needed [19,26].

Preterm Birth Prevention

Prophylactic cerclage placement in a multiple gestation pregnancy without a prior history of cervical insufficiency has not been proven helpful [21]. A recent systematic review of cerclage placement in high-risk twin pregnancies showed no benefit however; the number of women available for analysis was insufficient [27]. A more recent study using short cervical length as indication for cerclage noted some benefit for the subgroup analysis with cervical length less than 15 mm before 24 weeks [28]. Evidence is not sufficient to recommend its use at present [21].

Routine hospitalization and/or bedrest for uncomplicated twin pregnancies has shown no benefits.

Likewise prophylactic tocolytics show no effectiveness and prophylactic pessaries in low-risk twin pregnancies have not been helpful [29,30]. A recent addition to the literature studying 2,287 twin pregnancies suggests that with a vaginal probe cervical length less than 25 mm, possible benefit may occur with pessary placement [31].

Progesterone treatment in unselected twin pregnancy has also not shown clear benefit and is not currently recommended [21]. A recent meta-analysis looking at intramuscular and vaginal progesterone suggested that further research into the subgroup with cervical lengths less than 25 mm may show some benefit in this population [32].

Preterm Labor Management

Prevailing evidence suggests that acute tocolysis for 48 hours is helpful in both the singleton and multiple gestation situations. Caution should be used to avoid fluid overload as multifetal gestations are more prone to pulmonary edema in this setting. First line agents should include calcium channel blockers and nonsteroidal anti-inflammatories [21,33].

Antenatal corticosteroid use for singleton deliveries between 24 and 34 weeks has been well established to decrease necrotizing enterocolitis, neonatal death, respiratory distress syndrome and intraventricular hemorrhage. Similar usage patterns are routinely given to multifetal gestations although their efficacy has not been clearly delineated [21,34]. A 2010 Cochrane Database review did not show significant difference between singleton and multiple gestation subgroups [35].

Preterm Premature Rupture of Membranes

Preterm premature rupture of membranes (PPROM) is not uncommon with multifetal gestations and its frequency increases with increasing plurality. Management is similar to singletons (see Chapter 23). Some studies have indicated a shorter latency period for twin pregnancies when ROM occurs after 30 weeks of gestation [36].

Early Gestation Management of High Order Multiples

Multifetal Reduction

Multifetal reduction involves a first trimester or early second trimester procedure, which reduces one or more fetuses from a high order multifetal pregnancy, typically triplets and above [37]. A Cochrane Database review notes pregnancy reduction appears to be associated with a reduction in "pregnancy loss, antenatal complications, births before 36 weeks, cesarean birth" [38]. In terms of twins reduced to singletons, a recent study notes this reduced the risk of late preterm birth and birthweight less than the 10%ile but not the risks of more severe complications such as early preterm birth (PTB) and birthweights less than the 5th percentile [37].

Selective Termination

Selective termination occurs when fetal reduction is applied due to an anomalous fetus. Risks with this procedure are higher due to the usually later EGA at which the anomaly is diagnosed (i.e. 18–22 weeks vs. 10–12 weeks EGA). This risk includes a higher unintended loss rate for the unaffected fetus, which increases with increasing fetal number (i.e. 2.4% for twin gestation vs 11.1% for higher order multiples) [39].

Antepartum Considerations

Aneuploidy Screening

Overall aneuploidy risks are increased in multiple gestations so that a 33-year-old patient with twins has similar aneuploidy risks to her 35-year-old singleton counterpart [20]. Thus there are increased indications for screening multiple gestations but there are also limitations to the data obtained. For example, with second trimester quad screens, the detection rate for trisomy 21 was 71% if both twins were affected and 60% when only one was affected. This was also associated with a 10.8% false-positive rate [40].

As to first trimester screening, 75–80% of Down syndrome pregnancies can be identified with a 5% false-positive rate. Triplet pregnancies could consider screening based on nuchal translucency and maternal age alone. Noninvasive prenatal testing (NIPT) is a potential tool that holds promise in this patient population but is not yet recommended [21,41].

Discordant Fetal Growth

Discordant growth becomes concerning when the difference reaches 20–25%. This is calculated by dividing the difference in fetal weights by the weight of the larger fetus. Specific concerns with monochorionic gestations are discussed earlier in this chapter. This is not as of concern if there are no TTTS concerns and both fetuses remain appropriate for gestational age. It becomes more concerning when one fetus is growth restricted and increased surveillance in those pregnancies is warranted, including weekly nonstress tests (NSTs)/ amniotic fluid indexes (AFIs), Doppler flow studies and q2-3 week growth scans. Management and delivery plans must balance the risk of intrauterine fetal demise of the growth restricted twin with the risk of prematurity for the co-twin [21].

Death of One Fetus

Vanishing Twin

This refers to the spontaneous reduction of one fetus in the first trimester [21]. This phenomenon increases with the number of gestational sacs: 36% for twins, 53% for triplets and 65% for quads. Effects for the ongoing fetus are a trend toward lower birthweight and lower gestational age at birth. However, for twins to singletons, this did not reach clinical significance and for triplets to twins, the earlier delivery was less than 36 weeks [42].

Second and Third Trimester Loss

This occurs in up to 5% of twin gestations and 17% of triplets. The key predictor of morbidity is chorionicity: the risk of death to the co-twin is 15% in MC gestations and 3% in DC gestations [43]. As noted earlier, MC twins are also at risk for neurologic problems. Care needs to be individualized for each patient.

Antenatal Testing

Dichorionic/Diamniotic Gestations

These conditions should prompt a first trimester scan to determine chronicity. The anatomy scan should occur around 18–22 weeks and this should check for anomalies, amniotic fluid, placentation and presentation of each twin. Most centers then do routine growth scans every 4–6 weeks if no complications arise. Indications for weekly surveillance with biophysical profile (BPP) or nonstress tests (NSTs) remain unclear, with some authors noting uncomplicated pregnancies should not do this while others indicates there can still be consideration for its use [21,44].

Monochorionic Gestations

The first trimester scan should establish chorionicity. The second ultrasound assessment should occur at 16 weeks and continue every 2 weeks to check for sing of TTTS. Full growth parameters should be done at least every 4 weeks. The use of middle cerebral artery MCA Dopplers to check for TAPS syndrome has not yet been standardized [45].

Timing of Delivery with Uncomplicated Gestations

Uncomplicated DI/DI gestations can undergo delivery at 38 weeks gestation. For MC/DA gestations, these should undergo delivery between 34 and 37 6/7 weeks and uncomplicated MC/MA gestations should undergo delivery by 32–34 weeks estimated gestational age (EGA) [21].

Labor and Delivery Considerations

Monoamniotic gestations should undergo cesarean section due to the risk of cord entanglement. When the presenting fetus is breech, cesarean section is also recommended. Laboring breech/ vertex twins can be at risk for chin to chin locking, which can be very complicated [46]. If the second fetus is breech and the gestational age is less than 32 weeks, then cesarean section is recommended. Given the decreased frequency of higher multiple vaginal delivery experience, it is generally recommended that higher order gestations undergo cesarean section.

Multifetal pregnancies that are good candidates for vaginal delivery include diamniotic twins greater than 32 weeks with twin A in the vertex presentation. A previous low transverse cesarean section patient who is otherwise a good vaginal birth after cesarean (VBAC) candidate should be considered for vaginal twin delivery. To safely accomplish vaginal twin delivery, there should be an obstetrician skilled in vaginal twin deliveries and breech extraction. Anesthesia must be immediately available and neuro axial anesthesia at the time of delivery greatly assists the delivery of the second twin. The operating room must also be immediately available so that conversion to emergency cesarean section is possible [21].

Higher Order Multiples

Triplet and higher order pregnancies carry significantly higher risks for preterm delivery and maternal and perinatal morbidity. Such pregnancies should be managed in centers or in consultation with practitioners who are well versed in caring for higher order gestations. Access to advanced neonatal care is important as the pregnancy progresses.

No consensus exists for the timing of antenatal testing in higher order gestations as little data is available. It is reasonable to begin testing in these gestations earlier than one would for twins but this is based more on expert opinion and standard clinical practice due to the lack of available data [47].

Some authorities feel that vaginal delivery of triplets can be safely accomplished by experienced hands [48]. Due to the complications of monitoring in labor and delivery as well as a lack of higher order mulifetal gestations, most authorities advocate cesarean delivery for triplets and above. A recent review of triplet gestation morality is consistent with this approach [49].

Concluding Remarks

Multifetal gestations have increased over the past three decades with a small downward trend recently. They require special care and attention starting with the first trimester scan. Clinicians must remember to always search for multiple gestations during the first ultrasound. Chorionicity is key for the ability to stratify risks in multifetal pregnancies. Special attention should be given to maternal nutritional status as well. Care of these patients is very rewarding, but great care must be taken to ensure a successful outcome.

References

1. J.A. Martin, B.E. Hamilton, M.J. Osterman, "Three decades of twin births in the United States, 1980–2009." *NCHS Data Brief* 2012; 80:1–8.
2. J.A. Martin, B.E. Hamilton, S.J. Bentura, "Births: Final date for 2009." *Natl Vital Stat Rep* 2011; 60:1–17.
3. J.G. Bromer, B. Ata, M. Seli, C.J. Lockwood, E. Seli, "Preterm deliveries that result from multiple pregnancies associated with assisted reproductive technologies in the USA: a cost analysis." *Current Opin Obstet Gynecol* 2011; 23:168–73.
4. J. Hall, "Twinning." *Lancet* 2003; 362: 735.
5. J.S. Chow, "Frequency of a monchorionic pair in multiple gestations: Relationship to mode of conception." *J Ultrasound Med* 2001; 20:757–760.
6. K.J. Moise, A. Johnson, "There is NO diagnosis of twins." *Am J Obstet Gynecol* 2010; 203: 1–2.
7. B. Peterson, K.B. Nelson, L. Watson, F. Stanley,"Twins, triplets, and cerebral palsy in births in Western Australia in the 1980s." *BMJ* 1993; 307:1239–43.
8. B. Luke, M.B. Brown, "The changing risk of infant mortality by gestation, plurality, and race: 1989–1991 versus 1999–2001." *Pediatrics* 2006; 118(6):2488–97.
9. J.A. Martin, B.E. Hamilton, P.D. Sutton, et al. "Births: Final date for 2006." *Natl Vital Stat Rep* 2009; 57(7): 1–102.
10. A.I. Scher, B. Petteronw, E. Blair, et al. "The risk of mortality of cerebral palsy in twins: A collaborative population-based survey." *Pediatr Res* 2002; 52(6): 671–81.
11. S.V. Glinianaia, J. Rankin, C. Wright, "Congential anomalies in twins: A register-based study." *Human Reproduc* 2008: 23(6): 1306–11.
12. S.P. Emery, M.O. Bahtiyar, K.J. Moise, "Management of complicated monochorionic gestations: Consensus statement for The North American Fetal Therapy Network." *Obstet Gynecol* 2015; 126(3):575–84.
13. R.A. Quintero, W.J. Morales, M.H. Allen, et al. "Staging for twin–twin transfusion syndrome." *J Perinatol* 1999; 19(8):550–5.
14. D. Roberts, J.P. Neilson, M.D. Kilby, S. Gates, "Interventions for the treatment of twin–twin transfusion syndrome." *Cochrane Database Syst Rev* 2014; 30(1):1. CD 002073.
15. E. Lepoire, J.M. Middeldorp, D. Oepkes, "Twin anemia-polycythemia sequence in two monochorionic twin pairs without oligo-polyhydramnios syndrome." *Placenta* 2007; 28(1):47–51.
16. T. Van Mieghem, R. De Heus, R.L. Lewis, et al. "Prenatal management of monoamniotic twin pregnancies." *Obstet Gynecol* 2014; 124(3):498–506.
17. A. Shub, S.P. Walker, "Planned early delivery versus expectant management for monoamniotic twins." *Cochrane Database Syst Rev* 2014; 4. Art no: CD00820.
18. I. Blickstein, S. Perlman, "Single fetal death in twin gestations." *J Perinat Med* 2013; 41: 65–69.
19. B. Luke, M.B. Brown, "Contemporary risks of maternal morbidity and adverse outcomes with increasing maternal age and plurality." *Fertility Sterility* 2007; 88(2):283–93.
20. B. Luke, M.B. Brown, "Maternal morbidity and infant death in twin vs triplet and quadruplet pregnancies." *Obstet Gynecol* 2008; 198(401):e1-401.e10.
21. ACOG, "Multifetal gestations: twin, triplet, and higher order multi-fetal pregnancies. Practice Bulletin No. 144." *Obstet Gynecol* 2014; 123;1118–32.
22 S. McDonald, K. Murphy, J.Beyene, A. Ohlsson, "Perinatal outcomes of in vitro fetilization twin: A sytematic review and meta-analysis." *Am J Obstet Gynecol* 2005; 193:141–52.
23. A. Lynch, R. McDuffie Jr, J. Murphy, et al. "Preeclampsia in multiple gestations: The role of assisted reproductive technologies." *Am J Obstet Gynecol* 2002; 99(3):445–51.

24. ACOG, "Perinatal risks associated with assisted reproductive technology: ACOG Committee Opinion 324." *Obstet Gynecol* 2005; 106:1143–6.

25. W. Goodnight, R. Newman, "Optimal nutrition for improved twin pregnancy outcome." *Obstet Gynecol* 2009; 114:1121–34.

26. A. Conde-Agudelo, J.M. Belizan, G. Lindmark, "Cervical vaginal fetal fibronectin for prediction of spontaneous preterm birth in multiple pregnancies: A systematic review and meta-analysis." *J Maternal-Fetal Neonatal Med* 2010; 23(12):1365–76.

27. T.H. Rafael, V. Berghella, Z. Alfirevic, "Cervical stitch(cerclage) for preventing preterm birth in multiple pregnancy." *Cochrane Database Syst Rev* 2014; 9. Art No: CD009166.

28. A. Roman, B. Rochelson, N.S. Fox, et al. "Efficacy of ultrasound-indicated cerglage in twin pregnancies." *Am J Obstet Gynecol* 2015; 212(788): e.1–6.

29. W. Yamasmit, S. Chaithongwongwatthana, J.E. Tolosa, et al. "Prophylactic oral betamemetics for reducing preterm birth in women with a twin pregnancy." *Cochrane Database Syst Revi* 2010; 9. Art No. CD004733.

30. S. Liem, E. Schuit, M. Hegeman, "Cervical pessaries for prevention of preterm birth in women with a multiple pregnancy (ProTWIN): A multicenter, open-labe randomized controlled trial." *Lancet* 2013; 382:1341–49.

31. M Goya, J de la Calle, L Pratcorona, et al. "Cervical pessary to prevent preterm birth in women with twin gestation and sonographic short cervix: a multicenter randomized controlled trial (PECEP-twins)." *Am J Obstetric Gynecol* 2016; 214: 145–52.

32. E. Schuit, S. Stock, L. Rode, et al. "Effectiveness of progestogens to improve perinatal outcome in twin pregnancies: An individual participant data meta-analysis." *BJOG* 2015; 122:27–37.

33. D.M. Hass, D.M. Caldwell, P. Kirkpatrick, et al. "Tocolytic therapy for preterm delivery: Systematic review and network meta-analysis." *BMJ* 2012; 345:e6226.

34. A.K. Msan, I.M. Usta, F.G. Mirza, A.H. Nassar, "Use of antenatal corticosteroids in the management of preterm delivery." *Am J Perinatol* 2015; 32(6):417–26.

35. L.W. Doyle, C.A. Crowther, P. Middleton, S. Marrett, D. Rouse, "Magnesium sulphate for women at risk for preterm birth for neuroprotection of the fetus." *Cochrane Database Syst Rev* 2009; 1. Art.No. CD 004661.

36. R.M. Ehanispoor, N. Aurora, D.C. Lagrew, et al. "Twin versus singleton pregnacies complicated by preterm premature rupture of the membranes." *J Maternal Fetal Neonatal Med* 2012; 25(6): 658–61.

37. ACOG. "Multifetal pregnancy reduction: ACOG Committee Opinion 553." *Obstet Gynecol* 2013; 121:405–10.

38. J.M. Dodd, T. Dogwell, C.A. Crowther, "Reduction in the number of fetuses for women with a multiple pregnancy." *Cochrane Database Syst Rev* 2015; 11. Art No. CD 003932.

39. K.A. Eddleman, J.L. Stone, L. Lynch, R.L. Berkowitz, "Selective termination of anomalous fetuses in multifetal pregnancies: Two hundred cases at a single center." *Am J Obstet Gynecol* 2002; 187:1168–72.

40. A. Garchet-Beaudron, S. Dreaux, N. Leporrier, et al. "Second-trimester Down syndrome maternal serum marker screening: A prospective study of 11,040 twin pregnancies." *Prenat Diagn* 2008; 28:1105–9.

41. ACOG, "Cell-free DNA screening for fetal aneuploidy: ACOG Committee Opinion 640." *Obstet Gynecol* 2015; 126:e31–37.

42. R.P. Dickey, S.N. Taylor, P.Y. Lu, "Spontaneous reduction of multiple pregnancies: incidence and effect on outcome." *Am J Obstet Gynecol* 2002; 186:77–83.

43. S.C. Hillman, R.K. Morris, M.D. Kilby, "Co-twin prognosis after single fetal death: A systematic review and meta-analysis." *Obstet Gynecol* 2100; 118(4):928–40.

44. C. Signore, r.K. Freeman, C.Y. Spong, "Antenatal testing – A reevaluation: Executive summary of a Eunice Kennedy Shriver National Institute of Child Health and Human Development Workshop." *Obstet Gynecol* 2009; 113(3): 607–71.

45. M.O. Bahtiyar, S.P. Emery, J.S. Dashe, "The North American Fetal Therapy Network Consensus Statement: Prenatal Surveillance of Uncomplicated Monochorionic Gestations." *Obstet Gynecol* 2015; 125(1):118–23.

46. D.J. Kreis, R.T. Miller, "Interlocked twins: Report of a case of chin-to-chin locking." *Am J Obstet Gynecol* 1958; 76(6):1334–7.

47. R Newman, E Ramsey Unal, "Multiple gestations" in *Obstetrics: Normal and Abnormal Pregnancies*, Philadelphia: Elsevier, 2012; 673–705.

48 S Alran, O Sibony, D Luton, et al. "Maternal and neonatal outcome of 93 consecutive triplet pregnancies with 71% vaginal delivery." *Acta Obstet Gynecol Scand* 2004; 83:554–9.

49. AM Vintzileos, CV Ananth, E Kontopoulos, JC Smulian, "Mode of delivery and risk of stillbirth and infant mortality in triplet gestations: United States, 1995 through 1998." *Am J Obstet Gynecol* 2005; 192:464–9.

Premature Rupture of Fetal Membranes Preterm and at Term

Julia Lagow

Introduction

This chapter will review the diagnosis of premature rupture of membranes (PROM), as well as general management options for PROM in preterm and term pregnancies. Treatment options for PROM and preterm premature rupture of membranes (PPROM) are guided predominantly by balancing gestational age at the time of diagnosis against maternal and fetal risk factors such as intraamniotic infection and neonatal complications of prematurity. Individualized treatment plans are the hallmark of care for patients with PROM.

Scope of the Problem

Premature rupture of membranes (PROM), or rupture of membranes before the onset of labor, occurs in 20% of all pregnancies.[1] Prior to 37 weeks gestation, this is defined as preterm premature rupture of membranes (PPROM).[2] PROM predisposes a pregnancy to the neonatal complications of preterm delivery as well as maternal (chorioamnionitis and endometritis) and neonatal (early onset sepsis) infection.[3–5] Individualized treatment plans are the hallmark of care for patients with PROM, ranging from expectant management to induction of labor.

Term Premature Rupture of Membranes

At term, 8% of pregnancies experience PROM.[2] The greatest maternal complication is intrauterine infection. This risk increases with the length of time from rupture to delivery.[2] One randomized trial reports 50% of women at term with PROM who were managed expectantly delivered within 5 hours of rupture; 95% had delivered within 28 hours.[6]

Preterm Premature Rupture of Membranes

Preterm PROM is responsible for 30–40% of all preterm deliveries.[7] One-half of women will deliver within one week of PPROM regardless of management.[5] Expectant inpatient management is the mainstay of care for PPROM after viability. This can result in long hospital stays for the patient prior to delivery as well as extended NICU admissions for baby after delivery. During the intrapartum period, patients with preterm PROM are at risk for cesarean delivery related to malpresentation, prolapse of the umbilical cord for fetuses in the non-vertex position or nonreassuring fetal heart rate tracing related to cord compression from oligohydramnios. Risks to the fetus are associated with prematurity at the time of delivery. The most common of these is neonatal respiratory distress syndrome.[2] Other neonatal complications of prematurity observed in patients with preterm PROM are intraventricular hemorrhage, necrotizing enterocolitis and sepsis.[8] Risk factors for PROM are seen in Box 23.1.

Previable Premature Rupture of Membranes

Rupture of membranes between 14 and 24 weeks gestation occurs in less than 1% of pregnancies.[2] Survival rates are greatly increased when rupture occurs after 22 weeks gestation.[9]

Similar to PROM at other gestational ages, intrauterine infection (13–60%), placental abruption (4–12%) and retained placenta are common maternal complications from previable PROM. Maternal sepsis occurs infrequently, in approximately 1% of reported cases. Patients are higher risk for these complications the lower their gestational age at the time PROM is diagnosed.[5]

Pulmonary hypoplasia is a fetal complication commonly seen with previable PROM and correlates with a high risk for mortality.[9] The gestation at which rupture occurs and the level of remaining amniotic fluid determine the likelihood and severity of pulmonary hypoplasia. The risk of mortality decreases if rupture occurs after 23–24 weeks. This is likely due to alveolar growth at this gestational age that is appropriate to support the fetus after delivery.

Box 23.1 Risk factors for preterm premature rupture of membranes

- History of PROM
- History of preterm labor from other causes
- Second or third trimester vaginal bleeding
- Decreased cervical length
- Tobacco use
- Sexually transmitted infections
- Illicit drug use
- Low body mass index
- Lower socioeconomic status

Other complications include skeletal abnormalities from positional restrictions of the fetus due to low levels of residual amniotic fluid. These often resolve in the postnatal period.

Etiology of Premature Rupture of Membranes

PROM at term can be part of a physiologic process caused by uterine contractions and a physical weakening of membranes.

Preterm PROM occurs frequently without obvious cause or connection to known risk factors. The most common risk factor for PROM is intraamniotic infection. This risk increases at earlier gestational ages; 13–60% of pregnancies with preterm PROM and 1% of pregnancies with term PROM.[2,10] At the time of diagnosis, patients with PROM should be evaluated for clinical signs of intraamniotic infection, as this may drastically change their management plan. Uterine fundal tenderness, leukocytosis, maternal or fetal tachycardia, fever and purulent discharge are indicators of possible infection.[8] Patients who have experienced preterm PROM or preterm labor are at high risk for recurrence in future pregnancies. Other risk factors for preterm PROM include second and third trimester bleeding, decreased cervical length, tobacco use, sexually transmitted infections, illicit drug use, low body mass index, and lower socioeconomic status.[11–14]

Diagnosis of Premature Rupture of Membranes

Suspicion for rupture of membranes occurs when a patient reports loss of fluid or a diagnosis of oligohydramnios or anhydramnios is made by ultrasound. Physical exam combined with laboratory testing can confirm the diagnosis. Sterile speculum exam should be used to minimize introduction of infection. During sterile speculum exam, the provider attempts to visualize fluid in the vagina; this is known as pooling. The provider may also ask the patient to cough or perform Valsalva maneuvers in order to watch for fluid leaking from the cervix into the vagina. The cervix and vaginal mucosa should also be inspected for any abnormalities or lesions, as this may play a role in further management. A wet prep, cultures for gonorrhea, chlamydia and group beta strep should be obtained to minimize need for repeat examination.

The pH of any vaginal fluid may be measured to make a distinction between amniotic fluid and normal vaginal discharge. The normal pH of the vagina ranges between 4.5 and 6.0. Amniotic fluid will alter this level to a pH of 7.1–7.3. The presence of blood, semen or vaginal infection could falsify this measurement. It is also recommended to avoid lubricating gel during the sterile speculum exam, as this may also provide an erroneous result. Nitrazine paper or swab will change from yellow to a deep blue in the presence of an alkaline environment. See Figure 23.1.

Amniotic fluid can also be differentiated from vaginal secretions on microscopic examination. When allowed to dry on a slide, amniotic fluid will produce a pattern known as ferning, or arborization (see Figure 23.2). Measurement of amniotic fluid volume by ultrasound may provide additional support for the diagnosis.

If the diagnosis remains in question, definitive diagnosis can be accomplished with instillation of dye into the amniotic cavity. This is traditionally performed via amniocentesis. Indigo carmine dye is injected through the maternal abdomen into the amniotic fluid under ultrasound guidance. A tampon or pad is then used to observe for leakage of blue fluid from the vagina. A tampon in recommended as maternal urine could become blue as well. This diagnostic option may become obsolete as pharmaceutical companies are no longer producing indigo carmine dye. Finally, commercial testing kits are available.

Some authors have described the use of fetal fibronectin to evaluate for PROM. While a positive test does not confirm the diagnosis, a negative test is considered a sensitive result for intact membranes.[15] Other test kits detect the presence of amniotic proteins. Amnisure® tests for the concentration of placental

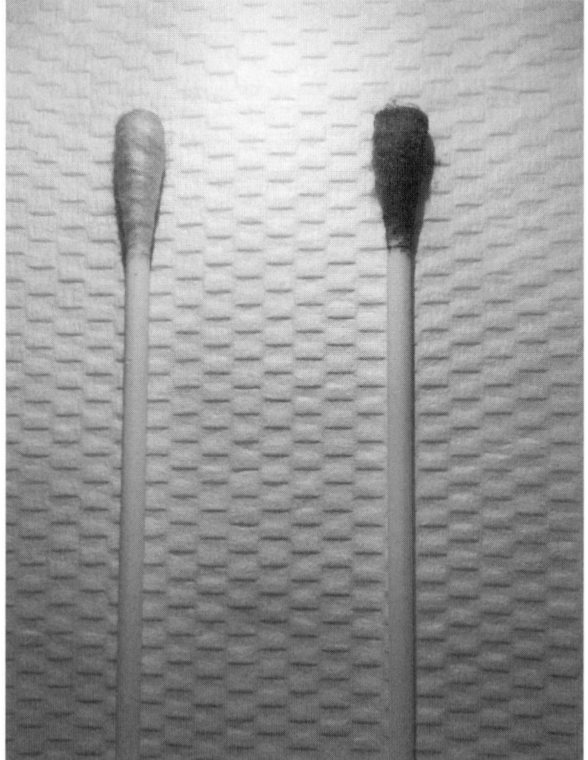

Figure 23.1 Nitrazine.

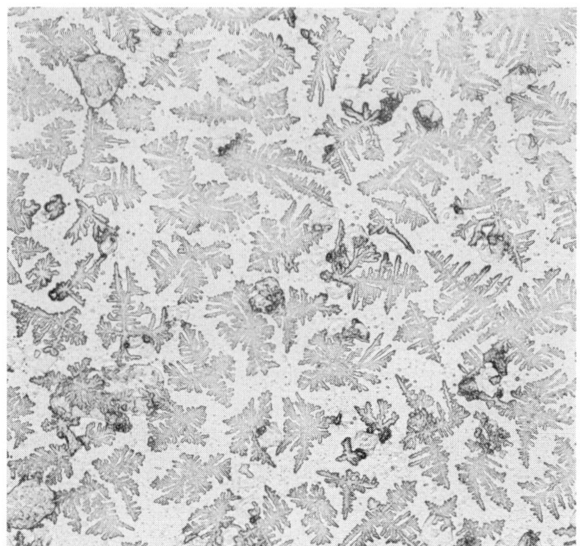

Figure 23.2 Ferning.

alpha-microglobulin-1 (PAMG-1). Amniotic fluid contains a higher concentration of PAMG-1 than vaginal secretions.[16] These testing options should be used as adjuncts to the above diagnostic methods.[2] False-positive rates of up to 31% have been identified in laboring patients with no clinical signs of rupture of membranes.[17,18]

Management of Premature Rupture of Membranes

Term and Near Term Rupture of Membranes

Gestational age is the primary factor in determining management once PROM is confirmed. Under ideal circumstances, this information is based on early ultrasonographic dating or documented last menstrual period. Other significant factors include any concern for infection or placental abruption. Evaluation of fetal status with fetal heart rate monitoring and assessment for the presence of uterine activity with tocometry should be initiated once the diagnosis of PROM is established. Fetal presentation and group B *Streptococci* (GBS) status should be obtained and prophylaxis initiated if indicated.

In early term and term pregnancies, induction of labor should be considered in those patients who do not experience spontaneous labor shortly after diagnosis. A period of expectant management is considered acceptable for those patients who wish to defer induction.[2] Cesarean delivery is used only for standard obstetrical indications. No indication for the routine use of antibiotics with PROM at term exists with the exception of GBS status.[13,19,20] One meta-analysis suggests that routine prophylactic antibiotics in term PROM can eliminate the role that latency plays in increased infection rates for mother and fetus.[21]

PROM at 34–37 Weeks Gestation

Pregnancies between 34 weeks 0 days and 36 weeks 6 days gestation account for 40–60% of preterm PROM.[7] Management of these patients should follow the recommendations for term pregnancies. Tocolysis has been used in order to administer corticosteroids to patients who present in preterm labor at these gestational ages. This practice has not, however, been shown to be of benefit in patients with PPROM. Furthermore, no significant improvement in overall neonatal outcomes has been noted with expectant management.[2] Increased rates of intraamniotic infection, lower umbilical cord gas pH as well as longer maternal hospitalization occur with delayed delivery in this group.[8] A recent international randomized controlled trial reevaluates the option of expectant management as these gestational ages.[22]

PPROM at 24–34 Weeks

PROM between 24 weeks 0 days and 33 weeks 6 days gestation is expectantly managed on an inpatient basis. As the onset of infection can occur rapidly, home management of a pregnancy with a viable fetus and PROM is not recommended.[2] Indications for delivery in this group are similar to other gestations; compromised fetal status, placental abruption and clinical signs of infection or labor. Demonstration of fetal lung maturity may also be used as an indicator to move toward delivery. The use of tocolytics in preterm PROM differs between specialists. Current data is of little use to formulate a recommendation due to limited use of latency antibiotics and corticosteroids in these studies. As no improvement is noted in neonatal outcomes, tocolysis is not recommended. Antenatal corticosteroids are recommended as a single course for preterm PROM between 24 weeks 0 days and 34 weeks 0 days gestation. The lower threshold of this range varies by institution. The use of antenatal corticosteroid therapy reduces neonatal mortality. It has also been shown to decrease respiratory distress, intraventricular hemorrhage and necrotizing enterocolitis.[4,23,24] The use of magnesium sulfate for neuroprotection against cerebral palsy has been recommended when delivery appears eminent prior to 32 weeks gestation. GBS prophylaxis is also appropriate where indicated. Clinicians should assess patients for potential placental abruption at least daily given the increased risk of this complication in patients with PPROM.

No single antibiotic protocol has been deemed optimal, as several show reduction in maternal and neonatal infections. Antibiotic therapy also increases latency from rupture to delivery; helping to decrease neonatal complications that occur more frequently at early gestational ages. To see these benefits, a seven-day course is recommended. Traditionally, 48 hours of intravenous antibiotics is followed by five days of oral antibiotics. A multicenter trial demonstrated doubling of the latency period for patients who received seven days of antibiotics in comparison with the placebo group.[14] One option is a course beginning with intravenous ampicillin and erythromycin followed by an oral course of amoxicillin and erythromycin. Other regimens use azithromycin in place of erythromycin.[25,26] Beta-lactam antibiotics (amoxicillin clavulanate) are avoided in favor of macrolides as the former are associated with increased rates of necrotizing enterocolitis in neonates. See Table 23.1.

Table 23.1 Latency Antibiotic Seven-Day Regimens in PROM

Protocol	IV	Oral
NICDH	Ampicillin 2 grams IV q 6 h for 48 h and Erythromycin 250 mg IV q 6 h for 48 h	Amoxicillin 250 mg PO q 8 h for 5 days and Enteric-coated Erythromycin 333 mg PO q 8 h for 5 days
Alternative	Ampicillin 2 grams IV q 6 h for 48 h and Azithromycin 500 mg IV daily for 48 h	Amoxicillin 250 mg PO q 8 h for 5 days and Azithromycin 500 mg PO daily for 5 days

PPROM Prior to 24 Weeks Gestation

Prior to 24 weeks gestation, the management plan for previable PROM requires extensive counseling of the patient. All options should be discussed with special emphasis placed on anticipated neonatal outcomes. Expectant management and induction are possible management options at the time of diagnosis. Outpatient management is appropriate for those previable PROM patients who are asymptomatic. Careful review of infection and bleeding precautions should be provided. Prior to viability, corticosteroids, GBS prophylaxis, magnesium sulfate for neuroprotection and tocolysis are not recommended. These management options, along with a transition to hospitalization, may be reconsidered as early as 23 weeks gestation. Antibiotics for latency could be a consideration as early as 20 weeks gestation.[2] See Box 23.2.

Induction of Patients with PROM

The preferred agent for induction of labor in patients with PROM is controversial. This is due to limited studies evaluating this specific group of patients. The goal of induction method selection in patients with PROM is to minimize the time from initiation to delivery. Decreasing the latency from induction to delivery has been shown to decrease the incidence of maternal and neonatal infections.[21] Oxytocin infusion is the induction method of choice with a favorable cervix (Bishop score of 8 or greater). Method of induction appears most controversial for those patients with PROM and an unfavorable cervix. Both oral and vaginal preparations

Box 23.2 Management of premature rupture of membranes by gestational age

Prior to 24 weeks gestation
- Expectant management vs. induction of labor
- Thorough counseling of patient
- Offer antibiotics as early as 20 weeks gestation
- Consider transition to inpatient management around 23 weeks gestation
- *Not* recommended before viability:
  - Corticosteroids
  - GBS prophylaxis
  - Magnesium Sulfate for neuroprotection
  - Tocolysis

24 weeks 0 days to 33 weeks 6 days gestation
- Expectant management
- Single course of corticosteroids
- GBS prophylaxis if indicated
- Antibiotics

34 weeks 0 days to 36 weeks 6 days gestation
- Delivery
- GBS prophylaxis if indicated

After or at 37 weeks 0 days gestation
- Delivery
- GBS prophylaxis if indicated

of prostaglandins may be helpful in the setting of an unfavorable cervix in order to expedite delivery.[27] Prostaglandins have been shown to be equally as effective for induction of labor as oxytocin. However, they are associated with higher incidence of chorioamnionitis.[6] Osmotic dilators for mechanical cervical ripening in PROM have been cautioned against, as studies have shown increased rates of peripartum infection.[28–34] There is no current body of data on which to base a recommendation for mechanical methods of cervical ripening such as Foley balloon or double balloon catheter. These mechanical options may be used with or without concurrent oxytocin infusion to expedite delivery. Again, cesarean delivery is used only when required by standard obstetrical indications.

Special Considerations

Patients with a History of PROM

Patients with history of PROM are at higher risk for recurrence of PROM and preterm delivery. They should be presented with management options similar to those offered to patients with a history of preterm delivery from other causes. These options include initiating progesterone therapy between 16 and 24 weeks gestation, cervical length screening prior to 24 weeks gestation and cervical cerclage for those with a cervical length less than 25 mm.[30] Studies report these interventions reduce the recurrence of preterm delivery, though outcomes in patients with PROM were not evaluated as an isolated study group.

Second Trimester Amniocentesis

PROM is seen in about 1% of all second trimester amniocentesis performed for prenatal diagnosis.[2] These patients have a greater chance to reaccumulate normal levels of amniotic fluid than their counterparts who experience spontaneous rupture. They are often managed on an outpatient basis with frequent reassessment of amniotic fluid volume by ultrasound.

Cervical Cerclage in Place

There is no single plan of care recommended for the management of preterm PROM with cervical cerclage in place.[2] If a cerclage does remain in place, no additional antibiotic regimen is recommended past a seven-day course or that required for GBS prophylaxis.[2] Removal or retention of cervical cerclage is based on presence of clinical infection or concern for imminent delivery.

Herpes Simplex Virus

The risk of vertical transmission should be a consideration for patients with PROM and a history of herpes simplex virus (HSV). Neonatal HSV infection from a primary outbreak has been demonstrated in between 30% and 50% of affected pregnancies; the risk is 3% from a recurrent outbreak. A meticulous sterile speculum exam should be performed with appropriate lighting at the time of admission and again at the time of induction or anticipated delivery to evaluate for the presence of HSV lesions. Expectant management with the addition of acyclovir therapy is recommended for a pregnancy prior to 34 weeks gestation with recurrent disease. When delivery is indicated, cesarean delivery is recommended in the presence of prodromal symptoms or active lesions. Management recommendations are less clear in the setting of primary outbreak. Acyclovir therapy should be administered and cesarean delivery performed for active lesions at the time delivery is indicated.

Human Immunodeficiency Virus

Individual plans of care should be created for patients with human immunodeficiency virus (HIV) and preterm PROM. No available data exist by which to make optimal management recommendations for these patients. Current data finds that for patients with (1) low viral loads who are (2) compliant with antiretroviral medications during pregnancy and (3)receive antepartum and intrapartum zidovudine, there is no correlation between vertical transmission and length of rupture.[2]

Concluding Remarks

Optimal gestational age for delivery with PROM remains controversial. Careful consideration must be taken to create individual plans of care. Accurate assignment of gestational age is essential in creating appropriate management plans for patients with PROM. Risks of prematurity as well as maternal and fetal risk factors must be weighed when creating management strategies for PROM. Changes in maternal and fetal condition should guide changes in the care plan.

References

1. Harger J, Hsing A, Tuomala R, Gibbs R, Mead P, et al. Risk factors preterm premature rupture of fetal membranes: A multicenter case–control study. *Am J Obstet Gynecol* 1990;163:130–7.
2. Premature Rupture of Membranes. Interim Update Practice Bulletin 160. American College of Obstetricians and Gynecologists. *Obstet Gynecol* 2016; 127(1):e39–51.
3. Moore R, Mansour J, Redline R, Mercer B, Moore J. The physiology of fetal membrane rupture: Insight gained from the determination of physical properties. *Placenta* 2006;27:1037–51.
4. Roberts D, Dalziel S. Antenatal corticosteroids for accelerating fetal lung maturation for women at risk of preterm birth. *Cochrane Database Syst Rev* 2006;3:CD004454. DOI 10.1002/14651858.
5. Mercer B. Preterm premature rupture of membranes. *Obstet Gynecol* 2003;101(1):178–93.
6. Hannah M, Ohlsson A, Farine D, Hewson S, Hodnett E, et al. Induction of labor compared with expectant management for prelabor rupture of membranes at term. TERMPROM Study Group. *N Engl J Med* 1996;334:1005–10.
7. Saccone G, Berghella V. Antibiotic prophylaxis for term or near-term premature rupture of membranes: Metaanalysis of randomized trials. *Am J Obstet Gynecol* 2015;212:627.e1–9.
8. Packard R, Mackeen A. Labor induction in the patient with preterm premature rupture of membranes. *Semin Perinatol* 2015;39:495–500.
9. Waters T, Mercer B. The management of preterm premature rupture of membranes near the limit of fetal viability. *Am J Obstet Gynecol* 2009;201:230–40.
10. Mercer B, Crocker L, Boe N, Sibai B. Induction versus expectant management in premature rupture of membranes with mature amniotic fluid at 32 to 36 weeks: A randomized trial. *Obstet Gynecol* 1993;169(4):775–82.
11. Mercer B, Goldenberg R, Meis P, Moawad A, Shellhaas C, et al. The Preterm Prediction Study: Prediction of preterm premature rupture of membranes through clinical findings and ancillary testing. The National Institute of Child Health and Human Development Maternal-Fetal Medicine Units Network. *Am J Obstet Gynecol* 2000;183:738–45.
12. Berkowitz G, Blackmore-Prince C, Lapinski R, Savitz D. Risk factors for preterm birth subtypes. *Epidemiology* 1998;9:279–85.
13. Cararach V, Botet F, Sentis J, Almirall R, Perez-Picanol E. Administration of antibiotics to patients with rupture of membranes at term: A prospective, randomized, multicentric study. Collaborative Group on PROM. *Acta Obstet Gynecol Scand* 1998;77:298–302.
14. Mercer B, Miodovnik, Thurnau G, et al. Antibiotic therapy for reduction of infant morbidity after preterm premature rupture of the membranes: A randomized controlled trial. *J Am Med Assoc* 1997;278(12):989–95.
15. Abdelazim I. Fetal fibronectin (Quick Check fFN test®) for detection of premature rupture of fetal membranes. *Arch Gynecol Obstet* 2013;287(2):205–10. DOI: 10.1007/s00404-012-2548-3.
16. Cousins L, Smok D, Lovett S, Poeltler D. AmniSure placental alpha macroglobulin-1 rapid assay versus standard diagnostic methods for detection of rupture of membranes. *Am J Perinatol* 2005;22(6):317–20.
17. Mi Lee S, Romero R, Park J, et al. The clinical significance of a positive Amnisure test in women with preterm labor and intact membranes. *J Matern Fetal Neonatal Med* 2012;25(9):1690–8.
18. Lee S, Lee J, Seong H, et al. The clinical significance of a positive Amnisure testing women with term laborwith intact membranes. *J Maternal Fetal Neonatal Med* 2009;22(4):305–10.
19. Flenady V, King J. Antibiotics for prelabour rupture of membranes at or near term. *Cochrane Database*

Syst Rev 2002;3:CD001807. DOI 10.1002/14651858. CD001807.

20. Ovalle A, Martinez M, Kakarieka E, Gomez R, Rubio R, et al. Antibiotic administration in patients with preterm premature rupture of membranes reduces the rate of histological chorioamnionitis: A prospective, randomized, controlled study. *J Matern Fetal Neonatal Med* 2002;12:35–41.
21. Kacerovsky M, Musilova I, Andrys C, et al. Prelabor rupture of membranes between 34 and 37 weeks: The intraamniotic inflammatory response and neonatal outcomes. *Am J Obstet Gynecol* 2014;210:325.e1-10.
22. Morris J, Roberts C, Bowen J, Patterson J, Bond D, et al. Immediate delivery compared with expectant management after preterm pre-labour rupture of membranes close to term (PPROMT trial): A randomized controlled trial. *Lancet* 2016 Jan 30;387(10017):444–52. doi: 10.1016/S0140-6736(15)00724-2. Epub 2015 Nov 10.
23. Vidaeff A, Ramin S. Antenatal corticosteroids after preterm premature rupture of membranes. *Clin Obstet Gynecol* 2011;54:337–43.
24. Harding J, Pang J, Knight D, Liggins G. Do antenatal corticosteroids help in the setting of preterm rupture of membranes? *Am J Obstet Gynecol* 2001;184:131–9.
25. Kenyon S, Boulvain M, Neilson J. Antibiotics for preterm rupture of membranes. *Cochrane Database Syst Rev* 2010;8:CD001058. DOI 10.1002/14651858. pub2.
26. Kenyon S, Taylor D, Tarnow-Mordi W. Broad-spectrum antibiotics for preterm, prelabour rupture of fetal membranes: The ORACLE I randomized trial. ORACLE Collaborative Group. *Lancet* 2001;357:979–88.
27. Jha N, Sagili H, Jayalakshmi D, Lakshminarayanan S. Comparison of efficacy and safety of sublingual misoprostol with intracervical dinoprostone gel for cervical ripening in prelabour rupture of membranes after 34 weeks of gestation. *Arch Gynecol Obstet* 2015; 291:39–44. DOI 10.1007/s00404-014-3383-5.
28. Krammer J, Williams M, Sawai S, O'Brien W. Pre-induction cervical ripening: A randomized comparison of two methods. *Obstet Gynecol* 1995;85(4):614–18.
29. Kazzi G, Bottoms S, Rosen M. Efficacy and safety of laminaria digitata for preinduction ripening of the cervix. *Obstet Gynecol* 1982;60(4):440–3.
30. Berghella V, Rafael T, Szychowski J, Rust O, Owen J. Cerclage for short cervix on ultrasonography in women with singleton gestations and previous preterm birth: A meta-analysis. *Obstet Gynecol* 2011;117:663–71.
31. Ofman G, Vasco N, Cantey J. Risk of early-onset sepsis following preterm, prolonged rupture of membranes with or without chorioamnionitis. *Am J Perinatol* 2015; DOI 10.1055/S-0035-1556758.
32. Treadwell M, Bronsteen R, Bottoms S. Prognostic factors and complication rates for cervical cerclage: A review of 482 cases. *Am J Obstet Gynecol* 1991;165:555–8.
33. Arias F, Tomich P. Etiology and outcome of low birth weight and preterm infants. *Obstet Gynecol* 1982;60:277–81.
34. Garite T, Freeman R. Chorioamnionitis in the preterm gestation. *Obstet Gynecol* 1982;59:539–45.

Preterm Delivery

Roxanne A. Vrees

Introduction

Preterm birth is defined as birth occurring between 20 0/7 and 36 6/7 weeks of gestation (1). Spontaneous preterm birth includes all births that occur as a result of preterm labor, cervical insufficiency and preterm premature rupture of membranes. Although fewer than 10% of women who meet clinical criteria for preterm labor will deliver within 7 days, it is important to note that there are many conditions that necessitate preterm delivery for maternal and fetal indications (1,2). In contrast, term births are broken into four categories. These include (a) early term (37 0/7 through 38 6/7 weeks gestation), (b) full term (39 0/7 through 40 6/7 weeks gestation, (c) late term (41 0/7 through 41 6/7 weeks) and (d) post-term (42 0/7 weeks of gestation and beyond) (3). While all deliveries occurring between 38 and 42 weeks are considered term, the risks of perinatal, neonatal and infant morbidity and mortality are lowest among infants who are born during the "full term" interval (2). Additionally, the rate of neonatal complications is inversely correlated with gestational age such that infants born prior to 32 weeks have the greatest risk of death and adverse health outcomes (2). The diagnosis of preterm labor is largely based on clinical findings including regular uterine contractions (four or more in 20 minutes or eight or more in 1 hour) in conjunction with cervical dilation and/or effacement and intact membranes; or an initial presentation with regular contractions and advanced cervical dilatation defined as >/=2 cm occurring between 20 0/7 and 36 6/7 weeks gestation. From a historical perspective, there were a variety of interventions thought to prevent preterm births in women presenting with preterm labor. These included bed rest, hydration, prolonged use of antibiotics and tocolytic therapy, home uterine monitoring and abstinence from intercourse. However, none of these interventions have been found to be clinically effective at preventing preterm labor and some are clearly associated with adverse effects (4–6). Presently, the pharmacologic agents that have shown improved neonatal outcomes include antenatal corticosteroids and magnesium sulfate for fetal neuroprotection. This chapter will review the diagnosis and management strategies for preterm labor as well as the evidence to support their use in current clinical practice.

Scope of the Problem

Preterm births in the United States have increased by 30% since 1981 and pose a significant public health problem related to both immediate and long-term sequelae (7). According to the most current estimates, preterm births result in a minimum annual expenditure of $26.2 billion in the United States. The overall economic burden to society includes costs related to prolonged care in neonatal intensive care units as well as the chronic conditions resulting from prematurity, including cerebral palsy, visual and hearing impairments, learning disabilities and behavioral problems. Approximately two-thirds of the annual cost is related to medical care, 85% of which will occur in early infancy. Additional costs include maternal delivery at $1.9 billion, $611 million for early intervention programs,$5.7 billion for loss of household and labor productivity and $1.1 billion for the four major disabilities seen in preterm infants(cerebral palsy, mental retardation, impaired vision and hearing loss) (7). It is important to note that the total cost per preterm delivery does not include medical care beyond early childhood or costs related to caregivers (7). Furthermore, beyond neonatal life, preterm birth remains the most frequent cause of infant death in the United States and was responsible for one-third of infant deaths in the 2002 (8). In addition to the significant financial burden of preterm births, significant racial and ethnic disparities exist. The highest rates of preterm births are seen in African American women, with 17.8% of births in this population being affected (7).

Furthermore, concerning trends have also been seen among certain groups with the most notable increases among American Indian, white and Hispanic groups between 2001 and 2003. In contrast, Asian and Pacific Islander women have the lowest rates of preterm birth with 10.5% of births affected.

The growing trends and disparities among racial and ethnic groups is of concern and cannot be explained solely by socioeconomic status or high-risk maternal behaviors. Multidisciplinary research is clearly needed to better define the scope of the problem, examine the multiple etiologies and disparities, identify the full impact from a public health and policy standpoint and improve maternal and neonatal outcomes.

Pathogenesis

The etiology of preterm labor is largely unknown but several associations between biological, environmental and socioeconomic factors have been identified (see Box 24.1). Medical conditions such as chronic hypertension, diabetes and underlying infections are often associated with indicated preterm birth (7). History of prior preterm birth remains one of the strongest clinical risk factors for preterm birth (9). In fact, a history of preterm birth is reported to represent a 1.5- to 2-fold increased risk of preterm birth in a subsequent pregnancy; the total number of prior preterm deliveries and gestational age at prior delivery further augment that risk (10). Risk factors for preterm labor and biologic conditions that have been implicated are seen in Box 24.1 (10–12). Despite known risk factors for preterm labor and subsequent preterm birth, epidemiologic scoring systems have not been found to demonstrate sufficient predictive value and are thus not clinically reliable. Several biologic markers have also been proposed for use in predicting preterm birth risk. These include home uterine activity monitoring, measuring of salivary estriol levels and screening and treatment of asymptomatic bacterial vaginosis. However, there is no current data to support the use of these biologic markers in clinical practice.

Box 24.1 Factors associated with preterm labor

- Chronic hypertension
- Diabetes
- Underlying infections
  - Acute of chronic inflammatory states in uterus or mother
- Decidual hemorrhage
  - Abruption
- Mechanical strain
  - Uterine over-distention
  - Cervical insufficiency
- Hormonally mediated by maternal or fetal stress
- Low pre-pregnancy weight (BMI <19.8)
- Substance abuse
- Non-white race
- Age <17 or >35
- Vaginal bleeding that persists beyond first trimester
- Short inter-pregnancy interval (<18–23 months)
- Smoking
- Low socioeconomic status

Screening and Prevention

A variety of factors have been implicated in preterm labor. However, very few strategies exist to stratify risk for preterm delivery in patients who meet clinical criteria for preterm labor. Importantly, predicting risk of subsequent preterm delivery is only useful when interventions to improve outcomes exist and are available. The presence of fetal fibronectin (fFN) and a shortened cervix have both been associated with preterm birth (13–15). Shortening of the cervix can occur for a variety of reasons including congenital, pathologic (e.g. inflammatory) and iatrogenic factors (16). Regardless of the etiology, however, cervical length represents a measurable marker for risk of preterm birth in both unselected and high-risk patients (17–19). Transvaginal cervical ultrasonography, when performed by a trained and qualified provider, is a reliable and reproducible method for determining cervical length (20). The most commonly utilized definition of a shortened cervix is a measurement less than 25 mm, usually prior to 24 weeks gestation, and up to 28 weeks in some studies (2). Several studies have evaluated the clinical utility of fFN alone or in conjunction with cervical length measurement as a predictive model in symptomatic women. Observational studies have shown that knowledge of fFN status and cervical length are helpful in the triage of at risk patients. One study evaluating the presence of either a shortened cervix less than 25 mm at less than 35 weeks gestation or a positive fFN demonstrated a strong association with preterm birth, especially in women with a prior history of preterm delivery (21,22). Furthermore, these results were particularly useful in decreasing the assessed risk of preterm birth in women with classic risk factors and negative results of either one or both tests (23). However, randomized trials have not been performed to date and neither a positive fFN status nor cervical length alone possess significant positive predictive value and should not be used in isolation to exclusively guide management in a patient with acute symptoms (24). Of note, modalities such as fetal fibronectin screening, testing for bacterial vaginosis and home uterine monitoring have not been shown to improve perinatal outcomes and are therefore not recommended for primary screening strategies (25,26).

Box 24.2 Criteria for cerclage placement

- Cervical insufficiency
  - History or clinical signs and symptoms consistent with cervical insufficiency
  - Physical examination demonstrating painless cervical dilation in second trimester
- History of a prior preterm birth at less than 34 weeks gestation with a current singleton pregnancy
- Shortened cervical length (<25 mm) prior to 24 weeks gestation

Prediction and Prevention

Women with a prior history of spontaneous preterm birth are more likely to experience a subsequent preterm delivery and should be evaluated for risk of preterm birth. The initial evaluation should include a detailed medical and obstetric history, identification of potential risk factors and determination of clinical indication for prophylactic interventions such as cervical cerclage and progesterone supplementation. It is critical to differentiate between prior spontaneous versus indicated preterm birth as the approach to each will vary significantly. Additionally, any modifiable risk factors (e.g. smoking) should be addressed as these can alter a woman's risk during the current pregnancy. Women with a prior spontaneous preterm singleton birth should be offered progesterone supplementation starting at 16 weeks to reduce the risk of a subsequent spontaneous preterm birth (27–29).

Cerclage placement is an additional tool available for the prevention of subsequent preterm birth and may be appropriate for certain women based on the criteria seen in Box 24.2 (30). While cerclage and supplemental progesterone have both been shown to reduce recurrent preterm birth in select patients, no data supports an additive effect in reducing risk of preterm birth when used in combination (31). Similarly there is no data to support adding an additional form of progesterone supplementation to women already receiving a particular formulation once a shortened cervix has been identified. Furthermore, despite the proven benefit of progesterone supplementation for prevention of preterm birth in women who have had a prior history of spontaneous preterm delivery, progesterone has not been evaluated for use as a tocolytic agent and should not be used in this fashion. While women with a prior history of spontaneous preterm birth are at greatest risk for recurrent preterm delivery, many women with no prior history or any identifiable risk factors will also experience spontaneous preterm birth. This raises the question of whether low-risk women should also be screened for a risk of preterm birth. The concept of universal cervical length screening is supported by the fact that two large randomized trials have demonstrated a significant reduction in preterm birth in women with a shortened cervix who receive vaginal progesterone (32–34). Additionally, initial analyses of cost-effectiveness suggest that universal cervical length screening is a cost-effective strategy to prevent spontaneous preterm birth (34–36). However, a more recent study has demonstrated that the specificity of universal cervical length screening is increased from 62.8% to 96.5% when a risk-based approach is utilized (34). Currently, universal cervical length screening for all low-risk patients or screening in high-risk populations only are both considered viable options and practitioners are encouraged to weigh risks and benefits of missed opportunities for intervention against the costs of unnecessary screening (3).

Management

It is extremely difficult to predict which women who present with signs and symptoms of preterm labor will ultimately go on to deliver a preterm infant. Current estimates indicate that approximately 30% of preterm labor will spontaneously resolve (37) and 50% of women hospitalized for preterm labor will go on to deliver at term (38–40). Non-pharmacologic agents such as intravenous hydration, avoidance of orgasm and bedrest that were once thought to prevent spontaneous preterm birth in women who present with preterm labor symptoms have not been shown to be effective. Additionally, these interventions add

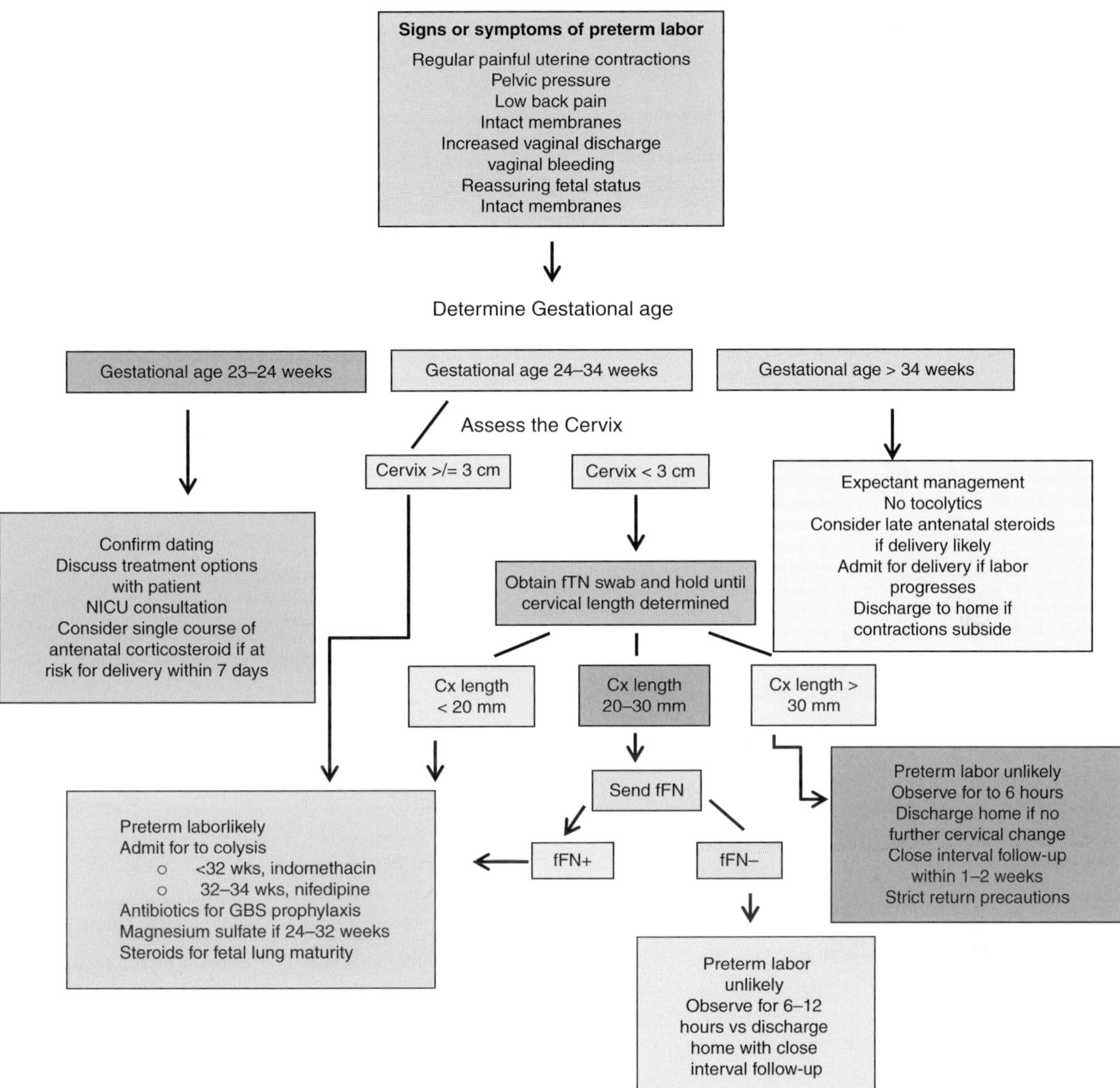

Figure 24.1 Proposed algorithm for the evaluation and management of preterm labor.

additional risks including venous thromboembolism, physical deconditioning and lost wages (4–6). An algorithm for the management of preterm labor is provided in Figure 24.1

Current treatment strategies that have been shown to be clinically effective include short-term tocolytic therapy, corticosteroids to promote fetal lung maturation and magnesium sulfate for neuroprotection. Tocolytic drugs function to inhibit myometrial activity and a variety of agents have been used to inhibit uterine contractions. These include ethanol, magnesium sulfate, calcium channel blockers, oxytocin antagonists, nonsteroidal anti-inflammatory drugs (NSAIDs) and beta-mimetic agonist (41). First-line tocolytic agents as listed in Table 24.1 include beta-adrenergic receptor agonists, calcium channel blockers and prostaglandic synthetase inhibitors for short-term pregnancy prolongation (i.e. up to 48 hours). Tocolytic therapy is typically effective for up to 48 hours (41) and should be reserved for women in whom a 48-hour delay would benefit the neonate. The short-term prolongation of pregnancy resulting from tocolytic use enables transfer

Table 24.1 Common Tocolytic Agents and Side Effects

Agent	Dosage	Contraindications	Maternal Side Effects	Neonatal Side Effects
Magnesium sulfate	4-6 g bolus for 20 minutes, then 2–3 g/hour	Myasthenia gravis Caution with significant renal impairment	Flushing Lethargy Nausea Headache Muscle weakness Respiratory depression Pulmonary edema Cardiac arrest	Hypotonia Lethargy Respiratory depression Bone deminieralization (prolonged use)
Beta-adrenergic	Terbutaline 0.25 mg subcutaneously every 20 minutes to 3 hours (hold for pulse >120 bpm)	Cardiac arrhythmias	Palpitations Tachycardia Tremor/Nervousness Hyperglycemia Hypokalemia Hypotension Pulmonary edema Myocardial ischemia Cardiac arrhythmias Maternal death	Tachycardia Hyperinsulism Fetal hyperglycemia Neonatal hypoglycemia Ileus Myocardial and septal hypertrophy Myocardial ischemia
Calcium channel blockers	Nifedipine 30 mg po load or 20 mg po q 20 minutes × 3 doses, then 10-20 mg po q4-6 hours	Cardiac disease Severe renal disease Maternal hypotension (BP <90/60) Concomitant use with magnesium sulfate	Flushing Headache Dizziness Nausea Transient hypotension Rebound tachycardia	None known
Prostaglandin synthase inhibitors	Indomethacin 50–100mg po/pr loading dose and 25–50 mg po q6 hours × 48 hours	Significant renal or hepatic impairment Gestational age >32 weeks	GI bleeding Nausea Heartburn Gastritis	Constriction of fetal ductus arteriosus Pulmonary hypertension Intraventricular hemorrhage Hyperbilirubinemia Necrotizing enterocolitis Oligohydramnios from reversible decline in renal function

to a tertiary care facility as well as administration of corticosteroids and magnesium sulfate. There is no data, however, to suggest that tocolytics in and of themselves provide direct benefit to neonatal outcomes. Maintenance tocolytic therapy is not effective for preventing preterm birth, does not improve neonatal outcomes and is not recommended in clinical practice.

The administration of tocolytic agents is not recommended prior to neonatal viability as the maternal risk of medication side effects far outweighs the small potential benefits in this perinatal population with very high rates of morbidity and mortality. Similarly, tocolytics are not recommended beyond 34 weeks gestation since the maternal and fetal risks associated with these interventions outweigh the risks associated with preterm birth at this gestational age. Contraindications for tocolytic therapy are seen in Box 24.3 (1).

One of the most beneficial interventions for improvement of neonatal outcomes among women who deliver preterm is the administration of antenatal corticosteroids. A single course of corticosteroids is recommended for pregnant women who present with preterm labor between 24 and 34 weeks of gestation

Box 24.3 Contraindications to tocolytic therapy

- Previable fetal status
- Gestational age >34 weeks
- Intrauterine fetal demise
- Non-reassuring fetal status
- Lethal fetal anomaly
- Pre-eclampsia with severe features
- Intraamniotic infection
- Maternal bleeding with hemodynamic instability
- Preterm premature rupture of membranes
- Maternal contraindications for tocolysis based on specific agent used

and can be considered for women at 23 weeks of gestation who are deemed to be at risk of preterm delivery within 7 days (1,42,43). Additionally, a single repeat course of antenatal corticosteroids should be considered in women who received a prior course of antenatal corticosteroids at least 7 days previously and who are considered at risk for preterm birth prior to 34 weeks (44). Regularly scheduled or multiple (i.e., more than two courses) of antenatal corticosteroids is not recommended.

Dexamethasone and betamethasone are the two most well-studied antenatal corticosteroids and both have been shown to decrease neonatal mortality (45,46). Acceptable dosing regimens include betamethasone two 12 mg intramuscular doses given 24 hours apart or dexamethasone four 6 mg doses administered every 12 hours. While the complete dose of corticosteroid therapy connotes the greatest neonatal benefit, there is a significant reduction in neonatal morbidity and mortality following just a single dose; therefore administration of a first dose should still be given even if an additional dose is unlikely (44).

Magnesium sulfate is a nonspecific calcium channel blocker than can be used in obstetrics for the indications seen in Box 24.4 (47). Pooled data from various clinical trials have demonstrated a reduction in both risk and severity of cerebral palsy when magnesium sulfate is administered to women with anticipated preterm birth prior to 32 weeks. Additionally, in line with the Food and Drug Administration (FDA) re-classification of magnesium sulfate use in pregnancy from a Category A to Category D drug, prolonged use of magnesium sulfate injection(i.e., >5–7 days) is not recommended (47–49). While there is a clear role for magnesium sulfate therapy in obstetrics, this medication should be

Box 24.4 Indications for Magnesium sulfate therapy

- Prevention of seizures in preeclamptic women
- Treatment of seizures in eclamptic women
- Short-term prolongation of pregnancy (</= 48 hours) in women at risk of preterm delivery within 7 days
- Fetal neuroprotection in women <32 weeks gestation with an anticipated early preterm delivery

used with caution and providers should be familiar with identification and management of potential complications. Maternal side effects following magnesium sulfate therapy range from mild symptoms such as flushing, nausea, diaphoresis and decreased deep tendon reflexes to more severe symptoms including muscle weakness, respiratory depression and cardiac arrest. Furthermore, magnesium sulfate is contraindicated in patients with myasthenia gravis and should be avoided in patients receiving calcium channel blocker therapy due to suppression of heart rate and left ventricular systolic pressure (1). While magnesium toxicity is quite rare in women with normal renal function, toxicity can be lethal and severity is directly correlated with maternal serum levels. Early signs of toxicity include loss of deep tendon reflexes at 7–10 mEq/L, respiratory paralysis at 10–13 mEq/dL, altered cardiac contractility at >15 mEq/L and maternal cardiac arrest with levels exceeding 25 mEq/L. Acute management of magnesium toxicity includes discontinuing the infusion, administration of 1 g of calcium gluconate intravenously over 5–10 minutes, supportive management and serial surveillance of serum levels.

Inflammation and intrauterine infection are commonly cited potential etiologies for contractions and preterm labor. Given this association, the role of antibiotics in preterm labor has come into question. A meta-analysis of eight randomized controlled trials comparing antibiotic use to placebo in patient with confirmed preterm labor, found no difference with respect to pregnancy prolongation, prevention of preterm birth, neonatal sepsis or respiratory distress syndrome (50).

Importantly, however, antibiotics for latency in the setting of preterm premature rupture of membranes (see Chapter 23) and group B *Streptococci* prophylaxis remains the standard of care.

Concluding Remarks

Preterm birth remains a large and growing public health problem with significant social, financial and emotional sequelae. While the primary etiology remains unclear, a complex and interrelated array of psychosocial, biological and environmental factors clearly play a role. A better understanding of the various causes, investigation of the disparities among certain racial and ethnic groups and further research regarding prediction and prevention strategies are needed.

References

1. Management of Preterm Labor. ACOG Practice Bulletin No. 159. American College of Obstetricians and Gynecologists. *Obstet Gynecol* 2016 Oct;128(4):e155–64. doi: 10.1097/AOG.0000000000001711.
2. Prediction and Prevention of Preterm Birth. ACOG Practice Bulletin No. 130. American College of Obstetrician and Gynecologists. *Obstet Gynecol* 2012 Oct;120(4):964–73.
3. Management of Late-Term and Postterm Pregnancies. ACOG Practice Bulletin No. 146. American College of Obstetricians and Gynecologists. *Obstet Gynecol* 2014;1–4.
4. Kovacevich GJ, Gaich SA, Lavin JP, Hopkins MP, Crane SS, Stewart J, et al. The prevalence of thromboembolic events among women with extended bed rest prescribed as part of the treatment for premature labor or preterm premature rupture of membranes. *Am J Obstet Gynecol* 2000;182:1089–92.
5. Sosa C, Althabe F, Belizan JM, Bergel E. Bed rest in singleton pregnancies for preventing preterm birth. *Cochrane Database Syst Rev.* 2004; Issue 1. Art. No.:CD003581. DOI:10.1002/14651858. CD003581,pub2.
6. Maloni JA. Antepartum bed rest for pregnancy complications: Efficacy and safety for preventing preterm birth. *Biol Res Nurs* 2010;12:106–24.
7. Institute of Medicine. *Preterm birth: Causes, Consequences and Prevention.* Washington, DC: National Academies Press; 2007.
8. Callaghan WM, MacDorman MF, Rasmussen SA, Win C, Lackritz EM. The contribution of preterm birth to infant mortality rates in the United States. *Pediatrics* 2006;18(4):1566–73.
9. Spong CY, Prediction and prevention of recurrent spontaneous preterm birth. *Obstet Gynecol* 2007;110:405–15
10. McManemy J, Cooke E, Amon E, Leet T. Recurent risk for preterm delivery. *Am J Obstet Gynecol* 2007;110:405–15.
11. Hickey CA, Cliver SP, McNeal SF, Goldenberg RL. Low pregravid body mass index as a risk factor for preterm birth: Variation by ethnic group. *Obstet Gynecol* 1997;89:206–12.
12. Zhong Y, Cahill AG, Macones GA, Zhu F, Odibo AO. The association between prepregnancy maternal body mass index and preterm delivery. *Am J Perinatol* 2010;27:293–8.
13. Peaceman AM, Andrews WW, Thorp JM, Cliver SP, Lukes A, Iam JD, et al. Fetal fibronection as a predictor of preterm birth in patients with symptoms: A multicenter trial. *Am J Obstet Gynecol* 1997;177:13–8
14. Swamy GK, Simhan HN, Gammill HS, Heine RP. Clinical utility of fetal fibronectin for predicting preterm birth. *J Reprod Med* 2005;50;851–6.
15. Skoll A, St. Louis P, Amiri N, Delisle MF, Lalji S. The evaluation of the fetal fibronectin test for prediction of preterm delivery in symptomatic patients. *J Obstet Gynaecol Can* 2006;182:439–42.
16. Romero R, Yeo L, Miranda J, Hassan SS, Conde-Agudelo A, Chaiworapongsa T. A blueprint for the prevention of preterm birth: Vaginal progesterone in women with a short cervix. *J Perinat Med* 2013;41(1):27–44.
17. Iams JD, Goldenberg RL, Meis PJ, et al. National Institute of Child Health and Human Development Maternal Fetal Medicine Unit Network. The length of the cervix and the risk of spontaneous premature delivery. *N Engl J Med* 1996;334(9):567–72.
18. Owen J, Yost N, Berghell V, et al. National Institute of Child Health and Human Development, Maternal Fetal Medicine Units Network. Mid-trimester endovaginal sonography in women at high risk for spontaneous birth. *JAMA* 2001;286(11);1340–8.
19. Fuchs IB, Henrich W, Osthues K, Dudenhausen JW. Sonographic cervical length in singleton pregnancies with intact membranes presenting with threatened preterm labor. *Ultrasound Obstet Gynecol* 2004;24:554–7.
20. Sonek JD, Iams JD, Blumenfeld M, Johnson F, Landon M, Gabbe S. Measurement of cervical length in pregnancy: Comparison between vaginal ultrasonography and digital examiniation. *Obstet Gynecol* 1990;76:172–5.
21. Giles W, Bisits A, Know M, Jadsen G, Smith R. The effect of fetal fibronectin testing on admission to a tertiary maternal-fetal medicine unit and cost savings. *Am J Obstet Gynecol* 2000;182;439–42.
22. Joffe GM, Jacques D, Bemis-Heys R, Burton R, Skram B, Shelburne P. Impact of the fetal fibronectin assay on admission for preterm labor. *Am J Obstet Gynecol* 1999;180:581–6.

23. Goldenberg RL, Culhane JF, Iams JD, Romero R. Epidemiology and causes of preterm birth. *Lancet* 2008;371:75–84.

24. Berghella V, Hayes E, Visintine J, Baxter JK. Fetal fibronectin testing for reducing the risk of preterm birth. *Cochrane Database Syst Rev* 2008; Issue 4. Art. No.:CD006843. DOI: 10.1002/14651858. DC006843.

25. Dyson DC, Danbe KH, Bamber JA, Crites YM, Field DR. Maier JA, et al. Monitoring women at risk for preterm labor. *N Engl J Med* 1998;338:15–19.

26. Andrews WW, Sibai BM, Thom EA, Dudley D, Ernest JM, McNellis D, et al. Randomized clinical trial of metronidiazole plus erythromycin to prevent spontaneous preterm delivery in fetal fibronectin-positive women. National Institute of Child Health & Human Development Maternal Fetal Medicine Unit Network. *Obstet Gynecol* 2003;101:847–55.

27. Meis PJ, Klebanoff M, Thom E, Dombrowski MP, Sibai B, Moawad AH, et al. Prevention of recurrent preterm delivery by 17 alpha-hydroxyprogesterone caproate. National Institute of Child Health & Human Development Maternal Fetal Medicine Units Network. *N Engl J Med* 2003;348:2379–85.

28. Tita AT, Rouse DJ. Progesterone for preterm birth prevention: An evolving intervention. *Am J Obstet Gynecol* 2009;200:219–24.

29. Use of progesterone to reduce preterm birth. ACOG Committee Opinion No. 419. American College of Obstetricians and Gynecologists. *Obstet Gynecol* 2008;112:963–5.

30. Cerclage for the Management of Cervical Insufficiency. ACOG Practice Bulletin No. 142. American College of Obstetricians and Gynecologists. *Obstet Gynecol* 2014 Feb;123(2 Pt 1):372–9. doi: 10.1097/01.AOG.0000443276.68274.

31. Berghella V, Figueroa D, Szychowski JM, Owen J, Hankin GD, Iam JD, et al. 17-alpha-hydroxyprogesterone caproate for the prevention of preterm birth in women with a prior preterm birth and a short cervical length. Vaginal Ultrasound Trial Consortium. *Am J Obstet Gynecol* 2010;202:351:1–6.

32. Fonseca EB, Celik E, Parra M, Singh M, Nicolaides KH. Fetal Medicine Foundation Second Trimester Screening Group. Progesterone and the risk of preterm birth among women with a short cervix. *N Engl J Med* 2007;357:462–9.

33. Hassan SS, Romero R, Vidyadhari D, Fusey S, Baxter JK, Khandelwal M, et al. Vaginal progesterone reduces the rate of preterm birth in women with a sonographic short cervix: A multicenter, randomized, double-blind, placebo controlled trial. *Ultrasound Obstet Gynecol* 2011;38:18–31

34. Midder ES, Tita AT, Grobman, WA. Second-trimester cervical length screening among asymotomatic women, an evaluation of risk-based strategies. *Obstet Gynecol* 2015;126:61–5.

35. Werner EF, Han CS, Pettker CM, Buhimschi CS, Copel JA, Funai EF, et al. Universal cervical-length screening to prevent preterm birth: A cost-effectiveness analyses. *Ultrasound Obstet Gynecol* 2001;38:32–7

36. Cahil AG, Odibo AO, Caughey AB, Stamilio DM, Hassan SS, Macones GA, et al. Universal cervical length screening and vaginal progestereone to prevent preerm birth: A decision and economic analysis. *Am J Obstet Gynecol* 2010;202:548:1–8.

37. Lewit EM, Baker LS, Corman H, Shiono PH. The direct cost of low birth weight. *Future Child* 1995;5:35–56

38. Ferguson JE 2nd, Dyson DC, Schutz T, Stevenson DK. A comparison of tocolysis with nifedipine or ritodrine: Analysis of efficacy and maternal, fetal and neonatal outcome. *Am J Obstet Gynecol* 1990;163:105–11.

39. Bracero LA, Leikin E, Kirshenbaum N, Tejani N. Comparison of nifedipine and ritodrine for the treatment of preterm labor. *Am J Perinatol* 1991;8:365–9.

40. Hearne AE, Nagey DA. Therapeutic agents in preterm labor: Tocolytic agents. *Clin Obstet Gynecol* 2000;43:787–801.

41. Anotayanonth S, Subhedar NV, Neilson JP, Harigopal S. Betamimetics for inhibiting preterm labor. *Cochrane Database Syst Rev* 2004; Issue 4. Art. No:CD004352. DOI: 10.1002/14651858,CD004352,pub2.

42. Magnesium Sulfate Use in Obstetrics. The American College of Obstetricians and Gynecologist Committee on Obstetric Practice Society for Maternal-Fetal Medicine. Committee Opinion No. 652.

43. Periviable Birth. Obstetric Care Consensus No. 3. American College of Obstetricians and Gynecologists. *Obstet Gynecol* 2015;126:82–94.

44. Antenatal corticosteroids revisited: Repeat courses. NIH Consensus Statement 2000;17(2):1–18.

45. Crowther CA, McKinlay CJ, Middleton P, Harding JE. Repeat doses prenatal corticosteroids for women at risk of preterm birth for improving neonatal health outcomes. *Cochrane Database Syst Rev* 2015; Issue 7. Art. No.:DC003935,DOI:10,1002/14651858. CD003935.

46. Antenatal corticosteroid therapy for fetal maturation. Committee Opinion No. 475. American College of Obstetricians and Gynecologists. *Obstet Gynecol* 2011; 117:422–4.

47. Magnesium sulfate use in Obstetrics. Committee Opinion No. 652. The American College of Obstetricians and Gynecologists Committee on Obstetric Practice Society for Maternal-Fetal Medicine. *Obstet Gynecol* 2016 Jan;127(1):e52–3. doi: 10.1097/AOG.0000000000001267.

48. Crowther CA, Hiller JE, Doyle LW, Haslam RR. Effect of magnesium sulfate given for neuroprotection before preterm birth; a randomized controlled trial. Australasian Collaborative Trial of Magnesium Sulphate (ACTO$MgSO_4$) Collaborative Group. *JAMA* 2003;290:2669–76.

49. Rouse DJ, Hirtz DG, Thom E, Varner MW, Spong CY, Mercer BM, et al. A randomized controlled trial of magnesium sulfate for the prevention of cerebral palsy. Eunice Kennedy Shriver NICHD Maternal Fetal Medicine Units Network. *N Engl J Med* 2008;359:895–905.

50. King JF, Flenady V, Papatsonis D, Dekker G, Carbonne B. Calcium channel blocker for inhibiting preterm labour. *Cochrane Database Syst Rev* 2003; Issue 1. Art. No.: CD002255.DOI: 10.1002/14651858. CD002255;10.1002/14651858.

Second Trimester Pregnancy Loss

Frances Casey

Introduction

Second trimester pregnancy loss, also known as a mid-trimester loss, is a loss that occurs between 12 and 24 weeks gestation. Variations in presentation and causative factors make a mid-trimester loss challenging to evaluate. Challenges also exist in the creation of recommendations for patients with histories of second trimester loss who desire childbirth. Spontaneous second trimester abortion overlaps with preterm delivery and preterm premature rupture of membranes (discussed in Chapters 23 and 24). Given the impact of second trimester loss, it is imperative to conduct a thorough, systematic review in order to identify modifiable factors for a patient's future pregnancy.

Scope of the Problem

Mid-trimester loss affects 2–3% of pregnancies (1) and includes fetal demise (1–2%) and spontaneous abortion (affecting 0.5–1%). Overlap also occurs with stillbirth (defined as in utero death > 20 weeks gestation), which occurs in <0.5% of pregnancies. Rates of fetal mortality are highest for women of youngest and oldest reproductive age. The rate for teenagers (younger than 15) and for women older than 45 is more than twice the rate for women aged 25–29. The fetal mortality rate for non-Hispanic white women in the United States is roughly equivalent to the rate for Asian and Pacific Islanders. The rate for non-Hispanic black women is more than twice the rate for non-Hispanic white women. The fetal mortality rate for American Indian and Alaskan natives is one-third higher than the rate for non-Hispanic white women (2). Obesity and severe obesity are associated with fetal deaths due to placental disease, hypertension, fetal anomalies and umbilical cord abnormalities (3).

Etiology

When a systematic approach is taken to evaluate second trimester demise, a diagnosis is possible in upward of 70% of cases (4). This systematic approach can be divided into maternal, placental and fetal causes. Overlap exists between with the investigation for second trimester spontaneous abortion and the investigation for second trimester fetal demise.

Maternal causes may include medical diagnoses (based on patient's history), cervical insufficiency, uterine anomalies, infection, and antiphospholipid antibody syndrome. Specific medical conditions in pregnancy that may contribute to a demise (such as diabetes, hypertension, autoimmune disorders or thrombophilia) are discussed elsewhere but will determine targeted labs (examples include HgbA1c, complete blood count (CBC), liver function tests (LFTs), creatinine, and coagulation studies) as a part of the patient's workup.

Cervical Insufficiency

Cervical insufficiency describes an inability of the uterine cervix to retain a pregnancy in the absence of the signs and symptoms of clinical contractions, labor or both in the second trimester. Typically cardiac activity is still present in cases of cervical insufficiency. Reported incidence varies due to differences in categorization. Painless dilation in the absence of other clear pathology (bleeding, infection, ruptured membranes) is necessary for the diagnosis (5). For classification purposes, a diagnosis should include cervical length, dilation and clinical presentation (6).

Congenital Anomalies

Uterine congenital anomalies are associated with a sevenfold increase in preterm birth prior to 34 weeks and a threefold increase in preterm premature rupture of membrane (PPROM) (7). Uterine congenital anomalies are less associated with fetal demise in the second trimester. Major uterine anomalies (unicornuate, bicornuate and didelphys) are associated with earlier gestational ages at time of preterm birth as compared to minor fusion defects (septate, arcuate, t-shaped) (8).

Infections

Infections may account for more than 20% of second trimester pregnancy loss, but this diagnosis can be challenging given that maternal infection may be asymptomatic. Currently recommendations included evaluation for syphilis and parvovirus when infection is suspected but evaluation for other infections may be tailored for patients with clinical or histologic evidence of specific processes. Infections in pregnancy may be viral, bacterial or polymicrobial in nature. See Box 25.1 for additional information on infections in the second trimester.

Box 25.1 Infections and second trimester loss

- Chorioamnionitis plays a significant role in preterm birth and PPROM. A retrospective review of placental histology from cases of mid-trimester loss demonstrated evidence of chorioamnionitis in 94% of cases <24 weeks and 40% of cases 24–28 weeks. Organisms associated with chorioamnionitis include anaerobic streptococci, enterococci, coliforms, staphylococci, *Fusobacterium* spp, *Mycoplasma* spp, *Ureaplasma* spp, and Group B streptococci (1).
- Bacterial vaginosis is a risk factor for preterm birth and PPROM (9). Bacterial vaginosis is an imbalance of vaginal flora with a reduction in normal lactobacillus and an overgrowth of mixed anaerobic flora including *Gardnarella vaginalis*, *Mycoplasma hominis*, and *Mobiluncus* species. A high level of BV-related vaginal flora may be associated with mid-trimester pregnancy loss (10).
- Parvovirus B19 has a seroprevalence of 50–70% in adults. The virus can be vertically transmitted with an infection rate of 30%. Fetal death in the second trimester is often associated with hydrops fetalis but this may not be associated with later fetal demise (11).
- Cytomegalovirus (CMV) is highly prevalent with seropositivity rates in adult women ranging between 40–90%. Fetal abnormalities associated with CMV infection may not be present in cases of fetal demise. Higher rates of placental transmission occur with a primary infection but can still occur with reactivation or re-infection (12).
- Other viruses such as Epstein–Barr (13) Herpes simplex, enterovirus and coxsackie have been implicated in cases of fetal demise and evaluation for these should be tailored to the patients circumstance.
- Syphilis, caused by the spirochete bacterium *Treponema pallidum*, has a known association to fetal demise. Antenatal screening and treatment of maternal infection are estimated to have reduced syphilis-related demise by 80% (14).
- *Listeria monocytogenes* is a gram-positive bacillus with an incidence associated with pregnancy 13 times higher than the general population. One in five pregnancies complicated by listeriosis results in spontaneous abortion or fetal demise. Most cases are associated with maternal ingestion of raw or undercooked meats or seafood, unpasteurized soft cheese or unwashed raw produce (15).
- Group B *Streptococcus,* a gram-positive coccus, is known to infect newborns through maternal rectovaginal colonization. The association with fetal demise has not been adequately delineated. However, available studies report an absolute rate ranging from 0.04 to 0.9 per 1,000 births (16).

Antiphospholipid Antibody Syndrome

A fetal demise in the second trimester is sufficient to satisfy the clinical criteria for antiphospholipid antibody syndrome (APS). A diagnosis, however, requires a combination of clinic and laboratory criteria (including repeat testing 6–12 months apart to confirm positive findings). Antiphospholipid antibody testing includes lupus anticoagulant, IgG and IgM for both anti-cardiolipin and anti-B2-glycoprotein antibodies. Testing for this syndrome is particularly important for cases in which placental insufficiency, intrauterine growth restriction or severe preeclampsia is suspected, as patients with these findings are more likely to be positive.

Placenta

Placental causes of second trimester fetal demise may include placental insufficiency, abruption, umbilical cord thrombosis, velamentous cord insertion and vasa previa or twin–twin transfusion in cases of multiple gestations. Umbilical cord knots may be present in up to 30% of normal pregnancies and so should be interpreted with caution (17). Placental histology can be supportive of infectious causes.

Genetic

At least 20% of demise in the second trimester may be attributable to chromosomal or genetic abnormalities; this may be an underestimate due to incomplete evaluations (4). Patients experiencing a mid-trimester fetal demise should be offered autopsy evaluation and karyotype. Microarray may be useful in cases where cytogenetic evaluation is normal. Centers experienced with evaluation can identify abnormalities in cases of induction or dilation and evacuation (D&E) (18).

Presentation

A thorough history and physical examination will help guide further evaluation of a mid-trimester loss. History of the patient's experience will help guide physical exam and subsequent diagnostics. It is possible for a patient to have multiple causal factors. Some considerations are seen in Box 25.2.

Diagnosis

A detailed physical exam will be guided by the patient's presenting circumstance, medical, gynecologic and obstetric history. Key historic elements are seen in Box 25.3.

Box 25.2 **Key historic elements in second trimester loss**

- Leaking of fluid-evaluation for PPROM, infection
- Vaginal bleeding-preterm dilation, evaluate for contributing factors: hypertension, substance abuse, trauma, abnormal placentation
- Pressure sensation-cervical insufficiency if painless, preterm labor if painful
- Fetal movement-patient's perception of decrease in fetal movement
- Contributing illnesses such as infection exposure or a history of maternal disease
- Specific history of pelvic infections prior to and during current pregnancy
- Last menstrual cycle to provide gestational age dating
- History of cervical LEEP or cone
- Prior history of preterm birth
- Prior history of chromosomal abnormality or diagnosis of fetal abnormality in current pregnancy

Box 25.3 **Physical exam in patients with second trimester loss**

Vital signs

Attention should be paid to fever, tachycardia, tachypnea or hypo/hypertension, as these may be indicative of underlying medical disease, infection or substance abuse.

Physical Exam

- General appearance – evaluate for acute pain, distress, and anxiety
- Cardiac and respiratory – evaluate for abnormalities in heart rate or oxygenation
- Abdominal exam – evaluate for tenderness, fundal height, indications of trauma
- Vaginal exam – evaluate for discharge, bleeding, infection, rupture of membranes, cervical dilation

Box 25.4 **Potential laboratory studies in second trimester loss**

- Complete blood count
- Renal and liver profiles
- Thyroid stimulating hormone
- Hemoglobin A1c
- Urinalysis
- Wet mount or cultures to evaluate infection, rupture of membranes
- Urine toxicology

Ultrasound evaluation will determine presence or absence of fetal cardiac activity, amniotic fluid level, placental location and growth with respect to expected dating by last menstrual cycle. Transvaginal ultrasound can provide further information about placental or vessel location with respect to the internal os (when vasa previa, marginal, low-lying or placenta previa, accreta or percreta are suspected). Transvaginal sonogram can also be used to evaluate the length of the cervical canal, funneling of membranes into the cervical canal and cervical dilation when cervical insufficiency is suspected.

A checklist for the evaluation of intrauterine demise may be helpful in ensuring equivalent workup for every patient. Some tests tailored for individual maternal conditions. Box 25.4 lists tests that may be warranted in all cases of second trimester loss, while Box 25.5 lists cases that's that may be specifically indicated for second trimester fetal demise (19).

Box 25.5 Studies recommended for evaluation of fetal demise

Parvovirus B19
Syphilis
Analysis of fetus including weight, length and head circumference
Amniocentesis for karyotype (highest yield)
If patient declines amniocentesis, karyotype may be performed on the placental block below the cord insertion site, umbilical cord segment or fetal tissue under low oxygen tension such as costochondral or patellar tissue
Gross and histologic evaluation of placenta, umbilical cord, and fetal membranes
Autopsy (may be brain sparing), if patient declines, may offer fetal magnetic resonance imaging or radiographic studies (fetogram)
Kleihauer–Betke (particularly in cases of maternal trauma)
Antiphospholipid antibodies (consider in cases of growth restriction or placental insufficiency)

Management

Sharing bad news with a patient and her family must be treated with great respect. Studies have demonstrated that parents who felt they were treated with sensitivity had mostly positive memories even though they felt devastated by their loss compared to only bad memories if they felt staff members were insensitive, especially blunt or unsupportive. Providers should allow sufficient time for parents to ask questions, understand what is known and unknown, express sympathy, balance honesty with sensitivity and avoid medical terminology. Using the parent's own terminology for their baby-perhaps their baby's name is more appropriate than referring to a fetus. Shock and anger is an understandable grief reaction and should be managed with sympathy rather than as a personal affront (20).

Management of second trimester fetal demise may require induction of labor or D&E by a trained provider. Cases of septic abortion must be evacuated immediately to prevent maternal progression to septic shock. Early recognition of sepsis with initiation of antibiotics and intravenous fluids is imperative for prevention of maternal morbidity and mortality.

Dilation and evacuation is associated with a low risk of complications in trained hands as compared to induction of labor (21). Cervical preparation is required to decrease the risk of cervical injury and complications but mechanical dilation may be possible in emergent cases. Cervical preparation for cases early in the second trimester may be achieved with misoprostol, a prostaglandin E1 analogue, 400 micrograms placed buccally or vaginally at least 3 hours prior to the procedure. Studies have demonstrated safe use of misoprostol for cervical ripening to 20 weeks gestation but use of misoprostol alone in later second trimester cases is associated with a need for further dilation and increased procedure time (22). Hygroscopic osmotic dilators facilitate cervical preparation later in the second trimester. Two types of dilators are available in the United States: laminaria made from dehydrated *Laminaria japonica* and Dilapan-S, a synthetic polyacrylate-based hydrogel. Laminaria continue to dilate 12–24 hours, while Dilapan achieves maximum expansion at 6 hours. A combination of misoprostol and osmotic dilators may be used for cases above 19 weeks (23).

The use of prostaglandins to induce labor in the second trimester is recommended. The majority of oxytocin receptors develop in the late second to early third trimester and thus comparisons of prostaglandin to high-dose oxytocin protocols demonstrate faster induction to delivery intervals with prostaglandins (24). Available evidence supports the use of misoprostol to induce nonviable pregnancies prior to 24 weeks gestation, including in patients with a prior cesarean delivery. A wide range of misoprostol dosing has been described but increased frequency shortens delivery intervals. Most recommendations agree on a regimen of 400 mcg vaginally or buccally every 3 hours. A vaginal loading dose of 600–800 mcg followed by 400 mcg every 3 hours may be more effective. The addition of mifepristone (if available) 200 mg 24 hours prior to induction significantly shortens the induction-to-delivery interval. Surgical management is rarely required for placental removal. Spontaneous delivery should be allowed to occur with additional dosing of misoprostol as scheduled (23).

The decision to perform dilation and evacuation versus induction of labor is based on the patient's desires, availability of a trained provider and urgency of the situation. No differences in grief resolution have been found for patients undergoing a D&E versus induction. A patient should be allowed to choose the method most appropriate for her individual needs and values (17). It is imperative that a patient and her family's decisions regarding holding the infant, options for burial/cremation and desire for mementos (pictures, handprints/footprints, blanket for the baby

Table 25.1 Stillbirth Worksheet

MRN:		
Gestational age at time of loss:		
Describe autopsy results or circle not performed:		
Describe placental pathology or circle not performed:		
Describe karyotype or circle not performed:		
Results of Kleihauer–Betke or circle not performed:		
Circle the most likely cause(s) of fetal death:		
Placental	**Congenital/Developmental**	**Uterine/cervical anomalies**
Growth restriction	Fetal Aneuploidy – Type:	Cervical insufficiency
Aneuploidy – Mosaicism	Gene disorder	Preterm labor
Umbilical cord prolapse	Dysmorphology – describe:	Premature rupture of membranes
Abruption		
Infarction		
Vasa previa		
Velamentous insertion		
Thrombin deposition		
Umbilical cord lesion/true knot		
Strangulation from umbilical cord		
Twin–twin transfusion		

Source: Adapted from Silver RM, Heuser CC. Stillbirth workup and delivery management. *Clin Obstet Gynecol*. 2010;53(3):681–90.

to be wrapped in) be honored, as this is impactful for mental health. Mementos may be obtained in D&E cases as well as induction. Some studies have shown that honoring a patient's decision not to see/hold a dead infant is equally important as this type of interaction may worsen depression and post-traumatic stress (25). Social support services and pastoral care should be individualized based on the patient's needs. Counseling services and close follow-up are imperative for further assessment of depression and anxiety. Twenty percent of patients experiencing loss continue to have diagnostic levels of depression and anxiety a year after the loss (26).

A checklist for describing fetal evaluation at time of D&E or induction, autopsy, pathology, karyotype and laboratory results is helpful for postpartum discussion and further recommendations (17) (see Table 25.1).

Subsequent Pregnancy Recommendations

Subsequent pregnancy recommendations will include modification of maternal risk factors if such are identified. Specific findings at the time of fetal demise may support subsequent pregnancy recommendations. Findings of genetic abnormalities may warrant earlier testing. Cell-free DNA (non-invasive prenatal) screening may be offered as early as ten weeks but still requires a subsequent diagnostic test for confirmation. Findings of maternal conditions may warrant weight loss, medications, surgery or repeat testing prior to a subsequent pregnancy.

Some findings will not be modifiable and over 30% will remain unexplained despite a thorough evaluation. Counseling for all cases of fetal demise, including those in which the diagnosis is undetermined, should include reassurance of close and frequent follow-up in a subsequent pregnancy given the heightened anxiety and psychological toll that a prior pregnancy loss can exert (27). A study of women in a subsequent pregnancy with a history of pregnancy loss receiving psychological support through weekly medical evaluations with frequent ultrasound exams as compared to routine prenatal care demonstrated a 40% increase in live births. As these patients are prone to heightened depression, anxiety, grief and guilt, it is imperative that care providers pay attention to the patient's physical, mental and emotional well-being in a subsequent pregnancy (19).

Well-designed studies have not demonstrated an increase in cervical insufficiency or preterm birth following a mid-trimester D&E (28). Optimal pregnancy timing following a mid-trimester loss has not been well established. Unlike the known adverse pregnancy outcomes with short interpregnancy intervals following a term birth, less is known about optimal pregnancy intervals following other pregnancy outcomes. Studies to date demonstrate no adverse outcomes for a short interpregnancy interval (< 6months) following a miscarriage up to 14 weeks gestation. One study including 5% women with a prior pregnancy loss at 14–19 weeks gestational age did not show any difference in live birth rates or obstetric complications for women conceiving <3 months as compared to women conceiving >3 months from their last pregnancy loss (29). In a study on post medical abortion patients, an increase in small for gestational age diagnoses in infants conceived <6 months with mifepristone was found. Data is insufficient to make recommendations post-surgical abortion but best estimate for interpregnancy interval recommendation based on limited data is 3–6 months. Evaluations post stillbirths have demonstrated an inherent risk of subsequent stillbirth regardless of interpregnancy interval (30). Further data stratified by gestational age is required prior to making recommendations post stillbirth.

For patients suffering loss caused by cervical insufficiency, counseling should include management options for a subsequent pregnancy. These patients should begin progesterone therapy starting at 16 weeks gestation with cervical length assessments every two weeks until 23 weeks gestation and may benefit from placement of a cervical cerclage if cervical length is less than 25 mm (31).

A patient with a second trimester loss will benefit from a follow up phone call/contact a week post delivery. A subsequent visit 4–6 weeks post delivery is also recommended and may include a consult with a maternal-fetal medicine specialist. This visit should include a review of the findings and probable diagnosis with suggestions for future pregnancies based on these findings. Assessment of the patient's psychological and emotional needs should also take place at this visit (32).

Concluding Remarks

Close follow-up for mid-trimester loss with a synopsis of modifiable risk factors is crucial in assisting patients with their healing. It is important to respect physical, mental and emotional health as anxiety, depression, guilt and grief may last well beyond the postpartum time period.

References

1. McNamee KM, Dawood F, Farquharson RG. Mid-trimester pregnancy loss. *Obstet Gynecol Clin North Am.* 2014;41(1):87–102.
2. MacDorman MF, Gregory EC. Fetal and perinatal mortality: United States, 2013. *Natl Vital Stat Rep.* 2015;64(8):1–24.
3. Bodnar LM, Parks WT, Perkins K, Pugh SJ, Platt RW, Feghali M, et al. Maternal prepregnancy obesity and cause-specific stillbirth. *Am J Clin Nutr.* 2015;102(4):858–64.
4. VanderWielen B, Zaleski C, Cold C, McPherson E. Wisconsin stillbirth services program: A multifocal approach to stillbirth analysis. *Am J Med Genet A.* 2011;155A(5):1073–80.
5. American College of O, Gynecologists. ACOG Practice Bulletin No.142: Cerclage for the management of cervical insufficiency. *Obstet Gynecol.* 2014;123(2 Pt 1):372–9.
6. Sneider K, Langhoff-Roos J, Sundtoft IB, Christiansen OB. Validation of second trimester miscarriages and spontaneous deliveries. *Clin Epidemiol.* 2015;7:517–27.
7. Hua M, Odibo AO, Longman RE, Macones GA, Roehl KA, Cahill AG. Congenital uterine anomalies and adverse pregnancy outcomes. *Am J Obstet Gynecol.* 2011;205(6):558 e1–5.
8. Fox NS, Roman AS, Stern EM, Gerber RS, Saltzman DH, Rebarber A. Type of congenital uterine anomaly and adverse pregnancy outcomes. *J Maternal-Fetal Neonatal Med.* 2014;27(9):949–53.
9. Guerra B, Ghi T, Quarta S, Morselli-Labate AM, Lazzarotto T, Pilu G, et al. Pregnancy outcome after early detection of bacterial vaginosis. *Eur J Obstet Gynecol Reprod Biol.* 2006;128(1–2):40–5.
10. Nelson DB, Bellamy S, Nachamkin I, Ness RB, Macones GA, Allen-Taylor L. First trimester bacterial vaginosis, individual microorganism levels, and risk of second trimester pregnancy loss among urban women. *Fertil Steril.* 2007;88(5):1396–403.
11. Tolfvenstam T, Papadogiannakis N, Norbeck O, Petersson K, Broliden K. Frequency of human parvovirus B19 infection in intrauterine fetal death. *Lancet.* 2001;357(9267):1494–7.
12. Naing ZW, Scott GM, Shand A, Hamilton ST, van Zuylen WJ, Basha J, et al. Congenital cytomegalovirus infection in pregnancy: A review of prevalence, clinical

features, diagnosis and prevention. *Aust N Z J Obstet Gynaecol.* 2016;56(1):9–18.

13. Tomai XH. Stillbirth following severe symmetric fetal growth restriction due to reactivation of Epstein-Barr virus infection in pregnancy. *J Obstet Gynaecol Res.* 2011;37(12):1877–82.
14. Ishaque S, Yakoob MY, Imdad A, Goldenberg RL, Eisele TP, Bhutta ZA. Effectiveness of interventions to screen and manage infections during pregnancy on reducing stillbirths: A review. *BMC Public Health.* 2011;11 Suppl 3:S3.
15. Committee on Obstetric Practice ACoO, Gynecologists. Committee Opinion No. 614: Management of pregnant women with presumptive exposure to Listeria monocytogenes. *Obstet Gynecol.* 2014;124(6):1241–4.
16. Nan C, Dangor Z, Cutland CL, Edwards MS, Madhi SA, Cunnington MC. Maternal group B Streptococcus-related stillbirth: A systematic review. *BJOG.* 2015;122(11):1437–45.
17. Silver RM, Heuser CC. Stillbirth workup and delivery management. *Clin Obstet Gynecol.* 2010;53(3):681–90.
18. Gawron LM, Hammond C, Ernst LM. Perinatal pathologic examination of nonintact, second-trimester fetal demise specimens: The value of standardization. *Arch Pathol Lab Med.* 2013;137(8):1083–7.
19. Practice Committee of the American Society for Reproductive M. Evaluation and treatment of recurrent pregnancy loss: A committee opinion. *Fertil Steril.* 2012;98(5):1103–11.
20. Henley A, Schott J. The death of a baby before, during or shortly after birth: Good practice from the parents' perspective. *Semin Fetal Neonatal Med.* 2008;13(5):325–8.
21. Bryant AG, Grimes DA, Garrett JM, Stuart GS. Second-trimester abortion for fetal anomalies or fetal death: Labor induction compared with dilation and evacuation. *Obstet Gynecol.* 2011;117(4):788–92.
22. Maurer KA, Jacobson JC, Turok DK. Same-day cervical preparation with misoprostol prior to second trimester D&E: A case series. *Contraception.* 2013;88(1):116–21.
23. ACOG Practice Bulletin No. 135: Second-trimester abortion. *Obstet Gynecol.* 2013;121(6):1394–406.
24. Borgatta L, Kapp N, Society of Family P. Clinical guidelines. Labor induction abortion in the second trimester. *Contraception.* 2011;84(1):4–18.
25. Hughes P, Turton P, Hopper E, Evans CD. Assessment of guidelines for good practice in psychosocial care of mothers after stillbirth: A cohort study. *Lancet.* 2002;360(9327):114–8.
26. Badenhorst W, Hughes P. Psychological aspects of perinatal loss. *Best Prac Res.* 2007;21(2):249–59.
27. Geller PA, Kerns D, Klier CM. Anxiety following miscarriage and the subsequent pregnancy: A review of the literature and future directions. *J Psychosom Res.* 2004;56(1):35–45.
28. Jackson JE, Grobman WA, Haney E, Casele H. Mid-trimester dilation and evacuation with laminaria does not increase the risk for severe subsequent pregnancy complications. *Int J Gynaecol Obstet.* 2007;96(1):12–5.
29. Wong LF, Schliep KC, Silver RM, Mumford SL, Perkins NJ, Ye A, et al. The effect of a very short interpregnancy interval and pregnancy outcomes following a previous pregnancy loss. *Am J Obstet Gynecol.* 2015;212(3):375 e1–11.
30. Bigelow CA, Bryant AS. Short interpregnancy intervals: An evidence-based guide for clinicians. *Obstet Gynecol Surv.* 2015;70(7):458–64.
31. Committee on Practice Bulletins-Obstetrics TACoO, Gynecologists. Practice bulletin no. 130: Prediction and prevention of preterm birth. *Obstet Gynecol.* 2012;120(4):964–73.
32. Rowland A, Goodnight WH. Fetal loss: Addressing the evaluation and supporting the emotional needs of parents. *J Midwifery Womens Health.* 2009;54(3):241–8.

Third Trimester Fetal Loss

Erin C. Rebele

Introduction

Fetal or neonatal death impacts over 2.6 million women worldwide per year.[1] In the United States, the number of stillbirths was 23,595 in 2013. Fetal death after 28 weeks until term accounts for 24.9% of all perinatal deaths.[2] This impact of stillbirth is not confined to the mother, but is felt throughout the family unit. The impact includes medical factors, psychological factors, and socioeconomic factors, each of which will be addressed in this chapter.

Stillbirth may result from aberrations in the maternal, placenta, or fetal units. The diagnostic workup involves evaluating each of these units and identifying potential causes from them. In up to 40% of cases, however, the underlying cause may not be identified.[3]

Providers must be educated in risk factors for stillbirth in order to determine which patients might require additional antenatal testing or treatment. Risk factors are addressed in this chapter. Patients who experience a stillbirth often report that they felt their provider did not provide adequate attention to their concerns prior to the event. The treatment of patients after diagnosis is also of paramount importance, as a proportion of patients report that they did not feel the quality of care was good after stillbirth. Many felt that providers failed to spend enough time with them.[4]

The aim of this chapter is to familiarize the reader with risk factors for stillbirth, key elements of the medical history and physical examination of affected patients, the laboratory and pathologic evaluation after stillbirth, treatment aims for delivery and postpartum, and management of future pregnancies. The socioeconomic impact on families will also be addressed.

Scope of the Problem

Perinatal death refers to death of a fetus or neonate less than 1 year of age. Perinatal death after 20 weeks can be divided into 20–27 weeks (25.2%), >28 weeks (24.9%), <28 days of life 33.8%, and 28 days through 1 year (16.1%).[2]

As mentioned, in 2013, there were 23,595 fetal deaths in the United States of which 11,721 were after 28 weeks gestation. The rate of fetal death has been relatively unchanged from 2006 to 2011 and showed a slight decrease in 2012.[2]

This equates to a rate of 5.96 per 1,000 live births and fetal deaths. The rate of fetal loss among non-Hispanic white women was 4.88. For Hispanic and American Indian women, this rate was 27% and 7% higher. The highest rate of fetal death is amongst non-Hispanic Black women and was twice that of the general population at 10.53 per 1,000 live births.[2]

Economic consequences after stillbirth are due to cost of evaluation, psychosocial impact on parents, and increased potential cost of management of future pregnancies.[4]

This chapter will utilize data on stillbirth rates, management, and socioeconomic issues primarily from the United States. It should be noted, however, that stillbirth is an important issue in the global health arena. A recent article in the *Lancet* shows that stillbirth rates are declining slowly and that the main area of focus should be in low and middle-income countries.[5]

Additionally, there has been concern that in the years following the adoption of awaiting 39 weeks for induction of labor, a small corresponding increase in stillbirth was noted in the United States in 2013.[6] Further studies are needed to fully elucidate this issue.

Diagnosis

Fetal death refers to a delivery in which the fetus shows no signs of life. These signs include breathing, heart rate, pulsating umbilical cord, or movement of voluntary muscle.[3] Reporting for fetal death is not standardized but is suggested to include fetuses weighing over 350 g or 20 weeks gestation.

Fetal death is often preceded by a maternal perception of decreased fetal movement. Providers must review kick counts routinely in the third trimester with pregnant women. Patient education by providers is increasingly important in light of recent findings that the majority of information online (70%) regarding decreased fetal movements and kick counts is erroneous or provides information that is contrary to evidence-based recommendations.[7]

Often diagnosis of third trimester loss is made prior to delivery by failure to find fetal heart tones with auscultation. The diagnosis is commonly confirmed with ultrasound visualization of lack of fetal cardiac activity. Anecdotally, many institutions prefer that two providers make this diagnosis for confirmation purposes, though this is not noted to be a defined policy.

Intrapartum stillbirth occurs after onset of labor but prior to delivery. Appearance of the skin is often used as a surrogate for timing of the stillbirth if fetal heart tones had not been recently detected. Softening and breakdown of the skin, also known as skin maceration, occurs within 6 to 12 hours of fetal death. Fresh skin appearance usually indicates intrapartum demise.[8]

Box 26.1 Risk factors for stillbirth in the United States[3]

- Racial factors [2]
  - Non-Hispanic Black (11.25/1,000)
  - American Indian and Alaskan Native (6.22/1,000)
  - Hispanic White (5.22/1,000)
  - Non-Hispanic White (4.88/1,000)
  - Asian and Pacific Islander women (4.79/1,000)
- Medical comorbidities
  - Diabetes mellitus (6–35/1,000 with insulin)
  - Hypertension and preeclampsia (6–29/1,000)
  - Systemic lupus erythematosus (40–150/1,000)
  - Thyroid disorders (12–20/1,000)
  - Renal disorders (15–200/1,000)
  - Obesity (8/1,000 for BMI >35, 11/1,000 BMI >40)
- Infection
  - Parvovirus B19
  - Syphilis
  - Listeria
- Smoking
- Multiple gestation (19.6 per 1,000)
- Congenital and genetic anomalies
- Growth restriction
- Advanced maternal age (11–14/1,000 >35yo; 11–21/1,000 >40yo)
- Previous stillbirth (9–20/1,000)

Source: From Goldenberg RL, Farrow V, McClure EM, Reddy UM, Fretts RC, Schulkin J. Stillbirth: Knowledge and practice among U.S. obstetrician-gynecologists. *Am J Perinatol*. 2013 Nov;30(10):813–20.

Risk Factors

A study by Goldenberg et al. in 2013 revealed distressing data regarding the knowledge base of obstetricians regarding stillbirth. This study, albeit limited by sample size, revealed only 30% of providers were well aware of established risk factors for stillbirth.[9]

In middle and high-income countries, data is collected regarding underlying risk factors for stillbirth. However, this data has failed to determine a consistent underlying cause. It should be appreciated that both modifiable and non-modifiable risk factors for stillbirth exist.[8]

Non-modifiable risk factors for stillbirth include non-Hispanic black race, nulliparity, and advanced maternal age. Modifiable risk factors include obesity, smoking, drug use, and alcohol use.[3]

The most recent rates of stillbirth by ethnicity are detailed in Box 26.1. The disparity is likely multifactorial and ongoing research is occurring in this field. Some risk factors are more prevalent in non-Hispanic black women; these likely are at least a component of the increased risk of stillbirth in this population. These risk factors include diabetes mellitus, hypertension, placental abruption, and premature rupture of membranes.[3]

One important risk factor for stillbirth is maternal obesity, which is becoming more problematic with the obesity epidemic in America. The risk for stillbirth persists after controlling for maternal medical conditions such as diabetes mellitus, hypertension, and pre-eclampsia. This has led to a recommendation for antenatal testing for obese mothers.[9]

Advanced maternal age (AMA) is a significant risk factor for stillbirth; these patients experience an up to 30% increase in risk for term intrauterine fetal death (IUFD). In a recent study of causative factors for AMA women in Europe, the only factor that was consistently associated with IUFD was the presence of congenital anomalies. In this study, the rate of unexplained stillbirth in pregnancies complicated by AMA is primarily related to obstetrical complications and not AMA alone. Other obstetrical factors studied in this group included mechanical causes, maternal disease, and associated obstetrical factors such as polyhydramnios and premature rupture of membranes (PROM).[10]

Another risk factor is maternal substance abuse. An increased risk of stillbirth is present in women who use cannabis or other illicit drugs. Positive urine toxicology was associated with a two- to threefold increase in stillbirth.[11,12] Cannabinoids are the most frequently used drug of abuse in the United States. As cannabinoids become legalized, the number of pregnant women exposed in pregnancy will increase.[12] Opioid drugs are also increasingly abused in the United States. There was a trend toward an increased risk of stillbirth with opioid exposure; this could become important as abuse increases.[12] Also, smoking is a known risk factor for stillbirth. In one study, women who reported smoking one to nine cigarettes per day had a 1.77 odds ratio for stillbirth. There appears to be a dose-dependent response with tobacco. Interestingly, several recent studies have shown an association between second-hand smoke exposure and stillbirth.[12] Physicians should take care to evaluate the patient's use of these agents as well as their use in the home.

Mothers with a history of a prior live born growth-restricted infant delivered at less than 32 weeks have a higher risk for stillbirth than mothers with a history of term stillbirth. The rate of stillbirth in this population is up to twice that of mothers with a history of term stillbirth (4.84 vs. 7.19/1,000).[13]

History and Physical Examination of the Patient

Evaluation at the time of diagnosis should focus on identifying possible causes of stillbirth, particularly in light of planning for future pregnancies. It is important, however, to recognize that a substantial percentage of stillbirth remains unexplained even in light of full evaluation and testing.

The maternal history should be reviewed in detail looking for diagnoses that may be associated with stillbirth. A family history should be taken in detail as well. Confirmation of the gestational age should be ascertained. Maternal testing is discussed in the laboratory evaluation section later.[3] The important components of the maternal history are detailed in Box 26.2.

Box 26.2 Maternal history after stillbirth

- Obstetrical history
  - Recurrent spontaneous abortion (SAB)
  - Previous pregnancy outcomes
    - Anomalies, hereditary conditions
    - Growth restriction in prior pregnancies
    - Gestational hypertension/pre-eclampsia
    - Previous placental abruption
    - Previous fetal demise
  - Current pregnancy
    - Medical complications of pregnancy
    - Weight gain and BMI
    - Abdominal trauma
    - Preterm labor/PPROM
- Maternal medical history
  - Prior venous thromboembolism (VTE) or pulmonary embolism (PE)
    - Thrombophilia
    - Systemic lupus erythematosus
  - Significant medical problems (chronic hypertension, diabetes mellitus, cardiac disease)
  - Severe anemia
  - Tobacco, alcohol, drug use
- Family history
  - Recurrent spontaneous abortion (SAB)
  - VTE or PE
  - Congenital or genetic anomalies
  - Developmental delay
  - Consanguinity

Maternal physical examination should also include evaluation for signs of infection. Infection is a possible cause of stillbirth, though less so at term than in the second trimester (2% in third trimester vs 19% in second trimester). The most commonly implicated pathogens are parvovirus, cytomegalovirus, *Listeria monocytogenes*, and syphilis.[3] Signs of infection can include recent viral illness or fevers, rash, and fundal tenderness.

Laboratory Evaluation

Laboratory testing should be undertaken at the time of diagnosis. The maternal laboratory evaluation is detailed in Table 26.1. It should be noted that some tests have unproven benefit including maternal antinuclear antibody testing, serology for toxoplasmosis, rubella, cytomegalovirus (CMV), and herpes simplex virus (HSV). In these cases, the testing may be

Table 26.1 Laboratory Evaluation of Stillbirth[3]

	Laboratory	Detailed Information
Fetal	Karyotype Acceptable specimens: - Amniotic fluid - Placental block below cord insertion site - Umbilical cord segment - Internal fetal tissue specimen	Optimally obtained by amniocentesis (84% yield), otherwise cord close to placenta (30%) FISH can also be performed Anomalies found: 8%
Maternal		
At time of demise	Type and screen CBC PT/PTT/fibrinogen Kleihauer–Betke or other test for fetal cells in maternal circulation Parvovirus B-19 IgG and IgM Syphilis Lupus anticoagulant Anticardiolipin Ab TSH Hemoglobin A1c	Consider testing for thrombophilia based on history Severe placental pathology, growth restriction, personal or family history of VTE (Factor V Leiden, prothrombin gene mutation, antithrombin III, and fasting homocysteine)
Postpartum	Protein C and protein S activity (selected case) Parental karyotype (if no yield from fetal karyotype)	
Selected cases	Glucose screeningToxicology screening	If not previously performed or LGA Drug use suspected

Abbreviations: FISH – fluorescence in situ hybridization; CBC – complete blood count; PT – prothrombin time; PTT – partia thromboplastin time; VTE – venous thromboembolism; LGA – large for gestational age.

falsely negative and may not fully represent a cause of fetal loss. In viral causes, diagnosis can be made more clearly by examination of the fetus rather than solely on maternal titers. TORCH titers are often sent in the setting of stillbirth; however, they may be of limited utility except in the setting of known maternal infection. Evaluation of the fetus and placenta will often provide better diagnostic capability for viral infection as a cause. It is the recommendation of some authors that TORCH titers only be selectively sent due to lack of benefit.[14]

Fetal causes may contribute to up to 25% of stillbirths. Fetal karyotypic abnormalities can be found in 8–13% of stillbirths and over 20% of fetuses with anatomic abnormalities or growth restriction. Single gene Mendelian disorders account for 1% of stillbirths. The most commonly diagnosed karyotypic abnormalities are monosomy X (23%), trisomy 21 (23%), trisomy 18 (21%), and trisomy 13 (8%).[3] Thus, it is recommended that karyotype be offered to all parents after stillbirth has been diagnosed. Amniocentesis, while a more invasive option for the mother, provides a much greater yield than evaluation of fetal tissue after delivery. An amniocentesis has an 85% yield rate, while fetal tissue has a 28% yield rate. The counseling of parents should reflect the difference as well as emphasize that despite the invasive nature of amniocentesis it may be the better option for some families.[3]

Additionally, structural anomalies such as congenital malformation may also contribute to stillbirth.[14] For this reason, autopsy should be offered to all families. If a family declines on religious grounds, then consideration should be given to photographs and radiographs in order to allow for evaluation by a genetics provider.

A workshop by the Eunice Kennedy Shriver National Institutes of Child Health and Human Development led to the creation of an Initial Causes of Fetal Death Screening, which is designed to assist providers in elucidating cause of stillbirth. This tool can be used at the time of evaluation, even when an extensive evaluation is not possible.[14]

Maternal infection is a contributor worldwide to stillbirth; however, in the United States, it accounts for only 5%. Parvovirus B19, Coxsackie virus A and B, CMV, and enteroviruses are all implicated; however, parvovirus is the main contributor in the United States. The lower genital tract is also a place of colonization of bacteria, and ascending infections play a role in maternal infection. The primary pathogens are *Escherichia coli*, Group B *Streptococcus*, and *Klebsiella*. More common bacteria such as *Ureaplasma*, *Mycoplasma*, *Gardnerella*, and *Enterococcus* have been noted in maternal infection; however, these infections are so prevalent among adult women that causation is not clear.[14] Two important bacterial infections are *Treponema pallidum* and *Listeria monocytogenes*. Some guidelines suggest third trimester screening for Treponema in women living in at risk areas or with risk factors for infection. Women should also be appropriately counseled during prenatal care on diet to avoid foods with a high risk of *Listeria* exposure, including avoidance of unpasteurized dairy, deli meats, and certain fruits.[3]

Pathology Evaluation

Since some portions of the evaluation can be performed prior to delivery, it is important that this be discussed before any induction of labor occurs. The most important components of evaluation are fetal autopsy, placental examination, and karyotype evaluation. Decisions should be made regarding autopsy and pathologic examination of the placenta. Families should be informed of the potential benefit as well as cost of these evaluations.[3] Table 26.2 outlines the important aspects of the pathology evaluation.

Chromosomal microarray is now preferred over karyotype as a method of assessment due to a broader diagnostic potential including assessment of microdeletions and microduplications. Microarray is able to detect abnormalities even in the face of inability to obtain live cells.[15]

Autopsy should be offered to all families. If the family declines autopsy, less invasive means can be undertaken such as X-ray, ultrasound, or magnetic resonance imaging (MRI). Photography can also be useful, especially if a geneticist is not available on staff.[3] All photographs or imaging should only be done with familial consent.

Twenty-five to thirty percent of stillbirths can be accounted for by abnormalities of the placenta or umbilical cord. Placental abruption and placental insufficiency are equally divided with abruption leading to 10–12% and insufficiency leading to 14% of stillbirths. In 5% of stillbirths, substantial maternofetal hemorrhage is the only finding.[14]

Cord accidents are often the attributed cause of fetal death; however, great care should be taken in assigning this as the cause. Nuchal cords may be found in up to 30% of normal deliveries. In order to attribute stillbirth to a cord accident, there should be evidence of obstruction or circulatory compromise on examination.[14]

Placental evaluation is important in the determination of potential stillbirth causes. Detection is also improved when the placenta is evaluated by a pathologist with specialized education in placental pathology.[17] It is one of the most frequently performed aspects of the evaluation of stillbirth as families are largely agreeable to it. However, placental assessment is difficult to standardize with inter-observer variation ranging from 25 to 91% in some studies.[17] Some changes are similar between fetal growth restriction and stillbirth and it is possible that assessment of these changes could lead to recognition of underlying

Table 26.2 Pathology Evaluation of Stillbirth[3]

	Evaluation	Detailed Information
Fetal autopsy	Parental consent should be obtained	In absence of consent, imaging studies may be substituted. Informative in 30% of cases
Placental examination	Signs of viral or bacterial infection Weight	Informative in 30% of cases.
Fetal inspection	Weight, head circumference, and length Photographs (if consent) - Frontal and profile of body, face, extremities, palms, abnormalities	Document any abnormalities Particularly helpful if geneticist not available on site.

cause of the stillbirth. Some concerning findings include increased presence of placental lesions in stillbirth; such lesions comprise diffuse terminal villous immaturity, inflammation, vascular degeneration in the chorionic plate, intra-placental thrombi, avascular villi, and parenchymal infarction. Term stillbirth is more associated with avascular villi and fetal vascular thrombi.[18] Placental lesions may be similar in live and stillbirths; however, the frequency with which they are noted is increased in stillbirth. This could reflect real pathologic change, but also observer bias in the setting of stillbirth.

Treatment

The diagnosis and management of a family recently informed of stillbirth is one of the greatest challenges in obstetrics. Care must be taken during the discussion of a cause and in provision of recommendations for further testing to ensure that the wishes of the parents as well as religious or cultural beliefs are observed. Providers should refer to the fetus by name if one had been given. Adequate time should be provided for the family to process the information.[3] Parents sometimes report that they subsequently re-evaluated decisions made around the time of diagnosis and delivery and felt frustration or injustice related to their decisions being influenced by insufficient information from birth attendants. Providers should recognize that the decision not to hold the stillborn baby is one of the most regretted decisions made around time of delivery. Also, induction started within 6 hours of diagnosis was associated with less anxiety than induction by 24 hours.[14]

Beliefs that the mother may become coagulopathic if delivery is not quickly undertaken are commonly held, but largely untrue. In the third trimester, labor induction is the preferred method of management. After 28 weeks gestation, induction should be managed by usual hospital protocols. While increased dosages of Cytotec may be appropriate for gestations less than 28 weeks, no evidence exists to support safety of this regimen in the third trimester.[3]

In women with a prior cesarean section, induction is still the preferred method of delivery. The plan for induction should be thoroughly reviewed with the patient and consent must be obtained. Cesarean delivery for fetal demise should be reserved for unusual circumstances due to increased risk of maternal morbidity without fetal benefit. The data on patients with a prior classical cesarean section is limited; therefore management should be on an individualized basis for this subgroup of patients.[3]

Following delivery, the parents and family should be allowed ample time with the fetus as desired. Providers should allow for cultural and religious ceremonies as appropriate. It is important to remember the stillborn infant as a member of the patient's family and to treat him or her accordingly. The baby should never be referred to as someone replaceable or less than a person.[4] There are conflicting reports that reflect the individualized nature of grief; some parents may take comfort in holding their infant, while there have also been studies that have shown attachment disorders with future children and increased anxiety associated with seeing the infant after delivery. The plan should be individualized to what the parents feel comfortable with at the time of delivery. Reviews have shown that the opportunity to see and hold the stillborn infant, make memories – which could include photos or mementos – and the completion of an evaluation may provide the family with closure surrounding the event.[4] All parents should be offered mementos of their baby, including locks of hair, hand, and footprints or impressions, clothing, and photographs.[14]

Perception of quality of care is also important after a stillbirth. A perception of suboptimal care can lead to friction between the parents and provider. One study showed that providers felt that aspects of quality of care were present more often than parents. Both parents and providers felt that they were not able to spend enough time together after the event. A focus on interaction is important for patients to believe that their concerns about their child are being taken seriously, as many believe that their concerns are not being heard prior to an adverse event.[16]

Psychosocial Ramifications

Grief and coping following a stillbirth is similar to that following loss of a child after delivery, but parents often feel that this grief is marginalized due to societal beliefs regarding its legitimacy. Stillbirth has been associated with subsequent depression, anxiety, posttraumatic stress disorder, anger, and agoraphobia. Parents who have experienced loss may voluntarily isolate themselves from their normal social activities, thus compounding their sense of isolation. Coping strategies can include taking time to themselves, increased or decreased involvement in religious activities, and a change in sexual activity. Some parents may cope by increasing their engagement in exercise and healthy activities, work, and social media, as well as activism with the community of women who have lost pregnancy.[1,4]

Fathers have a significant response to the stillbirth. They often, however, feel as though their grief is marginalized and deemed illegitimate. Often grieving styles may differ between mothers and fathers and this may lead to friction within the relationship including arguments, infidelity, and physical violence. Fathers also feel societal pressure to be the "rock" of the family and partner, and therefore feel increased pressure to keep their grief private. This may lead to increased substance abuse and also problems with employment.[1,4]

Some parents may also note a feeling of increased intimacy within their relationship, as they have been through a unique life event together. Sexual relationships are often changed for better or for worse after a stillbirth. Significant feelings can be related to the relationship's resumption of intimacy and conception of future pregnancies. Parents may experience increased or decreased interest in intercourse. Women also have complex body image changes after delivery; a woman may want to get back to the pre-pregnancy state as soon as possible to avoid looking as though she just delivered while another may want to retain the postpartum body to feel closer to her pregnancy. Women may express the sentiment that "my body failed me," which can complicate postpartum body image.[1,4]

Financially, the family may experience a decrease in revenue around the time of a stillbirth. Often, time away from work is required for the family to recover. Chronic pain and fatigue may also impact the ability to work outside of the home. Additionally, mothers have reported feeling unwelcome upon return to work. The parent may avoid work in order to avoid being confronted with other's expectations of their grief. There is also increased cost related to hospital bills and funeral expenses.[1]

Future Pregnancies

Following a stillbirth, parents may experience both internal and external pressure to either delay a future pregnancy or to pursue a pregnancy quickly.[4] It is important to set reasonable expectations with the family that the cause of stillbirth may never be identified. This can make future pregnancies more stressful for the parents, and this should be openly discussed with the family. The risk of recurrent stillbirth before 37 weeks is 7.8–10.5/1,000 and after 37 weeks is 1.8/1,000 live births.[13] Parents who have experienced stillbirth may experience hyper-vigilance surrounding subsequent pregnancies and the children of these pregnancies.[4] Box 26.3 outlines the important considerations for treatment of the subsequent pregnancy.[3]

Antenatal testing may be established at 32–34 weeks in subsequent pregnancies. It should be considered that antenatal testing has a false-positive rate and that acting on this may result in a 1.5% iatrogenic

Box 26.3 Management of subsequent pregnancies[3]

- Preconception or initial prenatal visit
  - Detailed maternal history
  - Review results of previous evaluation and determine risk of recurrence
  - Encourage lifestyle changes
    - Smoking cessation
    - Weight loss in obese women at preconception visit
    - Referral to genetic counseling as appropriate
    - Labs
    - Diabetes screen if indicated
    - Thrombophilia workup and antiphosphlipid antibody syndrome (APLS) evaluation if indicated
- First trimester
  - Dating ultrasound
  - First trimester genetic screen if desired
- Second trimester
  - Ultrasound for anatomic survey at 18–20 weeks
  - Maternal serum-alpha fetoprotein (MSAFP) or quad screen as desired
- Third trimester
  - Serial ultrasound for fetal growth restriction after 28 weeks gestation
  - Kick counts starting at 28 weeks
  - Antenatal testing starting at 32 weeks or 1–2 weeks prior to stillbirth
- Delivery
  - Elective induction of labor (IOL) at 39 weeks gestation
    - Must document fetal lung maturity (FLM) if delivering before 39 weeks without indication

preterm delivery rate. This will also increase the cost of the pregnancy as well as potential morbidity associated with iatrogenic induction and preterm delivery.[3]

Kick counts may be recommended; however, there is inadequate data on their efficacy and information on the internet that many patients access has been found to be insufficient. If kick counts are recommended, clear instructions should be given to the patient.[5]

If a patient was diagnosed with a thrombophilia during her stillbirth evaluation, then she has a 3.6-fold increase in stillbirth risk in a subsequent pregnancy. Care should be taken to solely attribute the prior stillbirth to the thrombophilia without other evidence of placental insufficiency. Discussion should be undertaken prior to subsequent pregnancies about the possibility of using folic acid, low-dose aspirin, or enoxaparin.[19]

The use of aspirin without evidence of thrombophilia has been discussed; however, there is insufficient data at this time to routinely recommend aspirin in subsequent pregnancies. Theoretically, aspirin is postulated to improve uteroplacental circulation, decrease the risk of placental thrombosis, infarction, and insufficiency.[19]

The delivery plan should be reviewed with the family throughout the pregnancy. Delivery mode should be based on usual indications. Induction of labor may be considered after 39 weeks and should be based on maternal anxiety, cervical ripeness, and cause of the previous stillbirth. If delivery prior to 39 weeks is considered, fetal lung maturity should be assessed.[19]

Of paramount importance for these patients is support throughout the subsequent pregnancy. This can be a time fraught with great joy as well as anxiety and depression. Women who experienced pregnancy after stillbirth reported that they felt they could not enjoy the pregnancy as much. These patients experience higher rates of depression and psychological symptoms.[4] Fathers will often desire more involvement with obstetrical care in subsequent pregnancies.[1] Both parents may experience a range of emotion from normal joy at pregnancy and optimism to fear, anxiety, and depression. An important part of their care will be for providers to show support for them through this time.

Concluding Remarks

Third trimester pregnancy loss is one of the most difficult life events for patients and their families. It is important to offer emotional support during this time and to provide the patient with resources given the psychosocial and financial impact of this event on the family. A thorough history, combined with a laboratory and pathologic evaluation may provide some answers regarding cause, but unfortunately 15–40% of stillbirths do not have a clear origin despite extensive workup.[14] Future pregnancies may be informed by the testing at the time of the loss; however, antenatal testing and delivery at 39 weeks is recommended.[3] Provider education should focus on knowledge of risk factors and possible interventions in a subsequent pregnancy. Ideally access to adequate prenatal care and health care services as well as contraception services are optimal methods with which to decrease the rate of stillbirth.[15]

References

1. A.E.P. Heazell. Stillbirths: Economic and psychosocial consequences. *Lancet* 2016; 387: 604–16.
2. National Vital Statistics Reports. Fetal and Perinatal Mortality: United States, 2013.
3. American College of Obstetricians and Gynecologists. Management of Stillbirth. ACOG Practice Bulletin No. 102. Washington, DC: ACOG; 2009.
4. C. Burden. From grief, guilt pain and stigma to hope and pride – A systematic review and meta-analysis of mixed-method research of the psychosocial impact of stillbirth. *BMC Pregnancy and Childbirth* 2016; 16: 9.
5. J.F. Froen. Stillbirths: progress and unfinished business. *Lancet* 2016; 387: 574–86.
6. J. M. Nicholson. US term stillbirth rates and the 39-week rule: A cause for concern? *American Journal of Obstetrics and Gynecology* 2016 May;214(5):621.e1–9. doi: 10.1016/j.ajog.2016.02.019. Epub 2016 Feb 12..
7. K. Farrant. Online information for women and their families regarding reduced fetal movements is of variable quality, readability, and accountability. *Midwifery.* http://dx.doi.org/10.1016/j.midw.2015.12.013
8. J.E. Lawn. Stillbirths: rates, risk factors, and acceleration toward 2030. *Lancet.* 387: 587–603.
9. R.L. Goldenberg, et al. Stillbirth: knowledge and practice among U.S. obstetrician-gynecologists. *American Journal of Perinatology*. 2013; 30 (10): 813–20.
10. American College of Obstetricians and Gynecologists. Obesity in Pregnancy. ACOG Practice Bulletin No. 156. Washington, DC: ACOG; 2015.
11. K.F. Walker. Causes of antepartum stillbirth in women of advanced maternal age. *European Journal of Obstetrics & Gynecology and Reproductive Biology* 2016; 197: 86–90.

12. M.W. Varner. Association between stillbirth and illicit drug use and smoking during pregnancy. *Obstetrics and Gynecology* 2014; 123: 113–25.
13. A. Gordon. Stillbirth risk in a second pregnancy. *Obstetrics and Gynecology* 2012; 119: 509–17.
14. A.G. Eller. Stillbirth at Term. *Obstetrics and Gynecology.* 2006; 108: 442–7.
15. D.J. Dudley. A new system for determining causes of stillbirth. *Obstetrics and Gynecology* 2010; 116: 254–60.
16. V. Flenady. Stillbirths: Recall to action in high-income countries. *Lancet* 2016; 387: 691–702.
17. H. Pinar. Placental findings in singleton stillbirths. *Obstetrics and Gynecology* 2014; 123: 325–36.
18. I. Ptacek. Quantitative assessment of placental morphology may identify specific causes of stillbirth. *BMC Clinical Pathology* 2016; 16: 1.
19. U.M. Reddy. Prediction and prevention of recurrent stillbirth. *Obstetrics and Gynecology* 2007; 110: 1151–64.

Antepartum Hemorrhage

Jessica R. Jackson and Julie DeCesare

Introduction

Antepartum hemorrhage is defined as bleeding occurring from 24 0/7 weeks gestation onward, from or into the genital tract. An identifiable cause for antepartum hemorrhage is only found in 50% of cases. In the other 50%, the cause is either indeterminate or unknown.[1,2] Blood loss is often underestimated by clinicians. Additionally, the blood loss may be significantly less than the actual amount of hemorrhage, such as in a concealed abruption.[3] Proper education regarding causes, management, and outcomes related to antepartum hemorrhage are imperative and will be discussed in this chapter. Management strategies regarding massive blood loss in obstetrics is described in detail in the chapter on postpartum hemorrhage, and will not be addressed in this chapter.

Scope of the Problem

Antepartum hemorrhage complicates 3–5% of all pregnancies and is one of the leading causes of perinatal and maternal morbidity worldwide.[3] Multiple causes of antepartum hemorrhage exist. This chapter will focus on the top four causes of antepartum hemorrhage, which include of placenta previa, placenta accreta, placental abruption, and vasa previa.[4] It is important to consider that, while the rates of abruption and vasa previa have stayed constant, the rates of placenta previa and placenta accreta have significantly risen over the last 20 years, in parallel with the overwhelming rise in cesarean delivery.[5]

Etiology

Placenta previa, placenta accreta, placental abruption, and vasa previa, as the top four causes of hemorrhage, will be described in detail. However, the astute clinician must always consider additional causes of bleeding from the lower genital tract during the antepartum period, such as cervicitis and genital trauma. Box 27.1 has a comprehensive list of other causes of antepartum hemorrhage.

Placenta Previa

Definition: Placenta previa is defined as a placenta implanted either over or very close to the internal cervical os. Placenta previa has been classically characterized by distance from the internal cervical os (see Box 27.2).[6] However, modern transvaginal ultrasound now allows for specific measurement of exact distance from the cervical os, causing this older classification to become somewhat outdated.[7]

Risk Factors: Risk factors are many and include prior cesarean delivery, with the risk of previa increasing with increasing number of prior cesareans.[8] Advanced maternal age, multiparity, multiple gestation, cigarette smoking, cocaine use, prior placenta previa, and otherwise unexplained elevated alphafetoprotein (MSAFP) have also been identified as risk factors.[9–12]

Diagnosis: The classic clinical presentation of placenta previa is painless vaginal bleeding that occurs in the late second or early third trimester.[13] In the developed world, however, most placenta previas are diagnosed via routine screening transabdominal ultrasound. In general, ultrasound diagnosis of all forms of abnormal placentation is approximately 90%.[14]

Many previas diagnosed in early pregnancy resolve with advancing gestation. An evaluation of 8,650 cases of placenta previa diagnosed at 20–23 weeks gestation demonstrated that only 10–20% persisted into the late third trimester.[15,16] The effect of gestational age on persistence of previa has been evaluated specifically in twin gestations. A retrospective cohort study from 2012 that included 120 cases of previa diagnosed in twins showed a higher likelihood of persistence with advancing gestation (19.2% at 20–23 weeks, compared to 50% at 24–27 weeks, and 92.5% at 32–35 weeks).[17] The placenta does

Box 27.1 Secondary causes of antepartum hemorrhage [4]

Cervicitis
Infections of the genital tract
Trauma
Tumors – benign
Tumors – malignant (cervical cancer most common)

Box 27.2 Placenta previa classification [5]

Low-lying placenta

Placenta is implanted in the lower uterine segment. The placental edge is close to the internal os but does not reach it.

Marginal placenta previa

Edge of the placenta is at the margin of the internal os

Partial placenta previa

Placenta partially covers the internal os

Complete placenta previa

Placenta completely covers internal os

not actually migrate, but rather undergoes a process called "trophotropism," in which it grows toward the area of the uterus with the best blood supply. This area is typically the uterine fundus. Consequently, the placental portion closest to the cervix regresses and atrophies, resulting in a resolution of the previa.[18]

Transvaginal ultrasound is useful, particularly in the third trimester, in confirming the diagnosis. Although theoretical concern may exist for disturbance of the placenta with the transvaginal ultrasound probe, this procedure is considered safe and more accurate than transabdominal approaches.[19,20] Ghourab studied the significance of thickness of placental edge detected at 28–32 weeks gestation, when predicting placental migration from the cervical os. The placental edge was defined as thick if the thickness was 1 cm or greater, within 1 cm from the edge, the angle between the basal and chorionic plate exceeded 45 degrees. All other placental edges were defined as thin. Placental migration was seen in 29.6% of thin placentas, whereas only 5.8% of thick placentas migrated. Thick placentas were also associated with a significantly higher rate of antepartum hemorrhage, cesarean delivery, adherent placenta, and low birth weight.[21]

Outcomes: One of the most devastating outcomes of placenta previa is catastrophic hemorrhage, which can result in morbidity and mortality for both mother and fetus. For this reason, planned delivery via scheduled cesarean is recommended during the late preterm period, between 36 0/7 to 37 6/7 weeks gestation, before the onset of labor.[22] Several studies have investigated the utility of serial transvaginal ultrasound for delivery timing in patients with placenta previa. A recent expert review by Vintzileos et al. proposed guidelines for management of asymptomatic patients with placenta previa, based on ultrasound findings such as cervical length, distance between internal cervical os and placenta, and placental edge thickness. Within this algorithm, patients with a diagnosis of placenta previa undergo transvaginal ultrasound with cervical length and measurement of placental thickness every 1–2 weeks. Patients are considered candidates for conservative outpatient management until delivery at 37–38 weeks if cervical length remains greater than 30 mm and placental thickness remains less than or equal to 1 cm. If cervical length falls less than 30 mm or placental thickness becomes greater than 1 cm, consideration should be given to antenatal steroid administration and increased surveillance for bleeding. If cervical length falls less than 10–15 mm, consideration should be given to in-patient management with delivery by 34–35 weeks gestation.[23] Although this algorithm has not been formally adopted by mainstream obstetric societies, it has been proposed as an alternative to delivery of every placenta previa at 36–37 weeks gestation.

Placenta Accreta

Definition: Placenta previa may also be associated with another form of abnormal placentation, called placenta accreta (a general term to describe the abnormal growth of all or part of the placenta into the uterine wall, becoming inseparable). Although the two can exist independently of each other, the presence of previa should prompt evaluation for accreta.

Risk Factors: Women at greatest risk for accreta are those with a prior uterine scar and a placenta previa. The risk of accreta is approximately 11%, in a patient with placenta previa and a history of one cesarean section. The risk of accreta in a patient with placenta previa rises to 40%, 61%, and 67% after two, three, and four or more cesareans, respectively. The risk of placenta accreta without prior uterine surgery, but with a current placenta previa is 1–5%.

Diagnosis: Placenta accreta is often diagnosed with ultrasonography. Characteristic findings include loss of the normal hypoechoic boundary between the placenta and the bladder, irregularly shaped placental lacunae (vascular spaces), thinning of the myometrium overlying the placenta, loss of the retroplacental "clear space," protrusion of the placenta into the bladder, increased vascularity within the uterine serosa–bladder interface, and turbulent blood flow through the lacunae on Doppler ultrasound. The most predictive ultrasonographic sign of accreta is the presence and increasing number of lacunae within the placenta at 15–20 weeks gestation (sensitivity 79% and positive predictive value 92%). See Figure 4.4 in Chapter 4 for an example of placenta accreta on ultrasound.

Outcomes: Without proper management, placenta accreta may result in catastrophic hemorrhage that can be fatal for the mother. Management of accreta is complex, but key management points include antenatal diagnosis with ultrasound, transfer of patient to a tertiary care center with adequate access to an appropriately sized blood bank, multidisciplinary team planning for delivery, and consideration for planned cesarean hysterectomy. Delivery should be planned before the onset of labor, at 34 weeks, without amniocentesis for fetal lung maturity.[24]

Placental Abruption

Definition: Placental abruption is defined as separation of the placenta from its implantation site before delivery. Placental abruption is also known as *abruptio placentae* in Great Britain.[25] Placental abruption may be complete or partial. Although the pathophysiology of placental abruption is not completely understood, key mechanisms appear to be impaired placentation, placental insufficiency, intrauterine hypoxia, and uteroplacental underperfusion. Ultimately, the abruption results from rupture of a maternal decidual artery, which causes dissection of blood at the decidual–placental interface, around the placental margin, or behind the membranes. Placental abruption accounts for 25% of antepartum hemorrhage cases.[26]

Risk Factors: The biggest risk factor for placental abruption is a history of placental abruption (recurrence risk 19–25% in women with history of two abruptions). Other risk factors include hypertension, intrauterine growth restriction, premature rupture of membranes, intra-amniotic infection, advanced maternal age, non-vertex fetal presentations, pregnancy following assisted reproductive techniques, low body mass index, abdominal trauma, cigarette smoking, and cocaine/amphetamine misuse. A finding of intrauterine hematoma identified on first trimester ultrasound is associated with subsequent placental abruption.[3]

Diagnosis: Placental abruption is a clinical diagnosis. The classic presentation is abdominal pain, uterine tenderness, contractions, and vaginal bleeding, although patients may also be asymptomatic. Vaginal bleeding is present in 70–80% of cases, and the degree of bleeding is indicative of the degree of abruption. In a concealed abruption, the blood pools behind the placenta and does not exit the uterine cavity; vaginal bleeding may therefore be absent.[27]

A recent study by Glantz showed that ultrasound detection of placental abruption is unreliable. The study included 149 patients who underwent sonography at 24 weeks gestation or greater for vaginal bleeding or rule out abruption. Ultrasound findings were correlated to placental findings at delivery. Sensitivity, specificity, and positive and negative predictive values of sonography were found to be: 24%, 96%, 88%, and 53%, respectively.[28] Traditionally, ultrasound diagnosis of placental abruption is estimated to be about 50% accurate. In fact, ultrasound findings may be relatively normal, even in cases of clinically significant abruption. If abnormal, ultrasound may demonstrate a hypoechoic, subchorionic thickened area at the margin of the placenta. Indeed, the most common site of separation is at the edge of the placenta. This is sometimes called a "marginal abruption" or "marginal hematoma."[29]

One interesting phenomenon that can be associated with abruption is the chronic abruption oligohydramnios sequence (CAOS). The syndrome was first described in 1998 by Elliot et al. as being characterized by (1) clinically significant vaginal bleeding in the absence of placenta previa or other identifiable source, (2) amniotic fluid volume initially documented as normal, and (3) oligohydramnios eventually developing, without evidence of membrane rupture. In this initial study, delivery was demonstrated to occur in patients with CAOS around 28 weeks gestation.[30]

Although the clinicopathological course of acute placental abruption has been well described, the pathophysiology of chronic abruption is still unclear. Acute abruption has been described as arterial bleeding that leads to the collapse of spiral arteries, which increases the risk of rapidly expanding placental dissection. This is a life-threatening emergency for both the mother and the fetus. On the other hand, it has been proposed that chronic abruption, such as that seen in CAOS, is the result of slow venous bleeding. The resulting increased venous pressure disturbs venous return from reservoirs that are the space between the chorionic membrane and chorionic plate at the edge of the placenta, resulting in chronic abruption and vaginal bleeding.[31]

Outcomes: In most cases, delivery occurs within seven days of placental abruption.[32] Outcomes for chronic abruption oligohydramnios sequence have been described in a small number of studies. Kobayshi et al, described increased rates of adverse outcomes in cases of CAOS when compared to cases of first trimester vaginal bleeding without CAOS. These adverse outcomes included lower neonatal birth weight, higher incidence of small for gestational age and chronic lung disease infants, and higher rates of preterm delivery. Additionally, prolonged and recurrent episodes of bleeding were predictive of CAOS development.[33]

In general, placental abruption has been associated with poor outcomes. For the mother, abruption has been associated with hemorrhagic shock, Couvelaire uterus (blood from the hemorrhage is trapped under the uterine peritoneum causing the uterus to appear dusky purple), and disseminated intravascular coagulation. For the fetus, abruption has been associated with low birth weight, preterm birth, severe birth asphyxia, and perinatal death. In particular, placental abruption associated with hypertension of pregnancy has been linked to higher incidence of disseminated intravascular coagulation, blood transfusion, and perinatal mortality when compared to placental abruption without hypertension. Also, placental abruption associated with Couvelaire uterus has been associated with a higher incidence of severe birth asphyxia than placental abruption without Couvelaire uterus.[34]

Anath et al. evaluated placental abruption in twin gestations. It was found that a birth weight discordance greater than or equal to 20% among the same sex, and greater than or equal to 40% for different sex twins, conferred an increased risk of placental abruption. The risk of abruption with growth discordance persisted, although at a lower level, with a growth discordance less than 5%.[35]

Vasa Previa

Definition: Vasa previa is defined as fetal blood vessels that are unprotected by the umbilical cord run

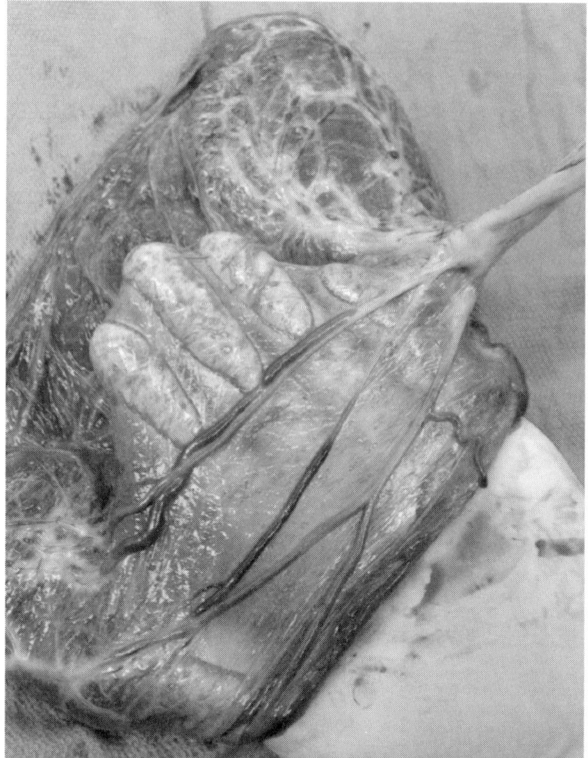

Figure 27.1 Concealed abruption.

through the amniotic membranes and traverse the cervix. It the membranes rupture, the fetal vessels may also rupture, leading to fetal hemorrhage, exsanguination, and possibly death. An example is seen in Figure 27.1. Vasa previa complicates approximately 1:2,500 deliveries. Two types of vasa previa exist: type I and type II. Type I occurs when there is a velamentous cord insertion between the umbilical cord and the placenta; the fetal vessels run unprotected through the membranes and traverse the cervix or lie in close proximity to it. Type II occurs when the placenta is multilobed or contains a succenturiate lobe, and fetal vessels that connect the two lobes traverse the cervix.

Risk Factors: There are two major risk factors for vasa previa: velamentous cord insertion (most common) and succenturiate placental lobe or bilobed placenta. Approximately 60% of women with vasa previa have a low-lying placenta identified on routine screening ultrasound. Other risk factors include in vitro fertilization and multiple gestation.[36]

Diagnosis: Vasa previa may be suspected when mother presents with painless vaginal bleeding and fetal distress or death following membrane rupture. Sometimes

Box 27.3 Antepartum screening for vasa previa

At the time of mid-trimester ultrasound, placental location should be documented, and the relationship between the placenta and cervical os evaluated.

The placental cord insertion site should be documented when technically possible.

A follow-up ultrasound should be performed at 32 weeks gestation for women with diagnosis of placenta previa or low-lying placenta,

If vasa previa is suspected, transvaginal ultrasound with color and pulsed Doppler should be used to facilitate the diagnosis.

The diagnosis of vasa previa is confirmed if an arterial vessel is visualized over the cervix, and Doppler demonstrates a heart rate equivalent to the fetal heart rate.

Box 27.4 Management recommendations for antepartum diagnosis vasa previa

If rupture of membranes occurs at a viable gestational age, cesarean section should be performed.

Antepartum hospitalization and corticosteroid administration between 28 and 32 weeks gestation should be considered.

Scheduled cesarean delivery should be considered between 34 and 37 weeks gestation.

Delivery should occur via cesarean section, at a center capable of performing neonatal blood transfusion

vasa previa may be diagnosed on digital examination of the cervix, but vasa previa is often diagnosed via ultrasonography. Most vasa previas are incidentally discovered during transvaginal ultrasound evaluation of low-lying placenta. Presence of an accessory placenta lobe or velamentous cord insertion should raise suspicion of vasa previa. Notably the risk of vasa previa is negligible if the umbilical cord inserts normally into the central portion of the placental plate. On gray scale ultrasound, vasa previa appears as echolucent parallel lines traversing the cervix. Color flow and pulsed Doppler may be used to demonstrate blood flow within these vessels. Differential diagnosis includes a normal loop of umbilical cord floating through the lower uterine segment over the cervical os. In this case, the loop of cord should move away from the cervix with maternal repositioning.[37]

The Society for Maternal Fetal Medicine recommends that the algorithm seen in Box 27.3 be followed for all pregnancies to facilitate the diagnosis of vasa previa.[38]

Outcomes: If membranes rupture and subsequent rupture of the vasa previa occurs, outcomes can be catastrophic, including fetal death. In one retrospective study, when vasa previa was not diagnosed prenatally, it was associated with a perinatal mortality of approximately 56%, whereas fetal survival was 97% in cases diagnosed prenatally.[39] For this reason, the Society for Maternal Fetal Medicine has provided recommendations for pregnancies with diagnosed vasa previa. which are seen in Box 27.4.[40]

Special Antenatal Considerations for Bleeding During Pregnancy

Prevention of RhD Alloimmunization

One concern with antepartum bleeding is alloimmunization of the fetus. This occurs when an Rh-negative mother is exposed to blood from an Rh-positive fetus. The mother then makes antibodies against the fetal Rh antigen. In subsequent pregnancies, the mother's antibodies may attack fetal red blood cells containing the Rh antigen. This can lead to fetal anemia, high output cardiac failure, hydrops, and death. Rh alloimmunization can be drastically decreased by administration of anti-D immune globulin. In patients with second and third trimester hemorrhage, the risk of alloimmunization is unclear. Particularly complex is the management of the patient with intermittent or persistent vaginal bleeding. The American College of Obstetricians and Gynecologists recommends that administration of anti-D immunoglobulin be considered in cases of second and third trimester vaginal bleeding.[41]

Optimization of Outcomes of Premature Birth

Any time premature birth is anticipated, it is important to remember that neonatal outcomes can be improved through administration of antenatal corticosteroids for fetal lung maturity and use of magnesium sulfate for prevention of cerebral palsy. Administration of these two therapies is recommended between 24 and 34 weeks gestation, but may be considered as early as 23 weeks gestation.[42]

Concluding Remarks

Antepartum hemorrhage is a leading cause of morbidity and mortality for both mother and baby. Four major causes of antenatal hemorrhage are placenta previa, placenta accreta, placental abruption, and vasa previa. Consideration should be given to prevention of alloimmunization and optimization of outcomes of prematurity.

References

1. Krishna A, Chandraharan E. Management of massive obstetric hemorrhage. *Current Women's Health Review*. 2011; 7: 136–142.
2. Bhandari S, Raja EA, Shetty A, Bhattacharya S. Maternal and perinatal consequences of antepartum haemorrhage of unknown origin. *BJOG*. 2014; 121 (1): 44–52.
3. Royal College of Obstetricians and Gynaecologists. Green top guideline number 63, 1st ed. Antepartum Hemorrhage. 2001; p. 1–23.
4. King Edward Hospital for Women Perth, Australia. Antepartum Hemorrhage. *Clinical Guidelines: Obstetrics and Midwifery*. 2015; B2.3: 1–12.
5. The American College of Obstetricians and Gynecologists. Committee Opinion. Placenta Accreta. No 529 July 2012, reaffirmed 2015.
6. Cunningham, Leveno, Bloom, Hauth, Rouse, Spong, eds. *Williams Obstetrics*, 23rd ed. New York: McGraw Hill. 2010.
7. Silver R. Abnormal placentation: placenta previa, vasa previa, and placenta accrete. *Obstet Gynecol*. 2015; 126 (3): 654–668.
8. Getahum D, Oyelese Y, Salihu HM, Ananth CV. Previous cesarean delivery and risks of placenta previa and placental abruption. *Obstet Gynecol*. 2006; 107: 771–778.
9. Cunningham, Leveno, Bloom, Hauth, Rouse, Spong, eds. *Williams Obstetrics*, 23rd ed. New York: McGraw Hill. 2010.
10. Ananth CV, Wilcox AJ, Savitz DA, Bowes WA, Luther ER. Effect of maternal age and parity on the risk of uteroplacental bleeding disorders in pregnancy. *Obstet Gynecol*. 1996; 88: 511–516.
11. Macones GA, Sehdev HM, Parry S, Morgan MA, Berlin JA. The association between maternal cocaine use and placenta previa. *Am J Obstet Gynecol*. 1997; 177: 1071–1078.
12. Ananth CV, Demisse K, Smulian JC, Vintzileos AM. Placenta previa in singleton and twin births in the United States, 1989 through 1998: A comparison of risk factor profiles and associated conditions. *Am J Obstet Gynecol*. 2003; 188: 275–281.
13. Cunningham, Leveno, Bloom, Hauth, Rouse, Spong, eds. *Williams Obstetrics*, 23rd ed. New York: McGraw Hill. 2010.
14. D'Antonio F, Bhide A. Ultrasound in placental disorders. *Best Prac Res Clin Obstet Gynaecol*. 2014: 28: 429–442.
15. Silver R. Abnormal placentation: Placenta previa, vasa previa, and placenta accrete. *Obstet Gynecol*. 2015; 126 (3): 654–668.
16. Becker RH, Vonk R, Mende BC, Ragosch V, Entezami M. The relevance of placental location at 20–23 gestational weeks for the prediction of placenta previa at delivery: Evaluation of 8650 cases. *Ultrasound Obset Gynecol*. 2001; 17: 496–501.
17. Kohari KS, Roman AS, Fox NS, Feinberg J, Saltzman DH, Klauser CK, Rebarber A. Persistence of placenta previa in twin gestations based on gestational age at sonographic detection. *J Ultrasound Med*. 2012; 31 (7): 985–989.
18. Dashe JS, McIntire DD, Ramus RM, Santos-Ramos R, Twickler DM. Persistence of placenta previa according to gestational age at ultrasound detection. *Obstet Gynecol*. 2002; 99: 692–697.
19. Leerentveld RA, Gilberts EC, Arnold MJ, Wladimiroff JW. Accuracy and safety of transvaginal sonographic placental localization. *Obstet Gynecol*. 1990; 11: 257–61.
20. Timor-Tritsch IE, Yunis RA. Confirming the safety of transvaginal sonography in patients suspected of having placenta previa. *Obstet Gynecol*. 1993; 81: 742–744.
21. Ghourab S. Third-trimester transvaginal ultrasonography in placenta previa: does the shape of the lower placental edge predict clinical outcome? *Ultrasound Obstet Gynecol* 2001;18:103–108.
22. ACOG committee opinion number 560: Medically-indicated late-preterm and early-term deliveries. *Obstet Gynecol*. 2013; 121 (4): 908–910.
23. Vintzileos A, Ananth C, Smulian J. Using ultrasound in the clinical management of placental implantation abnormalities. *Am J Obstet Gynecol*. 2015; 4(S): S70-S77.
24. The American College of Obstetricians and Gynecologists.Committee Opinion. Placenta Accreta. No 529 July 2012, reaffirmed 2015.
25. Cunningham, Leveno, Bloom, Hauth, Rouse, Spong, eds. *Williams Obstetrics*, 23rd ed. New York: McGraw Hill. 2010.
26. Tikkanen M. Etiology, clinical manifestations, and prediction of placental abruption. *Acta Obstet Gynecol Scand*. 2010; 89 (6): 732–740.

27. Tikkanen M. Etiology, clinical manifestations, and prediction of placental abruption. *Acta Obstet Gynecol Scand.* 2010; 89 (6): 732–740.

28. Glantz C, Purnell L. Clinical utility of sonography in the diagnosis and treatment of placental abruption. *J Ultrasound Med.* 2002; 32: 837–840.

29. Callen, P. *Ultrasound in Obstetrics and Gynecology*, 5th ed. Amsterdam: Elsevier. 2008.

30. Elliott JP, Gilpin B, Strong TH Jr, Finberg HJ. Chronic abruption-oligohydramnios sequence. *J Reprod Med.* 1998; 43: 418–422.

31. Kobayashi A, Minami S, Tanizaki Y, Shiro M, Yamamato M, et al. Adverse perinatal and neonatal outcomes in patients with chronic–abruption oligohydraminos sequence. *J Obstet Gynaecol Res.* 2014; 40 (6): 1618–1624.

32. Naftolin F, Khudr G, Benirschke K, Hutchinson DL. The syndrome of chronic abruptio placentae, hydrorrhea, and circumvallate placenta. *Am J Obstet Gynecol.* 1973; 116: 347–350.

33. Kobayashi A, Minami S, Tanizaki Y, Shiro M, Yamamato M, et al. Adverse perinatal and neonatal outcomes in patients with chronic-abruption oligohydraminos sequence. *J Obstet Gynaecol Res.* 2014; 40 (6): 1618–1624.

34. Pitaphrom A, Sukcharoen N. Pregnancy outcomes in placental abruption. *J Med Assoc Thal.* 2006; 86 (10): 1572–1578.

35. Anath CV, Demissie K, Hanley ML. Birth weight discordancy and adverse perinatal outcomes among twin gestations in the United States: The effect of placental abruption. *Am J Obstet Gynecol.* 2003; 188 (4): 954–960.

36. Sinkey R, Odibo A, Dasche J. Society for maternal fetal medicine consult series #37: Diagnosis and management of vasa previa. *Am J Obstet Gynecol.* 2015; 213 (5): 615–619.

37. D'Antonio F, Bhide A. Ultrasound in placental disorders. *Best Prac Res Clin Obstet Gynaecol.* 2014: 28: 429–442.

38. Sinkey R, Odibo A, Dasche J. Society for maternal fetal medicine consult series #37: Diagnosis and management of vasa previa. *Am J Obstet Gynecol.* 2015; 213 (5): 615–619.

39. Oyelese Y, Catanzarite V, Prefumo F, Lashley S, Schachter M, et al. Vasa previa: The impact of prenatal diagnosis on outcomes. *Obstet Gynecol.* 2004; 103 (5 Pt 1): 937–942.

40. Sinkey R, Odibo A, Dasche J. Society for maternal fetal medicine consult series #37: Diagnosis and management of vasa previa. *Am J Obstet Gynecol.* 2015; 213 (5): 615–619.

41. The American College of Obstetricians and Gynecologists. Practice bulletin number 4: Prevention of Rh D alloimmunization. May 1999, reaffirmed 2013.

42. The American College of Obstetricians and Gynecologists. Obstetric care consensus summary: Periviable birth. *Obstet Gynecol.* 2015; 126 (5): e82–94.

Postpartum Hemorrhage

Julie DeCesare

Introduction

The incidence of postpartum hemorrhage ranges from 1 in 100 or as high as 1 in 20 [1]. It is estimated that 140,000 women worldwide die of postpartum hemorrhage each year, which works out to one every four minutes [2].

Obstetrical hemorrhage is one of the three leading causes of pregnancy-related mortality worldwide. Women in the United States have a greater lifetime risk of dying from causes related to pregnancy than in 40 other countries. Maternal morbidity and mortality is trending in the wrong direction in the United States; it is increasing rather than decreasing. Severe morbidity is 50 times more common than death [3].

This chapter will review the risk factors for maternal hemorrhage, including the evaluation, recognitions and medical and surgical management options for obstetrical hemorrhage in the postpartum period.

Scope of the Problem

The incidence of maternal hemorrhage is increasing in the United States. A population-based study demonstrated that the rate of postpartum hemorrhage increased 26% between 1994 and 2006 [4].

In addition to being a top cause of pregnancy-related mortality, hemorrhage is considered to be the most preventable cause of maternal mortality, and early recognition was found to be the key factor in preventing morbidity and death from this complication. In a review by Berg et al. [5], almost 90% of maternal deaths due to hemorrhage were felt to be preventable if the diagnosis was made and the patient received adequate treatment in a more timely fashion.

Definition and Etiology

The universally accepted definition of postpartum hemorrhage is greater than 500 cubic centimeters (cc) of estimated blood loss for a vaginal delivery, greater than 1,000 cc for a cesarean delivery, and greater then 1,500cc for a cesarean hysterectomy. Current methods for visual estimation for blood loss are known to be inaccurate. Alternate methods, including change in hematocrit (10%), quantification methods (which rely on weight based measurements) or vital sign triggers have all been proposed as more accurate methods to diagnosis hemorrhage.

Postpartum hemorrhage can be classified as primary or secondary. A primary hemorrhage occurs within 24 hours of delivery, and a secondary hemorrhage occurs from 24 hours through 6 weeks postpartum. The most common etiology for primary postpartum hemorrhage is atony, followed by retained placenta (including placenta accreta), maternal clotting disorder and uterine inversion. The most common causes of secondary hemorrhage, or delayed postpartum hemorrhage, are sub-involution bleeding at the placenta site, retained placenta (including placenta accreta), infection or maternal clotting disorder.

Maternal Physiology

Physiological changes occur in the maternal system in anticipation of the blood loss associated with parturition. As a result, most women can tolerate the anticipated blood loss of 500 to 1,000 cc without major systemic impacts. Maternal blood volume expansion starts as early as 6 weeks gestation and increases on average 40–50% (range 20–100%) in pregnancy. The peak expansion is in the third trimester, usually at 30 to 34 weeks gestation, with no further volume expansion occurring in the final weeks of gestation. Hormonal influences in pregnancy play an important part in causing this volume expansion; however, the exact mechanism is unknown [6].

Parallel to the plasma volume expansion is an increase in erythrocyte mass. This expansion starts in the first trimester (10 weeks gestation) and continues to rise until parturition. The increase in erythrocytes mass starts later the plasma volume expansion; it results in the condition known as physiological anemia of pregnancy. This condition peaks at 30 to 34 weeks gestation and is minimized by the continued increase in erythrocyte mass, which occurs until term. Maternal erythrocyte volume increases by 18% in pregnancy, but can increase as much as 30% with supplemental iron [7]. Thus supplemental iron in pregnancy is an important factor in the prevention of complications from postpartum hemorrhage, especially for patients with baseline anemia.

Risk Factors

Multiple risk factors (Box 28.1) are linked to maternal hemorrhage; these can be classified in terms of the following broad categories; overdistention of the uterus, placenta problems, maternal factors, disease states, iatrogenic causes and intrapartum complications. See Box 28.1 for additional information [8–10]. As the incidence of postpartum hemorrhage continues to rise, recognition of these risk factors can alert the clinician to anticipate and prepare the obstetrical team for the possible hemorrhage. Furthermore, a complex and multifactorial relationship exists between trends in modern obstetrical practice and its impact on the increasing risk of maternal hemorrhage.

The increased incidence of postpartum hemorrhage in the United States appears to be most strongly associated with an increase in uterine atony. Many of the risk other factors related to hemorrhage are related to uterine atony, and risk assessment for these factors is especially clinically relevant [3]. Overdistention of the uterus caused by macrosomia, polyhydramnios, uterine fibroids or multiple gestations are four of such factors that directly increase rates of atony and thus result in more postpartum hemorrhage. Note that other factors, such as the rise in cesarean section (C-section), have an indirect impact on hemorrhage rates by the resulting increase in abnormal placentation through placental disorders such as placenta accreta [11].

Widespread and indiscriminate use of oxytocin as part of routine obstetrical practice is common in obstetrical practice today [12]. Data exists that this has contributed to the rise in maternal hemorrhage. A case-controlled study by Grotegut et al. involving over 12,000 patients, linked doses of oxytocin to severity of postpartum hemorrhage [13]. Judicious use of oxytocin as well as reserving use for specific clinical indications would theoretically reduce hemorrhage risk [14]. A Norway birth registry study involving over 300,000 patients demonstrated that induction of pre-labor women and labor cesarean deliveries (CD) are strongly correlated to hemorrhage [15]. As maternal morbidity continues to rise, evidenced-based protocols to minimize oxytocin exposure should be emphasized.

Box 28.1 Risk factors for postpartum hemorrhage [8–10]

- Uterine overdistention
  - Hydraminous
  - Multiple gestation
  - Fibroids
  - Macrosomia
- Placenta factors
  - Previa
  - Acreta
  - Abruption
  - Vaso previa
  - History of retained placenta
  - Retained placenta
- Maternal factors
  - Advanced age
  - Hispanic ethnicity
  - Asian ethnicity
  - Grand multipara
  - Obesity
- Disease states
  - Pre-eclampsia
  - Hypertension
  - Clotting disorder
  - Diabetes
  - Anemia
- Iatrogenic
  - Induction of labor
  - Epidural anesthesia
- Intrapartum complications
  - Intraamniotic infection
  - Rapid labor
  - Arrest disorders/pitocin augmentation
  - Operative vaginal delivery
  - Vaginal laceration/episiotomy
  - Uterine inversion
  - Compound presentation

Early Recognition

Risk assessment is important in the management of hemorrhage and should start early in the prenatal

Obstetric Hemorrhage Initiative

ADMISSION HEMORRHAGE RISK FACTOR EVALUATION

Low (Clot only)	Medium (Type and Screen)	High (Type and Crossmatch)
No previous uterine incision Singleton pregnancy ≤4 previous vaginal births No known bleeding disorder No history of PPH	Prior cesarean birth(s) or uterine surgery Multiple gestation >4 previous vaginal births Chorioamnioitis History of previous PPH Large uterine fibroids Estimated fetal weight greater than 4 kg Morbid obesity (BMI >35) Induction Augmentation	Placenta previa, low lying placenta Suspected Placenta accreta or percreta Hematocrit < 30 AND other risk factors Platelets < 100,000 Active bleeding (greater than show) on admit Known coagulopathy

Active Management of Third Stage

☐ Oxytocin infusion: 30 units/500 ml ☐ Vigorous fundal massage for at least 15 seconds

Ongoing Quantitative Evaluation of Blood Loss

☐ Using formal methods, such as graduated containers, visual comparisons and weight of blood

Ongoing Evaluation of Vital Signs

Estimated Blood Loss: ____________________

Physician/Nurse Signature Date Time

SHHS N-05/14 21-7010-066

Figure 28.1 Sample risk assessment sticker.

Courtesy University of Florida, Department of Obstetrics and Gynecology at Sacred Heart Health System.

Box 28.2 Vital sign triggers indicative of postpartum hemorrhage

Systolic blood pressure (mmHg) <85
Diastolic blood pressure (mmHg) <45
Heart rate beats per minute >110
Oxygen saturation (%) <95
Oliguria (mL/h for 2 hours) <30

course. A simple risk assessment tool (Figure 28.1) should be completed on the patient in the antepartum intrapartum and postpartum period. Note that risk assessment is not a static measure, but should be performed often by all members of the obstetrical team as many factors develop within the course of labor.

Highest risk patients should have blood products available on the obstetrical unit during the intrapartum period, and the unit should be prepared to administer large quantities of blood products should the situation arise. As almost half of all patients who die from a postpartum hemorrhage have no risk factors; it is therefore necessary for all until who perform obstetrical service be prepared for such an event [16]. The concept of vital sign triggers (Box 28.2) is an important concept for all members of the obstetrical team to understand as they are critical in the early diagnosis of an evolving postpartum hemorrhage. A change in pulse by 15%, or an absolute value of greater than 110 is of concern for volume depletion and can be diagnostic for postpartum hemorrhage. When considering blood pressure, a decline by 15% or absolute values of less than 85/45 is diagnostic. As most gravid patients are young and relatively healthy, they can tolerate massive blood loss before hypovolemic shock is reached. See Box 28.2 for additional information on vital sign assessment.

Prevention

Active management of the third stage of labor (AMTSL) is a key component in the prevention of postpartum hemorrhage. Vigorous fundal massage and oxytocin administration are both evidence-based best practice recommendations for the reduction of hemorrhage [17,18]. Although it is common obstetrical practice in the United States to start oxytocin after delivery of the fetus, initiation of the medication at delivery of the fetal shoulder will promote the least blood loss.

Initial Evaluation

Performance of a pelvic exam is critical in the initial evaluation and management of postpartum hemorrhage. An empty bladder facilitates the exam, and a soft, boggy enlarged uterus is suggestive of atony. Vigorous uterine massage and manual compression of the uterus between a hand placed into the uterus and another placed abdominally should be the first intervention. This should be done while the obstetrician is calling for uterotonic agents. Concurrent assessment of the vagina and cervix for laceration should be performed as well as a uterine sweep for retained membranes or placental fragments.

Lacerations and genital tract hematomas are important causes of hemorrhage and commonly present several hours after delivery. Risk factors include primiparous patients and macrosomia. Lacerations must be identified and repaired. Thorough inspection of the vaginal sidewall and cervix must be performed before this diagnosis is excluded. On occasion, the cervix must be grasped with ring forceps, pulled into the visual field and traced circumferentially in order to complete a thorough inspection.

Hematomas can occur in the vulva, vagina/paravaginal space or the broad ligament. The incidence is 1 in 500 to 1 in 12,500 deliveries [19,20]. A hematoma on the vulva is usually visible on physician exam. Anatomically, the cephalad border is the levator plate. The understanding of this anatomical boundary is important as compression against the levator plate will limit the expansion of this type of hematoma. Treatment with ice and compression is the mainstay of therapy as most of the bleeding is venous in nature; these measures will stop most of such bleeding. If initial measures are not successful, or if the hematoma is larger than 5 cm, drainage or suturing may be employed as secondary therapeutic measures [2].

Vaginal hematomas usually present as rectal pain and anatomically are superior to the levator plate in the pelvis. They are caused by bleeding from the inferior branch of the uterine artery. Although a vaginal mass may be a clinical clue to the diagnosis, depending on the location of the bleed, a mass may not always be present. Clinicians must have a high index of suspicion, and more often the initial presentation is a patient with vague rectal pain, signs of hypovolemia and at firm uterine fundus. Treatment is supportive, correction of hypovolemia and uterine artery embolization [19].

Prolonged third stage of labor (greater than 30 minutes) is usually caused by retained placenta (a portion of the placenta is trapped behind a closed cervix) or adherent placenta (partial or complete accreta). Active management of the third stage of labor is important; this will decrease blood loss and shorten the second stage of labor. Actively managed patients have a third stage of 15.5 minutes versus 18 minutes in those without active management [20]. Risk of hemorrhage increases with increasing length of time for the third stage. Ultrasound can be useful as a diagnostic tool and should be deployed. Initial management involves manual extraction, intraumbilical oxytocin (30 units oxytocin in 30 units of saline), or nitroglycerin 200mcg IV [21]. If more conservative management fails, operative banjo curette can per performed in the delivery room to facilitate removal [22]. One must consider the possibility of accreta and the need for emergent hysterectomy, especially in patients with previous abdominal delivery.

Medical Management

Initial labs in a patient with postpartum hemorrhage include blood count, type and cross for blood products, prothrombin time, partial prothrombin time, and fibrinogen. Supportive care measures must be initiated; these include securing additional intravenous access, warming protocols to prevent hypothermia and placement of a Foley catheter to track volume status. Activation of the unit-based hemorrhage policy, and blood bank notification are also important initial management measures.

Two important guiding principles in the initial management of hemorrhage are resuscitation and treatment. In the resuscitation stage, transfusion should be per clinical signs especially pulse and blood pressure. As the hemorrhage continues to progress, transfusion is dictated by lab parameters, with a plan to prevent and reverse the process of disseminated intravascular coagulation (DIC). It is also important to remember other needed supportive measures when the patient is in this critical state including the correction metabolic acidosis, prevention of hypothermia and initiation of uterotonic agents.

Uterotonic agents are the mainstay for medical management as close to 90% of postpartum hemorrhages arise from uterine atony. Oxytocin is used in the active management of the third stage of labor, and additional dosing may be used. Methergergonovine (methergine) and or 15-methyl PGF 2 alpha (Hemabate) Methergergonovine 2mg IM can be used next; however, it should be avoided in patients with hypertension. The onset of medication is 3–5 minutes and can be dosed every 2 to 4 hours, with a maximum of five doses. Except for the exclusion of patients with hypertension, this drug is well tolerated as a good option early in the course of a hemorrhage. Hemabate is an additional pharmacologic agent that is dosed as 250 micrograms. The time of onset for this drug is also 3–5 minutes, and it can be dosed every 20 minutes, with a maximum dosing of 6 minutes. Hemabate is highly effective; however it needs to be avoided in asthmatic patients. Its side effects include significant nausea, vomiting and diarrhea.

Additional uterotonic agents include misoprostol (cytotec) and dinoprostone (dinoprostee2). Dinopostone is an older agent with a significant side effect profile which is not currently in wide use. Misoprostol is gaining acceptance in the use of postpartum hemorrhage, due in part to its availability on most obstetrical units. It is also is being considered in low resource settings, due to the ease of administration and the low cost [23]. A recent Cochrane review showed that oral misoprostol had efficacy in the reduction of postpartum hemorrhage, but should not be used as a replacement for other first line agents such as oxytocin [24,25]. Several doing regiments and routes (rectal and oral) have been recommended; there is no consensus on which is preferable.

Recombinant factor 7a (rFVIIa) has been proposed as a newer method to treat refractory postpartum hemorrhage. Initially developed for treatment of hemophiliacs, at therapeutic doses, it causes activation of factor X on the surface of platelets and enhances the conversion of prothrombin to thrombin. This action subsequently causes enhanced clotting at the site of bleeding [26]. Although still considered experimental, its use in obstetrics is promising. In cases of refractory postpartum hemorrhage, over 85% of patients had resolution of the hemorrhage after treatment [27]. The biggest barrier with this medication is the extremely high cost and the lack of availability on obstetrical units.

Tranexamic acid (Lysteda) is an antifibrinolytic drug, which, in essence, stabilizes fibrin and decreases bleeding. It was approved by Food and Drug Administration (FDA) in 2009 for use in heavy menstrual bleeding. Additionally, it has been used in prevention of blood loss in trauma patients [28]. Its relatively low cost, and the familiarity of use in gynecologic indications, make this a good alternative option in refractory postpartum hemorrhage. A recent Cochrane review concluded that tranexamic acid not only decreases blood loss in the face of postpartum hemorrhage, but also decreased the amount of blood products needed in postpartum hemorrhage management [29].

Tamponade Techniques

Atony is the source of most postpartum hemorrhages. Initial treatment approach includes compression of the atonic enlarged uterus. This can be accomplished with one hand in the vagina while compressing the uterus between the second hand on the abdomen. This technique can be employed while the obstetrical team is alerted to the presence of an impending hemorrhage. Additional measures include packing or mechanical compression devices. Packing with a large gauze soaked in thrombin (5,000 units in 5 ml of saline) placed into the uterine cavity can be therapeutic [2]. Mechanical compression can be accomplished with the use of a large Foley catheter, as expansion of the Foley balloon in the uterine cavity will cause compression of the uterus.

The Bakri balloon and ebb (Belfort–Dildy Obstetrical Tamponade System) are two devices engineered on the same basic principles as the Foley catheter, but have modifications specific for obstetrical compression purposes. The Bakri balloon can be filled to a maximum of 500 cc, which is much larger than what an average Foley balloon can accommodate. One of the problems with the Bakri balloon is that if the cervix is parous and dilated, the balloon may slip out and not provide effective compression against the uterine wall. A cerclage-like stich can be placed in the dilated cervix, but this can be technically challenging in a bleeding patient. The "ebb" or Belfort–Dildy Obstetrical Tamponade System is essentially a Bakri balloon with a second balloon in the vagina. This duel balloon system prevents slippage of the device, and in theory enhances uterine compression [30].

Surgical Management

Surgical management of uterine hemorrhage should be reserved for those cases in which medical or

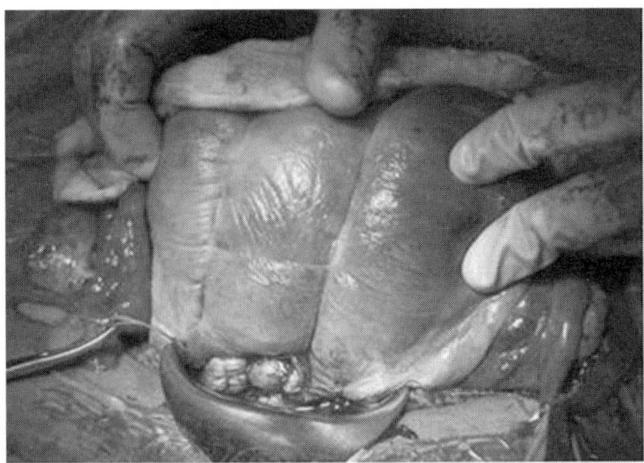

Figure 28.2 Uterus after B-lynch procedure. Image courtesy of Dipak Delvadia, DO, Clinical Associate Professor, Associate Residency Director, Department of Obstetrics and Gynecology, Drexel University College of Medicine.

compression methods have failed. Uterine curettage should not be performed for uterine atony, but only in cases of suspected retained products of conception. If the obstetric care provider plans to move to the operating room (OR) after a vaginal delivery, a midline skin incision is recommended for optimal exposure. All the major blood vessels which supply the uterus may be sutured to control blood flow to the uterus. Ligation of the uterine artery via the O'Leary stitch, followed by ligation of the uterine–ovarian plexus, the infundulopelvic ligament (containing the ovarian vessels) and the hypogastric arteries in a sequential fashion will each decrease the blood supply to the uterus. Hypogastric artery ligation is a technically challenging procedure, and should be performed by an advanced gynecologic surgeon only. Pregnancy has been reported after ligation of all the major blood vessels in the pelvis due to the rich arcade of collateral blood vessels. Newer suturing techniques, including the B-lynch suture or square suturing have gained popularity as surgical options to control postpartum hemorrhage. The B-lynch technique causes a fan-like compression of the large and atonic uterus and is held in place by absorbable suture. Square suturing places large, absorbable suture through the anterior and poster surface of the uterus in a square like fashion (see Figure 28.2). Both of these techniques have reported normal uterine cavities in subsequent pregnancies; however, there have been case reports of uterine synechiae and pyometra as complications [31,32].

The decision to move forward with a hysterectomy is a complex one. In a clinically unstable patient, this procedure may be lifesaving or may lead to further hemorrhage. Certainty if abnormal placentation is encountered, hysterectomy is the procedure of choice. Placenta accreta is most common when placenta previa presents in the face of a previous C-section. The risk increases with each additional C-section and is thought to be 11% if there are two previous C-sections with a previa, and 40% if there are three previous C-sections with a previa [33]. Performance of a supracervical hysterectomy may be indicated to shorten operative time.

Special Therapeutic Options

Uterine artery embolization (UAE) deserves special mention as a treatment option for postpartum hemorrhage. This procedure uses fluoroscopy to identify bleeding pelvic vessels and stops the bleeding by placement of hemostatic agents. UAE may be utilized prior to laparotomy if there is hemorrhage after a vaginal delivery. It can also be used in conjunction with massive hemorrhage during an abdominal delivery [34]. Since this procedure takes place outside of the labor and delivery unit, the patient must be stabilized for transfer to the radiology unit. Additionally, UAE is not available at many smaller facilities that provide obstetrical services.

Other measures, including cell saver technology and autologous maternal transfusion, can be strategies implemented prior to delivery in cases in which there is a high index of suspicion for massive blood loss.

Postpartum Hemorrhage Related to Special Circumstances

Uterine inversions are a rare cause of postpartum hemorrhage. A large Canadian study looked at the incidence of uterine inversion over a 40-year period and found the incidence to be 1 in 3,737 following spontaneous vaginal delivery (SVD), and 1 in 1860 following C- section [35]. The clinical picture is a postpartum hemorrhage with a large vaginal mass and lack of palpation of the uterine fundus abdominally. Uterine inversion can be caused by very aggressive traction on the uterine placenta during AMTSL. Risk factors for this condition are macrosomic infants, magnesium sulfate, adherent placenta, nulliparity and fundal insertion of the placenta [36]. The treatment is to quickly replace the everted fundus with manual pressure. If this in unsuccessful, uterine relaxants, such as terbutaline,

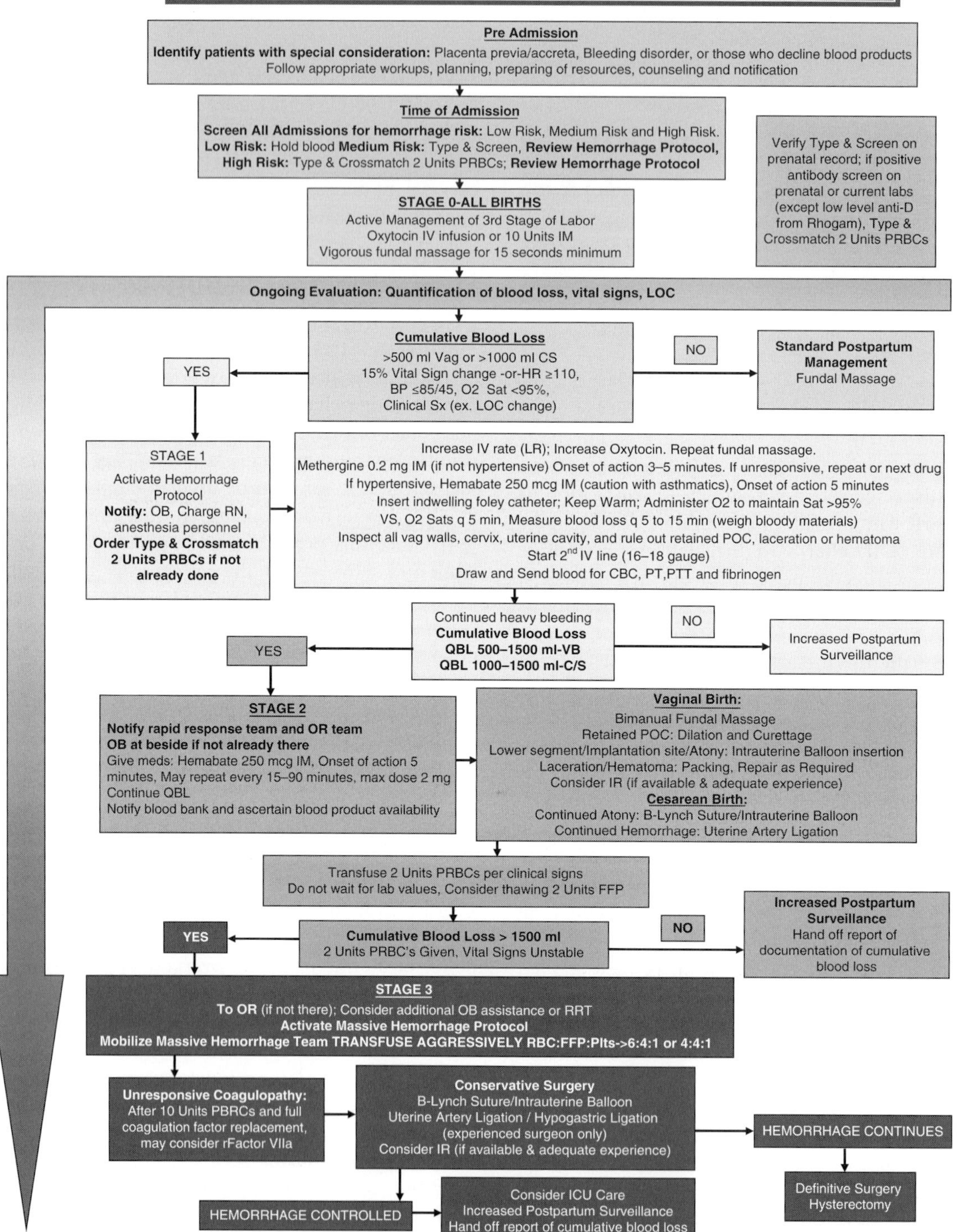

Figure 28.3 FPQC Care Guidelines. Figure reproduced with permission from Florida Perinatal Quality Collaborative (2015). Florida Obstetric Hemorrhage Initiative Toolkit: A Quality Improvement Initiative for Obstetric Hemorrhage Management. http://health.usf.edu/publichealth/chiles/fpqc/ohi. University of South Florida College of Public Health [43].

magnesium sulfate, nitroglycerine or general anesthesia, may be employed to promote replacement of the fundus [2]. Laparotomy is the last resort for replacement of the inverted uterus. The Huntington technique is employed when the round ligaments are grasped at laparotomy to pull the everted uterus back into place. Use of an obstetrical vacuum on the everted fundus to pull it back into place has also been described [36].

Uterine rupture is another rare cause of postpartum hemorrhage. The overall incidence of uterine rupture is reported to be 1% [36]. The most common risk factor is previous C-section, and the risk of rupture goes up proportionally to the number of previous C-sections. After previous C-section, trauma is the second strongest risk factor for uterine rupture.

Blood Replacement Products

Replacement of lost blood components is essential in postpartum hemorrhage management. Combat medicine in recent wars has taught much about the trauma response to massive hemorrhage. The principle of whole blood out, whole blood in (when available) is critical for proper resuscitation. Furthermore, early and aggressive crystalloid replacement may in fact enhance bleeding by increasing hydrodilution of clotting factors [37]. Traditional transfusion guidelines focusing primarily on replacement with packed red blood cells (PRBC) have been replaced with transfusion guidelines that recommend ratios of 1 unit PRBC to 1 unit of fresh frozen plasma to 1 unit of platelets [38]. Best practice guidelines includes a hospital wide massive transfusion protocol (MTP). This protocol should be available to the obstetrical providers in the case of a massive hemorrhage.

Quality Improvement

Maternal hemorrhage is one of the most preventable causes of maternal morbidity and mortality. Organized and deliberate quality improvement programs in maternal hemorrhage can reduce the morbidity [39]. Standardized unit-based guidelines have also been shown to improve care and reduce maternal consequences of hemorrhage [40]. Numerous guidelines exist and national societies are working together to decrease maternal effects of hemorrhage; state quality collaborative efforts have also been instrumental in this change [41]. The California Maternal Quality Collaborative (CMCC) has had a maternal hemorrhage quality collaborative in place since 2008. At that time, the maternal mortality in California was similar to the rate in the rest of the United States at 14–16 per 100,000. In 2012, the maternal mortality rate in the United States continued to rise and was 18 per 100,000, whereas in California the rate fell to 6.3 per 100,000 [42]. The Florida Perinatal Quality Collaborative (FPQC) stages of maternal hemorrhage is a simple graphic that illustrates a comprehensive maternal hemorrhage quality program (Figure 28.3) The escalation of the interventions based on the stages makes this a very useful tool when implementing a program, and creating culture change within a unit.

Box 28.3 Standardized Unit Based Maternal Safety Bundle [40]

Readiness (every facility)

1. Hemorrhage cart
2. Immediate access to hemorrhage medications (kit or equivalent)
3. Establish a response team
4. Protocols for emergency release of blood products and for massive transfusion
5. Unit education on protocols: Regular unit-based drills with debriefs

Recognition and prevention (every patient)

6. Assessment of hemorrhage risk
7. Measurement of cumulative blood loss
8. Active management of third stage of labor

Response (every hemorrhage)

9. Obstetric hemorrhage emergency management plan
10. Support program for patients, families and staff

Reporting and systems learning (every unit)

11. Establish a culture of huddles and debriefs
12. Multidisciplinary review of serious hemorrhages
13. Monitor outcomes and process metrics

Further recommendations, developed by National Partnership for Maternal Safety, put forth a comprehensive call to action for all obstetrical units to develop a standardized unit based maternal safety bundle. The key domains include readiness, recognition, response and reporting, with individual elements within the domains (Box 28.3). Adoption of the principles of the elements across all obstetrical units is the goal. Some smaller obstetrical units may not be able to adopt all of these recommendations, however through risk assessment it is anticipated that the highest risk patients can be sent to facilities with expanded capabilities to manage such complex situations.

Concluding Remarks

The consequences of maternal hemorrhage can be devastating. Clinical understating must start with identification of risk factors and early recognition of hemorrhage, active management of the third stage of labor and proper use of medications, including traditional uterotonics as well as an understanding of the newer antifibrinolytic agents. Invasive procedures, ranging from simple compression balloons to emergent hysterectomy, all must be employed as part of a deliberate and organized approach to hemorrhage.

References

1. M. Lu, M Fridman, L Korst. Variations in the incidence of postpartum hemorrhage across hospital in California. *Matern Child Health J* 2005;9:297.
2. ACOG Practice Bulletin. Clinical management guidelines for obstetrician-gynecologists number 76, October 2006: Postpartum hemorrhage (reaffirmed in 2015). *Obstet Gynecol* 2006;108: 1039–1047.
3. Y. Oyelese, C. Ananth. Postpartum hemorrhage: Epidemiology, risk factors, and causes. *Clinical Obstet Gynecol* 2010; 53(1):147–156.
4. W. Callaghan, E. Kuklina, C. Berg. Trends in postpartum hemorrhage: United States, 1994–2006. *Am J Obstet Gynecol* 2010;202(4):353.e1–6.
5. C. Berg, M. Harper, S. Atkinson, E. Bell, H. Brown, M. Hage, A. Mitra, K. Moise, W. Callaghan. Preventability of pregnancy-related deaths: Results of a state-wide review. *Obstet Gynecol* 2005; 106(6):1228–1234.
6. M Gordon, Maternal physiology, in S. Gabbe, J. Niebyl, H. Galan, E. Jauniaux, M, Landon, J. Simpson, D. Driscoll, editors. *Obstetrics: Normal and Problem Pregnancies*, 6th edition. Philadelphia: Elsevier Health Sciences, 2012.
7. J. Pritchard. Changes in blood volume during pregnancy and delivery. *Anesthesiology* 1965;26:393.
8. C. Combs, E. Murphy, R. Laros. Factors associated with postpartum hemorrhage with vaginal birth. *Obstet Gynecol* 1991;77:69–76.
9. L. Wetta, J. Szychowski, S. Seals, M. Mancuso, J. Biggio, A. Tita. Risk factors for uterine atony/postpartum hemorrhage requiring treatment after vaginal delivery. *Am J Obstet Gynecol* 2013 Jul; 209(1):51.e1–51.e6.
10. E. Magann, S. Evans, M. Hutchinson, R. Collins, B. Howard, J. Morrison, J. Postpartum hemorrhage after vaginal birth: An analysis of risk factors. *South Med J* 2005;98(4):419–420.
11. R. Silver. Abnormal placentation: Placenta previa, vasa previa, and placenta accreta. *Obstet Gynecol* 2015 Sep;126(3):654–668.
12. S. Clark, K Simpson, G Knox. Oxytocin: New perspectives on an old drug. *Am J Obstet Gynecol* 2009;200:35.e16.
13. J. Belghiti, G. Kayem, C. Dupont C, R. Rudigoz R, M. Bouvier-Colle M, Deneux-Tharaux C, Oxytocin during labour and risk of severe postpartum haemorrhage: A population-based, cohort-nested case–control study. *BMJ Open* 2011;1:e000514.
14. C. Grotegut, M. Paglia, L. Johnson. Oxytocin exposure during labor among women with postpartum hemorrhage secondary to uterine atony. *Am J Obstet Gynecol* 2011; 204:56.e1–6.
15. I. Al-Zirqi, S. Vangen S, Forsén L, et al. Effects of onset of labor and mode of delivery on severe postpartum hemorrhage. *Am J Obstet Gynecol* 2009;201:273.e1-9.
16. S. Clark. Obstetric hemorrhage – Expert opinion *Semin Perinatol* 2015; 15:176–7.
17. G. Westhoff, A. Cotter, J. Tolosa. Prophylactic oxytocin for the third stage of labor to prevent postpartum hemorrhage. *Cochrane Database Syst Rev* 2013;10;93.
18. D. Leduc, V. Senikas, A. Lalonde, C. Ballerman, A. Biringer, M. Delaney, L. Duperron, I. Girard, D. Jones, L. Lee, D. Shepherd, K. Wilson. Active management of the third stage of labour: Prevention and treatment of postpartum hemorrhage. Clinical Practice Obstetrics Committee; Society of Obstetricians and Gynaecologists of Canada *J Obstet Gynaecol Can* 2009;31(10):980–993.
19. S. Mawhinney, R. Holman.Puerperal genital haematoma: A commonly missed diagnosis. *Obstet Gynaecol* 2007;9:195–200.
20. Z. Saleem, H. Rydhstrom. Vaginal hematoma during parturition: A population-based study. *Acta Obstet Gynecol Scand* 2004; 83: 560–2.
21. W. Prendiville, D. Elbourne, S. McDonald. Active versus expectant management in the third stage of labour *Cochrane Database Syst Rev* 2000;3:CD000007.
22. A. Weeks. The retained placenta. *Best Prac Res Clin Obstet Gynaecol* 2008;22(6)1103–1117.
23. V Hundley, B Avan, C Sullivan, W Graham. Should oral misoprostol be used to prevent postpartum haemorrhage in home-birth settings in low-resource countries? A systematic review of the evidence. *Br J Obstet Gynecol* 2013; 120(3):277–285; discussion 86–87.
24. Ö Tunçalp, G Hofmeyr, A. Gülmezoglu. Prostaglandins for preventing postpartum haemorrhage *Cochrane Database Syst Rev* 2012;15;8.

25. A. Garrigue, F. Pierre. Misoprostol: Off-label use in the treatment of post-partum hemorrhage. *J Gynecol Obstet Biol Reprod* 2014;43(2):179–189.

26. M. Hoffman, D. Monroe. A cell-based model of hemostasis. *Thromb Haemost* 2001;85:958–965.

27. M. Franchini, M. Franchi, V. Bergamini, Montagnana M, Salvagno GL, Targher G, Lippi G. The use of recombinant activated FVII in postpartum hemorrhage. *Clin Obstet Gynecol* 2010;53(1):219–227.

28. K. Ker, I. Roberts, H. Shakur, T. Coats. Antifibrinolytic drugs for acute traumatic injury. *Cochrane Database Syst Rev* 2015 May 9;5.

29. N. Novikova, G. Hofmeyr, C. Cluver. Tranexamic acid for preventing postpartum haemorrhage. *Cochrane Database Syst Rev* 2015;6:CD007872.

30. G Dildy, M Belfort, C Adair. Initial experience with a dual-balloon catheter for the management of postpartum hemorrhage. *Am J Obstet Gynecol* 2014;210:136.e1–6.

31. H. Holtsemaa, R. Nijlanda, A. Huismanb, J. Donya, P. van den Berga The B-Lynch technique for postpartum haemorrhage: An option for every gynaecologist. *Eur J Obstet Gynecol Reproduc Biol* 2004;11(1):39–42.

32. J. Cho, H. Jun, C. Lee, Hemostatic suturing technique for uterine bleeding during cesarean delivery.*Obstet Gynecol* 2000;96(1):129–130.

33. R. Silver, M. Landon, D. Rouse, K. Leveno, C. Spong, E. Thom, A. Moawad, S. Caritis, M. Harper, R. Wapner, Y. Sorokin, M. Miodovnik, M. Carpenter, A Peaceman, M. O'Sullivan,B. Sibai, O.Langer, J. Thorp, S.; Ramin, B. Mercer, Maternal morbidity associated with multiple repeat cesarean deliveries. *Obstet Gynecol* 2006;107(6):1226–1232.

34. R. Winograd Uterine artery embolization for postpartum hemorrhage. *Best Pract Res Clin Obstet Gynaecol* 2008 Dec;22(6):1119–1132.

35. T. Baskett. Acute uterine inversion: A review of 40 cases. *Obstet Gynaecol Can* 2002;24(12):953–956.

36. F. Mirza, S. Gaddipati. Obstetric emergencies. *Semin Perinatol* 2009;33(2)97–103.

37. B. Ickx. Fluid and blood transfusion management in obstetrics. *Eur J Anaesthesiol* 2010; 27;1031–1035.

38. L. Pacheco MD, G. Saade, A. Gei, and G. Hankins. Cutting-edge advances in the medical management of obstetrical hemorrhage. *Am J Obstet Gynecol* 2011;205(6):526–532.

39. L. Shields, S Wiesner, J. Fulton, B. Pelletreau. Comprehensive maternal hemorrhage protocols reduce the use of blood products and improve patient safety. *Am J Obstet Gynecol* 2015;212:272–280.

40. E. Main, D. Goffman, B. Scavone, L. Low, D. Bingham, P. Fontaine, J. Gorlin, D. Lagrew,B. Levy. National Partnership for Maternal Safety: Consensus Bundle on Obstetric Hemorrhage. *Obstet Gynecol* 2015;126(1):155–162.

41. L.Shields, K. Smalarz, L. Reffigee, S, Mugg, T. Burdumy, M. Propst. Comprehensive maternal hemorrhage protocols improve patient safety and reduce utilization of blood products. *Am J Obstet Gynecol* 2011;205(4):368.e1–368.

42. California Maternal Quality Collaborative. www.cmqcc.org/focus-areas/maternal-mortality. Accessed January 20, 2016.

43. Florida Perinatal Quality Collaborative (2015). Florida Obstetric Hemorrhage Initiative Toolkit: A Quality Improvement Initiative for Obstetric Hemorrhage Management. http://health .usf.edu/publichealth/chiles/fpqc/ohi. University of South Florida College of Public Health. Accessed January 20, 2016.

Postpartum Infection

David Churchill and Mahmoud Moussa

Introduction

Sepsis is a major cause of mortality around the world. Over the last 15 years, there has been an increased focus on understanding the pathophysiological processes and improving the management of the infection in pregnant and postpartum women. Infection is a major cause of maternal mortality in both developed and developing countries. Most of the deaths occur in postnatal women although the origin of the infection may have occurred in the antenatal period. When infection is diagnosed, the need for treatment is urgent. Two key components of therapy are antibiotics and intravenous fluids. If treatment is not forthcoming in a timely way, then disease may progress to septic shock, multi-organ failure and death.

Scope of the Problem

The most common causes of infection and sepsis post delivery are endometritis, urinary tract infections, surgical wound infections, mastitis and breast abscesses.

Data from the United States has shown that the overall mortality rate from sepsis has fallen (from 27.8% to 17.9% between 1979 and 2000). The incidence of the disease has, however, risen by 8% per year over the same time period. These trends are not specific to North America have been replicated around the world.[1] The same trends are true in pregnancy and the puerperium, where sepsis remains a significant cause of maternal mortality. Data published in 2014 shows that the proportion of maternal deaths caused by sepsis is roughly the same in developed and developing countries despite the widely differing opportunities for access to healthcare for their citizens.[2]

Data from two large epidemiology studies, one in the United States and one from the UK, show that the incidence of severe sepsis and septic shock in pregnancy is between 4.9 and 5.6/10,000 and for sepsis overall, 10/10,000.[3]

In the 2014 report produced by Mothers and Babies Reducing Risk through Audits and Confidential Enquiries across the UK (MBRRACE-UK) it was noted that there was a decline in the maternal mortality from sepsis, and specifically, a statistically significant fall in genital tract sepsis. Sepsis nevertheless was still the second highest direct cause of maternal death in these countries between 2009 and 2012.[4]

Definitions

Formerly sepsis was defined as a combination of two or more clinical criteria from the systemic inflammatory response syndrome (SIRS) in the presence of, or a strong suspicion for, an infection. As understanding of the process progressed, the disease became classified as severe sepsis when it was associated with organ dysfunction, lactic acidosis, altered mental state, or hypotension. It was called septic shock when persistent hypotension was present. The definitions were revised in February 2016 by the European Society of Intensive Care Medicine (ESICM) and the Society of Critical Care Medicine (SCCM).[5]

The driving factors for the change were that the causes for SIRS also include pancreatitis, trauma, burns, and surgery, and the elements of the syndrome were poor prognostic indicators for mortality. The new definitions dispense with SIRS and define sepsis as "life threatening organ dysfunction caused by a dysregulated host response to infection." Formerly this was called severe sepsis. Septic shock is a subset of sepsis associated with underlying circulatory and cellular/metabolic abnormalities profound enough to substantially increase mortality. The clinical parameters that specify the criteria for these diagnoses arise out of the sequential organ failure assessment (SOFA)

Box 29.1 The sequential organ failure assessment criteria (SOFA)

- Respiration $PaO_2/Fi\ O_2$
- Coagulation – platelet count
- Liver – bilirubin
- Cardiovascular – mean arterial pressure (MAP) and use of inotropes
- Central nervous system (CNS) – Glasgow coma score
- Renal – creatinine and urine output

Quick SOFA

- Respiration rate ≥ 22/min
- Altered mental state / consciousness Glasgow Coma Scale (GCS) <15
- Low blood pressure – systolic < 100 mmHg

score, which has been found to be more efficient at predicting mortality.[6] See Box 29.1.

SIRS is, however, still useful as a clinical tool for identifying women who have significant disorders in pregnancy when the most frequent cause is likely to be infection. While the definition of sepsis may therefore change, retaining the concept of SIRS helps understand the nature of the pathophysiological insult in women with serious illnesses.

Risk Factors

Common risk factors have been identified for severe sepsis. Ethnicity (Black or other ethnic minority group), low socio-economic status, primigravidity, diabetes, hypertension and the mode of delivery are all independent risk factors. In addition, the United Kingdom Obstetric Surveillance Study (UKOSS) identified primiparity, operative delivery, a febrile illness and/or treatment with antibiotics within the two weeks prior to presentation as additional risk factors. This study also reported that with a greater number of risk factors, the risk of sepsis was incremental.

Clinical Management

The key to the successful management of a woman with sepsis is early diagnosis and prompt systematic intervention. Once treatment has been initiated, ongoing monitoring of the patient's condition with charting of the progress of vital physiological signs is mandatory. If continuing deterioration of the patient is documented, then alternative actions must be taken in a timely way to restore the patient to health.

Box 29.2 Sepsis Six care bundle

3 in

- Take an arterial blood gas and give high flow oxygen if required
- Take blood cultures
- Take blood for hemoglobin and lactate levels

3 out

- Commence intravenous antibiotics
- Start intravenous fluid resuscitation
- Measure the urine output hourly

Source: Adapted from The UK Sepsis Trust 2013.

Once the diagnosis of sepsis is made, the application of a "care bundle," such as the Sepsis Six care bundle with its three-in and three-out approach, will ensure systematic deployment of life sustaining treatments as well as prepare the patient for ongoing monitoring.[7] See Box 29.2.

Some controversy exists over whether the application of care bundles and a goal-oriented approach to treating patients with sepsis improves outcomes. One study found non-compliance with 6- and 24-hour sepsis bundles in a UK hospital was associated with a more than twofold increase in mortality.[8] Additionally, a randomized trial of early goal-directed therapy (EGDT) of early septic shock applied in emergency departments did not improve outcomes for these patients.[9]

Clear evidence of benefit, therefore, has yet to be proven. But notwithstanding the controversy, a sepsis care bundle will ensure the early and optimal delivery of care to these patients while the clinician then develops the ongoing clinical strategy to identify the infection and deal with it in the most efficient way possible. Discovery of the correct diagnosis and implementation of the right treatments is the important factor rather than the bundles themselves. The two key elements of early treatment are the administration of antibiotics and circulatory support with intravenous fluids.

Antibiotics

Time to administration of antibiotics is critical to reduction of the risk of death. The concept of golden hour has been developed since it has become known that every hour's delay in the administration of antibiotics from the time of diagnosis results in an 8% increase in mortality.[10]

Decisions on antibiotic selection are difficult because sensitivities and resistances of bacteria to specific antibiotics varies from locality to locality. The decision also depends on the most likely organism(s) causing the infection. The principle of first starting with a combination of broad-spectrum antibiotics, before narrowing the antibiotic spectrum once the microbiological culture results are known, is the best approach. Advice from local microbiologists is important. Local experts will have knowledge of the current status with respect to organism resistance in the region. All hospitals should have antibiotic policies that reflect the local rates of resistance.

Box 29.3 Causes of fever and infection after delivery

- Wound infections including abdominal and perineal wounds
- Urinary tract infections – cystitis, pyelonephritis
- Endometritis including infected retained products
- Post caesarean section pelvic abscess
- Mastitis
- Breast abscess
- Septic thrombophlebitis
- Drug reactions and *Clostridium difficile*
- Anesthetic complications

Fluid Management

No definitive evidence guides decisions on which type of fluid is the best to use when supporting the circulation of patients with sepsis. Concern has been raised over the issue of hyperchloremia possibly causing acute kidney injury resulting from infusions of large volumes of sodium chloride. Controversy continues about whether albumin or artificial plasma expanders or crystalloid are better in maintaining an expanded circulation persist.[11,12] The current view is to support the circulation with a buffered crystalloid solution rather than saline and if a plasma expander is required then to use a colloid solution. If fluid boluses of 30 ml/kg over 30 minutes, followed if necessary by continuous infusions of 20 ml/kg/hour, fail to maintain a satisfactory circulatory blood pressure (a mean arterial pressure (MAP) > 65 mmHg or a central venous pressure (CVP) > 8 mmHg), then inotropic support will be required. The inotropic drug of choice is norepinephrine as dopamine has been found to be associated with a higher mortality.[13]

Causes of Postnatal Sepsis

The main sources of postpartum infections are the genitourinary tract, breast, surgical sites and drug-related gastrointestinal disorders. Although other causes occur they are rare in comparison. See Box 29.3.

Endometritis

Endometritis is often recognized early and resolves with a course of oral antibiotics but it can have deadly consequences, especially when the infecting organism is the group A *Streptococcus* (GAS), *Streptococcus pyogenes*. The causative organisms are by no means limited to GAS. The infection is most commonly made up of a mixture of two or three anaerobic and/or aerobic species arising from the genital tract. Other organisms include *Staphylococci*, *Clostridia*, *Escherichia coli*, bacterial vaginosis, among others.

Risk factors for the development of endometritis include chorioamnionitis, prolonged labor and prolonged rupture of membranes, thick meconium, operative vaginal delivery and group B *Streptococcus* colonization.

The clinical features of endometritis are fever, lower central abdominal pain, offensive lochia, a tender uterus on examination, a general feeling of ill health and malaise. Some women may describe symptoms of a urinary tract infection or diarrhea if there is more widespread pelvic inflammation. With some species of bacteria, necrosis may develop within the endometrium and myometrium, which is the most severe form of the disease.

If endometritis is untreated, toxic shock syndrome may develop with symptoms that could include a high fever above 38°C and rigors or sometimes a low temperature < 35°C. Other signs of toxic shock syndrome may include increasingly severe pain, vomiting, diarrhea, altered mental state and in the later stages a depressed level of consciousness, persistent hypotension and multi-organ dysfunction, including renal failure.

Investigation of Patients with Suspected Endometritis

The diagnosis of endometritis is largely made on clinical findings. Hematological, biochemical and microbiological investigations, however, help to confirm the diagnosis and are also valuable to track the resolution or deterioration of the disease process in response to treatment. All patients should therefore have a full blood count, C-reactive protein, urea, creatinine, electrolytes and lactate measurements. In addition, blood and urine should be taken for cultures. Swabs from all potential sites of infection should be assessed as part of a broad differential diagnosis including infections other than endometritis. This assessment includes a swab of the throat to look for GAS.

It should be remembered that treatment must *not* be deferred until the results of blood cultures are known. In about 50% of cases, organisms will not be cultured even in the presence of florid sepsis.

When the source of infection is believed to be endometritis, it may be important to image the uterus for retained products of conception, which may be precipitating cause of the intrauterine infection. An ultrasound will usually be adequate, but in cases of severe sepsis, a CT scan may be required to exclude a necrotizing process.

Source control in all cases of sepsis is mandatory. The management is as outlined earlier with fluids and antibiotics, but relying on antibiotics is often insufficient in severe disease and courts disaster. Surgical excision or drainage may be required to ensure the full resolution of sepsis. In severe cases where there is necrotizing fasciitis or myometritis, excision of the necrosed tissue including possibly a hysterectomy will be necessary and is very often life-saving.

Mastitis and Breast Abscesses

Mastitis

Mastitis occurs in 2–10% of lactating mothers. It is usually unilateral and is associated with fever, myalgia and systemic flu like symptoms. This distinguishes it from breast engorgement, which is bilateral and not usually associated with systemic disturbance. With mastitis, an area of the affected breast is painful, swollen and erythematous, and there is often palpable axillary lymphadenopathy on the affected side. In addition to the usual investigations, culturing the breast milk may help in guiding the choice of antibiotic.

The most common organism causing mastitis is *Staphylococcus aureus*, although *S. pyogenes*, *E. coli* and bacteroides are also possibilities. The condition usually responds to simple antibiotics such as penicillin, cephalosporin or clindamycin.[14]

Antibiotics will require time to take effect, but during this interval symptomatic relief can be provided with cold compresses, non-steroidal analgesics and complete emptying of the breast by whatever method is least distressing to the mother. The mother may continue to breastfeed during treatment but the baby's pediatrician should be notified that the neonate will be exposed to antibiotic medication. Prior to the availability of microbiological cultures the antibiotics of choice are amoxicillin/clavulanic acid and metronidazole if anaerobic infection is suspected. An alternative drug to amoxicillin/clavulanic acid is cephalexin or in penicillin-sensitive patients clindamycin.

A failure in response raises the possibility of methicillin-resistant *S. aureus* (MRSA). While some MRSA infections will respond to clindamycin, severe infections will require empirical treatment with vancomycin. It is recommended that if there is no improvement in the patient's condition within 48 hours, ultrasound imaging of the breast is undertaken to examine for any evidence of a deep-seated abscess.

Breast Abscess

Breast abscesses are an uncommon problem, occurring in less than 1% of lactating women. The incidence does rise with lactational mastitis to around 3%.[15] Smoking is as a significant risk factor for the development of breast abscesses, with an odds ratio of 8.[16]

In addition to the symptoms associated with lactational mastitis, on exam, a palpable tender fluctuant mass will be palpable. Ultrasound helps to guide aspiration of the abscess in more difficult cases where there may be multiple locules of purulent material. Surgical drainage is required if the overlying skin shows evidence of breaking down, or if there is a poor response to needle aspiration. The antibiotic options are the same as with mastitis unless cultures reveal an organism with different sensitivities.

Urinary Tract Infections

The incidence of urinary tract infection postpartum is said to be between 2% and 3% but the rate is influenced by vaginal procedures, catheterization and epidural anesthesia.[17]

Urinary catheters should be removed as soon as possible to reduce the risk, but in women who do develop symptoms, antibiotics are usually successful in eliminating the infection. Sepsis is most likely to occur with the development of acute pyelonephritis. If any signs of flank or renal angle tenderness develop, then consideration should be given about admitting the woman to the hospital and treating her with intravenous antibiotics and fluids. If admission is not accepted, then close out-patient follow-up will be necessary.

Surgical Site and Wound Infections

Cesarean section and episiotomy wounds, as well as wounds resulting from vaginal and perineal trauma, are sources of potential infection and sepsis. The rate of infection in low transverse cesarean wounds is about 5%.[18]

The current trend for early discharge means that most wound infections are now diagnosed in the community as they tend to develop 4 to 5 days post surgery. The most common organisms are *Streptococci*, affecting early wound infections, i.e. within 48 hours and *Staphylococci*, *E. coli* and proteus in later infections. When there is no identifiable abscess, treatment with antibiotics and close follow-up form the best management. For early wound infections, amoxicillin/clavulanic acid or a combination of cephalexin and metronidazole are good first-line antibiotics while waiting for the results of cultures. Clindamycin is a good choice for those who are allergic to penicillin and where the suspicion is that a group A *Streptococcus* may be the causative organism. If *Staphylococcus* is suspected, then flucloxacillin can be used. If an abscess develops and there is no spontaneous discharge of the pus, then surgical drainage should be performed to avoid a prolonged course before healing of the wound. At times, the wound must be opened and allowed to heal by secondary intention.

Necrotizing fasciitis is an extremely dangerous infection, which may progress very rapidly. It may initially look like a simple wound infection. Necrotizing fasciitis occurs in a small number of women post caesarean section.[19] In addition to the therapies described above, aggressive debridement of all the affected tissues is mandatory, as antibiotics alone will not be effective. Delay in therapy is associated with increased mortality. Without surgery, the mortality is 100% for necrotizing fasciitis.[20]

Perineal infections in tears or episiotomy wounds are associated with a prolonged second stage of labor, instrumental deliveries and third and fourth degree tears. They usually result in breakdown of the skin and subcutaneous tissues and can be treated conservatively with drainage, debridement and regular cleansing, allowing healing by secondary intention. Large defects may need to be re-sutured when the wound is clean and covered with pink granulation tissue. Antibiotics are usually reserved for women with associated cellulitis.

Septic Pelvic Thrombophlebitis

Septic pelvic thrombophlebitis (SPT) is one of two conditions, deep septic pelvic thrombophlebitis (DSPT) or ovarian vein thrombosis (OVT). The incidence is reported to be 1 in 9,000 for vaginal deliveries and 1 in 800 for cesarean deliveries.[21] They may occur in tandem; the underlying pathology of both conditions is thrombosis of pelvic veins. The etiology involves endothelial damage caused by trauma to the pelvic veins during delivery in association with venous stasis resulting from the low pressures in the pelvic vessels, especially in the ovarian vein and the hypercoaguable state induced by pregnancy are the causes of the thrombosis.

SPT of either variety usually presents within one week of delivery or surgery. DSPT causes a fever without an obvious source, which persists despite antibiotic therapy. OVT, in addition to the fever, is associated with abdominal and pelvic pain localized to the affected side radiating to the back. There may also be mild gastrointestinal or urinary symptoms and when the patient is examined pelvic tenderness is usually elicited. In severe cases, a pelvic examination may not be tolerated, but in cases of OVT a mass may be palpable. Given the constellation of symptoms the condition is often confused with endometritis.

Investigation of SPT is difficult. There are no specific laboratory tests to positively diagnose the condition. Leukocytosis may be observed and be persistent and blood cultures may be negative. However, these investigations are useful in ruling out other causes for the sepsis. Imaging is equally problematic and both computed tomography (CT) and magnetic resonance (MR) scanning have been used. Both have their limitations and cannot be exclusively relied upon to diagnose the thromboses, although more success has been recorded with detection of OVT than DSPT. CT scanning is preferred to MR imaging. There is, however, a note of caution. Thirty asymptomatic women 4 days after a vaginal delivery agreed to undergo screening using magnetic resonance venography and it was discovered that 20 of them had evidence of non-obstructing venous thrombosis.[22]

Because of the limitations outlined earlier, the conditions have largely become diagnoses of exclusion.

The treatment of choice for the condition includes antibiotics and anticoagulation. By the time the diagnosis is made, the woman will have usually been on broad-spectrum antibiotics for some time. In such a case, the advice of a microbiologist may be required but the antibiotic choices are likely to include piperacillin or meropenem or a third-generation cephalosporin with the addition of metronidazole. The anticoagulant of choice is a low molecular weight heparin such as enoxaparin at 1mg/kg every 12 hours. A return to a normal temperature after 48 hours of treatment with anticoagulation helps to confirm the diagnosis, although some studies have reported a longer period of time (up to 5 days) for the fever to resolve.[23] Anticoagulation will also help to reduce the risk of the extension of the thrombosis into the pelvic veins and prevent pulmonary emboli.

SPT is a very difficult diagnosis to make. Diagnosis relies upon clinician awareness of the possibility and frequently involves making the diagnosis by exclusion.

Concluding Remarks

Sepsis can be a deadly condition if not treated quickly and thoroughly. It is responsible for a high level of maternal mortality in both the developed and developing world. Although the number of deaths have fallen, the overall incidence and severity of sepsis in the general population is increasing. This rise is due to increases in the number of patients older than 65 years, immunecompromise and multiple medical co-morbidities. For women in the postnatal period, the main causes of sepsis are infections such as endometritis, mastitis, breast abscesses and surgical site infections including perineal trauma wounds. Rapid treatment with antibiotics, intravenous fluid support for the circulation and surgical control for the source of the infection, if known, are key components of successful management.

References

1. Martin GS, Mannino DM, Eaton S, Moss M. The epidemiology of sepsis in the United States from 1979 through 2000. *N Engl J Med.* 2003;348:1546–54.
2. Kassebaum NJ, Bertozzi-Villa A, Coggeshall MS, et al. Global regional and national levels and causes of maternal mortality during 1990–2013: A systematic analysis for the global burden of disease study 2013. *Lancet.* 2014;384:980–1004.
3. Acosta CD, Knight M, Lee HC, Kurinczuk JJ, Gould JB, Lyndon A. The continuum of maternal sepsis severity: Incidence and risk factors in a population based cohort study. *PLoS ONE.* 2013;8(7): e67175. doi:10.1371/journal.pone.0067175
4. Churchill D, Rodger A, Clift J, Tuffnell D. on behalf of the MBRRACE UK Sepsis Chapter Writing Group. Think Sepsis. In Knight M, Kenyon S, Brocklehurst P, Neilson J, Shakespeare J, Kurinczuk JJ (Eds.) *On behalf of MBRRACE-UK Saving Lives, Improving Mothers' Care – Lessons learned to inform future maternity care from UK and Ireland Confidential Enquiries into Maternal deaths and Morbidity 2009–12. Oxford: National Perinatal Epidemiology Unit.* University of Oxford 2014: pp. 27–43.
5. The Third International Consensus Definitions for Sepsis and Septic Shock (Sepsis-3) *JAMA.* 2016;315(8):801–10.
6. Jones AE, Trzeciak S and Kline JA. The sequential organ failure assessment score for predicting outcome in patients with severe sepsis and evidence of hypoperfusion at the time of emergency department presentation.*Crit Care Med.* 2009;37:1649–54.
7. UK Sepsis Trust (2013). "Clinical Tools." http://sepsistrust.org/info-for-professionals/clinical-tools/.
8. Goa F, Melody T, Daniels DF, et al. The impact of compliance with 6-hour and 24-hour sepsis bundles on hospital mortality in patients with severe sepsis: A prospective observational study. *Critical Care.* 2005;9:R764-R770.
9. Yealy DM, Huang T, Barnato AE, et al. On behalf of the ProCESS Investigators. A randomized trial of protocol-based care for early septic shock. *N Engl J Med.* 2014;370:1683–93.
10. Kumar A, Roberts D, Wood KE, Light B, et al. Duration of hypotension before initiation of effective antimicrobial therapy is the critical determinant of survival in human septic shock. *Crit Care Med.* 2006,34;1589–1596.
11. Patel A, Laffan MA, Waheed U, Brett SJ. Randomised trials of human albumin for adults with sepsis: A systematic review and meta-analysis with trial sequential analysis of all-cause mortality. *BMJ.* 2014;349:g4561.
12. Caironi P, Tognoni G Masson S, et al. ALBIOS Study Investigators. Albumin replacement in patients with severe sepsis or septic shock. *NEJM.* 2014;370:1412–21.
13. Dellinger RP, Levy MM, Rhodes A, et al. Surviving Sepsis Campaign Guidelines Committee including the Pediatric Subgroup. Surviving sepsis campaign: International guidelines for the management of severe sepsis and septic shock: 2012 *Crit Care Med.* 2013;41:580–637.
14. Jahanfar S, Ng CJ, Teng CL Antibiotics for mastitis in breastfeeding women. *Cochrane Database Syst Rev.* 2013 Feb 28;(2):CD005458. doi: 10.1002/14651858.CD005458.pub3.

15. Amir LH, Forster D, McLachlan H, Lumley J. Incidence of breast abscess in lactating women: Report from an Australian cohort. *BJOG*. 2004;111(12):1378.

16. Gollapalli V, Liao J, Dudakovic A, Sugg SL, Scott-Conner CE, Weigel RJ.Risk factors for development and recurrence of primary breast abscesses. *J Am Coll Surg*. 2010;211(1):41.

17. Stray-Pedersen B, Solberg VM, Torkildsen E, Lie S, Velken M, Aaserud J, Kierulf KA, Blakstad M, Ulshagen K, Sandstad B. Postpartum bacteriuria. A multicenter evaluation of different screening procedures and a controlled short-course treatment trial with amoxycillin. *Eur J Obstet Gynecol Reprod Biol*. 1989;31(2):163.

18. Olsen MA, Butler AM, Willers DM, Devkota P, Gross GA, Fraser V. Risk factors for surgical site infection after low transverse cesarean section. *J Infect Control Hosp Epidemiol*. 2008;29(6):477.

19. Sarsam SE, Elliott JP, Lam GK. Management of wound complications from cesarean delivery. *Obstet Gynecol Surv*. 2005;60(7):462.

20. Anaya DA, Dellinger EP. Necrotizing soft-tissue infection: Diagnosis and management. *Clin Infect Dis*. 2007;44(5):705

21. Wysokinska EM, Hodge D, McBane RD. Ovarian vein thrombosis: Incidence of recurrent venous thromboembolism and survival. *Thromb Haemost*. 2006;96(2):126.

22. Khalil H, Avruch L, Olivier A, Walker M, Rodger M. The natural history of pelvic vein thrombosis on magnetic resonance venography after vaginal delivery. *Am J Obstet Gynecol*. 2012 Apr;206(4):356.

23. Brown TK, Munsick RA. Puerperal ovarian vein thrombophlebitis: A syndrome. *Am J Obstet Gynecol*. 1971;109(2):263.

Chapter

30 The Obstetric Patient with Trauma

Felicity Plaat and Charles Cox

Introduction

Trauma is the most common cause of deaths among young adults worldwide. It is in addition a major cause of death and morbidity in the obstetric population (1). Trauma complicates between 6% and 8% of pregnancies in the United States (2). Data from trauma registries in the United States and United Kingdom suggest that the incidence is on the increase. In the UK between 2009 and 2013, there were 152 traumatic deaths in the obstetric population [8% of the total), most involving suicide, followed by homicide and accidents (3).

Fetal mortality exceeds maternal mortality fivefold (1). The incidence of spontaneous abortion, stillbirth, preterm rupture of membranes, preterm birth, uterine rupture and placental abruption are increased in women who may have suffered sometimes minor trauma.

The most common threat to fetal well-being is maternal compromise and thus the most effective way to treat the fetus is to resuscitate the mother.

A multidisciplinary approach is essential in the management of trauma and all the more so when a pregnant patient is involved. It is essential to take into account the anatomical and physiological effects of pregnancy for assessment of trauma, the fetal response to asphyxia and the types and mechanism of injury in the obstetric population.

Unfortunately, little high-grade scientific evidence exists for the management of trauma; most knowledge is based on animal studies, retrospective clinical reviews, expert opinion and consensus statements.

Management of the trauma patient with a potentially viable fetus is particularly challenging and controversial aspects include the use of ionizing radiation and the role of perimortem cesarean section.

Scope of the Problem

In the United States, trauma is the leading non-obstetric cause of death in the obstetric population. Five to eight percent of women experience trauma while pregnant although less than 1% will require hospital admission. Of those that are admitted, however, one-third will deliver during the admission (4). In the UK, 1% of female trauma victims are pregnant; this group has a higher mortality than their non-pregnant counterparts.

Fetal death exceeds maternal mortality by approximately 3 to 1. The incidence of trauma related fetal deaths is estimated to be 3.7 per 100,000 live births. Fetal survival in one UK cohort was 56%, with fetal death most common in the second trimester (5). Fetal demise was most commonly associated with placental abruption. Penetrating trauma, although much less common than blunt, is associated with a much higher fetal and maternal mortality: 73% and 66% respectively (1). The injury severity score (ISS), developed for the non-pregnant trauma patient, is a good predictor of maternal death; prediction of fetal outcome is much less certain. Even minor maternal trauma is associated with increased placental abruption and preterm labor. In one study >50% of fetal deaths occurred to women who showed no signs of injury following trauma (ISS=0) (6).

The initial assessment of injury severity is not accurate at predicting placental abruption and fetal death. Relatively minor injuries may be associated with adverse pregnancy outcomes and ISS are not accurate in predicting placental abruption or fetal death (7).

The most common cause of trauma in the obstetric population is domestic violence. It is 40 times more common than the second leading cause – road traffic accidents. A US study estimated that 15% of pregnant women were victims of domestic violence (8). Other studies put the incidence at double this figure. What is not in question is that significant underreporting is a major problem for understanding of domestic violence. In the UK, 5% of all women who died were

Table 30.1 Trauma Deaths in the UK

	2000–2002	2003–2005	2006–2008	2009–2013*
Total deaths**	391	432	344	1048
Trauma deaths (% of all deaths)	51 [13]	83 [19]	58 [17]	152 [15]
Suicide	28	37	29	101
Homicide	11	19	11	36
Accidents (including RTAs)	12	27	18	15

* Including direct, indirect, late (<1 year post partum) and coincidental deaths.

** Figures only available for the five year period.

known to be victims of domestic abuse. Of these, a quarter died due to homicide. The most common cause of trauma, however, among those who died was suicide. The majority (>80%) of these patients with death by suicide used violent means such as hanging, jumping from a height or being hit by a train. These high levels of violent means in pregnant women compare with 60–65% of suicides in non-pregnant women (3). See Table 30.1 lists the trauma deaths in the UK.

Changes in Pregnancy Affecting Management of Trauma

Both anatomical and physiological changes in pregnancy will impact the assessment and management of the patient with trauma. The avoidance of aorto-caval compression is of primary importance. All patients with a pregnancy beyond 20 weeks (i.e. with the uterus above the pelvic brim) must be kept in the lateral or tilted position or have the uterus manually displaced from the inferior vena cava (see below). One of the recommendations from a recent report into maternal deaths in the UK was that all ambulance staff should be trained in the relief of aorto-caval compression during transfer of all pregnant women (3).

Airway and Respiratory Changes Affecting the Management of the Pregnant Trauma Patient

Because the pregnant patient is at increased risk of aspiration, early tracheal intubation is indicated. Providers should avoid securing the airway using the nasal route because of the risk of potentially catastrophic epistaxis due to engorged mucus membranes found in pregnancy.

Compared to the non-pregnant patient, difficulty maintaining the airway and intubating the trachea is increased 10- to 12-fold. This will be aggravated by the placement of a cervical spine collar; cervical spine collars are commonly required following blunt trauma and falls. Cervical spine trauma should be excluded as early as possible to allow the collar to be removed to facilitate airway maneuvers.

Oxygen demand by the pregnant patient increases by 20%. This intensifies the adverse impact of even minor falls in hemoglobin due to the related reduction in oxygen-carrying capacity.

An increase in minute ventilation (which is up by 40%) and decreased functional residual capacity (a 20% fall occurs) makes the pregnant patient particularly susceptible to hypoxemia. Even brief episodes of maternal hypoxemia can cause fetal acidosis, hypoxemia and compromise. All pregnant trauma patients should be given high flow oxygen as part of their initial management. Hyperventilation must be avoided because the resultant alkalosis causes vasoconstriction and shifts the oxygen dissociation curve to the right, further reducing fetal oxygenation.

The respiratory alkalosis caused by increased ventilation in pregnancy reduces bicarbonate, which is the blood's buffering capacity against acidosis of whatever type.

Cardiovascular and Hematologic Changes Affecting the Management of the Pregnant Trauma Patient

Plasma volume increases by 45% and there is an associated increase in cardiac output of 25% (1.5 L/min). The increase in cardiac output is due to both an increase in stroke volume and heart rate (increase of 5–10 beats per minute). Due to a fall in systemic vascular resistance, systemic blood pressure and central venous pressure remain within the normal range. There is a smaller increase in red cell mass compared to the plasma volume; this leads to the anemia of pregnancy (Hb 95–150 g/L) A hematocrit of 32–34% is normal for pregnancy.

Because of the increase in cardiac output and oxygen-carrying capacity, the pregnant patient is remarkably resilient to hypovolemia: she will present few signs before 2–3 liters of blood have been lost. Systolic blood pressure is therefore unreliable as an assessment tool since hypotension is a late sign. Early signs of shock include fetal heart rate changes as well as an increase in maternal respiratory rate. Conversely, tachycardia and increased respiratory rate should not be dismissed as normal for pregnancy in the case of trauma.

Uterine blood flow has no autoregulation: it is dependent on maternal blood pressure. Maternal hypovolemia will decrease not only if maternal blood pressure falls but also because there will be an alpha-adrenergic induced shift of blood volume centrally.

The risk of thromboembolic complications is increased four- to fivefold in pregnancy. A hypercoagulable state results from increased coagulation factors and decreased fibrinolytic activity. The increased venous stasis in the lower extremities compounds the risk. Trauma is also associated with hypercoagulability. In the immobilized trauma patient, in whom hemorrhage has been excluded, consideration should be given to thromboprophylaxis in the form of low molecular weight heparin and compression stockings or sequential compression devices. Conversely, the risk of developing disseminated intravascular coagulation in the presence of shock is also increased and early use of an anti-fibrinolytic drug is indicated.

Abdominal and Gastrointestinal Changes Affecting the Management of the Pregnant Trauma Patient

All trauma patients should be managed as if they have a full stomach and are thus at risk of aspiration. The pregnant patient is at even greater risk due reduced lower esophageal sphincter tone caused by mechanical effects of the enlarging uterus and effect of progesterone on smooth muscle. The conscious patient should be placed in the semi-recumbent position as soon as spinal injury has been excluded. If tracheal intubation is required, a rapid sequence induction of general anesthesia should be used to reduce the risk of aspiration.

Pregnant patients have reduced peritoneal sensitivity and may not demonstrate signs of abdominal injury such as rebound tenderness and guarding. If intraperitoneal injury is suspected, early ultrasound imaging should be used since computed tomography (CT) of the abdomen delivers a potentially damaging dose of radiation to the fetus (see imaging in pregnancy below).

Before 12 weeks gestation, because the uterus is still a pelvic organ, it is relatively protected from abdominal trauma. Displacement of intra-abdominal organs cephalad by the enlarging uterus provides some protection. Bowel injury is less common in the pregnant compared to non-pregnant patient.

Renal and Pelvic Changes Affecting the Management of the Pregnant Trauma Patient

Increased glomerular filtration is associated with a 30% increase in renal blood flow at term. This results in lowered serum creatinine (30–69mmol/L) and urea (1.1–3.9 mmol/L). Normal non-pregnant laboratory values may actually indicate compromised renal function in a pregnant patient.

By 28 weeks gestation, progesterone-induced widening of the symphysis pubis and sacroiliac joints can be noted. This should not be confused with pelvic fractures. When pelvic fractures occur, they may be associated with fetal skull fractures. Fetal skull fractures are associated with a 25% fetal mortality rate (9).

Imaging in Pregnancy

Magnetic resonance imaging (MRI) and ultrasound are the preferred methods of imaging in pregnancy (10).

When indicated, the appropriate imaging technique should not be withheld due to concerns about fetal radiation exposure. Those patients for which a CT scan or X-ray is the best imaging modality should receive that test. The levels of radiation, which the fetus is exposed to during diagnostic imaging, poses far less of a threat than the risk of undiagnosed maternal injury. If ionizing radiation is used, the abdomen should be shielded whenever possible. A small increase in the risk of childhood leukemia is present with any exposure to ionizing radiation.

The standard technique for detecting intra-abdominal blood and cardiac tamponade is focused assessment with sonography for trauma (FAST). It has been shown to be as sensitive and specific in pregnant as in non-pregnant patients (11) and has largely replaced peritoneal lavage and abdominal CT.

Principles of Pre-Hospital Care for the Pregnant Trauma Patient

All female victims of trauma of reproductive age should be assumed to be pregnant and a specific obstetric history taken.

As previously noted, aortocaval compression (ACC) significantly reduces maternal cardiac output and uterine blood flow. It is essential that measures are taken to minimize ACC in any woman who is at >18–20 weeks gestation or visibly pregnant. In essence, if the uterus is palpable above the umbilicus, then the patient must not be allowed to assume the supine position. If spinal immobilization with a spinal board is required, ACC can be reduced by tilting the entire board 15–30 degrees or by manual displacement of the uterus. The latter is the technique of choice during cardiac arrest and is probably the most effective in most situations (12). See Figure 30.1.

It is easy to underestimate the effects of trauma on both the woman and the fetus. Maternal systolic blood pressure will be maintained in the presence of 2–3 L blood loss. A non-tender abdomen does not exclude maternal abdominal injury. Even minor maternal trauma may result in serious fetal compromise. A raised pulse rate should not be put down to pregnancy: hemorrhage must be excluded as a cause.

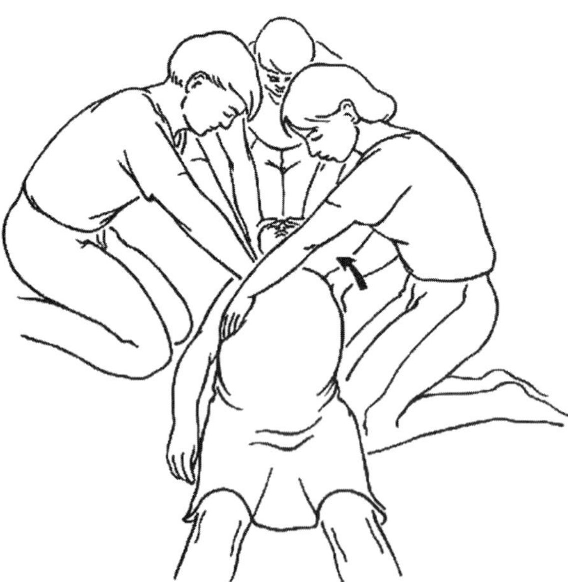

Figure 30.1 Two-handed manual uterine displacement to the left. Reproduced with permission from Paterson-Brown S, Howell C, editors. The MOET Course Manual Managing Obstetric Emergencies and Trauma, 3rd edition. Cambridge: Cambridge University Press; -2014: 108.

All trauma victims should be given supplementary oxygen 10–15 L/minute via a non-rebreathing bag. This is especially important in the pregnant patient with her increased oxygen demand and important to decrease the risk of fetal hypoxemia and acidosis.

Although the risk of aspiration is high in the pregnant patient, it is even higher when tracheal intubation fails (13). Thus in the pre-hospital setting, unless trained personnel are present, the airway should be secured with a second generation supra-glottic airway. This device provides limited protection against aspiration, incorporates a bite block and requires limited skill to insert.

The gravid uterus displaces the diaphragm 4 cm cephalad. Therefore, intercostal drains and thoracotomies should be undertaken in the third or fourth intercostal space, anterior to the midline (14).

Because of the absence of autoregulation of uterine blood flow, if hypovolemia is suspected, there should be aggressive fluid resuscitation preferably with blood (O-negative blood can be used if cross-matched/group specific blood is not yet available). For the same reason, hypotensive resuscitation is contraindicated if the fetus is viable (15).

If hemorrhage is suspected, early use of an antifibrinolytic agent such as tranexamic acid is recommended. In non-pregnant trauma patients, Tranexamic acid given within 3 hours of injury reduces the severity of hemorrhage and need for transfused blood significantly (16). Antishock garments may be used in the pregnant patient but the abdominal portion should be left open (17).

The obstetric trauma patient should be transferred to a level 1 trauma center with co-located obstetric and neonatal services. Figure 30.2 describes advanced life support for the obstetric patient.

Managing Traumatic Cardiac Arrest

Cardiac arrest from any cause, let alone trauma, is extremely rare in the obstetric population and guidelines for management are based on consensus opinion based on case reports and series. Although cardiopulmonary resuscitation was introduced into clinical practice in 1961, it took 30 years for it to be used in the obstetric population. In a review of reports of cardiac arrest in the

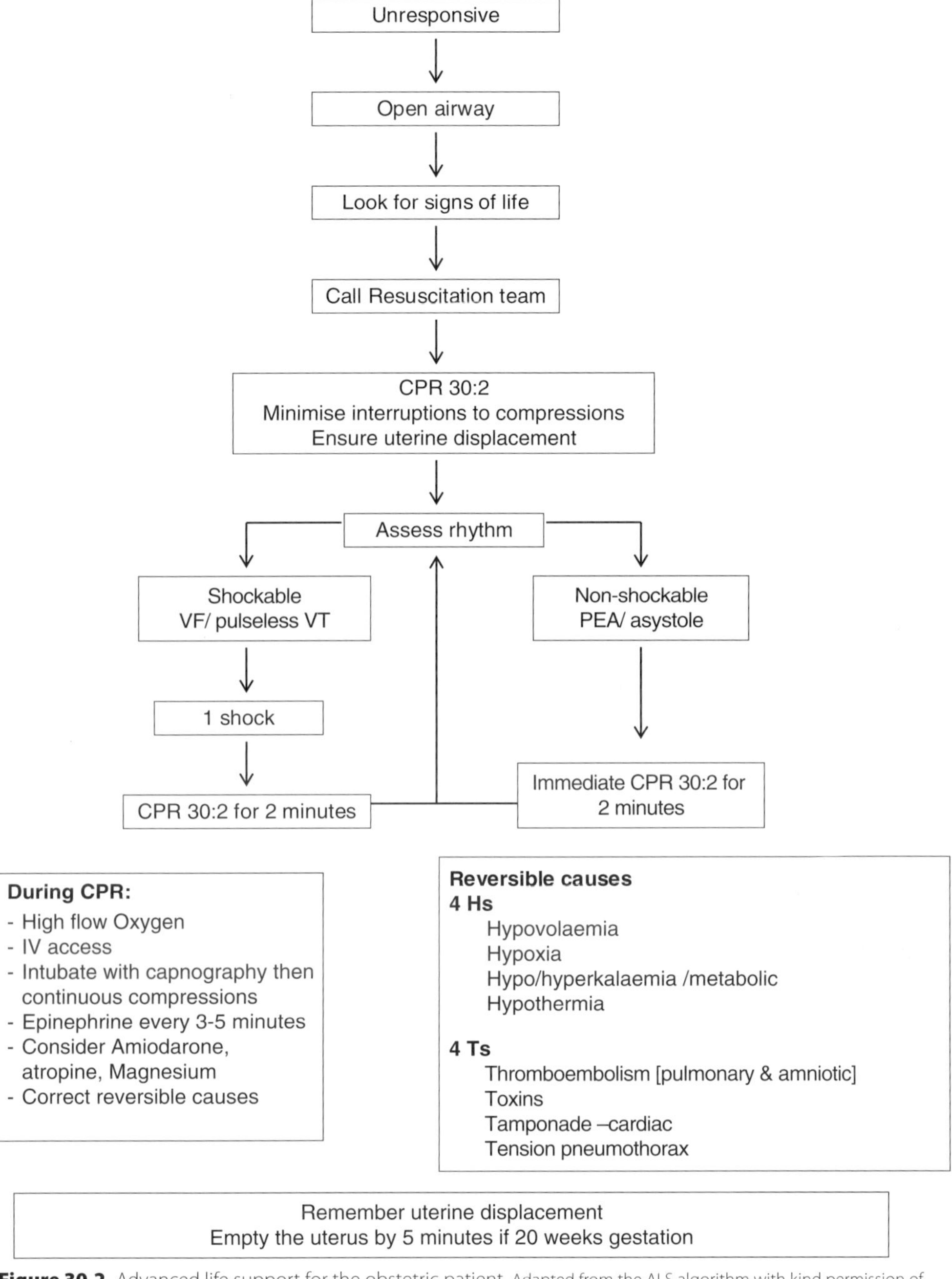

Figure 30.2 Advanced life support for the obstetric patient. Adapted from the ALS algorithm with kind permission of the Resuscitation Council UK.

obstetric population spanning 30 years, trauma was the most common cause (14). Guidelines on the management of the collapsed obstetric patient contain few recommendations specific to obstetric patients (12).

Guidelines for adult basic and advanced resuscitation should be followed. The main modifications are provided in Box 30.1.

Perimortem Cesarean Section

Authorities recommend that perimortem caesarean section should be undertaken in the undelivered obstetric patient when there has been no return of spontaneous circulation following cardiac arrest. There is, however, no consensus on the lower limit of gestation

Box 30.1 Modifications indicated for cardiac resuscitation of the pregnant patient

Manual lateral displacement of the uterus > 20 weeks is done to minimize aortocaval compression (ACC). ACC, by interfering with venous return, decreases the efficacy of cardiac compressions. Tilting the patient should be avoided if possible as it reduces the efficacy of external cardiac compressions (see Figure 30.1).

Early tracheal intubation is recommended but difficulty should be anticipated and intubation should be attempted only by an experienced operator. A second generation supra-glottic device should be inserted if airway patency and mask ventilation are difficult. Also, 100% oxygen must be given.

It is recommended that hand position is slightly higher on the sternum for compressions than in the non-pregnant patient to adjust for diaphragmatic elevation.

Intravenous access should be above the diaphragm.

Defibrillation and the drug and doses recommended for the non-pregnant population are the same as in the obstetric population. It must be noted that a different spectrum of reversible causes should be considered in pregnant patients, as these may also occur in the traumatized patient (see Figure 30.2).

When cardiac arrest is secondary to trauma, resuscitative thoracotomy should be considered within 5 minutes of blunt trauma and 10 minutes of penetrating trauma. The aim of resuscitative thoracotomy is to relieve cardiac tamponade, control intrathoracic haemorrhage, allow open cardiac massage and enable the thoracic aorta to be temporarily clamped to preserve blood flow to heart and brain, until surgical control of haemorrhage can be achieved. If appropriate facilities and personnel are present, this should be undertaken at the same time as perimortem cesarean section.

when this should be performed, the timing, or even the reason for undertaking the procedure. The Eastern Association for the Surgery of Trauma (EAST) guidelines state that "perimortem Cesarean section should be considered in any moribund pregnant woman >24 weeks gestation within 20 minutes of death and ideally within 5 minutes of cardiac arrest" (18).

Twenty-four weeks is the generally agreed gestation at which there is fetal viability. The limited evidence presently suggests that the quicker the delivery occurs following maternal cardiac arrest, the greater the chance the neonate will survive neurologically intact. On the other hand, the American Heart Association advises, "When the gravid uterus is large enough to cause maternal hemodynamic changes due to aortocaval compression, emergency Caesarean section should be considered, regardless of fetal viability" and recommends that preparation for perimortem section are begun as soon as cardiac arrest is diagnosed (12).

In the UK, perimortem cesarean section is performed primarily to "significantly improve the chance of successful [maternal] resuscitation." This is due both to more complete relief of aortocaval compression and also due to the effect of auto-transfusion that follows evacuation of the uterus. Perimortem cesarean section should be started if there is no return of spontaneous circulation at 4 minutes with delivery by 5 minutes (19). To emphasize the rationale for undertaking the procedure it is sometimes referred to as resuscitative hysterotomy (20).

There is evidence that the 4-minute deadline is largely unachievable and good results in terms of maternal and fetal outcome are possible with longer arrest to delivery intervals (14). One of the predictors of both maternal and fetal survival is an in-hospital, witnessed arrest. This is unlikely to be the case in traumatic cardiac arrest. In the pre-hospital environment, it is vital that there is a contingency plan, should the procedure be followed by signs of life in mother and or fetus.

Once the decision has been reached to perform cesarean section, speed is of the essence and the procedure should carried out without moving the patient to the operating room. Bleeding will not be a problem while in cardiac arrest and anesthesia will not be required at this stage. Vertical abdominal incision and uterine incision with blunt dissection is recommended as the quickest approach (unless the operator is more familiar with a transverse incision), as this minimizes the risk to adjacent organs. It is essential to continue cardiopulmonary resuscitation during the procedure. Following delivery, immediate closure of the uterus and peritoneum is not required: packing, pressure and compression can be used until the required surgical skill is available. Oxytocin should not be used due to its potent cardiovascular effects in the face of profound maternal cardiovascular instability. Antibiotics should be given as soon as possible.

Primary Survey of Pregnant Trauma Patients

For those patients not yet in a diagnosed state of extremis, a primary survey is undertaken to identify and treat threats to life in order of urgency. These threats are the same in pregnant and non-pregnant patients: The airway must be maintained and secured, breathing confirmed/established, oxygen given, and the circulation maintained. ACC must be minimized at all times.

Should a woman require general anesthesia, shortly before delivery, a neonatologist should be summoned as the neonate may need resuscitation due to the effects of drugs that cross the placenta (including muscle relaxants), as well as hypoxia secondary to maternal compromise.

Secondary Survey

The secondary survey involves a complete history and physical examination along with diagnostic adjuncts such as ultrasound, X-rays and CT scan. Again priorities remain the same as for the non-pregnant woman but the gestation and status of the fetus should be established. Gestational age should be documented in the pregnancy records. The obstetric history may be useful. Ultrasound should be used to establish fetal viability and gestation.

An initial estimate of fetal well-being is made during the secondary survey. An early sign of fetal hypoxia is a fetal tachycardia (>150 bpm), which may reflect maternal hypovolemia. Fetal bradycardia indicates more severe/ prolonged hypoxia [< 110 bpm]. Indications for delivery include the need to facilitate other surgery, such as exploratory laparotomy. Whether delivery should be undertaken purely for fetal factors will depend on the condition of the woman.

Pelvic and rectal inspection and examination are part of the secondary survey in pregnant trauma patients. Fluid leakage or bleeding may herald onset of labor or abruption. Abruption frequently accompanies maternal trauma. A tender and/ or hard uterus are concerning signs consistent with abruption. Obvious trauma to the perineum should be noted and if fractures of the pelvis are suspected, the patient's pelvis may need evaluation from the orthopedic point of view.

Vaginal examination must be performed if assault or abuse is suspected. A sterile speculum examination should be performed before a bimanual exam to take swabs and identify any lacerations in the vagina. These may be the result of abuse, trauma or underlying pelvic fractures. If vaginal injury or pelvic fracture is considered possible, it may be appropriate to undertake the examination under anesthesia.

Fetal Monitoring

Fetal monitoring is important to assess both fetal and maternal well-being. Ultrasound is also useful in confirming gestational age and identifying the position of the placenta. The advantages of ultrasound include repeatability, portability and avoidance of radiation exposure. Its sensitivity in detecting placental abruption immediately after trauma has not been established and it cannot be considered reliable for that indication.

Cardiotocography (CTG) records the fetal heart rate and uterine contractions. Because the sympathetic and parasympathetic systems of a pre-term fetus are still developing, the interpretation of CTGs in the premature fetus is even more challenging than in a mature fetus. Interpretation would not normally be undertaken until 25–26 weeks. At more advanced gestations, a rise in the fetal heart rate, decelerations of the fetal heart after a contraction and loss of variability in the heart rate are considered signs of fetal distress.

The majority of pregnant victims of major trauma who are at more than 20 weeks gestation will experience uterine irritability (contractions). If this uterine irritability lasts for more than 24 hours, the outcome for the fetus is usually poor.

A Kleihauer–Betke test (KBT) should be performed in all pregnant trauma patients at more than 12 weeks of gestation. A positive KBT test is one a marker of preterm labor and may be a sign of placental abruption. A negative test however does not exclude abruption. KBT will determine the dose of anti-D Rh immunoglobulin needed to prevent maternal sensitization, by establishing the number of fetal cells in a given volume of maternal blood. The standard dose of Rhogam (300 micrograms) covers only 15 ml of fetal red cells or 30 ml of fetal whole blood. The KBT test can estimate the volume of fetal red cells involved in the feto-maternal hemorrhage and thereby allow calculation of the correct Rhogam dose.

Specific Types of Injury

Blunt Trauma

Blunt trauma is the predominant type suffered by pregnant women. Motor vehicle accidents are by far the most common cause and comprise 55% to 70% of blunt trauma events. Violence, abuse and falls make up the rest (21). Maternal hemorrhage and brain injury are the predominant causes of maternal death.

The presence of the gravid uterus means that the type of abdominal injury found in pregnant females is different from their non-pregnant counterparts. Uterine rupture involving the fundus is commonly the result of blunt trauma to the abdomen. Traumatic uterine rupture is almost invariably associated with fetal death, although it is associated with maternal demise in only 10% of the cases, due to the associated intra-abdominal and orthopedic injuries.

Damage to the small bowel and bladder are frequently associated with pelvic injuries. In addition, in the pregnant trauma victim, the risk of trauma to the fetal head when a cephalic presentation exists must be assessed. Vaginal delivery remains a possibility only if a pelvic fracture does not narrow the pelvic contours and is not unstable or displaced. In these cases, cesarean delivery is indicated.

Pregnant women are more prone to falls than their non-pregnant counterparts. The incidence appears to increase as pregnancy progresses. The severity of injury varies but can include fetal loss. In one study, the incidence of falls equaled that of women in their seventies (22).

Penetrating Trauma

Penetrating trauma is much less common in pregnancy. The outcomes for the fetus and the pregnant woman are markedly different. Because the woman's intra-abdominal contents are displaced cephalad by the gravid uterus, damage to intra-abdominal organs is less common. In contrast, the fetus is at risk of fatal injury. Direct injury or to the umbilical cord and/ or placenta may cause fetal fatalities.

The management of penetrating trauma does not differ in pregnant patients. Stab wounds to the thorax or abdomen should be explored if the woman is obviously bleeding, is hemodynamically unstable or damage to an organ is suspected. Traumatic pneumothorax, hemothorax or free air under the diaphragm should be excluded on chest x-ray.

Gunshot wounds usually require an exploratory laparotomy. Anterior and posterior radiographs should be used to identify the bullet trajectory. The uterus itself should be examined. The uterus may need to be emptied to facilitate inspection of the other abdominal organs. Penetrating uterine injury at less than 25 weeks' gestation may be treated conservatively. Cesarean section is indicated in severe maternal hemorrhage or fetal death in association with a uterine laceration that would contraindicate labor. Fetal death is not itself an indication for cesarean section as the fetus is usually expelled naturally.

Burns

Burns are relatively rare in pregnant patients in the developed world. Mortality is related to the extent of the area burned. Management is the same as for the non-pregnant patient but relief of ACC should be undertaken. In the assessment of the area burned, the pregnant abdomen will account for more than 9% of the body surface area.

If any evidence of smoke inhalation or airway damage (such as singed nasal hair, soot in mouth/ nose, hoarseness, stridor) is present, early intubation is required. In cases of carbon monoxide intoxication, serial carboxyhemaglobin levels should be measured. Carboxyhemoglobin crosses the placenta and can cause fetal carboxyhemoglobinaemia. The treatment is hyperbaric oxygen therapy. The safety of hyperbaric oxygen therapy in the pregnant patient and in the fetus has not been established but hyperbaric oxygen therapy had been used successfully in pregnant patients (23).

Both maternal and fetal mortality rise sharply once more than 50% of the patient's body surface area is affected and urgent cesarean delivery is usually indicated. When the afflicted body surface area is less than 30%, the outcome for both woman and the fetus is usually good.

Domestic and Sexual Abuse

The outcome of pregnancy is poor in women who suffer domestic abuse. These patients are often prevented from accessing antenatal care. Preterm labor, stillbirth, low birth-weight babies and antepartum hemorrhage are more common.

Identification of at-risk women in pregnancy may be difficult due to poor antenatal attendance or the continuous presence of the partner. Strategies to enable the woman to speak freely and safely, including the provision of non-related interpreters, should be organized locally.

Effects of Trauma on Pregnancy

Feto-maternal haemorrhage, abruption, preterm labour and the need for emergency cesarean section are all outcomes of maternal trauma.

As previously mentioned, uterine activity is very common following trauma. However, tocolytic agent are rarely if ever indicated in the trauma victim as in the hemodynamically compromised patient they cause vasodilation and will exacerbate maternal hypotension and can cause pulmonary edema.

In normal pregnancy, labor and delivery, there is transfer of fetal blood into the maternal circulation. Trauma may directly increase this amount but feto-maternal haemorrhage can also result from placental abruption and rupture of the membranes. If the mother is Rhesus-negative, she may develop Rhesus-positive antibodies if the fetus is Rhesus-positive, which may lead to isoimmunization in subsequent pregnancies. KBT will guide the appropriate dose of anti-D to be given.

Placental abruption involves separation of placental lining from the uterus after 20 weeks of gestation. It may complicate even minor degrees of maternal trauma and must always be considered and evaluated. Abdominal pain with or without vaginal blood loss, with a rising fundus (due to blood collecting in the uterus) are signs of abruption. The only signs, however, may be those of fetal distress. Traumatic placental abruption is associated with a high fetal mortality (20–40%). This can also have severe consequences for the mother. Placental abruption can be associated with massive blood loss that may be hidden (concealed abruption) and associated disseminated intravascular coagulopathy. Urgent delivery is often required.

Uterine rupture is a rare outcome of blunt trauma (<1%). The risk increases with gestation. Fetal mortality is extremely high. The woman may complain of severe abdominal or chest pain and/or shoulder-tip pain (from diaphragmatic irritation by blood). Palpitable fetal parts and loss of uterine contours may be evident on abdominal palpation. The only sign, however, may be fetal distress on fetal heart rate monitoring.

Emergency Cesarean Section

Maternal indications for emergency surgical delivery following trauma include control of hemorrhage in a hemodynamically unstable patient. The hemorrhage may be due to uterine rupture or placental abruption. Cesarean delivery may also be required to allow access to non-obstetric intra-abdominal hemorrhage.

Fetal distress alone is only an indication for surgical delivery following trauma if the gestation the gestational age is consistent with fetal viability and the mother is hemodynamically stable. In a series of 441 pregnant victims of trauma, 32 underwent cesarean section for either maternal or fetal indications. Of this, 72% women survived and 45% of the newborns survived. The authors concluded that, at beyond 26 weeks gestation, if the fetal heart is heard, regardless of the severity of maternal injury, the fetus is salvageable (24).

Concluding Remarks

Management of pregnant trauma patients requires a multidisciplinary team response, and immediate priorities for resuscitation are the same for the pregnant as for the non-pregnant patient. During resuscitation, it is important to realize that the fetus is an excellent monitor for maternal blood loss as placental blood flow is reduced early with maternal hypovolemia. Finally, obstetricians must remember that delivery of the fetus either alive or dead may be life-saving for the mother.

References

1. Petrone P, Talving P, Browder T et al. Abdominal injuries in pregnancy: A 155-month study at two level 1 trauma centers. *Injury* 2011;42(1):47–49.
2. Hill CC, Pickinpaugh J. Trauma and surgical emergencies in the obstetric patient. *Surg Clin North Am* 2008; 88(2): 421–440.
3. Knight M on behalf of the MBRRACE-UK homicide and domestic abuse chapter writing group. In Knight M, Kenyon S, Brocklehurst P, Neilson J, Shakespeare J, Kurinczuk JJ (eds). *On behalf of MBRRACE-UK. Saving lives, improving mothers' care – lessons learned to inform future maternity care from the UK and Ireland Confidential Enquiries into maternal deaths and morbidity 2009–12*. Oxford: National Perinatal Epidemiology Unit, University of Oxford, 2014.
4. Kuo C, Jamieson DJ, McPheeters ML, Meikle SF, Posner SF. Injury hospitalizations of pregnant women in the United States, 2002. *Am J Obstet Gynecol* 2007;196:161.e1–6.
5. Battaloglu E, McDonnell D, Chu J et al. Epidemiology and outcomes of pregnancy and obstetric complications in trauma in the United Kingdom. *Injury* 2016; 47: 184–187.
6. Poole GV, Martin JN, Perry KG, et al. Trauma in pregnancy: The role of interpersonal violence. *Am J Obstet Gynecol* 1996; 174: 1873–1877.
7. Schiff, MA, Holt, V. The Injury Severity Score in pregnant trauma patients: Predicting placental abruption and fetal death. *J Trauma* 2002;53(5):946–9.

8. AMA. Violence against women: Relevance for medical practitioners. *JAMA* 1992;267:3184–9.
9. Hill CC, Pickinpaugh J. Trauma and surgical emergencies in the obstetric patient. *Surgical Clinics North Am* 2008;88(2):421–40.
10. ACOG Committee Opinion. Number 656 Guidelines for diagnostic imaging during pregnancy and lactation. February 2016. www.acog.org. Resources and publications. Committee opinions.
11. Goodwin H, Holmes JF, Wisner DH. Abdominal ultrasound examination in pregnant blunt trauma patients. *J Trauma* 2001; 50(4):689–93.
12. Vanden Hoek TL, Morrison LJ, Shuster M et al. Cardiac arrest in special situations 2010 American heart Association guidelines for cardiopulmonary resuscitation and emergency cardiovascular care. *Circulation* 2010;122(18):S829–61.
13. Quinn AC, Milne D, Columb M, et al. Failed intubation in obstetric anaesthesia: A 2 year national case–control study in the UK. *Br J Anaesth* 2013;110(1):74–80.
14. Einav S, Kaufman N, Sela HY 2012; Maternal cardiac arrest and perimortem caesarean delivery: Evidence or expert based? *Resuscitation* 2012; 83(10):1191–200.
15. Plaat F, Shonfeld A. Major obstetric haemorrhage. Continuing education in anaesthesia, *Critical Care Pain Med* 2015;15(4):190–3.
16. Roberts I, Shakur H, Afolabi A et al. The importance of early treatment with tranexamic acid in bleeding trauma patients: An exploratory analysis of the CRASH-2 randomised controlled trial. *Lancet* 2011;377(9771);1096–101.
17. Mattox KL, Goetzl L. Trauma in pregnancy. *Crit Care Med* 2005; 33:S385–9.
18. Barraco RD, Chiu WC, Clancy TV et al. Practice management guidelines for the diagnosis and management of injury in the pregnant patient: The EAST practice management guidelines Working group. *Trauma* 2010;69(1):211–14.
19. Paterson-Brown S, Howell C, (eds). *Managing Obstetric Emergencies and Trauma*, 3rd ed. Cambridge University Press, Cambridge, 2014:109–120.
20. Faculty of Pre-Hospital Care Consensus statement guidelines for the Pre-hospital resuscitative hysterotomy/peri-mortem Caesarean section. Direct communication – FPHC Clinical Standards Committee 2016.
21. Ikossi DG, Lazar AA, Morabito D, et al. Profile of mothers ar risk: An analysis of injury and pregnancy loss in 1,195 trauma patients. *J Am Coll Surg* 2005;200:49–56.
22. Dunning K, LeMasters G, Levin L, et al. Fall in workers during pregnancy: Risk factors, job hazards and high risk occupations. *Am J Ind Med* 2003;44:664–72.
23. Elkharrat D, Raphael JC, Korach JM, et al. Acute carbon monoxide intoxication and hyperbaric oxygen therapy in pregnancy. *Intensive Care Med* 1991;17(5):289–92.
24. Morris JA, Rosenbower TJ, Jerkovitch GL, et al. Infant survival after caesarean section for trauma. *Ann Surg* 1996;223:481–91.

Post-term Pregnancy

Olukayode Akinlaja and William Gist

Introduction

Post-term pregnancy refers to an extended pregnancy, but the term is often used interchangeably by some clinicians with prolonged pregnancy. It was defined, however, in 1997 by the American College of Obstetricians and Gynecologists as a pregnancy at or exceeding 42 completed weeks from the first day of the last menstrual period or 294 days [1].

This definition assumes that ovulation occurs two weeks after the last menses but there is a known variation in the menstrual cycle. This may explain why a majority of infants delivered post term show no evidence of post maturity.

About 50% of pregnancies are delivered by the estimated date of confinement (EDD) but due to limitations in estimating the date of delivery and the variation in fetal maturation, only 4% of women deliver on their EDD [2].

The majority of post-term pregnancies have no known cause. Evidence suggests a biological predisposition, as post-term pregnancy tends to be repeated in mothers with prior post-term births. Bakketieg and Bergsjo in a study of 27,677 Norwegian births noted that a prior post-term birth is associated with a 10% to 27% incidence of subsequent post-term birth; this is increased to 39% with two prior successive post-term deliveries [3]. No clear-cut evidence exists for other maternal-associated factors but studies have linked age, socioeconomic class, nulliparity, male fetus, obesity, race, ethnicity and parity with post-term pregnancies [4,5].

Fetoplacental factors linked to post-term pregnancy include the X-linked recessive disorder-placental sulfatase deficiency, anencephaly and adrenal hypoplasia [6,7].

Scope of Problem

Incidence

In 2013, about 5.5% of pregnancies delivered at ≥42 weeks gestation and 8.5% at 41 weeks gestation compared to 2001 when 7% of live births in the United States were at 42 weeks gestation or more relative to the 12% that occurred at or before 36 weeks gestation [8].

Variations in the worldwide prevalence is attributed to (a) differences in obstetrics practices and (b) availability of routine first trimester ultrasound estimation of the EDD. The prevalence of post-term delivery is lower than when EDD is solely calculated based on the last menstrual period (LMP) as error with dating may occur [9,10].

The EDD is most accurately based on the crown rump length in the first trimester with an error margin of ± 7 days as illustrated in Table 31.1. Studies by Bennett and colleagues demonstrated that there tend to be fewer inductions for post-term indications when dating is done by first trimester ultrasound as compared to second trimester sonography [11].

Obstetrics practices such as the rate of elective induction of labor and scheduled cesarean section can also have an effect on the prevalence.

The use of techniques for stimulating uterine contractions before the onset of labor, also known as induction of labor, has been increasing. Induction rates have risen from 9.5% to 23.3% between 1990 and 2012 [8] due to various reasons ranging from medical and obstetric factors to the increased acceptance of induction of labor [15].

Historically, it is known that the perinatal mortality tends to increase beyond the expected due date and this cuts across antepartum, intrapartum and neonatal death with the most significant increases occurring intrapartum.

A review of 56,317 consecutive singleton pregnancies delivered at 40 or more weeks at Parkland Hospital showed that the rates of fetal distress and dystocia were significantly increased for post-term pregnancies. Additionally, there was a doubling of the incidence of neonatal seizures and deaths. Finally, more infants were admitted to the intensive care

Table 31.1 Ultrasonography Dating Accuracy

Parameter	Gestational Age	Accuracy	References
Mean sac diameter (MSD)	4.5 to 6 weeks	± 5 to 7 days	[12–14]
Crown rump length (CRL)	7 to 10 weeks 10 to 14 weeks 15 weeks	± 3 days ± 5 days ± 8.4 days	
Biparietal diameter (BPD), head circumference (HC), femur length (FL).	14 to 20 weeks 21 to 30 weeks > 30 weeks	± 7 days ± 14 days ± 21 to 28 days	

unit at 42 weeks gestation when compared to earlier deliveries [16].

Studies done in the United Kingdom also demonstrated that antepartum stillbirth rates increase after 40 weeks. Rates 0.86–1.08/1,000 live births between 40 and 41 weeks, 1.2–1.27/1,000 live births between 41 and 42 weeks, 1.3–1.9/1,000 live births between 42 and 43 weeks and 1.58–6.3/1,000 live births after 43 weeks have been reported [17].

Fetal hypoxia and asphyxia resulting from intrauterine infection, cord compression and placental insufficiency account for some of the excess perinatal mortality, while labor dystocia and increased rates of perineal trauma, postpartum hemorrhage, and cesarean deliveries are the associated maternal complications.

Sequelae of Post-term Pregnancy

Postmaturity Syndrome. Shime and colleagues reported that this syndrome tends to occur in about 10% of pregnancies between 41 and 43 weeks gestation [18]. These infants usually display advanced maturity features with wrinkled peeling skin, more prominent on the palms and soles and a thin body, suggestive of wasting. They usually appear older and alert with wide opened eyes.

Placental Dysfunction. A series of studies have suggested that there is no compromise to the placental function as post-term fetus do continue to grow and gain weight, leading to an increase in macrosomic infants at birth. A study by Nahum and colleagues demonstrated that there is no cessation of fetal growth until at least 42 weeks gestation [19].

Fetal Growth Restriction. This complication is frequently seen in post-term pregnancies and may account for some of the increased adverse effects. An analysis by Clausson and co-workers of about 700,000 births between 1991 and 1995 in the National Swedish Medical birth registry indicated that about one-third of the post-term stillbirths were growth restricted [20].

Fetal Distress and Oligohydramnios. As pregnancy advances beyond 42 weeks gestation, an associated decrease in the amniotic fluid volume occurs, leading to oligohydramnios and cord compression with consequent antepartum and intrapartum fetal distress.

Meconium aspiration syndrome, which is an unexplained respiratory distress in infants newly born through meconium-stained amniotic fluid, can result from the passage of meconium into an already decreased amniotic fluid volume due to hypoxemia-induced relaxation of the rectal sphincter tone [21].

Dysmaturity. Dysmaturity is also known as postmaturity syndrome. It is a term used to describe chronic intrauterine malnutrition related features in infants and occurs in about 20% of post-term infants [22].

Management

Post-term pregnancy is regarded as a high-risk condition by the American College of Obstetricians and Gynecologists and recommendations are as listed in Box 31.1.

Antepartum fetal testing to reduce perinatal morbidity and mortality is usually started at 41 weeks to identify fetuses at risk of intrauterine fetal asphyxia while induction of labor is usually commenced at 42 weeks gestation, especially in the setting of a favorable cervix. There is only limited evidence to justify either approach and there is an argument for allowing women with uncertain post-term pregnancy to be followed weekly without intervention in the absence of fetal jeopardy.

Box 31.1 Evaluation and Management of Post-term Pregnancy

1. Post-term pregnancy is defined as a pregnancy that has extended to or beyond 42 completed weeks.
2. Women with a post-term gestation who have an unfavorable cervix can either undergo labor induction or be managed expectantly.
3. Prostaglandin can be used for cervical ripening and labor induction.
4. Delivery should be effected if there is evidence of fetal compromise or oligohydramnios.
5. It is reasonable to initiate antenatal surveillance between 41 and 42 weeks despite lack of evidence that monitoring improves outcomes.
6. A nonstress test and amniotic fluid volume assessment should be adequate, although no single method has been shown to be superior.
7. Many recommend prompt delivery in a woman with a post-term pregnancy, a favorable cervix and no other complications.

Findings from the Maternal-Fetal Medicine Network trial of induction versus fetal testing as reported by Gardner et al. did not elicit any major difference between both management modalities. There were no perinatal deaths in any subgroup or associated increased rates of cesarean section in either management group [23]. Goeree and colleagues, in a cost-effectiveness study of Canadian data, found a mean cost per patient of $3,132 with fetal testing compared to $2,939 for labor induction [24]. Fetal testing is usually done twice weekly either with nonstress testing and amniotic fluid assessment or the biophysical profile, neither of which is superior [25]. The various techniques used for fetal testing include nonstress test, biophysical profile, modified biophysical profile, contraction stress test and fetal movement count. See Table 31.2 for clinician-based methods interpretation.

A meta-analysis of 22 trials by Boulvain et al. found that the frequency of post-term pregnancies was decreased by membrane stripping between 38 and 40 weeks with no increase in the incidence of maternal and neonatal infections or risk for cesarean delivery; the likelihood of spontaneous labor within 48 hours was increased [30].

This generally involves the digital separation of the membranes from the lower uterine segment during a cervical examination and is believed to induce uterine contractions by increasing the level of endogenous prostaglandin production. A prospective study that further compared GBS positive and negative groups found no significant difference in neonatal and maternal outcomes after membrane stripping [31].

Alexander and associates examined the effect of labor induction at 42 weeks gestation on rates of cesarean deliveries at Parkland Hospital. They concluded that patient intrinsic factors such as unfavorable cervix, nulliparity, and epidural analgesia accounted for the increased rates of cesarean deliveries rather than the act of labor induction itself [32].

A meta-analysis of randomized trials done in 2012 showed that labor induction resulted in a 70% reduction in perinatal mortality and a 40% reduction in meconium aspiration syndrome. No increase in cesarean delivery was found when compared to expectant management of pregnancy at 41weeks gestation [33]. See Figure 31.1 for an example of a fetal tracing seen in a post-term induction of labor.

Sanchez-Ramos and colleagues performed a meta-analysis and found a 22% cesarean section rate in expectantly managed pregnancies compared to the 20% seen in uncomplicated pregnancies induced at 41 weeks gestation. No differences in neonatal intensive care unit (NICU) admission or meconium aspiration were found [34]. The reduced cesarean delivery rate was confirmed by another meta-analysis done in 2009 [35]. The fetal heart rate tracing of a laboring patient with post dates gestation is seen in Figure 31.1.

Management of Macrosomia in Post-term Pregnancy

Although the majority of post-term pregnancies demonstrate appropriate growth, some clinicians argue for a reduction in macrosomia-associated maternal and fetal morbidity through the induction of labor. The incidence of macrosomia at more than 42 weeks gestation is about 2.2% compared to 1.4% between 37 and 41 weeks, a result of the growth afforded by the longer gestational period and macrosomic babies are prone to increased birth injury due to prolonged labor, shoulder dystocia and cephalopelvic disproportion.

The American Congress of Obstetricians and Gynecologists, however, recommends that an estimated fetal weight of 5,000 g is not a contraindication to vaginal delivery in the absence of maternal diabetes. Present

Table 31.2 Interpretation of Antenatal Fetal Testing Methods

Type	Techniques	Results	References
Nonstress test (NST)	Continuous FHR monitoring	Non-reactive: < 2 accelerations in a 40-minute period Reactive: ≥ 2 accelerations within a 20-minute period	[26]
Contraction stress test	Continuous FHR monitoring	Positive: Late decelerations following ≥ 50% of contractions. Negative: No late or significant variable decelerations Unsatisfactory: < 3 contractions in 10 minutes or difficult to interpret FHR tracing. Equivocal – Intermittent late decelerations or significant variable decelerations.	[27]
Biophysical profile	Ultrasound confirmation of the presence of five components within 30 minutes. - ≥ 1 episode of fetal breathing movements lasting ≥ 30 s - ≥ 1 episode of opening or closing of a hand or extremity extension with return to flexion - ≥ 3 discrete body or limb movements - Reactive NST - Maximum vertical AF > 2 cm	A score of 2 is assigned if the criteria is met and 0 if not. Maximum score is 10. Abnormal: ≤ 4/10 Normal: ≥ 8/10 Equivocal: 6/10	[28]
Modified biophysical profile	- Single deepest AF pocket - NST	Abnormal: Single deepest AF pocket ≤ 2 cm and a nonreactive NST Normal: Single deepest AF pocket > 2 cm and a reactive NST	[29]

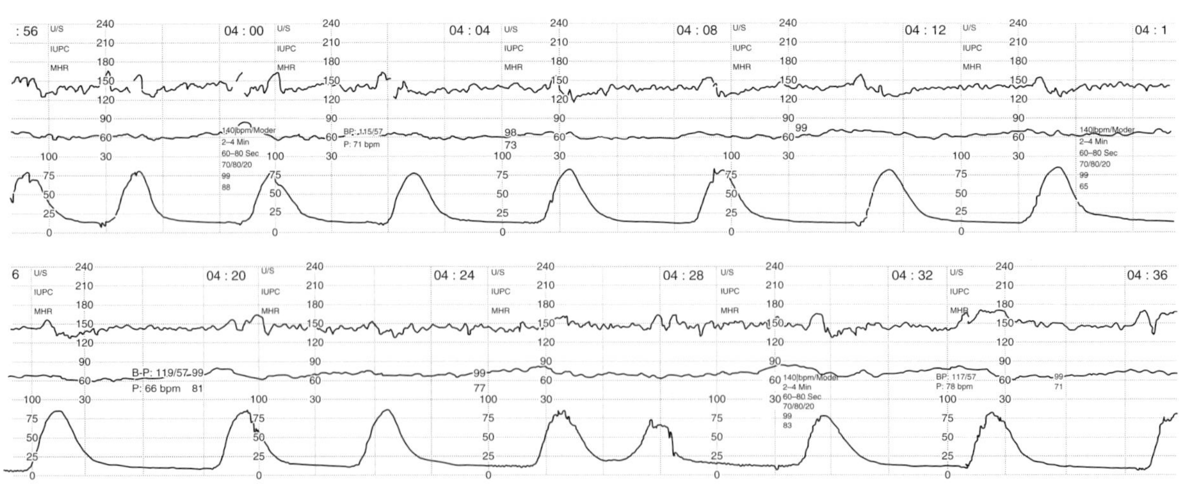

Figure 31.1 Post-term gestation patient in labor.

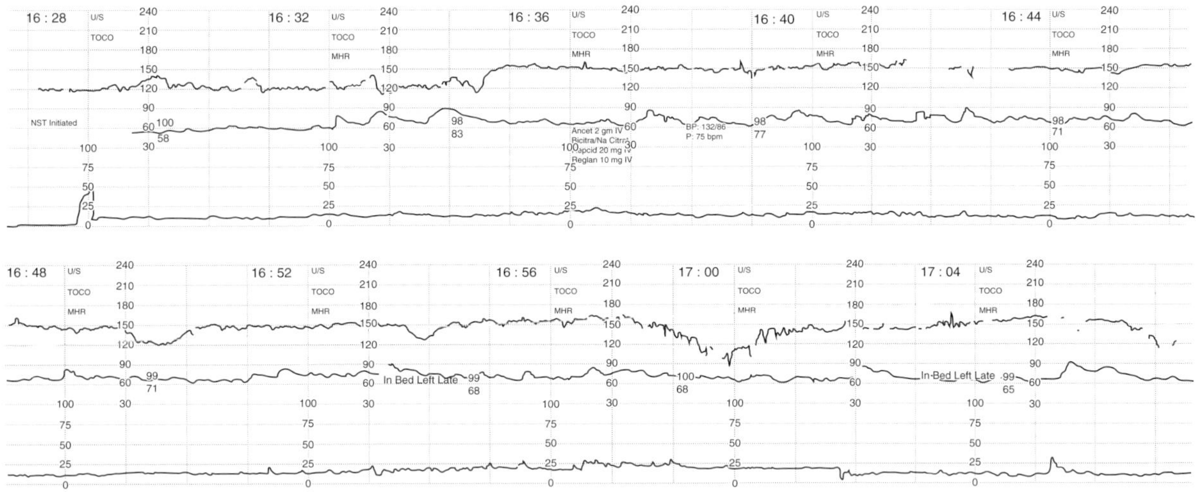

Figure 31.2 Fetal tracing in a post-term gestation patient with oligohydramnios.

evidence does not support an early labor induction policy for fetal macrosomia at term. Ultrasound estimation of fetal weight is not precise, while early induction or cesarean delivery does not necessarily reduce the morbidity associated with fetal macrosomia [36].

Management of Oligohydramnios in Post-term Pregnancy

A decrease in the amniotic volume can lead to an increased risk to the fetus and is associated with umbilical cord compression, abnormal fetal heart tracings and meconium stained amniotic fluid. Figure 31.2 illustrates a fetal tracing noted in the presence of oligohydramnios.

Oligohydramnios is defined on ultrasound evaluation as an absence of a vertical pocket of amniotic fluid greater than 2 cm or an amniotic fluid volume (AFI) less than 5 cm. Oligohydramnios in post-term pregnancy is presumed to be due to altered renal perfusion and decreased urinary output from fetal hypoxemia. Such oligohydramnios is associated with an increase in fetal tracing abnormalities in labor. Even in the presence of normal amniotic fluid volume, an abrupt development of oligohydramnios can occur [37].

The American College of Obstetricians and Gynecologists recommends delivery in post-term pregnancies with oligohydramnios [38].

The presence of normal amniotic fluid volume does not preclude abnormal outcomes in post-term pregnancies. See Figure 31.2 for a fetal heart rate tracing of a patient with oligohydramnios.

Intrapartum Management of Post-term Pregnancy

Post-term pregnancies are regarded as high risk due to the association with maternal, fetal and neonatal effects. It is thus imperative that patients with post-term gestation be advised to present to the hospital at the onset of labor. Continuous electronic monitoring of the fetal heart rate and contractions should be commenced and amniotomy done as needed. In the absence of other obstetric indications or fetal jeopardy, high likelihood exists for successful vaginal deliveries.

Long-Term Sequelae

The long-term effects for newborns that result from post-term pregnancies still need further investigation. Some studies have demonstrated outcomes that are comparable to term infants but others showed lower cognitive scores, increased risks of attention deficit disorder and cerebral palsy in post-term infants [39].

Concluding Remarks

Post-term pregnancies remain one of the most common reasons for labor induction in the United States and the importance of accurate dating of pregnancy cannot be overemphasized in order to avoid an overdiagnosis and when labor induction is chosen as a management option, assessment of the fetal presentation and size as well as the maternal pelvis and cervix should be conducted to confirm eligibility.

References

1. American College of Obstetricians and Gynecologists. Management of Postterm Pregnancy. Practice Bulletin No. 55, September 2004.
2. Jukic AM, Baird DD, Weinberg CR, et al. Length of human pregnancy and contributors to its natural variation. *Hum Reprod* 2013;28:2848.
3. Bakketeig LS, Bergsjo P. Post-term pregnancy: Magnitude of the problem. In Chalmers I, Enkin M, Keirse M (eds). *Effective Care in Pregnancy and Childbirth.* Oxford: Oxford University Press, 1991, p. 765.
4. Oberg AS, Frisell T, Svensson AC, LLiadou AN. Maternal and fetal genetic contributions to postterm birth: Familial clustering in a population-based sample of 475,429 Swedish births. *Am J Epidemiol* 2013;177: 531.
5. Morken NH, Melve KK, Skjaerven R. Recurrence of prolonged and post-term gestational age across generations: Maternal and paternal contribution. *Br J Obstet Gynaecol* 2011;118:1630.
6. Macdonald PC, Siiteri PK. Origin of estrogen in women pregnant with anencephalic fetus. *J Clin Invest* 1965;44:465.
7. Rabe T, Hosch R, Runnebaum B. Sulfatase deficiency in the human placenta: Clinical findings. *Biol Res Pregnancy Perinatol* 1983;4:95.
8. Births: Final Data for 2013. www.cdc.gov/nchs/data/nvsr64/nvsr64_01.pdf (Accessed on January 19, 2016).
9. Caughey AB, Nicholson JM, Washington AE. First vs. second trimester ultrasound: The effect on pregnancy dating and perinatal outcomes. *Am J Obstet Gynecol* 2008;198(703):e1.
10. Neilson JP. Ultrasound for fetal assessment in early pregnancy. *Cochrane Database Syst Rev* 2000; CD000182.
11. Bennett KA, Crane JMG, O'Shea B, et al. First trimester ultrasound screening is effective in reducing postterm labor induction rates: A randomized controlled trial. *Am J Obstet Gynecol* 2004;190:1077.
12. Hadlock FP, Harrist RB, Martinez-Poyer J. How accurate is second trimester fetal dating? *J Ultrasound Med* 1991;10: 557.
13. Hadlock FP, Shah YP, Kanon DJ, Lindsey JV. Fetal crown-rump length: Reevaluation of relation to menstrual age (5–18 weeks) with resolution real-time US. *Radiology* 1992;182:501.
14. Kurtz AB, Needleman L. *Ultrasound Assessment of Fetal Age*, 2nd ed. Philadelphia: WB Saunders Co., 1998.
15. Leduc D, Biringer A, Lee L, et al. Induction of labour. *J Obstet Gynaecol Can* 2013;35:840.
16. Alexander JM, McIntire DD, Leveno KJ. Forty weeks and beyond: Pregnancy outcomes by week of gestation. *Obstet Gynecol* 2000;96:291.
17. Myers ER, Blumrick R, Christian AL, et al. Management of Prolonged Pregnancy. Rockville (MD): Agency for Healthcare Research and Quality (US); 2002 May. (Evidence Reports/Technology Assessments, No. 53).
18. Shime J, Gare DJ, Andrews J, et al. Prolonged pregnancy: Surveillance of the fetus and the neonate and the course of labor and delivery. *Am J Obstet Gynecol* 1984;148;547.
19. Nahum GG, Stanislaw H, Huffaker BJ. Fetal weight gain at term: Linear with minimal dependence on maternal obesity. *Am J Obstet Gynecol* 1995;172:1387.
20. Clausson B, Cnattingius S, Axelsson O. Outcomes of post-term births: The role of fetal growth restriction and malformations. *Obstet Gynecol* 1999;94:758.
21. Fanaroff AA. Meconium aspiration syndrome: Historical aspects. *J Perinatol* 2008;28 Suppl 3:S3.
22. Mannino F. Neonatal complications of postterm gestation. *J Reprod Med* 1988;33:271–6 (Level III).
23. National Institute of Child Health and Human Development Network of Maternal-Fetal Medicine Units. A clinical trial of induction of labor versus expectant management in postterm pregnancy. *Am J Obstet Gynecol* 1994;170:716.
24. Goeree R, Hannah M, Hewson S. Cost-effectiveness of induction of labour versus serial antenatal monitoring in the Canadian Multicenter Postterm Pregnancy Trial. *Can Med Assoc J* 1995;152:1445.
25. Alfirevic Z, Walkinshaw SA. A randomized controlled trial of simple compared with complex antenatal fetal monitoring after 42 weeks of gestation. *Br J Obstet Gynaecol* 1995;102:638.
26. Evertson LR, Gauthier RJ, Schifirin BS, Paul RH. Antepartum fetal heart rate testing. I. Evolution of the nonstress test. *Am J Obstet Gynecol* 1979;133:29–33.
27. Freeman RK, Anderson G, Dorchester W. A prospective multi-institutional study of antepartum fetal heart monitoring. I. Risk of perinatal mortality and morbidity according to antepartum fetal heart rate test results. *Am J Obstet Gynecol* 1982;143:771–7.
28. Manning FA, Morrison I, Harman CR, Lange IR, Johnson JM. Fetal assessment based on fetal biophysical profile scoring. An analysis of perinatal morbidity and mortality. *Am J Obstet Gynecol* 1990;162:703–9.

29. Clark SL, Sabey P, Jolley K. Nonstress testing with acoustic stimulation and amniotic fluid assessment: 5973 tests without unexpected fetal death. *Am J Obstet Gynecol* 1989;160:694–7.

30. Boulvain M, Stan C, Irion O. Membrane sweeping for induction of labour. *Cochrane Database Syst Rev* 2005;CD000451.

31. Kabiri D, Hants Y, Yarkoni TR, et al. Antepartum membrane stripping in GBS carriers. Is it Safe? (The STRIP-G Study). *PLoS One* 2015;10:e0145905.

32. Alexander JM, McIntire DD, Leveno KJ. Prolonged pregnancy: Induction of labor and cesarean births. *Obstet Gynecol* 2001;97:911.

33. Gulmezoglu AM, Crowther CA, Middleton P, Heatley E. Induction of labour for improving birth outcomes for women at or beyond term. *Cochrane Database Syst Rev* 2012;6:CD004945.

34. Sanchez-Ramos L, Olivier F, Delke I, Kaunitz AM. Labor induction versus expectant management for postterm pregnancies: A systematic review with meta-analysis. *Obstet Gynecol* 2003;101:1312.

35. Caughey AB, Sundaram V, Kaimal AJ, et al. Systematic review: elective induction of labor versus expectant management of pregnancy. *Ann Intern Med* 2009;151:252.

36. American College of Obstetricians and Gynecologists. Fetal Macrosomia. Practice Bulletin No. 22, November 2000.

37. Clement D, Schifirin BS, Kates RB. Acute oligohydramnios in postdate pregnancy. *Am J Obstet Gynecol* 1987;157:884. The Cochrane Library. The Cochrane Collaboration; Issue 4, Oxford: Update Software, 1997.

38. Management of late-term and postterm pregnancies. Practice Bulletin No. 146. American College of Obstetricians and Gynecologists. *Obstet Gynecol* 2014;124:90–6.

39. El Marroun H, Zeegers M, Steegers EA, et al. Post-term birth and risk of behavioral and emotional problems in early childhood. *Int J Epidemiol* 2012;41:773.

Musculoskeletal Disorders

Sarah Shaffer and Colleen K. Stockdale

Introduction

Musculoskeletal discomfort and dysfunction in pregnancy present a unique challenge to the patient and practitioner. Symptoms are often non-specific and the cause is often difficult to elucidate due to the effects of pregnancy on the involved tissues. Limited studies evaluate prevention and treatment of low back pain in pregnancy, as well as other causes of musculoskeletal pain in pregnancy (1). Nonetheless, musculoskeletal disorders of pregnancy are common and worth the effort of a differential diagnosis to guide treatment.

Scope of the Problem

Many attempts have been made to quantify the prevalence of back and/or pelvic pain during pregnancy. Efforts to derive an estimate are complicated by the effect pregnancy has on all body tissues as well as posture and gain. They cause some symptomatology in most gravid patients, but are not necessarily disease processes. Various reports note musculoskeletal complaints to exist in the majority of obstetric patients – low back pain in 25% of a Scandinavian population (2) to 50% in US population (3) and "musculoskeletal pain" in 67% of an urban, underserved population of US women (4). It is disappointing to note, however, that limited studies evaluate prevention and treatment of low back pain in pregnancy and the same is true for other causes of musculoskeletal pain. Indeed, the contemporary study of US underserved women found 85% reported receiving no treatment for their back and/or pelvic pain and only 1% of the total study population was satisfied with treatment when it was rendered (4).

Back Pain

Scoliosis is a term denoting abnormal curvature of the spine, which is usually mild and diagnosed before or around puberty. Pregnancy does not appear to affect progression of spine curvature (5). Similarly scoliosis, especially when mild or treated, does not appear to have any effect on pregnancy outcome. Only women with severe curvatures causing morbidity prior to pregnancy are likely to need special consideration or management during pregnancy. Scoliosis, treated or untreated, does not limit administration of regional anesthesia in most cases (6) and does not appear to independently affect the risk of cesarean delivery (5).

Spondylosis, fracture of the L5 pars interarticularis, and spondylolisthesis, anterior displacement of the L5 vertebrae, diagnosed prior to pregnancy, have not been shown to worsen acutely during pregnancy nor to cause worsening low back or pelvic pain in pregnancy (7). However, one study did show that parous women with spondylolisthesis have an increased risk of degenerative spondylolisthesis in their later years compared to nulliparous women (8).

Disc herniation is a rare cause of back pain in pregnancy (9), especially acute back pain. A small study using MRI assessment suggests that disc herniations are common in reproductive age women; pregnancy does not increase the prevalence (10). This study suggests that outcomes for pregnant women are no different than non-pregnant patients; imaging indications are the same for both populations. Back or radiating leg pain can often be controlled conservatively. If symptomatic disc disease in pregnancy is associated with progressive neurologic deficits and bladder or bowel dysfunction, consultation with a specialist is indicated (11,12). Surgical treatment is not contraindicated by the pregnancy, but must be carefully considered.

Low back pain (LBP) in pregnancy is common. Pre-existing LBP is a risk factor for LBP in the current pregnancy as are LBP in prior pregnancies, multiparity, multiple gestation, obesity and de-conditioning. Regular exercise prior to pregnancy seems to prevent some degree of LBP in pregnancy. Symptoms usually worsen in the latter half of pregnancy, are aggravated by activity and relieved by rest. Radiation of pain down the back of the thighs and around to the pelvis or lower abdomen is not uncommon and disturbance of sleep may occur. True radicular pain or concomitant change in bowel or bladder continence are concerning findings.

The spine should be palpated to exclude areas of point tenderness. Bilateral evaluation of lower extremity range of motion, muscle strength, sensation and reflexes is indicated. LBP is worsened with lumbar spine extension produced by forward flexion at the waist while discogenic (and facet joint) pain is exacerbated by lumbar spine flexion with backward bending. Sacro-iliac joint pain is exacerbated by hip rotation among other tests described later in this chapter. Imaging is not required initially, unless neurologic symptoms are present, and is usually nondiagnostic. If imaging is deemed necessary, magnetic resonance imaging (MRI) is preferred for planning of therapeutic interventions such as epidural injection or surgery.

Treatment should be non-invasive unless concern exists for a pathologic cause of LBP in pregnancy. Oral analgesics, heat and ice therapy and activity modification are recommended. Women with other small children should be counseled on appropriate lifting posture and alternating arms when carrying children or heavy bags and car seats. Bed rest is no longer recommended for any pregnancy condition as decreased mobility in the pregnant woman adds a risk factor for development of venous thromboembolism. During normal periods of rest, lying in the left lateral recumbent position with the hips and knees flexed can provide some relief. A pillow placed between the knees while in this position for rest or sleeping can also reduce strain on the lower back. Wearing low-heeled shoes, sleeping on a firmer mattress, requesting help with heavy lifting and consideration of occupational duties should also be suggested in the appropriate circumstances.

Many different therapies have been studied for the relief of LBP in pregnancy, but the evidence for most interventions is moderate at best. Therapeutic considerations that may have some benefit include osteopathic manipulative medicine, chiropractic medicine, massage, physical therapy, pelvic belts and acupuncture. Exercise regimens including yoga, walking, swimming and water therapy have also been variously studied with improvement in some patients and no noted detrimental effects. Simple regimens of daily pelvic-tilt exercises and general stretching prior to sleep can provide significant relief. There is no proven benefit for epidural steroid injections for LBP in pregnancy. Non-radicular back pain usually improves significantly or resolves within several weeks of delivery.

Postpartum LBP can have unique causes and considerations. Specific risk factors for postpartum LBP include a history of LBP prior to or first occurring in the index pregnancy, inability to lose weight gained in the index pregnancy and obesity. Coccydynia, pain from the coccyx or sacro-coccygeal symphysis, may be caused by trauma during birth. Pain is acute in onset and easily localized to the coccyx limiting the ability to sit. Using a donut-shaped sitting pad can relieve some symptoms along with scheduled oral analgesics. LBP along with other pain syndromes can predispose or contribute to depression which is already an increased risk in the postpartum period (3).

Pelvic Girdle Pain

Unlike LBP in pregnancy, pelvic girdle pain, including that localized to the sacroiliac joints and pubic symphysis, has been reported to be significantly different in pregnant patients (13,14).

Sacroiliac joint pain and dysfunction is a common, but often overlooked, source of posterior pelvic pain in pregnancy. Risk factors include high parity, other anatomic sources of low back pain, obesity and physically strenuous work. Due to the size, shape and varying angles of the bilateral sacroiliac (SI) joints, pain character can vary widely from a sharp pain radiating from the SI joint down the posterior thigh to a dull, non-radiating pain in the ipsilateral gluteal region. Several tests may localize the pain to the SI joint including the "p4 test," which exerts pressure from the knee along the femur to the hip to localize pressure, and elicit pain, at the ipsilateral SI joint while stabilizing the pelvis with the patient in a supine position (13). The active straight leg raise test, with greater ease of hip flexion in the supine position with manual compression of the ipsilateral SI joint, is also easily employed in the pregnant patient (15,16). Relief of symptoms attributed to application of an appropriately sized and positioned pelvic belt has been described (17). The belt should be positioned to apply pressure over the bilateral SI joints posteriorly and the bilateral anterior superior iliac spines anteriorly; it should be worn consistently. Pregnancy exercises aimed at strengthening the muscles of the pelvic girdle have been reported to have short and long-term benefit (18). Oral analgesics, acupuncture, heat therapy or local injections may also be needed. During labor, prolonged positioning with hyperflexion at the hips or McRobert's maneuver should be avoided (19).

Osteitis pubis is non-infective inflammation and pain associated with bone resorption at the pubic symphysis and subsequent re-ossification. This disorder is often seen in elite athletes but can also be caused by the structural and physiologic changes of pregnancy. Pain, exacerbated by movement of the lower extremities, can become intense over just a few days. It radiates from the region of the pubic symphysis down to the inner thighs. This dysfunction is self-limited and can be managed with supportive pelvic binding (20) and activity modification. Acetaminophen and topical anesthetics can be added. Rarely ultrasound-guided local injections of steroids and anesthetics are required.

Pubic osteomyelitis is an infective inflammation of the pubic symphysis and pubic bones, which mimics osteitis pubis. It should be considered in every woman with pubic symphysis pain before during or after delivery. Strong suspicion for this condition should exist if pain is accompanied by an identifiable nidus of infection (e.g. abscessed tooth), which may cause bacteremia to seed an inflamed or damaged symphysis (21). Symptoms may be significantly delayed from the time of delivery (22). Rectus abdominus or thigh adductor muscle spasms may be noted due to altered posture caused by pain at the symphysis where these muscles insert. Imaging will show more destructive changes to the bone than are demonstrated with osteitis pubis. Ultrasound-guided aspiration and attempted culture of the infective organism should be attempted to guide intravenous antibiotic therapy; empiric antibiotics should be initiated while awaiting culture results. The most commonly identified organisms include *Staphylococcus aureus* and gram-negative rods (21). Antibiotic regimens may fail to adequately treat the patient; in such cases, significant improvement has been described with surgical debridement (22).

Pubic symphyseal separation is described in some sources synonymously with osteitis pubis, or on a spectrum of pubic symphysis changes in pregnancy that may become pathologic. It is best, however, considered a unique entity (23). Risk factors for separation or even frank rupture of the symphysis include history of damage to the pelvic girdle, precipitous delivery or rapid second stage of labor, use of McRobert's maneuver, regional anesthesia (24), multiparity and fetal macrosomia or malpresentation (25). Symptoms of separation, dislocation and rupture include pain in the region of the pubic symphysis with radiation to the legs, hips, and back along with edema and swelling. Pain is potentiated by weight bearing, walking or other activity utilizing the lower extremities. Tests to localize pelvic pain to the pubic symphysis include hip flexion with the lower leg in extension and pressure on the bilateral trochanters which compresses the symphysis. These tests should be used carefully to avoid causing severe pain (25). An audible "pop" or "crack" is often described in cases of acute symphyseal rupture. Imaging is required only if symphyseal rupture is suspected; separation can be diagnosed clinically (26).

Separation of the pubic symphysis is treated with pelvic binding and activity modification; complete bed rest is not advised. Modifications to activities of daily living include the avoidance of stair climbing and holding a child on one hip, keeping knees close together (e.g. exiting a car or bed) and standing on one leg to dress or reach for an object (19). Ambulatory supports (e.g. crutches, walker) along with physical and occupational therapy should be considered; these may be required for several weeks or months (27). Oral analgesics are usually required. Opiates may be used only with great caution. Local injections and use of a transcutaneous electrical nerve stimulation (TENS) unit have been reported to be helpful (25). Surgery is rarely needed and only routinely considered for cases of rupture with significant pelvic instability (23), associated with sacroiliac joint dysfunction and/or a minimum of 4 cm of separation; otherwise, even rupture can be treated as noted above over a longer period of time. Vaginal delivery is not precluded by pubic symphyseal separation or a history of rupture (27). During labor, prolonged positioning with hyperflexion at the hips or McRobert's maneuver should be avoided (19). Symptoms may recur in subsequent pregnancies although the rate of recurrence is difficult to determine and long-term impairment is uncommon.

Round ligament pain is commonly blamed for a majority pelvic pain in pregnancy. Discomfort is attributed to hypertrophy of the round ligaments of the uterus. The ligaments are composed of smooth muscle and course from the lateral uterus to the pelvic sidewall, through the inguinal canal, ending in the upper labium majus; pain can be perceived from innervation anywhere along this course. Pain may be worse on the right side as rotation of the uterus caused by the sigmoid colon puts greater stretch on the ipsilateral round ligament. Placing the patient in a left lateral reclining position and then gently pressing the fundus of the gravid uterus toward the right can re-create a sharp, shooting pain to the left inguinal region or labium majus on the left side, and vice versa. Alternatively, the patient can slowly roll from one side to the other to note recurrence of the pain. Round ligament pain can be treated with activity modification. Oral analgesics, heat therapy and stretching exercises designed to be safe in pregnancy may also provide relief. Rarely, varicosities of the round ligaments mimic benign round ligament pain or inguinal hernia presenting in pregnancy; imaging is required to differentiate these diagnoses (28,29).

Hip Joint Pain

Differential diagnosis includes osteonecrosis of the femoral head, transient osteoporosis as well as infectious arthritis. The latter requires needle aspiration of the involved joint with or without laboratory studies for inflammatory markers (30,31).

Osteonecrosis of the femoral head is labeled variously as ischemic, aseptic, non-traumatic or avascular osteonecrosis of the femoral head; it is a rare condition of uncertain cause. Ischemia of the femoral head may be temporary or permanent. Patients most commonly present in the third trimester with non-specific symptoms but often do not undergo imaging until the pain persists, worsens or recurs in the postpartum period (30–32). Pain radiating to the buttock, groin, thigh or knee region may be worse with weight-bearing. Decreased internal rotation of the involved hip in 15% of patients may occur (30,31). Gait change with worsening limp is also noted. Contributing factors may include remote or recent trauma to the hip joint, glucocorticoid exposure, hypercoagulable state of pregnancy, altered mechanics of the hip joint in pregnancy, excessive weight gain and increased mechanical load. The left hip is more commonly involved possibly due to excessive compression of the left common iliac vein by the right common iliac artery and the fetus. Bilateral lesions are very rare but have been described (33). Imaging of the hips is needed for diagnosis; plain radiographs may be utilized, although bony changes are not always seen initially. MRI is the preferred imaging study, with very specific findings for osteonecrosis described (34). Core tissue biopsy may assist with diagnosis (33). The disease is progressive and no treatments have been found to halt its advance. Limitation of weight-bearing is suggested along with anti-inflammatory (if the patient is less than 30 weeks gestation) and analgesic medications. Small case series describe core decompression and tissue graft performed in the postpartum period with favorable results (31,33). Without hip arthroplasty, the patient has an increased risk of secondary osteoarthritis of the affected hip and may require later treatment (35). High degree of suspicion, early consultation with a specialist and early imaging are suggested. No cases of recurrence in a subsequent pregnancy have been published.

Transient osteoporosis is a self-limiting condition with spontaneous resolution in the postpartum period. This disorder can initially present with symptoms much like osteonecrosis when the hip joint is affected. Vertebrae are the next most common bones to cause symptoms of low back pain and exhibit radiographic changes, including fractures (36). Pregnant patients in the third trimester complain of acute onset of pain during standing, weight-bearing, ambulation or other joint motion but deny history of trauma. Radiographs and MRI of the hip show demineralization of the femoral head and the acetabulum (the latter is unaffected in osteonecrosis), preservation of joint space and absence of chondral collapse (33). Radiographs of the spine may reveal vertebral fractures. Fractures related to this condition are rare but may be underdiagnosed as imaging is infrequently performed during pregnancy. Dual X-ray absorptiometry (DXA) scan can suggest the severity of the condition, but not true bone density loss as the availability of a pre-pregnancy DXA scan for comparison is rare (37). The etiology of transient osteoporosis is unknown (32,33). Treatment is conservative and guided by the patient's symptoms. Activity including weight-bearing ambulation should be strongly encouraged (37); physical therapy may preserve range of motion and prevent joint contractures (38). Bisphosphonates are not well studied in pregnancy and should not be used (39). Daily calcium and vitamin D intake has not been studied for prevention or treatment of this condition, but should be discussed with all pregnant patients, especially those who have advanced maternal age or altered diets or dietary restrictions limiting calcium intake. In most cases, symptoms of transient osteoporosis resolve slowly but completely within 6 to 12 months of delivery, although duration of recovery is affected by the duration of breastfeeding (37). Avoidance of lactation and breastfeeding have been recommended (36,37) especially in cases where fracture is diagnosed. Another study with serial imaging of patients with vertebral fractures attributed to transient osteoporosis noted that the increase in bone mass density (BMD) at the spine was significant between 8 and 18 months after the symptomatic pregnancy with further improvement noted at both the spine and hip at 24 and 48 months (36). The condition has been reported to recur, albeit sporadically, in subsequent pregnancies (40). If findings of osteoporosis are found in pregnancy or in the postpartum period, family history should be recorded and a secondary cause of osteoporosis pre-dating pregnancy should be considered (36).

Lower Extremity Pain

Leg cramps affect up to 30% of pregnant women, occur more frequently in latter part of pregnancy and at night with the calf muscles most commonly affected. The etiology is uncertain and few treatments have been tested in pregnant patients. Supplementation of several vitamins and minerals has been studied; definitive evidence of benefit is lacking (41). Various stretching exercises, especially prior to lying down at night, are also commonly described but have not been rigorously tested in a pregnant population.

Thigh pain may be related to lateral femoral cutaneous neuropathy (also termed meralgia paraesthetica), which is caused by compression or injury to this nerve and is unilateral 80% of the time. Symptoms include paresthesia, numbness or pain. Pregnant women may be twelve times more likely to suffer this neuropathy (42). This may be the most common neuropathy identified after labor and delivery (43). Cesarean delivery has not been shown to be a distinct risk factor (43). Hyperflexion of the hips during maternal pushing efforts may put pressure on the lateral femoral cutaneous nerve. Diagnosis is clinical; conduction studies of the lateral femoral cutaneous nerve are difficult and of little benefit. Modification of clothing and posture, including alternating sides when carrying older children, can relieve some symptoms prior to delivery. Use of nerve blocks in pregnant patients has not been described. In most cases, spontaneous and complete resolution occurs in the postpartum period.

Knee pain is not uncommon in pregnant patients and should be considered in relation to other comorbid conditions such as obesity. Postural changes, ligamentous laxity and related gait changes may all play a role in pregnancy-related knee pain. In general, bed rest should be avoided and, instead, exercise programs and physical therapy should be employed.

Patellofemoral pain syndrome can present in pregnancy with anterior knee pain due to abnormal tracking of the patella over the femoral condyles. Known risk factors for patellofemoral pain syndrome in pregnancy include altered muscle strength, altered range of motion, ligamentous laxity and alterations of gait. The pain is usually noted while sitting or when walking down stairs. Imaging is only useful to rule out radiologically visible pathology. Short-term "RICE" (rest, ice, compression, elevation) is recommended along with oral acetaminophen. Physical therapy or exercises targeted at strengthening the quadriceps are recommended.

Foot pain in pregnant women is increased compared to age-matched non-pregnant women. This has been variously attributed to weight gain, ligamentous laxity, increased peripheral edema and postural changes. In general, treatments include adequate foot hygiene, elevation, massage, stretching exercises and supportive, well-fitted shoes.

Tarsal tunnel syndrome is a focal compressive neuropathy of the posterior tibial nerve, and more rarely the deep peroneal nerve. It is thought peripheral edema or varicose veins can contribute to significant symptoms in the plantar margins of the foot which resolve after delivery. The diagnosis is made by nerve conduction studies and electromyography. Treatment in pregnant patients should be conservative as symptoms will likely resolve in the postpartum period. Oral analgesics with judicious use of antiinflammatory medications (antiinflammatory medications should not be used after 30 weeks gestation and earlier only if benefits clearly outweigh risks) are the mainstays of therapy, but can be supplemented with physical therapy mobilization exercises. Corticosteroid injections could also be considered. Surgery for a definitive point of nerve entrapment has not yet been described in a pregnant patient.

Plantar fasciitis is a degenerative condition of the plantar fascia that results in heel pain. Pregnancy is not an identified risk factor. Treatment is initially symptomatic; acetaminophen coupled with gentle daily stretching can often manage mild symptoms. Podiatric or physical therapy consultation can be considered if taping, orthoses or corticosteroid injections are needed. Most studies of investigational therapies exclude pregnant women.

Upper Extremity Pain

Median neuropathy (also termed carpal tunnel syndrome) can present initially in pregnancy and resolve afterward. The carpal tunnel is a small space; any cause of increased volume can compress the median nerve. Pregnancy, with its increased fluid volume and peripheral edema, may cause bilateral symptoms. Overuse injury is more often unilateral and may have been present to some degree prior to pregnancy. Numbness and tingling of the thumb, index, middle and radial ring finger are commonly noted along with pain during sleep when relaxation of the hand into a hyperextended position can exacerbate symptoms. Diagnosis can be made with several provocative clinical tests including, among others, Phalen's test and reverse Phalen's test; these elicit paresthesias in the median nerve distribution with prolonged flexion and extension of the wrist, respectively. Treatment is symptomatic. Wrist splints worn as needed throughout the day and night as well as during exacerbating activities afford up to 80% of pregnant women with relief. Electromyography of the median nerve in various studies shows improvement in nerve function that mirrors clinical improvement (3,40). For severe cases, local steroid injection can be considered in pregnancy. Surgery should be deferred to the postpartum period as median neuropathy attributable to pregnancy should resolve within a few weeks after delivery. This mononeuropathy may persist beyond pregnancy or recur with future pregnancies, possibly due to residual ischemic damage to the nerve (23,44).

Stenosing tendinopathy is caused by restriction of the abductor pollicis longus and extensor pollicis brevis tendons by the extensor retinaculum at the styloid process of the radius. The term tenosynovitis is not used here as inflammation is not always present. This disorder presents as a pain on the radial side of the wrist exacerbated by thumb and wrist movements. The pain may radiate along the forearm or into the thumb or be associated with a sensation of swelling. Grip and ability to hold objects securely, especially while moving the wrist, may also be described. The Finkelstein test is classically described as making a closed fist then gently bending the wrist in an ulnar direction which elicits characteristic discomfort. This diagnosis is not specific to pregnancy or the postpartum patient although fluid retention and local edema are suggested as contributing factors in pregnant patients. Stenosing tendinopathy, historically termed de Quervain tenosynovitis, is most often a repetitive use injury that can be seen in the reproductive-aged woman with childcare activities including positioning during breastfeeding or with hobbies like knitting and crocheting. Treatment includes oral analgesics along with activity modification and heat or ice therapy. A thumb spica splint provides some patients relief. If these measures fail and a component of inflammation is suspected, a judicious trial of non-steroidal anti-inflammatory drugs (NSAIDs) is suggested with discontinuation if there is no relief after 3–5 days. The use of NSAIDs in pregnancy is safe if employed prior to the 30th week of gestation after which NSAIDs exposure is associated with an increased risk of premature closure of the fetal ductus arteriosus and oligohydramnios (45) but should be used only if benefits clearly outweigh risks. Local steroid injection may be needed in severe cases but spontaneous resolution is the usual outcome. In some cases, spontaneous resolution is delayed until after the cessation of breastfeeding due to mechanical irritation of the tendons with breastfeeding actions.

Ulnar neuropathy, also called cubital tunnel syndrome, presents as numbness, tingling or discomfort in the ring and small fingers or grip weakness related to altered function of these digits. Transient symptoms in the distribution of the ulnar nerve are the second most common upper extremity neuropathy in pregnancy or the postpartum period. The cubital tunnel of the elbow is a common site of ulnar nerve compression, which may occur bilaterally in pregnancy related to edema. Other risk factors not specific to pregnancy, but occasionally exacerbated by pregnancy, include obesity, glucose intolerance or diabetes and hypertension. Oral analgesics and activity modification are recommended along with physical therapy, as needed.

Chest and Abdominal Pain

Abdominal wall laxity is caused by strain on all layers of the abdominal wall (46), not simply separation of the abdominal rectus muscle bellies from the linea alba. Abdominal wall laxity may occur apart from pregnancy or be acquired secondary to the anatomic and physiologic changes of pregnancy. Diagnosis is made by placing the patient in supine position and then asking her to engage her rectus abdominus muscles by starting to sit up; the appearance of a midline fusiform bulge is diagnostic, although body habitus may obscure this view. Midline abdominal wall laxity is not a ventral hernia although the two can coexist. Although abdominal wall laxity rarely causes functional limitation during pregnancy and does not place the fetus at any risk, it can be bothersome in appearance especially if it worsens during pregnancy or persists after childbearing has ended. A recent systematic review suggests exercise during or after pregnancy may improve bothersome abdominal wall laxity (47). Spontaneous improvement is common after delivery and surgical correction is not appropriate during pregnancy.

Desmoid tumors belong to the group of disorders termed musculoskeletal fibromatosis, benign proliferations of fibrous elements a muscle. Desmoid tumors can grow in an aggressive fashion but there is no reported metastatic disease. The most common sites include the mesentery, abdominal wall and retroperitoneum (48). Trauma to the involved muscle and hereditary conditions including Gardner syndrome, a subtype of familial adenomatous polyposis, are known risk factors. Pregnancy is still largely an anecdotal risk factor attributed to hyperestrogenism. There are few studies to support this supposition. One study notes estrogen receptor positivity in 33% of desmoid tumors surveyed, but there have been no robust investigations of the biologic implications of this finding (49). Patients will often note a palpable mass that is minimally symptomatic. Palpation of an abdominal mass can differentiate it from the uterus in most cases. Imaging of any new or changing mass is suggested with MRI recommended if a desmoid tumor is suspected. These tumors appear well-differentiated on imaging, but histology routinely shows them to be highly infiltrative of adjacent tissues. This explains the high risk of recurrence of desmoid tumors and other types of musculoskeletal fibromatosis. Resection of the tumor may be indicated if symptomatic or if growth impinges on vital structures. When a desmoid tumor is suspected or diagnosed in a pregnant patient, delay of surgery until the postpartum period is appropriate. Manageable patient discomfort is not an indication for surgery or preterm delivery. Reports of desmoid tumor regression attributed to various non-steroidal anti-estrogen medications exist but are not based on definite knowledge of the pharmacologic effect on the tumor nor have any large or randomized trials been performed (50). Spontaneous regression has also been reported.

Umbilical pain in pregnancy is rarely related to acute herniation, although assessment for strangulation or incarceration of abdominal contents in a patient with risk factors and/or acute symptoms is necessary. Other considerations include myofascial trigger points (see below), infected or impacted umbilical piercing (whether or not hardware is still in place) or a previously undiagnosed umbilical mass of which most are benign.

Painful rib syndrome has not been evaluated specifically in pregnancy. Nonetheless, rib pain can be persistent and extremely bothersome in pregnancy. Suggested risk factors include short torso or stature, large uterus (e.g. multiple gestation) and abdominal wall laxity. Tenderness of the lower ribs, more commonly noted on the right, can be reproduced with direct palpation by a single digit to the noted area. The pain is most often unilateral but can involve multiple costochondral joints. No study has been done to elucidate if this pain is actually a costochondritis induced by chronic strain from the enlarging uterus and stretching of the abdominal wall muscles. Oral analgesics and judicious use of NSAIDs (prior to the 30th week of gestation) can be considered along with local heat or ice therapy. Postural awareness and activity modification are important; women must be advised to identify and minimize exacerbating activities. Older children should not consistently be carried on one hip.

Thoracic outlet syndrome (TOS) is a constellation of symptoms caused by compression of nerves and/or vessels of the upper extremity as they pass under the first rib and behind the clavicle. Thoracic outlet syndrome is not specific to but can be exacerbated by pregnancy. Three types of TOS have been described – neurogenic, arterial and venous. Hypercoagulable states and regional edema are risk factors along with local trauma and repetitive arm motion or stress, including carrying children or car seats and diaper bags. Symptoms can vary widely but may mimic median nerve compression in pregnancy. Imaging with radiography can demonstrate a cervical rib, the most common anatomic cause of symptoms; MRI evaluation is rarely needed. Vascular imaging studies and electromyography can be performed in pregnancy, but should be discussed with a specialist. Oral analgesic, postural awareness, activity modification and appropriate adjustment of work duties are recommended for most patients. Neurogenic TOS may benefit from physical therapy. Identification of a thromboembolus would require anticoagulant therapy prior to delivery but any consideration of surgical therapy for a symptomatic cervical rib should be deferred to the post-partum period.

Soft Tissue Issues

Myofascial pain is associated with painful trigger points, palpable areas of muscle irritation that, depending on their location, cause characteristic referral patterns related to the nerve that is likewise irritated (51). Myofascial pain is localized or referred discomfort that can be reproduced with pressure applied to a trigger point. Localized hypoxia and inflammation appear to contribute to the release of inflammatory substances which sensitize muscle nociceptors (52). Myofascial pain should be considered with reports of discomfort at unusual location like the umbilicus or in the tendons and aponeuroses of various muscles; some authors note trigger points to be more common in postural muscles than dynamic muscles (51).

The diagnosis is made simply by palpating the localized area of muscle tautness with or without referral of discomfort in the distribution of the involved nerve. Extensive texts are published on mapping and treatment of trigger points. Initial treatment includes a variety of peripheral stimulation techniques aimed at release of the muscle trigger point. Sustained pressure, occasionally marketed as acupressure, can result in some degree of relief or complete resolution. Travell, who initially described trigger points, treated them with local injection of anesthetic. These lesions also respond to dry needling and localized cooling and stretching regimens (51). Other therapies with moderate level evidence include osteopathic manipulative medicine and electrical stimulation. One article addresses the use of local anesthetic injection to relieve pain from myofascial trigger points as an adjunct to epidural during labor (53). Consideration of vertebral misalignment and related somatic dysfunction is encouraged with recurrent or persistent myofascial pain.

Summary

Musculoskeletal disorders are an often overlooked and underdiagnosed cause of pain and dysfunction during pregnancy. While some causes of musculoskeletal pain are common and benign, it is essential to evaluate the patient thoroughly. A proper examination may negate the need for imaging. However, imaging to diagnose a pathologic disorder should not be avoided simply because the patient is pregnant. An accurate diagnosis will allow the indicated treatments to optimize outcomes. In most cases, the evaluation and management are the same for pregnant and nonpregnant patients.

References

1. Pennick V, Liddle SD. Interventions for preventing and treating pelvic and back pain in pregnancy. *The Cochrane Database of Systematic Reviews.* 2013;8:CD001139.
2. Gutke A, Ostgaard HC, Oberg B. Predicting persistent pregnancy-related low back pain. *Spine.* 2008;33(12):E386–93.
3. Borg-Stein JP, Fogelman DJ, Ackerman KE. Exercise, sports participation, and musculoskeletal disorders of pregnancy and postpartum. *Seminars in Neurology.* 2011;31(4):413–22.
4. Skaggs CD, Prather H, Gross G, George JW, Thompson PA, Nelson DM. Back and pelvic pain in an underserved United States pregnant population: A preliminary descriptive survey. *Journal of Manipulative and Physiological Therapeutics.* 2007;30(2):130–4.
5. Betz RR, Bunnell WP, Lambrecht-Mulier E, MacEwen GD. Scoliosis and pregnancy. *The Journal of Bone and Joint Surgery American volume.* 1987;69(1):90–6.
6. Ko JY, Leffert LR. Clinical implications of neuraxial anesthesia in the parturient with scoliosis. *Anesthesia and Analgesia.* 2009;109(6):1930–4.
7. Saraste H. Spondylolysis and pregnancy – A risk analysis. *Acta Obstetricia et Gynecologica Scandinavica.* 1986;65(7):727–9.
8. Sanderson PL, Fraser RD. The influence of pregnancy on the development of degenerative spondylolisthesis. *Journal of Bone and Joint Surgery British volume.* 1996;78(6):951–4.
9. Chan YL, Lam WW, Lau TK, Metreweli C, Chan DP. Back pain in pregnancy – Magnetic resonance imaging correlation. *Clinical Radiology.* 2002;57(12):1109–12.
10. Weinreb JC, Wolbarsht LB, Cohen JM, Brown CE, Maravilla KR. Prevalence of lumbosacral intervertebral disk abnormalities on MR images in pregnant and asymptomatic nonpregnant women. *Radiology.* 1989;170(1 Pt 1):125–8.
11. Garmel SH, Guzelian GA, D'Alton JG, D'Alton ME. Lumbar disk disease in pregnancy. *Obstetrics and Gynecology.* 1997;89(5 Pt 2):821–2.
12. Heckman JD, Sassard R. Musculoskeletal considerations in pregnancy. *Journal of Bone and Joint Surgery American volume.* 1994;76(11):1720–30.
13. Ostgaard HC, Zetherstrom G, Roos-Hansson E. The posterior pelvic pain provocation test in pregnant

women. *European Spine Journal: Official Publication of the European Spine Society, the European Spinal Deformity Society, and the European Section of the Cervical Spine Research Society*. 1994;3(5):258–60.

14. Cohen SP, Chen Y, Neufeld NJ. Sacroiliac joint pain: A comprehensive review of epidemiology, diagnosis and treatment. *Expert Review of Neurotherapeutics*. 2013;13(1):99–116.
15. Mens JM, Huis In 't Veld YH, Pool-Goudzwaard A. The active straight leg raise test in lumbopelvic pain during pregnancy. *Manual Therapy*. 2012;17(4):364–8.
16. Mens JM, Vleeming A, Snijders CJ, Koes BW, Stam HJ. Validity of the active straight leg raise test for measuring disease severity in patients with posterior pelvic pain after pregnancy. *Spine*. 2002;27(2):196–200.
17. Mens JM, Damen L, Snijders CJ, Stam HJ. The mechanical effect of a pelvic belt in patients with pregnancy-related pelvic pain. *Clinical Biomechanics*. 2006;21(2):122–7.
18. Stuge B, Laerum E, Kirkesola G, Vollestad N. The efficacy of a treatment program focusing on specific stabilizing exercises for pelvic girdle pain after pregnancy: A randomized controlled trial. *Spine*. 2004;29(4):351–9.
19. Mitchell DA, Esler DM. Pelvic instability – Painful pelvic girdle in pregnancy. *Australian Family Physician*. 2009;38(6):409–10.
20. Flack NA, Hay-Smith EJ, Stringer MD, Gray AR, Woodley SJ. Adherence, tolerance and effectiveness of two different pelvic support belts as a treatment for pregnancy-related symphyseal pain – A pilot randomized trial. *BMC Pregnancy and Childbirth*. 2015;15:36.
21. Eskridge C, Longo S, Kwark J, Robichaux A, Begneaud W. Osteomyelitis pubis occurring after spontaneous vaginal delivery: A case presentation. *Journal of Perinatology: Official Journal of the California Perinatal Association*. 1997;17(4):321–4.
22. Knoeller SM, Uhl M, Herget GW. Osteitis or osteomyelitis of the pubis? A diagnostic and therapeutic challenge: Report of 9 cases and review of the literature. *Acta Orthopaedica Belgica*. 2006;72(5):541–8.
23. Rommens PM. Internal fixation in postpartum symphysis pubis rupture: Report of three cases. *Journal of Orthopaedic Trauma*. 1997;11(4):273–6.
24. Cappiello GA, Oliver BC. Rupture of symphysis pubis caused by forceful and excessive abduction of the thighs with labor epidural anesthesia. *Journal of the Florida Medical Association*. 1995;82(4):261–3.
25. Snow RE, Neubert AG. Peripartum pubic symphysis separation: A case series and review of the literature. *Obstetrical & Gynecological Survey*. 1997;52(7):438–43.
26. Jain N, Sternberg LB. Symphyseal separation. *Obstetrics and Gynecology*. 2005;105(5 Pt 2):1229–32.
27. Culligan P, Hill S, Heit M. Rupture of the symphysis pubis during vaginal delivery followed by two subsequent uneventful pregnancies. *Obstetrics and Gynecology*. 2002;100(5 Pt 2):1114–7.
28. Bulbul E, Taskin MI, Yanik B, Demirpolat G, Adali E, Basbug M. Rare cause of bilateral groin swelling: Round ligament varicosities. *Pakistan Journal of Medical Sciences*. 2015;31(4):1012–4.
29. FF IJ, Boddeus KM, de Haan HH, van Geldere D. Bilateral round ligament varicosities mimicking inguinal hernia during pregnancy. *Hernia: Journal of Hernias and Abdominal Wall Surgery*. 2009;13(1):85–8.
30. Montella BJ, Nunley JA, Urbaniak JR. Osteonecrosis of the femoral head associated with pregnancy. A preliminary report. *Journal of Bone and Joint Surgery American volume*. 1999;81(6):790–8.
31. Pellicci PM, Zolla-Pazner S, Rabhan WN, Wilson PD, Jr. Osteonecrosis of the femoral head associated with pregnancy. Report of three cases. *Clinical Orthopaedics and Related Research*. 1984(185):59–63.
32. Lausten GS. Osteonecrosis of the femoral head during pregnancy. *Archives of Orthopaedic and Trauma Surgery*. 1991;110(4):214–5.
33. Ugwonali OF, Sarkissian H, Nercessian OA. Bilateral osteonecrosis of the femoral head associated with pregnancy: Four new cases and a review of the literature. *Orthopedics*. 2008;31(2):183.
34. Zurlo JV. The double-line sign. *Radiology*. 1999;212(2):541–2.
35. Cheng N, Burssens A, Mulier JC. Pregnancy and post-pregnancy avascular necrosis of the femoral head. *Archives of Orthopaedic and Trauma Surgery*. 1982;100(3):199–210.
36. Phillips AJ, Ostlere SJ, Smith R. Pregnancy-associated osteoporosis: Does the skeleton recover? *Osteoporosis International: a journal established as result of cooperation between the European Foundation for Osteoporosis and the National Osteoporosis Foundation of the USA*. 2000;11(5):449–54.
37. Kovacs CS, Ralston SH. Presentation and management of osteoporosis presenting in association with pregnancy or lactation. *Osteoporosis International: a journal established as result of cooperation between the European Foundation for Osteoporosis and the National Osteoporosis Foundation of the USA*. 2015;26(9):2223–41.
38. Ireland ML, Ott SM. The effects of pregnancy on the musculoskeletal system. *Clinical Orthopaedics and Related Research*. 2000;(372):169–79.

39. Suresh E, Pazianas M, Abrahamsen B. Safety issues with bisphosphonate therapy for osteoporosis. *Rheumatology*. 2014;53(1):19–31.

40. Thabah M, Ravindran V. Musculoskeletal problems in pregnancy. *Rheumatology International*. 2015;35(4):581–7.

41. Zhou K, West HM, Zhang J, Xu L, Li W. Interventions for leg cramps in pregnancy. *Cochrane Database of Systematic Reviews*. 2015;8:CD010655.

42. van Slobbe AM, Bohnen AM, Bernsen RM, Koes BW, Bierma-Zeinstra SM. Incidence rates and determinants in meralgia paresthetica in general practice. *Journal of Neurology*. 2004;251(3):294–7.

43. Redick LF. Maternal perinatal nerve palsies. *Postgraduate Obstetrics and Gynecology*. 1992;12:1–5.

44. Mondelli M, Rossi S, Monti E, Aprile I, Caliandro P, Pazzaglia C, et al. Long term follow-up of carpal tunnel syndrome during pregnancy: A cohort study and review of the literature. *Electromyography and Clinical Neurophysiology*. 2007;47(6):259–71.

45. Antonucci R, Zaffanello M, Puxeddu E, Porcella A, Cuzzolin L, Pilloni MD, et al. Use of non-steroidal anti-inflammatory drugs in pregnancy: Impact on the fetus and newborn. *Current Drug Metabolism*. 2012;13(4):474–90.

46. Brauman D. Diastasis recti: Clinical anatomy. *Plastic and Reconstructive Surgery*. 2008;122(5):1564–9.

47. Benjamin DR, van de Water AT, Peiris CL. Effects of exercise on diastasis of the rectus abdominis muscle in the antenatal and postnatal periods: A systematic review. *Physiotherapy*. 2014;100(1):1–8.

48. Dyrstad SW, Fowler AM, Jokerst CE, Baker JC, Hillen TJ, Menias C. Abdominal and pelvic tumors with musculoskeletal histology. *Current Problems in Diagnostic Radiology*. 2014;43(2):68–79.

49. Lim CL, Walker MJ, Mehta RR, Das Gupta TK. Estrogen and antiestrogen binding sites in desmoid tumors. *European Journal of Cancer & Clinical Oncology*. 1986;22(5):583–7.

50. Sturt NJ, Clark SK. Current ideas in desmoid tumours. *Familial Cancer*. 2006;5(3):275–85; discussion 87–8.

51. DeStefano L. *Greenman's Principles of Manual Medicine*. 4th ed. Philadelphia PA: Lippincott Williams & Wilkins; 2011.

52. Shah JP, Danoff JV, Desai MJ, Parikh S, Nakamura LY, Phillips TM, et al. Biochemicals associated with pain and inflammation are elevated in sites near to and remote from active myofascial trigger points. *Archives of Physical Medicine and Rehabilitation*. 2008;89(1):16–23.

53. Tsen LC, Camann WR. Trigger point injections for myofascial pain during epidural analgesia for labor. *Regional Anesthesia*. 1997;22(5):466–8.

Obesity in Pregnancy

Jasjit K. Beausang and Shontreal M. Cooper

Introduction

Obesity is an increasingly common medical problem, and it is often underrecognized and underaddressed. Because obesity carries significant risks to the health of the reproductive age woman and her children, it is imperative that evidence-based guidelines for the management of this condition in pregnancy are available to providers. Powerful barriers to the implementation of these guidelines exist in our medical and lay culture.

Scope of the Problem

Obesity is defined as the disease in which excess body fat has accumulated to such an extent that health may be adversely affected (1,2). Comorbidities associated with obesity in pregnancy include increased rates of infertility, pregnancy loss, congenital anomalies, cardiac and renal dysfunction, gestational diabetes, sleep apnea, macrosomia and paradoxically, growth restriction, operative and cesarean delivery, and stillbirth (1,3,4). Obesity confers increased premature mortality and cardiovascular risk for mothers (5).

According to most recent data from the National Center for Health Statistics, the current prevalence of overweight status in United States women above the age of 20 is 64.6% (6). As of 2011–2012, obesity prevalence in all women aged 20–39 was 31.8%, with prevalence disproportionately high in non-Hispanic Black women (56.6%) and Hispanic women (44.4%). In girls aged 12–19, the obesity rate is slightly lower at 20.7% (7). This data highlights the opportunity for prevention in the management of obesity.

Diagnosis is simple: the standard accepted criterion is the WHO classification according to body mass index (BMI) calculated as weight in kilograms divided by the square of height in meters (kg/m^2) (see Table 33.1). This index allows population-level examination of the effects of obesity, but is crude in the estimation of individual health risk; it appears that the adverse health effects vary with body fat content, fat distribution, and gender, variations that are not accounted for by the BMI (2). Nonetheless, BMI remains the standard metric that can be used to guide women's' care and is predictive of pregnancy outcomes (8).

Etiology

At the heart of this complex health problem is an energy imbalance: energy intake exceeds energy expenditure. Even a minor excess of energy intake over a long period of time can lead to a significant increase in weight, and human physiology favors maintenance of the new overweight status.

A gross estimate of energy intake via micronutrients is summarized in Table 33.2. In general, fat is a higher-density macronutrient than protein or carbohydrate, and exposure to high-fat foods can lead to overconsumption of calories. Specifically, however, trans fat, cholesterol, and saturated fat intake are associated with increased cardiovascular risks, while polyunsaturated fats decrease risk (9). Carbohydrate type and quantity influence caloric intake: foods high in fiber such a fruits, vegetables, legumes, and whole grains provide a low-energy density source, which is associated with more satiety and less weight gain (2). Simple carbohydrates, especially those in sugary drinks and processed foods, increase risk of passive overconsumption and should be limited to less than 10% of caloric intake (10). Protein intake is recommended at about 5.5 oz per day, but type of protein is also important. For example, processed red meat intake is associated with increased mortality (11).

Energy expenditure is characterized by a basal metabolic rate (BMR), dietary thermogenesis (energy released by digestion and absorption), and physical activity level. There is little variation in BMR in an individual, but physical activity levels can be modified

Table 33.1 World Health Organization BMI[a] Classification for individuals 20 Years Old or Greater with Institute of Medicine Recommended Gestational Weight Gain[b]

BMI[a]	Nutritional Status	Gestational Weight Gain (lb)[b]
<18.5	Underweight	28–40
18.5–24.9	Normal weight	25–35
25.0–29.9	Overweight/pre-obese	15–25
30.0–34.9	Obesity Class I	11–20
35.0–39.9	Obesity Class II	11–20
>40	Obesity Class III	11–20

[a] In units of kg/m^2.

[b] Singleton pregnancy.

Source: From World Health Organization. *Body Mass Index – BMI*. www.euro.who.int. Accessed February 1, 2016.

Institute of Medicine. *Weight gain during pregnancy: re-examining the guidelines*. www.ion.nationalacademies.org. Accessed February 1, 2016.

Table 33.2 Caloric Value of Macronutrients

Macronutrient	Atwater Value (kcal/g)
Carbohydrate	4
Fat	9
Protein	4
Ethanol	– (heat of combustion = 7)

* Atwater equivalent now uniformly used in food labeling.

Source: From National Academy of Sciences. Institute of Medicine. Food and Nutrition Board. *Dietary Reference Intakes for Energy, Fiber, Carbohydrate, Fat, Fatty Acids, Cholesterol, Protein, and Amino Acids.*

(12). Occupational work, household chores, and leisure-time physical activity comprise an individual's overall activity.

Societal factors play a role in the development of obesity. Socioeconomic status is inversely associated with obesity rates in mothers and children (13). Education, food culture, body image, legislation, industry, media, and consumer demand all influence food choices and risks of excessive intake.

Individual biological susceptibility mediates the response to a positive energy balance. BMI is thought to be approximately 40% heritable (40% of variation can be explained by genetics). There are eight well-established single gene causes of obesity, which are thought to account for about 10% of severe obesity in children. An individual's endocrine milieu strongly influences their tendency to gain weight, and adipose tissue is now seen as a major endocrine organ, secreting leptin, estrogen, and TNFalpha among many other hormones. Environmental exposures to endocrine disrupting compounds, such as Bisphenol A and organochlorine pesticides, have impacted, perhaps generationally, the signaling that determines energy balance. These effects are propagated by epigenetic changes (DNA methylation, histone modification) (14). We also know that maternal obesity is strongly linked with obesity and its adverse health outcomes in offspring, likely via in-utero epigenetic changes.

Finally, individual factors such as smoking cessation, excessive alcohol intake, and certain medications can facilitate weight gain and contribute to obesity (15).

Preconception Considerations

A patient who is considering pregnancy (or not reliably contracepting) is an ideal target for discussion of BMI as it relates to health outcomes for the patient and her family. She may be more receptive to change in the context of the health of her children. Yet, only 5% of women report receiving weight loss counseling in the preconception period (16).

Height, weight, and calculation of BMI should be incorporated into the vital signs assessment at each office visit. When a patient with elevated BMI is identified, this and the associated risks (maternal and fetal/neonatal) should be clearly communicated to her. Additional parameters should be measured to assess for the risk or existence of comorbidities such as hypertension, insulin resistance, or hyperlipidemia. Waist circumference should be measured, as well as blood pressure with a large cuff. Additional orders should include fasting lipid panel, hemoglobin A1C, thyroid studies, and screening for obstructive sleep apnea.

Once an overweight or obese patient is identified, a follow-up visit is necessary to thoroughly explore the factors contributing to her weight. A nonjudgmental attitude is essential and an open interviewing style helpful when encouraging patients to make a change. Motivational interviewing, a technique that aims to recognize a person's ambivalent feelings toward making a healthy change, assesses his or her readiness for change and guide him or her to a sustainable solution, is endorsed by American Congress of Obstetricians and Gynecologists (ACOG) as an effective means of communication with patients (17).

Patients need not strive to achieve a normal BMI prior to pregnancy. Even a 5–10% weight loss can improve hypertension, insulin resistance, and fertility. A 10% weight loss could reduce preeclampsia, gestational diabetes, and macrosomia risk during gestation (18). An intensive program initiated 6 months prior to planned conception can positively affect pregnancy outcomes. A sustained caloric deficit of about 500 kcal/day can result in a weight loss of 0.45 kg/week (0.9 lb). This deficit should be achieved by a combination of reduced energy intake and increased expenditure. Diets that have less fat content, lower energy density, incorporate portion size control, increased fresh fruit and vegetable intake, and minimization of processed foods are the most effective (19). Substantial patient education is required to achieve this type of diet; referral to a dietician is necessary. Patients can also be referred to comprehensive lifestyle modification programs, such as Weight Watchers or Jenny Craig, as these are cost-effective (20).

Increased physical activity (30–60 minutes of exercise five to seven times per week) is associated with sustained weight loss and less gestational weight gain during pregnancy (21). One hour of brisk walking daily can be sufficient, though including resistance exercise (weight training) further decreases fat mass (19).

Pharmaceutical intervention is best undertaken outside of pregnancy to avoid exposure to the fetus. Several Food and Drug Administration (FDA)-approved medications, including orlistat, phentermine-topiramate XR, and lorcaserin, are well-tolerated, effective and have relatively modest adverse effect profiles (22). These should be combined with thorough dietary and physical activity counseling for maximum efficacy and sustainability of weight loss. Over-the-counter supplements are not well-documented as efficacious, and their safety is not monitored; physicians should discourage their use. Patients using metformin to moderate insulin resistance in the treatment of polycystic ovarian syndrome (PCOS) may continue, as it results in lower gestational weight gain (but no reduction in birth weight) (23).

Surgical intervention for weight loss is indicated for patients with a BMI 40 or greater, or a BMI between 35 and 39.9 with comorbidities related to obesity, such as cardiovascular disease, diabetes, or sleep apnea. In this group of patients, weight loss and reduction in comorbidities outweighs surgical risk (24). This is discussed further later.

Counterintuitively, micronutrient deficits are common in obese women. Prepregnancy BMI is inversely correlated with serum 25-hydroxy-vitamin D (25(OH)D) levels in early pregnancy. Most vitamin D is synthesized in the skin in response to ultraviolet exposure. The Institute of Medicine (IOM) recommends a daily intake of 600 IU for most adults, including pregnant women. Serum 25(OH)D status should be assessed, especially in dark-skinned women, to correct deficiency. A recent Cochrane review has established that vitamin D supplementation in pregnancy does increase serum 25(OH)D levels and may reduce the risk of preterm birth and birth weight < 2,500g (25).

Folic acid supplementation is important for all women considering pregnancy, as it is protective against neural tube defects. Because of the increased rate of neural tube defects in obese women, a higher dose of folate can be recommended, from 1 mg/day up to 5 mg/day, though some analyses have showed the increased risk conferred by obesity to be independent of folate levels (26). In fact, red blood corpuscle (RBC) folate levels increase with increasing BMI, data that is yet of uncertain clinical significance (27). Calcium intake, via diary intake or supplementation, should also be discussed. Obese pregnant women are at higher risk of iron deficiency (28). Iron-deficiency anemia may be better corrected outside of pregnancy, given the constipating effects of iron supplementation, which can compound the constipation many women experience in early pregnancy.

Gestational Weight Gain

The caloric excess required for a normal weight woman with a singleton pregnancy is approximately 200–300 kcal per day. Appropriate weight gain guidelines have been in place since 2009, recommended by the IOM based on extensive review of literature. Many women do not follow these recommendations: 40% of normal-weight women exceed guideline-suggested weight gain, and overweight status is associated with a 60% risk of exceeding recommended gain. Excessive gestational weight gain (GWG) is more likely to occur in the first pregnancy and is correlated with postpartum weight retention. Excessive GWG itself is a predictor of macrosomia and large for gestational age (LGA) fetuses, preeclampsia, cesarean delivery, and childhood obesity in the offspring (29), and this independent effect persists in the population with gestational diabetes (30). Weight gain in the first trimester may be of most significance, as it is linked with increased rates of diabetes, hypertensive disease, and weight retention, as well as maternal cardiovascular health in the long term (31). Limiting GWG to IOM guidelines is therefore of critical importance. Exercise plays an important role in this; obese women in general tend to be less active than normal weight women and tend to decrease their activity levels during pregnancy. Many providers do not strongly emphasize the need for physical activity during gestation, but there is substantial evidence that it improves insulin resistance, limits weight gain, and even benefits the long-term health of the offspring (32). Especially for obese patients, providers should advocate for 30 minutes of moderate-intensity exercise daily.

Special Considerations by Trimester

First Trimester

The current estimate of unintended pregnancy in the United States is 51% (33); providers will therefore find that many considerations of the preconceptional period must be shifted to a patient's initial obstetric visit. Weight loss during pregnancy, however, cannot be safely recommended, though high-quality evidence is lacking. Gestational weight gain below the recommended amount is associated with small for gestational age (SGA) neonates and pre-term birth (34), even in obese women.

Late onset of prenatal care may be more common in the obese gravida; hyperandrogenism and menstrual irregularity could contribute by delaying diagnosis of pregnancy. An early fetal ultrasound should be obtained to increase the accuracy of pregnancy dating and assess for obesity-associated pregnancy outcomes. An increased rate of dizygous twinning is associated with increasing BMI (35). Congenital anomalies are more common in the obese gravida, including open neural tube defects (OR, 1.87; 95% confidence interval [CI], 1.62–2.15), congenital heart disease (OR, 1.30; 95% CI, 1.12–1.51; $P = .001$) (36), hypospadias, cystic kidney, pes equinovarus, omphalocele, and diaphragmatic hernia, and risks are dose-dependent (increase with increasing BMI) (37). Finally, miscarriage rate is increased in obese compared to normal-BMI patients (38).

At the first prenatal visit, if there is no diagnosed history of comorbid conditions such as hypertension, diabetes, obstructive sleep apnea, hyperlipidemia, thyroid conditions, or depression, screening for these conditions should be undertaken. Blood pressure measurements should be obtained at each visit with an appropriately sized cuff. Hemoglobin A1C, serum thyroid stimulating hormone (TSH), and fasting lipid profile are sufficient screenings, unless a clinically significant vitamin D deficiency is suspected. Questionnaire screening for depression (PHQ2 or PHQ9) (39) and sleep apnea (STOP-Bang) (40) is sensitive for detection of these treatable contributors to worsened obstetric outcome. Because the risk of preeclampsia doubles with each 5–7 kg/m^2 increase in pre-pregnancy BMI (independent of comorbid hypertension, diabetes, or multiple gestation) (41), consideration should be given to obtaining baseline liver function tests (LFTs), 24-hour urine protein measurement, and creatinine clearance. A baseline electrocardiogram may also be useful.

All pregnant women, regardless of BMI, should be offered aneuploidy screening as a routine. It is noted, however, that increasing BMI is associated with significantly decreased ability to obtain a nuchal translucency measurement (42) for use in conjunction with serum markers to screen for chromosomal abnormalities.

Second Trimester

The major challenge posed by the obese patient in the second trimester is accurate prenatal ultrasound. Completion rate of the routine anatomical survey decreases with increasing BMI. In one estimate, only 4% of comprehensive anatomical surveys were completed on the first attempt in patients with Class III obesity (43). Multiple visits can be required to complete the survey. Even with additional visits, detection of fetal anomalies is significantly decreased in obese women, and reduced to a mere 25% in Class III obese women. This confers a residual anomaly risk of 1% in obese women (compared to 0.4% in normal-weight women) (44). The optimal timing of anatomical survey is between 18 and 24 weeks, with better completion rates at more advanced gestational ages, but this must be weighed against a potential desire to terminate the pregnancy for severe defects. Local legislation about pregnancy termination should be reviewed (45).

Obesity and morbid obesity are linked with increased rates of gestational diabetes, OR 2.6 (95% CI 2.1–3.4) and 4.0 (95% CI 3.1–5.2), respectively (4). Gestational diabetes (GDM) screening should be performed early in obese women (24 weeks) and since the insulin resistance associated with pregnancy increases with gestational age, repeat screening, or monitoring of fasting and post-prandial capillary blood glucose should be considered at 28 weeks.

Third Trimester

Maternal overnutrition leads to fetal overgrowth (46). Conversely, the decreased vascular function of the obese state can lead to impaired placental function and fetal growth restriction (47). Due to these growth abnormalities and the inability to rely on fundal height measurements when the subcutaneous fat layer is thick, sonographic assessment of growth is indicated in the third trimester. The accuracy of this assessment is not changed by obesity; in one study, sonographic estimated fetal weight (EFW) was within 6% of actual birthweight for all BMI categories (48).

An increased risk of stillbirth is seen for obese mothers, conferred by obesity independent of age and comorbidities such as diabetes or hypertension (49). However, evidence for induction of labor for the prevention of stillbirth is weak, and we know that induction is more likely to fail in an obese parturient (50).

Antenatal testing in obese women, aimed at prevention of stillbirth, can be helpful in management of timing of delivery (51) and is thought to reduce perinatal death, but decrease in stillbirth is not proven (52).

Indicated preterm birth is more common in obese women, though spontaneous preterm birth may not be increased (53,54). Some data indicates decreased effectiveness of 17-hydroxyprogesterone caproate to prevent recurrent preterm birth in women with BMI > 35 (55).

Consideration should be given to an anesthesia consult prior to delivery. Safe and effective regional anesthesia relies on landmarks that become obscured in obese women. More attempts are required to place epidurals, and the rate of failed epidural increases with BMI category (56). It can be more difficult to avoid dural puncture and complications such as spinal headache may increase. Anesthesia providers may wish to use ultrasound guidance for spinal and epidural blocks. General anesthesia is required more often in obese patients (though this effect has decreased in the last 20 years) (57) and carries greater risks, as the soft tissue around the trachea and larynx is increased in obese women, and edematous in parturients. Difficult intubation can be anticipated, and equipment such as video laryngoscopy and fiber optic bronchoscopes should be available. Ventilation is more difficult in the supine and Trendelenburg positions due to the excess pressure from abdominal fat and contents on the diaphragm. Most anesthesia-related maternal deaths are related to failure to secure an airway (58) and obesity is found more frequently in this group. To reduce these complications, morbidly obese patients should be evaluated early in their admission for epidural or continuous spinal analgesia (58).

Intrapartum

Difficulties are encountered with fetal monitoring and tocometry in obese laboring patients. No strong guidelines exist for internal monitoring, though it may be needed on a case-by-case basis. Another option is the fetal electrocardiograph transduced from the maternal skin, which may be easier to maintain than standard ultrasound-based cardiotocogram (59–61).

Labor curves are slower in obese and overweight women. When maternal and fetal status permits, more time allowed in the active phase of labor will increase the rate of vaginal delivery (62). Active labor management is important, as providers may recommend cesarean delivery more frequently due to perception of logistic delay. Indeed, decision-to-incision times are longer for increasing BMI (63). Operative vaginal delivery is also increased, likely as a result of soft tissue dystocia (64). If macrosomia is not suspected, this may be an effective intervention in order to prevent the morbidity of cesarean delivery.

Induction of labor occurs more frequently in the obese gravida (3). Likely this is partly a result of the strong association with comorbidities such as preeclampsia and gestational diabetes. Also, increased pre-pregnancy BMI is associated with increased rates of post-term pregnancy. Less than half of obese women in one UK study labored spontaneously, compared to 69% in the general obstetric population (65). Failed induction of labor also increases with increasing BMI (50).

Macrosomia and its attendant risks of birth trauma are a significant risk to the neonates of obese gravidas (4,66). Maternal obesity and weight gain are independent contributors to the rate of large for gestational age neonates. Shoulder dystocia and brachial plexus injury rates are also increased, though the absolute rate remains low. In the neonates of obese women, low Apgars, and meconium aspiration are more frequent (67).

Accordingly, the cesarean rate increases with BMI category, and approaches 50% for the morbidly obese (64,68,69). Successful vaginal birth after cesarean is much less likely in obese women (13% when women weigh > 300 lb) (70). Because of the logistics of patient transfer in the event of an emergency, and high likelihood of cesarean delivery, some providers may consider elective prelabor cesarean delivery. Although this may be appropriate on an individual basis, overall, vaginal delivery should be attempted if no medical or obstetric contraindications exist.

Delivery Preparedness

Given the likelihood of encountering an obese patient on the labor floor, education and planning are necessary. Risks to the patient, health care providers, and neonates can and should be anticipated. Referral should be considered in the case of inadequate personnel or resources to manage the obese patient.

Table 33.3 Equipment and Supplies Useful in the Care of the Obese Parturient

Equipment	Details
Labor beds	Capacity up to 500 lb
OR Tables	With table extenders, Yello-Fins
Stretchers	Capacity up to 500 lb
Mechanical patient lifts	Hydraulic and wheeled
Bariatric wheelchairs	Wide seat/capacity 450 lb
Waiting room/Hospital room chairs	For support persons
Long instrument tray for C-section	Consider long instrument hysterectomy tray
Self-retaining retractors	Alexis O or Mobius
Large BP Cuffs	44–66 cm
Large sequential compression devices (SCDs)	Up to 32 in calf circumference
Long spinal needles	
Long IV cannulas	
Wedge for patient positioning	Slight reverse Trendelenberg
Fiberoptic bronchoscope	Awake intubation
Video laryngoscope	Improved visualization of glottis
Fetal electrocardiogram monitor	Invasive or non-invasive

Multidisciplinary team conference and handoff is absolutely essential, and patients whose pregnancy is complicated by morbid obesity should be reviewed at such a meeting in advance when possible. Table 33.3 lists equipment that should be available in units that regularly care for obese patients.

Intraoperative Considerations

In obese women, post-cesarean surgical site infection is estimated to occur in 16–30% of cases (71). Some study has been dedicated to surgical technique, wound management, and use of prophylactic antibiotics, but high-quality studies are lacking.

Consideration must be given to incision planning. The traditional Pfannenstiel incision provides best access to the lower uterine segment, but may result in an incision that is covered by a pendulous pannus, with greater exposure to microbes, especially anaerobes that thrive in this moist, low-oxygen environment. The patient may be restricted in her visualization and care of this incision, by mechanics or by pain. The pannus is likely to have poor arterial perfusion and venous drainage if it is dependent: evidence of this can be seen in the edema that often occurs at the most dependent aspect of the pannus. Diabetic vascular compromise and poor wound healing may further compound the problem. An incision above the pannus, while avoiding the anaerobic environment described above, may result in traversing a thicker subcutaneous layer, increasing the risk of seroma or hematoma, which may become superinfected. A vertical incision could be under more tension and therefore incur greater risk of separation/dehiscence. One analysis of the NICHD/MFMU registry revealed that in women with a prepregnancy BMI >40, the rate of incision complication, after multivariate regression analysis, was lower in the vertical incision group. Of note, the incision-to-delivery time was also shorter in this group (72), whereas other studies indicate that the operative time, blood loss, and rate of classical hysterotomy are increased with vertical incision (73). Other incision types described in the literature for cesarean delivery of the obese include the Joel–Cohen incision, and supraumbilical transverse and vertical paramedian incisions (74,75).

Use of a negative-pressure wound device (NPWD) has been shown in randomized trials to decrease the incidence of surgical site infection (SSI) in non-cesarean wound types (abdominal and extremity) by about half. Extrapolating that data to apply to cesarean wounds, a preliminary analysis indicates NPWD to be cost-effective (71).

In a single retrospective cohort study, panniculectomy at the time of cesarean delivery was a feasible means of decreasing post-operative wound infection (76).

First-line use of cefazolin antibiotic prophylaxis in cephalosporin-tolerant women is recommended by the ACOG. Antibiotics should be administered within 60 minutes prior to incision and therapeutic levels maintained for about 3–4 hours. Because of the increased volume of distribution and drug clearance in obese patients, a higher dose of cephalosporin should be considered, but no specific dose recommendation is given by ACOG (77). Pharmacologic data showed that no woman weighing greater than 100 kg achieved adequate cefazolin levels in adipose tissue after a 2 g dose, whereas 100% of women 100–120 kg and 42.9% of women weighing > 120 kg achieved therapeutic levels after a 3 g dose (78). No difference in surgical site infections was found in a retrospective cohort study between 2 g or 3 g, though the study may have been underpowered (79). Current Clinical Practice Guidelines in Surgery recommend 3 g cefazolin in women > 120 kg undergoing cesarean delivery (80). Antibiotics should be redosed when there is excessive blood loss (>1500 mL) or prolonged operative time (two half-lives of the drug; 4 hours for cefazolin) (60).

Self-retaining retractors can be very useful for the obese patient and can save energy and injury to the delivery team, though they are not shown to reduce SSI (81). Any subcutaneous space > 2 cm should be closed (82) and skin should be closed with sutures rather than staples (83).

Adequate pain control is necessary for early ambulation and reduction of lung atelectasis after surgery. However, narcotic use should be judicious in patients who may suffer from undiagnosed obstructive sleep apnea, because the incidence of respiratory suppression is higher (58). Adjunctive pain control measures, such as IV acetaminophen, IV NSAIDs, and transversus abdominis plane (TAP) blocks should be employed after general anesthesia.

The Postpartum Period

Obesity confers an increased risk of hemorrhage, wound disruption and infection, and venous thromboembolism (VTE). Hemorrhage should be managed aggressively in the obese postpartum patient, as the risk of cesarean hysterectomy also increases with BMI.

Among the leading causes of maternal morbidity and mortality, VTE remains one of the strongest in the United States. Morbidly obese women are four times as likely to experience VTE in the postpartum period. The Royal College of Obstetricians recommends weight-based VTE chemoprophylaxis for 10 days after delivery in all patients with BMI > 40, and in patients with two persisting risk factors, such as obesity, age > 35, smoking, preeclampsia, post-partum hemorrhage > 1 L, among others. The Royal College of Obstetrics and Gynecology (RCOG) recommends 10 days of weight-based VTE chemoprophylaxis for all patients delivered by cesarean section, unless it was elective, in which case prophylaxis is prescribed if an additional risk factor is present (84). Low molecular weight heparin is safe, effective and easily administered by the patient herself. Sequential compression devices are effective prophylaxis for low-risk women undergoing vaginal and cesarean delivery.

For the patient with BMI > 50, intensive care unit (ICU) admission is found to be much more common. For obese women, the average length of hospital stay is increased.

Contraception is essential in the postpartum period, especially for overweight and obese women. Consideration should be given to the patient's comorbidities when choosing a contraceptive method. Long-acting reversible contraceptives (LARC), such as the intrauterine device (IUD) and implant, are effective in obese women (85,86) and should be a provider's first-line recommendation, both in terms of safety and efficacy. Combination oral contraceptives are more likely to fail in obese women (87), though as studied, the difference in failure rate was small when considering the overall typical-use failure rate of 9% for oral contraceptives. Depo-medroxyprogesterone is also safe and effective in obese women (88,89) and may provide a contraceptive bridge to interval placement of LARC. Tubal sterilization can be accomplished immediately postpartum in most obese women, regardless of the thickness of the adipose layer and should not be declined on the basis of BMI.

Breastfeeding initiation rates are lower in obese women, and they are less likely to continue (90,91). This may be a result of an endocrine-mediated delay in lactogenesis, mechanical difficulties due to large breast size and flattened areolae, or social-psychological reasons (92). Overweight and obese women may need more assistance and encouragement to establish a comfortable breastfeeding relationship. Lactation support should be provided for the first 6 months.

In the scheme of postpartum weight loss, breastfeeding can be helpful by creating an energy deficit of about 500 kcal/day. Exclusive breastfeeding is linked with greater postpartum weight loss than non-exclusive or no breastfeeding. A net weight change of –3.2 lb was sustained at one year postpartum in one cohort of women who breastfed exclusively for at least 3 months (93).

Postpartum body weight increases are common and occur even more frequently in overweight and obese women (94). These increases may be a result of failure to lose pregnancy weight, or weight gain after initial loss. Regardless of the cause, excessive weight gain and failure to lose pregnancy weight can lead to long-term weight gain (95), increasing obesity and its comorbidities later in life. Maternal obesity is strongly linked to obesity and cardiometabolic disease in offspring (96). Increasing maternal BMI is associated with higher body fat composition in offspring, even into later life (97). To reduce risks, patients should be encouraged to lose weight in the 6 months after delivery. A Cochrane review suggests that dietary modification impacts postpartum weight loss more than does exercise intervention, though exercise does confer cardiorespiratory benefits. Breastfeeding performance was not significantly impacted by the weight loss interventions studied (98). Therefore, there is a strong need for continued dietary counseling and education in the postpartum period.

Gastric Bypass

Surgical management of obesity is effective in reducing weight and comorbidities associated with obesity. This effect is best proven when preoperative BMI is greater than 40. Four types of surgery are used widely: Roux-en-Y bypass, vertical band gastroplasty, adjustable gastric band, and biliopancreatic diversion with duodenal switch. Weight loss occurs rapidly after surgery, with losses of 20–30 kilograms sustained over a 10-year period (24). Obese women may experience an unanticipated return to fertility in the first 12 months. Few bariatric surgeons discuss contraception with their reproductive-age patients (99), but this is imperative. It is recommended to defer pregnancy until 1 year after the procedure, both to optimize weight loss and minimize risks to the pregnancy.

Pregnancy outcomes are overall good after bariatric surgery. Gestational diabetes incidence is reduced (100). Risks of delivering an LGA infant are decreased, and pregnancies are significantly less likely to continue post-term. There may be an increased risk of SGA infants associated with bariatric surgery but no other adverse neonatal outcomes are associated (101). Nutritional deficiencies, especially in malabsorptive procedures, must be screened for and corrected (102). Serum iron, vitamin B_{12}, calcium, and vitamin D levels should be checked each trimester. Screening for gestational diabetes must be considered: the glucose load of standard testing can result in dumping syndrome (post-load diaphoresis, dizziness, tachycardia, nausea, loose stools, and hypoglycemia) in women with malabsorptive bypass. These women should be monitored instead with fasting and postprandial blood glucose monitoring.

Concluding Remarks

If current trends continue, in one conservative estimate, 2.16 billion people will be overweight in 2030, and 1.12 billion will be obese. Those overweight and obese will comprise about 57.8% of the world's population (103). As understanding of the causes of this pervasive condition progresses, the cyclic and progressive nature of the problem becomes clear. Obesity in parents results in genetic, epigenetic, and behavioral pressures on offspring, who then enter their childbearing years already facing the health challenges of obesity. Pregnancy provides a unique moment of opportunity to challenge this cycle and exert changes to improve the health of the mother and her children. For this reason, it is imperative that obstetric providers address this challenging medical and societal issue.

Barriers to the discussion and treatment of obesity are ample. Weight and body image can be closely linked to self-esteem, and many providers hesitate to challenge an obese patient's body image. Cultural and societal preferences may favor increased adiposity, and are among the most difficult factors to change. The overweight state has undergone some normalization in urban populations; since the majority is overweight, normal weight is perceived as too thin. Finally, many resource-poor urban areas do not offer accessibility to fresh produce and healthy foods; these "food deserts" lead residents to rely on fast, cheap pre-made food rather than cook at home.

Resources for patient education include nutrition.gov, a service of the National Agricultural Library of the United States Department of Agriculture (USDA). The Centers for Disease Control and Prevention (CDC) offers community and local-government-level resources to implement and measure the effects of obesity prevention programs. It is important to open the dialogue with patients about their perceptions of their weight, its health effects, and the ability to make sustainable dietary and physical activity changes. A non-judgmental, inquisitive approach will make the conversation about weight and obesity more fruitful for both parties.

References

1. Gynecologists ACOG Obesity in Pregnancy. American Congress of Obstetricians and Gynecologists; 2015.
2. World Health Organization. *Obesity: Preventing and Managing the Global Epidemic*. Geneva, Switzerland: 2000.
3. Sebire NJ, Jolly M, Harris JP, et al. Maternal obesity and pregnancy outcome: a study of 287,313 pregnancies in London. *International Journal of Obesity and Related Metabolic Disorders*. 2001;25:1175–82.
4. Weiss JL, Malone FD, Emig D, Ball RH, Nyberg DA, Comstock CH, et al. Obesity, obstetric complications and cesarean delivery rate–a population-based screening study. *American Journal of Obstetrics and Gynecology*. 2004;190(4):1091–7.
5. Lee KK, Raja EA, Lee AJ, Bhattacharya S, Bhattacharya Si, Norman JE, Reynolds RM. Maternal obesity during pregnancy assocates with premature mortality and major cardiovascular events in later life. *Hypertension*. 2015;66:938–44.
6. Centers for Disease Control and Prevention. Healthy weight, overweight, and obesity among adults aged 20 and over, by selected characteristics: United States, selected years 1988–1994 through 2009–2012. US Department of Health and Human Services; 2014.
7. Statistics NCfH. NCHS Obesity Data. Hyattsville, MD: NCHS, 2014.
8. McDonnold M, Mele LM, Myatt L, Hauth JC, Leveno KJ, Reddy UM, et al. Waist-to-hip ratio versus body mass index as predictor of obesity-related pregnancy outcomes. *American Journal of Perinatology*. 2016 May;33(6):618–24. doi: 10.1055/s-0035-1569986. Epub 2016 Jan 20.
9. Hu FB, Stampfer MJ, Manson JE, Rimm E, Colditz GA, Rosner BA, et al. Dietary fat intake and the risk of coronary heart disease in women. *New England Journal of Medicine*. 1997;337(21):1491–9.
10. 2015–2020 Dietary Guildelines for Americans. National Agricultural Library of the United States Department of Agriculture,. 8th ed. December 2015. Available at: https://health.gov/dietaryguidelines/2015/guidelines/, accessed April 26, 2017.
11. Larsson SC, Orsini N. Red meat and processed meat consumption and all-cause mortality: A meta-analysis. *American Journal of Epidemiology*. 2014;179(3):282–9.
12. Pate RR et al. Physical activity and public health. *Journal of the American Medical Association*. 1995;273(5):402–7.
13. Gibbs BG. Socioeconomic status, infant feeding practices, and early childhood obesity. *Pediatric Obesity*.9(2):135–46.
14. Burgio E, Lopomo A, Migliore L. Obesity and diabets: From genetics to epigenetics. *Molecular Biology Reports*. 2015;42:799–818.
15. Chiolero A, Faeh D, Paccaud F, Cornuz J. Consequences of smoking for body weight, body fat distribution, and insulin resistance. *The American Journal of Clinical Nutrition*. 2008;87:801–9.
16. Waring ME, Moore Simas TA, Rosal MC, Pagoto SL. Pregnancy intention, receipt of pre-conception care, and pre-conception weight counseling reported by overweight and obese women in late pregnancy. *Sexual and Reproductive Health*. 2015;6(2):110–1.
17. American Congress of Obstetricians and Gynecologists. Motivational Interviewing: A Tool for Change. ACOG Committee Opinion 2009.
18. Schummers L, Hutcheon JA, Bodnar LM, Lieberman E, Himes KP. Risk of adverse pregnancy outcomes by prepregnancy body mass index. *Obstetrics and Gynecology*. 2015;125:133–43.
19. Thompson WG, Cook DA, Clark MM, Bardia A, Levine J. Treatment of obesity. *Mayo Clinic Proceedings*. 2007;82(1):93–102.
20. Finkelstein EA. Meta- and cost-effectiveness analysis of commercial weight loss strategies. *Obesity*. 2014;22:1942–51.
21. Hayes L, Mcparlin C, Kinnuned TI, Poston L, Robson SC, Bell R. Change in level of physical activity during pregnancy in obese women: Findings from the UPBEAT pilot trial. *BMC Pregnancy and Childbirth*. 2015; 15(52):1–8.
22. Hainer V, Aldhoon-Hainerová I. Tolerability and safety of the new anti-obesity medications. *Drug Safety*. 2014;37:693–702.
23. Syngelaki A, Nicolaides KH, Balani J, Hyer S, Akolekar R, Kotecha R, Pastides A, Shehata H. Metformin versus placebo in obese pregnant women without diabetes mellitus. *New England Journal of Medicine*. 2016;374:434–43.
24. Maggard MA, Shugarman LR, Suttorp M, Maglione M, Sugerman HJ, Livingston EH, Nguyen NT, Li Z, Mojica WA, Hilton L, Rhodes S, Morton SC, Sheikelle PG. Meta-analysis: surgical treatment of obesity. *Annals of Internal Medicine*. 2005(142):547–99.
25. De-Regil LM, Palacios C, Lombardo LK, Pena-Rosas JP. Vitamin D supplementation for women during pregnancy (Review). *Cochrane Database of Systemic Reviews*. 2016(1):1–123.

26. Suarez L FM, Brender JD, Canfield M, Zhu H, Hendricks KA. Neural tube defects on the Texas–Mexico border: What we've learned in the 20 years since the Brownsville Cluster. *Birth Defects Research*. 2012;94:882–92.

27. Bird JK, Ronnenberg AG, Choi SW, Du F, Mason JB, Liu Z. Obesity is associated with increased red blood cell folate despite lower dietary intakes and serum concentrations. *The Journal of Nutrition*. 2015;145:79–86.

28. Garcia-Valdes L, Campoy C, Hayes H, Florido J, Rusanova I, Miranda MT, McArdle HJ. The impact of maternal obesity on iron status, placental transferrin receptor expression and hepcidin expression in human pregnancy. *International Journal of Obesity*. 2015;39:571–8.

29. Gesche J, Nilas L. Pregnancy outcome according to pre-pregnancy body mass index and gestational weight gain. *International Journal of Gynecology and Obstetrics*. 2015;129:240–3.

30. Berggren EK, Stuebe AM, Boggess KA. Excess maternal weight gain and large for gestational age risk among women with gestational diabetes. *American Journal of Perinatology*. 2015;32:251–6.

31. Walter JR, Perng W, Kleinman KP, Rifas-Shiman SL, Rich-Edwards JW, Oken E. Associations of trimester-specific gestational weight gain with maternal adiposity and systolic blood pressure at 3 and 7 years postpartum. *American Journal of Obstetrics and Gynecology*. 2015;212(499):e1-12.

32. Seneviratne S, McCowan LM, Cutfield WS, Derraik JGB, Hofman PL. Exercise in pregnancies complicated by obesity: Achieving benefits and overcoming barriers. *American Journal of Obstetrics and Gynecology*. 2015:442–9.

33. Finer LB, Zolna MR. Shifts in intended and unintended pregnancies in the United States, 2001–2008. *American Journal of Public Health*. 2014;104:S43–S8.

34. Kapadia MZ, Park CK, Beyene J, Giglia L, Maxwell C, and McDonald SD. Can we safely recommend getational weight gain below the 2009 guidelines in obese women? A systematic review and meta-analysis. *Obesity Reviews*. 2015;16:189–206.

35. Reddy UM, Branum AM, Klebanoff MA. Relationship fo maternal body mass index and height to twinning. *Obstetrics and Gynecology*. 2005;105(3):593–7.

36. Stothard KJ, Tennant PW, Bell R, Rankin J. Maternal overweight and obesity and the risk of congenital anomalies. *Journal of the American Medical Association*. 2009;301:636–50.

37. Blomberg MI, Källén B. Maternal obesity and morbid obesity: The risk for birth defects in the offspring. *Birth Defects Research*. 2010;88:35–40.

38. Boots C SM. Does obesity increase the risk of miscarriage in early conception: A systematic review. *Seminars in Reproductive Medicine*. 2011;29(6):507–13.

39. Kroenke K, Williams JB, Lowe B. The Patient Health Questionnaire Somatic, Anxiety, and Depressive Symptom Scales. *General Hospital Psychiatry*. 2010;32(4):345.

40. Chung F, Liao P, Sasaki E, Shapiro C, Sun Y. High STOP-Bang score indicates a high probability of obstructive sleep apnoea. *British Journal of Anaesthesiology*. 2012;108(5):768–75.

41. O'Brien TE, Chan WS. Maternal body mass index and the risk of preeclampsia: A systematic overview. *Epidemiology*. 2003;14:368–74.

42. Aagaard-Tillery KM, Malone FD, Nyberg DA, Collins J, Comstock CH, Hankins G, Eddleman K, Dugoff L, Wolfe HM, D'Alton ME. Influence of maternal BMI on genetic sonography in the FaSTER trial. *Prenatal Diagnosis*. 2010;30:14–22.

43. Thornburg LL, Ho M, Pressman EK. Fetal anatomic evaluation in the overweight and obese gravida. *Ultrasound in Obstetrics and Gynecology*. 2009;33:670–5.

44. Dashe JS, Twickler DM. Effect of maternal obesity on the ultrasound detection of anomalous fetuses. *Obstetrics and Gynecology*. 2009;113:1001–7.

45. Tsai P-JS, Zalud MD. Obesity and the challenges of ultrasound fetal abnormality diagnosis. *Best Practice and Research Clinical Obstetrics and Gynaecology*. 2015;29:320–7.

46. Siega-Riz AM, Moos M-K, Deierlein A, Mumford S, Knaack J, Thieda P, Lux L, Lohr KN. A systematic review of outcomes of maternal weight gain according to the Institute of Medicine recommendations: Birthweight, fetal growth, and postpartum weight retention. *American Journal of Obstetrics and Gynecology*. 2009;201(339):e1-14.

47. Campbell MK, Xie B, Kouniakis G, Huang W, Han V. Determinants of small for gestational age birth at term. *Paediatric and Perinatal Epidemiology*. 2012;26(6):525–33.

48. Cody F, Daly S, et al. The effect of maternal obesity on sonographic fetal weight estimation and perinatal outcome in pregnancies complicated by fetal growth restriction. *Journal of Clinical Ultrasound*.44(1):34–9.

49. Yao R, Park BY, Pereira L, Plante LA, Perinatal Research Consortium. Obesity and the risk of stillbirth: A population-based cohort study. *American Journal of Obstetrics and Gynecology*. 2014;210(5):457.e1-9.

50. Pevzner L, Rayburn WF, et al. Effects of maternal obesity on duration and outcomes of prostaglandin

cervical ripening and labor induction. *Obstetrics and Gynecology*. 2009;114(6):1315–21.

51. Flynn AM, O'Conor M. Unstressed antepartum cardiotocography in the management of the fetus suspected of growth retardation. *BJOG*. 2014;121(Suppl 7):14–8.

52. Bhutta ZA, Lawn JE, Rizvi A, Friberg IK, Weissman E, Buchmann E, Goldenberg RL. Stillbirths: What difference can we make and at what cost? *Lancet*. 2011;377(9776):1523–38.

53. Heslehurst N, Ells LF, Rankin J, Wilkinson J, Lang R, Brown TJ, Summerbell CD. The impact of maternal BMI status on pregnancy outcomes with immediate short-term obstetric resource implications: A meta-analysis. *Obesity Reviews*. 2008;9(6):635–83.

54. Marchi J, Dencker A, Olander EK, Begley C. Risks associated with obesity in pregnancy, for the mother and baby: A systematic review of reviews. *Obesity Reviews*. 2015;16:621–38.

55. Heyborne KD, Carey JC. Does 17-alpha hydroxyprogesterone caproate prevent recurrent preterm birth in obese women? *American Journal of Obstetrics and Gynecology*. 2015;213(844):e1–6.

56. Hood DD . Anesthetic and obstetric outcomes in morbidly obese parturients. *Anesthesiology*. 1993;79:1210–8.

57. Tonidandel A, D'Angelo R, Harris L, Tonidandel S. Anesthetic and obstetric outcomes in morbidly obese parturients: A 20-year follow up retrospective cohort study. *International Journal of Obstetric Anesthesia*. 2014;23(4):357–64.

58. Soens MA, Birnbach DJ, Ranasinghe JS, Van Zundert A. Obstetric anesthesia for the obese and morbidly obese patient: An ounce of prevention is worth more than a pound of treatment. *Acta Anaesthesiologica Scandinavica*. 2008;52(1):6–19.

59. Graatsma EM, van Egmond LAJ, Mulder EJH, Visser GHA. Fetal electrocardiography: Feasibility of long term fetal heart rate recordings. *British Journal of Obstetrics and Gynecology*. 2009;116:334–8.

60. Ghaffari N, Durnwald MD. The multidisciplinary approach to the care of the obese parturient. *American Journal of Obstetrics and Gynecology*. 2015:318–25.

61. Cohen WR, Ommani S, Hassan S, Mirza FG, Solomon M, Brown R, et al. Accuracy and reliability of fetal heart rate monitoring using maternal abdominal surface electrodes. *Acta Obstetricia et Gynecologica Scandinavica*. 2012;91(11):1306–13.

62. Vahratian A, Troendle JF, Savitz DA, Siega-Riz AM. Maternal prepregnancy overweight and obesity and the pattern of labor progression in term nulliparous women. *Obstetrics and Gynecology*. 2004;104:943–51.

63. Girsen AI, Naqvi M, Garabedian MJ, Lyell D. Body mass index and operative times at cesarean delivery. *Obstetrics and Gynecology*. 2014;124(4):684–9.

64. Weiss JL, Emig D, Ball RH, Nyberg DA, et al. Obesity, obstetric complications and cesarean delivery rate – A population-based screening study. *American Journal of Obstetrics and Gynecology*. 2003;190:1091–7.

65. Kobayashi N, Induction of labour and intrapartum care in obese women. *Best Practice and Research Clinical Obstetrics and Gynaecology*. 2015;29(3):394–405.

66. Ovesen P, Kesmodel U. Effect of prepregnancy maternal overweight and obesity on pregnancy outcome. *Obstetrics and Gynecology*. 2011;118:305–12.

67. Cedargren M. Maternal morbid obesity and the risk of adverse pregnancy outcome. *Obstetrics and Gynecology*. 2004;103:219–24.

68. Crane SS, Dye TD, et al. Association between pre-pregnancy obesity and the risk of cesarean delivery. *Obstetrics and Gynecology*. 1997;89(2):213–6.

69. Chu SY, Schmid CH, et al. Maternal obesity and risk of cesarean delivery: A meta-analysis. *Obstetrics Reviews*. 2007;8(5):385–94.

70. Lim CC . Obesity in pregnancy. *Best Practice and Research in Clinical Obstetrics and Gynaecology*. 2015;29:309–19.

71. Tuffaha HW, Chaboyer W, Gordon LG, Scuffham PA. Cost-utility analysis of negative pressur wound therapy in high-risk cesarean section wounds. *Journal of Surgical Research*. 2015;195:612–22.

72. Marrs CC, Sibai BM, et al. The relationship between primary cesarean delivery skin incision type and wound complications in women with morbid obesity. *American Journal of Obstetrics and Gynecology*. 2014;210(319):e1–4.

73. Brocato B, Gomez LM, Wan JY, Mari G. The effect of cesarean delivery skin incision approach in morbidly obese women on the rate of classical hysterotomy. *Journal of Pregnancy*. 2013;2013:3.

74. Hofmeyr J, Mathai M, Shah A. Techniques for cesarean section. *American Journal of Obstetrics and Gynecology*. 2009:431–44.

75. Houston M . Postoperative morbidity in the morbidly obese parturient woman: Supraumbilical and low transverse abdominal approaches. *American Journal of Obstetrics and Gynecology*. 2000;182:1033–5.

76. Fennimore R. Panniculectomy at the time of cesarean section and postoperative wound complication in morbidly obese women. *Journal of Reproductive Medicine*. 2015;60(11–12):535–9.

77. American College of Obstetricians and Gynecologists . Use of Prophylactic Antibiotics in Labor and Delivery. Practice Bulletin No 120. 2011.

78. Swank ML, Nicolaou DP, McNulty JA. Increased 3-gram cefazolin dosing for cesarean delivery prophylaxis in obese women. *American Journal of Obstetrics and Gynecology*. 2015;213(415):e1–8.

79. Ahmadzia HK, Joshi D, Liao C, Witter F, Heine RP, Coleman JS. Obstetric Surgical Site Infections: 2 grams compared with 3 grams of cefazolin in morbidly obese women. *Obstetrics and Gynecology*. 2015;126:708–15.

80. Bratzler DW, Olsen KM, Perl TM, Auwaerter PG, Bolon MK, et al. Clinical practice guidelines for antimicrobial prophylaxis in surgery. *American Journal of Health System Pharmacy*. 2013;70:195–283.

81. Childress KMSC, Ward DG, Berger K, Gross GA. A barrier retractor to reduce surgical site infections and wound disruptions in obese patients undergoing cesarean delivery: a randomized controlled trial. *American Journal of Obstetrics and Gynecology*. 2016;214(285):e1–10.

82. Dahike JD M, Rouse DJ, Berghella V, Baxter JK, Chauhan SP. Evidence-based surgery for cesarean delivery. *American Journal of Obstetrics and Gynecology*. 2013;209(4):294–306.

83. Mackeen AD, Fleisher J, Vogell A, Han C, Sendecki J, Pettker C, Leiby BE, Baxter JK, Sfakianaki A, Berghella V; CROSS Consortium. Suture compared with staple skin closure after cesarean delivery: A randomized controlled trial. *Obstetrics and Gynecology*. 2014;123(6):1169–75.

84. Royal College Obstetrics and Gynecology. Reducing the Risk of Venous Thromboembolism during Pregnancy and the Puerperium. GreenTop Guidlines: RCOG; 2015.

85. Xu H, Peipert JF, Zhao Q, Madden T, Secura GM. Contraceptive failure rates of etonogestrel subdermal implants in overweight and obese women. *Obstetrics and Gynecology*. 2012;120:21–6.

86. Bergisson NE, Secura GM, Madden T, Peipert JF. Preventing unintended pregnancy: The contraceptive CHOICE Project in review. *Journal of Women's Health*. 2015;24(5):349–53.

87. Yamazaki M, Sobhan M, Davis D, Kim M-J, Soule L, Willett G, Yu C. Effect of obesity on the effectiveness of hormonal contraceptives: An individual participant data meta-analysis. *Contraception*. 2015;92(5):445–52.

88. Segall-Gutierrez P, Liu X, Stanzcyk F, Azen S, Mishell DR Jr. Follicular development and ovulation in extremely obese women receiving depo-medroxyprogesterone acetate subcutaneously. *Contraception*. 2010;81(6):487–95.

89. Lopez LM, Chen M, Otterness C, Westfoft C, Edelman A, Helmerhorst FM. Hormonal contraceptives for contraception in overweight or obese women. *Cochrane Database of Systemic Reviews*. 2013(4).

90. Wojcicki JM. Maternal prepregnancy body mass index and initiation and duration of breastfeeding: A review of the literature. *Journal of Women's Health*. 2011;20(3):341–7.

91. Turcksin R, Bel S, Galjaard S, Devlieger R. Maternal obesity and breastfeeding intention, initiation, intensity and duration: A systematic review. *Maternal & Child Nutrition*. 2014;10(2):166–83.

92. Amir LH DS. A systematic review of maternal obesity and breastfeeding intention, initiation, and duration. *BMC Pregnancy and Childbirth*. 2007;7(9):1–14.

93. Jarlenski MP BW, Bleich SN, Barry CL, Stuart EA. Effects of breastfeeding on postpartum weight loss among U.S. women. *Preventive Medicine*. 2014;69:146–50.

94. Lipsky LM, Strawderman MS, Olson CM. Maternal weight change between 1 and 2 years postpartum: The importance of 1 year weight retention. *Obesity*. 2012;20(7):1496–502.

95. Rooney B SC. Excess pregnancy weight gain and long-term obesity: One decade later. *Obstetrics and Gynecology*. 2002;100(2):245–52.

96. Drake AJ RR. Impact of maternal obesity on offspring obesity and cardiometabolic disease risk. *Reproduction*. 2010;140(3):387–98.

97. Eriksson JG SS, Salonen M, Kajantie E, Osmond C. Maternal weight in pregnancy and offspring body composition in late adulthood: Findings from the Helsinki Birth Cohort Study. *Annals of Medicine*. 2015;47:94–9.

98. Amorim AA LY. Diet or exercise, or both, for weight reduction in women after childbirth. *Cochrane Database of Systemic Reviews*. 2013:CD005627.

99. Chor J, Chico P, Ayloo S, Roston A, Kominiarek MA. Reproductive health counseling and practices: a cross-sectional survey of bariatric surgeons. *Surgery for Obesity and Related Diseases*. 2015;11(1):187–92.

100. Johansson K, Cnattingius S, Näslund I, Roos N, Trolle Lagerros Y, Granath F, et al. Outcomes of pregnancy after bariatric surgery. *New England Journal of Medicine*. 2015;372(9):814–24.

101. Adams TO HA, Davidson LE, Laferrere B, et al. Maternal and neonatal outcomes for pregnancies before and after gastric bypass surgery. *International Journal of Obesity*. 2015;39:686–94.

102. Devlieger R GI, Jans G, Voets W, Vanholsbeke C, Vansant G. Micronutrient levels and supplement intake in pregnancy after bariatric surgery: A prospective cohort study. *PLoS One*. 2014;9(12):e114192.

103. Kelly T YW, Chen C-S, Reynolds K, He J. Global burden of obesity in 2005 and projections to 2030. *International Journal of Obesity*. 2008;32:1431–7.

Nausea and Vomiting of Pregnancy and Hyperemesis Gravidarum

Olukayode Akinlaja and William Gist

Introduction

Nausea with or without vomiting is commonly associated with early pregnancy. This can impact the quality of life of pregnant women despite its common consideration as part of first trimester pregnancy's physiology. Nausea of pregnancy is often labeled as morning sickness and follows preterm labor as the most common reason for hospitalization in pregnancy [1].

Hyperemesis gravidarum refers to severe vomiting unresponsive to antiemetics and simple dietary modification and it is associated with systemic effects. The diagnostic criteria include (1) pregnancy related vomiting that occurs greater than three times per day in conjunction with (2) a weight loss greater than 3 kg or 5% of body weight and (3) ketonuria unrelated to other causes [2].

The etiology is unknown but believed to be related to a placental product. Theories on etiology are seen in Box 34.1. A mobile app resource is the Association of Professors of Gynecology & Obstetrics WellMom: Managing Nausea and Vomiting of pregnancy, which can be downloaded from www.apgo.org/nvpapp.html.

Scope of the Problem

Nausea with or without vomiting tends to be more common in the younger primigravidas of Western nations but generally occurs in about 70–85% of all pregnancies. In contrast, hyperemesis gravidarum generally occurs between 0.3 to 3% of pregnancies [11]. It was reported by Borowski, et al. to be 1.6% at the Mayo clinic in 2003 [12]. The etiology is unknown. Risk factors include an increased association with multiple gestation, hydatidiform mole, acid reflux disease and a prior similar pregnancy history; the risk of recurrence is about 15% [13–15].

An increased incidence has also been noted in (1) women who experience nausea and vomiting related to estrogen-based medications, (2) younger age groups, (3) low pre-pregnancy body mass, (4) female fetus and (5) a history of motion sickness or migraines. Conversely, alcohol use, cigarette smoking and anosmia appear to be protective [7,15,16]. Hyperemesis gravidarum often persists throughout pregnancy and is associated with weight loss, electrolyte imbalance, dehydration and ketonemia. Fetal effects include an increased risk of preterm birth and low birth weight especially in the scenario of maternal weight gain of <15 lb [17].

Pregnancies with nausea and vomiting are generally associated with a lower rate of miscarriage compared to women without these symptoms whereas with hyperemesis gravidarum, there is an association with placental dysfunction and an increased risk of preterm delivery, small for gestational age fetuses and low birth weight infants [18].

Prevention measures include preconceptional intake of daily multivitamins with folic acid and adequate management of acid reflux disorders may help decrease the frequency and severity of nausea and vomiting during pregnancy [19].

Differential Diagnosis

Nausea and vomiting during pregnancy can result from many conditions both unrelated to pregnancy and related to pregnancy. See Box 34.2 for a list of differential diagnosis possibilities.

Diagnosis and Clinical Course

The onset of symptoms of nausea related to pregnancy is usually between 5 and 6 weeks gestation with peak around 9 weeks of gestation. Symptoms usually improve before 14 to 16 weeks and abate at 16–20 weeks. Even at 20 to 22 weeks, 10 to 25% of patients still experience symptoms. Unfortunately, in 15–20% of pregnancies, nausea does continue until the third

Box 34.1 Various theories associated with hyperemesis gravidarum etiology

- *Hormonal changes*

  Higher levels of serum human chorionic gonadotropin (hCG) has been observed in women with hyperemesis. This observation may account for the increased incidence of hyperemesis gravidarum seen in women with multiple gestation and hydatidiform mole. Serum concentration of hCG also peak in the first trimester, which corresponds to the time hyperemesis gravidarum, is typically seen. The existence of a significant correlation between the level of maternal hCG and the degree of nausea and vomiting, however, is doubtful [3].

  Another hormonal cause was postulated in a case of recurrent hyperemesis gravidarum in the absence of an elevated hCG in a mother and daughter pair due to the presence of a more hCG-sensitive thyrotropin receptor mutation [4].

  The high estrogen hypothesis is a third postulated hormonal etiology. A study by Schiff et al. did show a 1.5-fold increased tendency of having a female fetus with severe disease [5].
- *Psychological factors*

  Individual response to stress and the pregnancy have been proposed as contributing factors [6].
- *Abnormal gastrointestinal motility*

  Dysrhythmic gastric motility has been suggested as well as gastroesophageal reflux. These theories do not account for symptom improvement as pregnancy progresses [7].
- *Helicobacter pylori*

  Case reports have shown improvement in symptoms with treatment of infection. This observation requires confirmatory evidence as some recent studies report conflicting information [2,8–10].

trimester and even until delivery in 5% of cases [15,20]. Nausea and vomiting can occur at any time of the day and in most instances, vital signs, physical and laboratory examinations remain normal. Nausea and vomiting of pregnancy (NVP) rarely lead to electrolyte disturbances, ketonemia or significant weight loss.

Box 34.2 Differential diagnosis for severe nausea in pregnancy

Non-pregnancy related

Pancreatitis
Intrahepatic cholestasis of pregnancy
Acute cholecystitis
Viral hepatitis
Cholelithiasis
Gastroesophageal reflux disorder (GERD)
Appendicitis
Gastroparesis diabeticorum
GI obstruction and thyroid disease

Pregnancy related

Preeclampsia
HELLP syndrome
Acute fatty liver of pregnancy
Pregnancy-related conditions tend to be associated with emesis occurring in the latter half of pregnancy in combination with other clinical and laboratory findings.

In contrast, women with hyperemesis gravidarum often experience frequent vomiting, which can be prolonged, severe and associated with orthostatic hypotension, weight loss and starvation-induced acidosis, physical signs of dehydration and laboratory abnormalities. These patients often need hospitalization for stabilization. See Box 34.3 for standard evaluation parameters. See Box 34.4 for possible laboratory abnormalities.

Persistent, severe nausea and vomiting refractory to outpatient management, severe dehydration, starvation-related ketonemia, electrolytes derangements, acid–base abnormalities and other associated complications necessitate inpatient admission for hydration and treatment.

The Motherisk-PUQE scoring index and the Rhodes index have been used in research, with higher scores pointing to a need for serum electrolyte check and evaluation for dehydration.

Severely ill patients may present with various degrees of renal impairment from pre-renal causes and in some instances, Wernicke encephalopathy, Beriberi, peripheral neuropathy, central pontine myelinolysis, hepatic failure and rhabdomyolysis. Complications associated with continuous retching such as Mallory–Weiss tears, pneumothorax,

Box 34.3 Standard evaluation parameters

- Measurement of weight
- Orthostatic blood pressure
- Heart rate check
- Serum electrolytes/urea and creatinine
- Urine ketones and specific gravity
- Obstetrical ultrasound for gestational age, number of gestation and to rule out hydatiditiform mole.
- Others include a complete blood count, liver function tests, thyroid function tests, amylase, lipase and calcium level.
- If liver disease is suspected, an ultrasound examination of the liver is indicated.

Box 34.4 Possible laboratory abnormalities

Electrolyte derangements such as hypokalemia, hypochloremic metabolic alkalosis and ketosis

Hemoconcentration leading to an increase in hematocrit level

Abnormal liver enzymes especially an elevation of alanine aminotransferase

Serum amylase and lipase may increase by up to fivefold

retinal detachment and pneumomediastinium may also occur [21]. Other serious complications related to hyperemesis gravidarum include vitamin K deficiency with associated coagulopathy as described by Robinson et al. [22].

Hyperemesis Gravidarum Associated Transient Hyperthyroidism

Mild hyperthyroidism may occur due to an elevated serum level of hCG, but this tends to resolve without any need for intervention. The most common cause of hyperthyroxinemia in pregnancy is the transient hyperthyroidism of hyperemesis gravidarum. This should be suspected when thyroid tests are in the hyperthyroid range, in conjunction with a sudden onset of severe nausea and vomiting in the absence of hypermetabolic symptoms predating pregnancy.

This condition is likely due to the high hCG level, which stimulates the thyroid stimulating hormone (TSH) receptor as hCG does have the same alpha subunit as TSH. Often a four to six times elevation of the free T4 (FT4) and total T4 (TT4) levels is present. The total T3 (TT3) and free T3 (FT3) are elevated in 40% of women with a T3/T4 ratio less than 20 [4,23].

The signs and symptoms of hypermetabolism are infrequent aside from mild heat intolerance and palpitations. Most cases spontaneously resolve between 14 and 20 weeks but in 15–25% of cases, the condition persists beyond 20 weeks gestation. Antithyroid medications, even when used to normalize the serum thyroid level, do not stop the associated hyperemesis and are not needed. The presence of goiter or ophthalmopathy is suggestive of Graves disease as compared to hCG-mediated transient hyperthyroidism and can be confirmed by a positive serum test for thyrotropin receptor antibodies (TRAb), which is usually detected in about 95% of patients with Graves disease [23,24].

Treatment

Treatment is largely supportive. Management should generally be aimed at reducing symptoms, minimizing the effects on the fetus, reversing consequences, reassurance and psychological support.

Non-pharmacologic Interventions

Dietary measures include the ingestion of small, frequent meals preferably liquids and protein instead of carbohydrates. The elimination of coffee and spicy, odorous, fatty and sweet foods is recommended. Cold carbonated drinks can be helpful for symptoms as well as hydration maintenance [25].

Triggers such as iron supplements, odors, heat and humidity should be avoided until symptoms resolve. Hypnosis, psychotherapy, acupuncture and acupressure with wristbands may give relief to some patients [26–28].

Pharmacologic Interventions

Ginger in the form of ginger supplements or ginger containing food such as ginger tea have been associated with mild improvement in randomized controlled studies [29].

Pyridoxine or vitamin B6 is a water-soluble vitamin that can be used alone or in conjunction with doxylamine succinate [26]. Pyridoxine has a good safety profile with minimal side effects and is usually given as 25 mg orally every 6 to 8 hours.

Anti-histamines including doxylamine, meclizine, dimenhydrinate, promethazine and diphenhydramine do significantly reduce pregnancy-related nausea and vomiting in controlled trials [30,31]. The mechanisms of action involve the inhibition of histamine at the H1 receptor and an indirect effect on the vestibular system by reducing stimulation of the vomiting center. Lightheadedness, dry mouth, constipation and sedation are some of the associated side effects.

A fixed dose drug combination of pyridoxine hydrochloride and doxylamine succinate has been proven to be moderately effective in the treatment of nausea and vomiting of pregnancy with no demonstrable increase in the incidence of birth defects and in 2013, the brand, Diclegis ® was approved in the United States by Food and Drug Administration (FDA) for the treatment of pregnancy-associated nausea and vomiting but studies need to be done to confirm its effectiveness in hyperemesis gravidarum [32–34].

Dopamine antagonists such as butyrophenones (droperidol), phenothiazines (Promethazine) and benzamides (metoclopramide) mediate the inhibition of gastric motility through their action on dopamine receptors in the stomach. They are usually used as second-line agents due to their safety profile not limited to promethazine-induced sedation and risk of dystonic reaction, tardive dyskinesia associated with metoclopramide and QT prolongation seen with high doses of droperidol [35].

Serotonin antagonists are mainly selective antagonists at 5-HT3 serotonin receptor and an example is ondansetron given at 4 to 8 mg orally every 8 hours, as needed or intravenously. Side effects include headache, constipation, drowsiness and fatigue. The use of this class of drugs for the treatment of nausea and vomiting of pregnancy has not been associated with congenital anomalies or other adverse effects but though effective in managing chemotherapy-induced nausea and vomiting, it is not superior to promethazine in controlling hyperemesis gravidarum [36].

Acid-reducing agents are used as adjuncts to antiemetics and include antacids, H2 receptor antagonists or proton pump inhibitors. They appear to be safe in pregnancy with a significant correlation demonstrated between reduction in reflux disease and a decline in NVP [19].

A trial of multiple medications may be required for severely afflicted patients before symptom improvement is achieved. The use of steroids such as oral methylprednisone has not been shown to be effective by multiple studies [37,38].

Inpatient Therapy

When patients fail outpatient treatment, in-patient therapy and hospitalization for hydration and medication is needed. Emotional support is required to deal with the stressful nature of the illness. At present, individualization of care with the aid of the hyperemesis impact of symptoms questionnaire has not been associated with any significant improvement in the quality of care [39].

Patients should be kept totally on nothing by mouth (NPO) for 24 to 48 hours. Hydration with up to 2 liters of lactated Ringers or saline solution over 3 to 6 hours is frequently needed in conjunction with appropriate electrolyte and vitamins replacement as shown in Figures 34.1 and 34.2. Dextrose 5% in 0.45% saline is commonly continued for one to two days with urine output maintained at about 100ml/h (see Figures 34.1 and 34.2).

Thiamine (vitamin B1) is replaced by administration of 100 mg intravenously with the initial rehydration fluids and then 100 mg daily for the next two to three days. This prevents the development of Wernicke encephalopathy.

Multivitamin (MVI) 10 ml, folic acid 0.6 mg and vitamin B6 25mg are given in every liter of fluid.

In the presence of hypocalcaemia, the clinician must correct the low magnesium level by giving 2 g (16 meq) magnesium sulfate as a 10% solution over 10 to 20 minutes; 1 g (8 meq) in 100 ml of fluid per hour

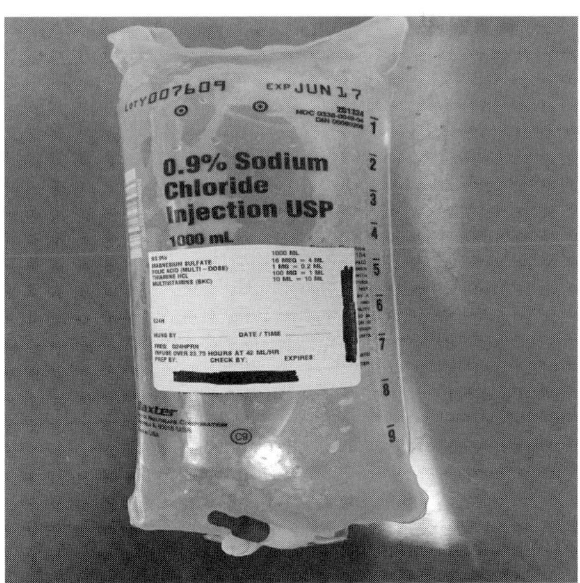

Figure 34.1 Saline 0.9% solution with multivitamins.

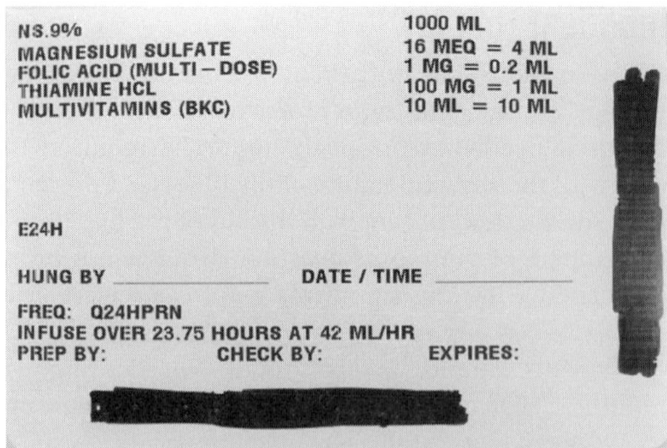

Figure 34.2 Magnesium and multivitamin content.

is then added to raise the magnesium level to more than 0.8 meq/l. If the serum calcium continues to be low, 1–2 g calcium gluconate in 50 ml of 5% dextrose solution over 10–20 minutes is infused [40].

Potassium chloride (20 mEq) is added to the intravenous fluid to replace potassium loss related to persistent vomiting and in the presence of low phosphorous level, 20 to 40 mmol/day of sodium phosphate is added to the intravenous fluid to attain a serum level greater or equal to 2 mg/dl [41].

When oral intake is resumed, dietary measures after the period of bowel rest will consist of either a BRAT (bananas, rice, apple sauce and toast) diet or full liquid diet. Diet is then advanced as tolerated.

Medications are given through non-oral routes until oral administration is tolerated. Severely afflicted patients and enteral (tube feeding) patients may require intravenous fluids as long as necessary.

Parenteral feeding has associated risks such as sepsis, thrombophlebitis, pericardial tamponade and significant hepatic disease. Parenteral nutrition is therefore only indicated after multiple failed attempts of antiemetic medication and enteral tube feedings. Successful nasojejunal enteral feeding has been described by Vaisman et al. [42].

Adverse effects of malnutrition such as Wernicke encephalopathy (vitamin B1 deficiency) and bleeding diathesis (vitamin K deficiency) are known to occur while esophageal tears and rupture, pneumothoraces, osmotic demyelination syndrome, hepatic insufficiency and acute tubular necrosis might result from persistent severe vomiting. Awareness of these conditions must be a part of the daily assessment of inpatients with hyperemesis gravidarum.

Psychologic Component

Many theories have related nausea and vomiting of pregnancy to either a conversion disorder or a response to stress but studies have yet to support these assumptions. The effectiveness of hypnotic therapy in some cases does make the possibility of psychological response such as conditioning feasible [43]. Interrelated psychological components have been found to play a role in the development of hyperemesis gravidarum and studies have indicated that affected women are at increased risk of psychological dysfunction in pregnancy and the related posttraumatic stress symptoms can be associated with breastfeeding, marital and financial problems [44,45]. Family and emotional support services may be needed due to the household disruption, burden placed on care givers and the financial impact of the maternal illness and psychiatric consultation might occasionally be needed [46].

Concluding Remarks

Hyperemesis gravidarum continues to be a debilitating problem in pregnancy and controversies still encompass its etiology.

Continuous education on the physical and psychological burden of hyperemesis gravidarum should be instituted in the medical community. The prompt intervention using the available pharmacological and non-pharmacological modalities in combination with the provision of emotional support is paramount.

References

1. Gazmararian JA, Petersen R, Jamieson DJ, Schild L, Adams MM, Despande AD, et al. Hospitalizations during pregnancy among managed care enrollees. *Obstet Gynecol* 2002;100:94–100.
2. Golberg D, Szilagyi A, Graves L. Hyperemesis gravidarum and *Helicobacter pylori* infection: A systematic review. *Obstet Gynecol* 2007;110:695.
3. Soulos M, Hughes C, Garcia J, et al. Nausea and vomiting of pregnancy: Role of human chorionic gonadotropin and 17-hydroxyprogesterone. *Obstet Gynecol* 1980;55:696.
4. Rodien P, Bremont C, Raffin-Sanson ML. Familial gestational hyperthyroidism caused by a mutant thyrotropin receptor hypertensive to human chorionic gonadotropin. *N Engl J Med* 1998;339:1823.

5. Schiff MA, Reed SD, Daling JR. The sex ratio of pregnancies complicated by hospitalization for hyperemesis gravidarum. *Br J Obstet Gynecol* 2004;111:27.
6. Buckwalter JG, Simpson SW. Psychological factors in the etiology and treatment of severe nausea and vomiting in pregnancy. *Am J Obstet Gynecol* 2002;186: S210.
7. Gill SK, Maltepe C, Koren G. The effect of heartburn and acid reflux on the severity of nausea and vomiting of pregnancy. *Can J Gastroenterol* 2009;23:270.
8. Jacobson GF, Autry AM, Somer-Shely TL, et al. *Helicobacter pylori* seropositivity and hyperemesis gravidarum. *J Reprod Med* 2003;48:578.
9. McKenna D, Watson P, Dornan J. *Helicobacter pylori* infection and dyspepsia in pregnancy. *Obstet Gynecol* 2003;102:845.
10. Mansour GM, Nashaat EH. Role of Helicobacter pylori in the pathogenesis of hyperemesis gravidarum. *Arch Gynecol Obstet* 2011;284:843.
11. Lee NM, Saha S. Nausea and vomiting of pregnancy. *Gastroenterol Clin North Am* 2011; 40:309.
12. Borowski KS, Ramsey PS, Williams L, et al. The impact of hyperemesis gravidarum on pregnancy outcome (abstract). *Obstet Gynecol* 2003;101:86S.
13. Basso O, Olsen J. Sex ratio and twinning in women with hyperemesis or pre-eclampsia. *Epidemiology* 2001;12:747.
14. Hou JL, Wan XR, Xiang Y, et al. Changes of clinical features in hydratidiform mole: Analysis of 113 cases. *J Reprod Med* 2008; 53: 629.
15. Goodwin TM. Hyperemesis gravidarum. *Obstet Gynecol Clin North Am* 2008;35:401.
16. Weigel MM, Weigel RM. The association of reproductive history, demographic factors, and alcohol and tobacco consumption with the risk of developing nausea and vomiting in early pregnancy. *Am J Epidemiol* 1988;127:562.
17. Dodds L, Fell DB, Joseph KS, et al. Outcomes of pregnancies complicated by hyperemesis gravidarum. *Obstet Gynecol* 2006;107:285.
18. Fell DB, Dodds L, Joseph KS, et al. Risk factors for hyperemesis gravidarum requiring hospital admission during pregnancy. *Obstet Gynecol* 2006;107:277.
19. Gill SK, Maltepe C, Mastali K, Koren G. The effect of acid-reducing pharmacotherapy on the severity of nausea and vomiting of pregnancy. *Obstet Gynecol Int* 2009;2009:585269.
20. Goodwin TM. Hyperemesis gravidarum. *Clin Obstet Gynecol* 1998;41:597.
21. Yamamoto T, Suzuki Y, Kojima K, et al. Pneumomediastinum secondary to hyperemesis gravidarum during early pregnancy. *Acta Obstet Gynecol Scand* 2001;80:1143.
22. Robinson JN, Banerjee R, Thiet MP. Coagulopathy secondary to vitamin K deficiency in hyperemesis gravidarum. *Obstet Gynecol* 1998;92:673.
23. Tagami T, Hagiwara H, Kimura T, et al. The incidence of gestational hyperthyroidism and postpartum thyroiditis in treated patients with Graves' disease. *Thyroid* 2007;17:767.
24. Vos XG, Smit N, Endert E, et al. Frequency and characteristics of TBII-seronegative patients in a population with untreated Graves' hyperthyroidism: A prospective study. *Clin Endocrinol (Oxf)* 2008;69:311.
25. Jednak MA, Shadigian EM, et al. Protein meals reduce nausea and gastric slow wave dysrhythmic activity in first trimester pregnancy. *Am J Physiol* 1999;27:G855.
26. Practice Bulletin No. 153. Nausea and vomiting of pregnancy. *Obstet Gynecol* 2015;126:e12.
27. Murphy A. Alternative therapies for nausea and vomiting of pregnancy. *Obstet Gynecol* 1998;91:149.
28. Heinrichs L. Linking olfaction with nausea and vomiting of pregnancy, recurrent abortion, hyperemesis gravidarum and migraine headache. *Am J Obstet Gynecol* 2002;186:S215.
29. Viljoen E, Visser J, Koen N, Musekiwa A. A systematic review and meta-analysis of the effect and safety of ginger in the treatment of pregnancy-associated nausea and vomiting. *Nutr J* 2014;13:20.
30. Magee LA, Mazzotta P, Koren G. Evidence- based view of safety and effectiveness of pharmacologic therapy for nausea and vomiting of pregnancy (NVP). *Am J Obstet Gynecol* 2002;186:S256.
31. Jewell D, Young G. Interventions for nausea and vomiting in early pregnancy. *Cochrane Database Syst Rev* 2003; Issue 4, Art. No.: CD000145. DOI: 10.1002/14651858. CD000145; 10.1002/14651858.CD000145.
32. McKeigue PM, Lamm SH, Linn S, Kutcher JS. Bendectin and birth defects: I. A meta-analysis of the epidemiologic studies. *Teratology* 1994;50:27.
33. Koren G, Clark S, Hankins GD, et al. Effectiveness of delayed-release doxylamine and pyridoxine for nausea and vomiting of pregnancy: A randomized placebo controlled trial. *Am J Obstet Gynecol* 2010;203:571. e1.
34. www.drugs.com/newdrugs/fda-approves-diclegis-pregnant-women-experiencing-nausea-vomiting-3749.html (Accessed on March 1, 2016).

35. Jackson CW, Sheehan AH, Reddan JG. Evidence-based review of the black-box warning for droperidol. *Am J Health Syst Pharm* 2007;64:1174.

36. Sullivan CA, Johnson CA, Roach H, et al. A pilot study of intravenous ondansetron for hyperemesis gravidarum. *Am J Obstet Gynecol* 1996;174:1565.

37. Duggar CR, Carlan SJ. The efficacy of methylprednisolone in the treatment of hyperemesis gravidarum: A randomized, double blind controlled study [Abstract]. *Obstet Gynecol* 2001;97:45S.

38. Safari HR, Fassett MJ, Souter IC, et al. The efficacy of methylprednisolone in the treatment of hyperemesis gravidarum: A randomized, double blind, controlled study. *Am J Obstet Gynecol* 1998;179:921.

39. Fletcher SJ, Waterman J, Nelson L, et al. Holistic assessment of women with hyperemesis gravidarum: A randomized controlled trial. *Int J Nursing Studies* 2015 Nov;52(11):1669–1677. doi: 10.1016/j.ijnurstu.2015.06.007

40. Akinlaja O. Nausea and vomiting in pregnancy-the bump in the road of motherhood. *Gynecol Obstet Res Open J.* 2015;2(4):85–88.

41. Lentz RD, Brown DM, Kjellstrand CM. Treatment of severe hypophosphatemia. *Ann Intern Med* 1978;89:941.

42. Vaisman N, Kaidar R, Levin I, et al. Nasojejunal feeding in hyperemesis gravidarum – A preliminary study. *Clin Nutr* 2004;23:53.

43. Buckwalter JG, Simpson SW. Psychological factors in the etiology and treatment of severe nausea and vomiting in pregnancy. *Am J Obstet Gynecol* 2002;186:S210.

44. McCarthy FP, Khashan AS, North RA, et al. A prospective cohort study investigating associations between hyperemesis gravidarum and cognitive, behavioral and emotional well-being in pregnancy. *PLoS One* 2011;6(11):e27678.

45. Christodoulou-Smith J, Gold JI, Romero R, et al. Posttraumatic stress symptoms following pregnancy complicated by hyperemesis gravidarum. *J Matern Fetal Neonatal Med* 2011;24(11):1307.

46. Deuchar N. Nausea and vomiting in pregnancy: A review of the problem with particular regard to psychological and social aspects. *Br J Obstet Gynaecol* 1995;102:6.

Hypertension in Pregnancy

Lauren Coyne and Colleen K. Stockdale

Introduction

The most commonly encountered forms of hypertension in pregnancy are gestational hypertension, preeclampsia–eclampsia (which can be further subdivided to preeclampsia with or without severe features and HELLP syndrome), chronic hypertension, chronic hypertension with superimposed preeclampsia, and postpartum hypertension. Gestational hypertension and preeclampsia are thought to a part of the same disease continuum with the natural history of the former evolving into the later if given adequate time for disease progression.

Scope of the Problem

Hypertensive disorders of pregnancy remain the leading cause of maternal and perinatal morbidity and mortality. Hypertensive disorders of pregnancy, pre-existing and those arising de novo, are the most common maternal complications of pregnancy and occur in up to 10% of all gestations. This hypertensive disease spectrum is second only to venous thromboembolism as leading cause of maternal mortality in the United States, accounting for 12% of all maternal deaths.[1–4] Maternal mortality is most often associated with complications of eclampsia, uncontrolled severe hypertension, and multisystem organ failure.[5] Perinatal mortality is twice as high in pregnancies affected by preeclampsia and 15% of preterm deliveries are a result of preeclampsia.[3,6–8] The etiology of these multisystem disorders remains unknown. Risk factors have been identified and include primigravida, previous pregnancy affected by preeclampsia, chronic hypertension with or without chronic renal disease, history of thrombophilia, multifetal gestation, in vitro fertilization, family history of preeclampsia, types I and II diabetes mellitus, obesity, systemic lupus erythematosus, and advanced maternal age (Box 35.1).[9] There also appears to be a poorly understood genetic component of disease development, with a threefold increased risk of preeclampsia in patients with an affected first degree relative.[10] Given the changing demographics of patients worldwide, with an increasingly high incidence of advanced maternal age and preexisting medical comorbidities such as chronic hypertension, obesity, and diabetes, it is estimated that the incidence of hypertensive disorders in pregnancy will continue to rise.[10] Despite the high incidence of these disorders, the ability to predict and prevent hypertensive disease in pregnancy has remained elusive. Diagnostic criteria, treatment recommendations, and long-term follow-up strategies are continually reviewed and revised so as to optimize both acute and long-term maternal-fetal outcomes.

Gestational Hypertension

Gestational hypertension, also termed pregnancy-induced hypertension, is defined as systolic blood pressure equal or greater than 140 mmHg and/or diastolic blood pressure equal or greater than 90 mmHg on at least two occasions at least 6 hours apart after the 20th week of gestation in a woman with no prior history of hypertension. By definition, no proteinuria or evidence of systemic findings are present in gestational hypertension. Gestational hypertension is the most commonly seen hypertensive disorder of pregnancy. The rate ranges from 6% to 17% in nulliparous patients and between 2% and 4% in multiparous patients.[11,12] The incidence increases with gestational age with 50% of cases being diagnosed near or at term.[10] The risk of gestational hypertension is higher in patients with a history of preeclampsia in previous pregnancies and with multifetal gestations.[11] While making this diagnosis, it is important to consider the possibility of an underlying history of undiagnosed chronic hypertension. Treatment and management recommendations are made while being mindful of the natural history of this disorder. Gestational

Box 35.1 Pregnancy-related hypertension risk factors[9]

Primigravid pregnancy
Previous pregnancy affected by preeclampsia
Chronic hypertension with or without chronic renal disease
History of thrombophilia
Multifetal gestation
In vitro fertilization
Family history of preeclampsia
Types I and II diabetes mellitus
Obesity
Systemic lupus erythematosus
Advanced maternal age

hypertension may progress to preeclampsia with rates dependent on gestational age at time of diagnosis. Up to 50% of patients diagnosed with gestational hypertension prior to 30 weeks gestation will later develop preeclampsia.[11] Twenty percent of patients with gestational hypertension will progress to preeclampsia.[10] Those that progress to preeclampsia will have a higher incidence of fetal demise, preterm delivery, and low birth weight compared to unaffected pregnancies or those with gestational hypertension alone.[10]

Management of patients with gestational hypertension is similar to those with preeclampsia without severe features and is dependent on gestational age, maternal and fetal status at time of evaluation, presence of labor, cervical Bishop score, and maternal wishes.[11] Most cases of gestational hypertension develop at 37 weeks or later and thus will tend to have outcomes similar to those with unaffected pregnancies.[11–14] Because of the similar management strategies, further management guidelines are included in the discussion of preeclampsia without severe features.

Preeclampsia–Eclampsia

Literature has used the terms preeclampsia, preeclamptic toxemia, and proteinuric pregnancy-induced hypertension synonymously. This disorder has classically been defined as elevated blood pressure with proteinuria after the 20th week of gestation. The incidence of preeclampsia has been found to range from 3 to 7% of pregnancies depending on the specific characteristics of the population being examined.[10] Preeclampsia is thought to develop from an interaction of maternal diseases, such as abnormal vasculature, renal or metabolic system disease, or cardiovascular predisposition, with placenta factors.[10] Earlier onset preeclampsia (prior to 34 0/7 weeks gestation) is seen in up to 20% of all cases and often has the most severe manifestations and sequelae including intrauterine growth restriction and poor placentation.[10,15] It is postulated that an immuno-placental maladaptation leads to subsequent sympathetic dominance within the cardiovascular system, elevated serum markers of endothelial dysfunction, inadequate trophoblastic invasion of the uterine spiral arteries, iatrogenic preterm delivery, and low birth weights.[10,16–18] Later onset, diagnosis after 34 0/7 weeks, preeclampsia is more common, occurring in 80% of affected pregnancies.[15] This phenomenon is more often seen with preexisting medical conditions previously discussed including chronic hypertension, renal disease, and obesity. Established fetal consequences such as low birth weight seen with earlier onset disease are not as often demonstrated with later onset cases.[10] There have been extreme early onset cases of preeclampsia prior to 20 weeks gestational age demonstrated in cases of trophoblastic disease such as hydatidiform mole or hydrops.[1]

Historically preeclampsia was a disease defined by hypertension and proteinuria in pregnancy. Modified definitions have eliminated the diagnostic requirement of proteinuria. Current diagnostic criteria emphasize blood pressure elevations and categorize patients based on the presence or absence of severe features.

The blood pressure criteria remain unchanged: greater than or equal to 140 mmHg systolic or greater than or equal to 90 mmHg diastolic on two occasions at least 4 hours apart after 20 weeks of gestation in a woman with previously normal blood pressure or greater than or equal to 160 mmHg systolic or greater than or equal to 110 mmHg diastolic. Proteinuria is described as a minimum of 300 mg of protein in a 24-hour urine collection or a urine protein/creatinine ratio of 0.3 (each measured as mg/dL). A urine dipstick value of 1+ can be used to diagnose proteinuria, but this test has poor reproducibility and therefore is utilized only in cases where no other diagnostic tools are available.[9] Proteinuria greater than 5 g and fetal growth restriction are no longer considered as diagnostic criteria.

Severe features of preeclampsia are seen in Box 35.2.

Box 35.2 Severe features of preeclampsia[9]

Systolic blood pressure greater than or equal to 160 mmHg or diastolic blood pressure greater than or equal to 110 mmHg on two occasions 6 hours apart while the patient is on the bed rest

Thrombocytopenia – platelet count less than 100,000/microliter

Impaired liver function – elevated liver enzymes to twice normal concentration

Severe persistent RUQ/epigastric pain unresponsive to medication and not accounted for by alternative diagnoses

Renal insufficiency – serum creatinine greater than 1.1 mg/dL or a doubling of serum creatinine in absence of other renal disease

Pulmonary edema

Now-onset cerebral or visual disturbances

Box 35.3 Fetal manifestations of preeclampsia[20]

Oligohydramnios

IUGR

Abnormal umbilical artery Doppler velocity

Decreased fetal middle cerebral artery resistance

Abnormal ductus venosus waveform

Stillbirth

Fetal manifestations of preeclampsia may be present with or without concomitant maternal manifestations of disease (Box 35.3). Most commonly seen fetal manifestations are oligohydramnios, intrauterine growth restriction (IUGR) seen in up to 30% of affected pregnancies,[19] abnormal umbilical artery Doppler velocimetry, decreased fetal middle cerebral artery resistance, an abnormal ductus venosus waveform, and/or stillbirth.[20]

Eclampsia is the occurrence of new onset grand mal seizure or coma during pregnancy or postpartum unrelated to other cerebral conditions with signs or symptoms of preeclampsia.[12] Common alternative etiologies for seizures include bleeding arteriovenous malformation, ruptured aneurysm, or idiopathic seizure disorder and these are more common when onset of seizure is greater than 72 hours postpartum or during the use of magnesium sulfate therapy.[12] Eclampsia can be preceded by severe headache and hyperlexia but up to 50% of patients will not have any preceding signs or symptoms.[5,9] The incidence of eclampsia has been estimated to be approximately 1/3,448 pregnancies.[5] It is seen more commonly in tertiary care centers, multi-fetal gestations, and in pregnancy with little to no prenatal care.[12] Cerebral imaging is not necessary for the diagnosis of eclampsia though it is indicated in patient with focal neurologic deficits and prolonged coma.[12] Eclampsia is associated with an increased risk of maternal death – 1.8% in developed countries and 14% in developing countries.[12] Pregnancies complicated by eclampsia are also more likely to be associated with placental abruption, disseminated intravascular coagulation (DIC), pulmonary edema, acute renal failure, aspiration pneumonia, and cardiopulmonary arrest.[12]

The primary goal of treating a patient presenting with eclampsia is maternal stabilization by prevention of maternal injury and support for cardiovascular functions.[12] The maternal bed should be padded and maternal oxygenation level should be evaluated. Maternal oxygen saturation should be adequately maintained during seizure episodes because hypoventilation and respiratory acidosis may develop.[12] Magnesium sulfate is the drug of choice for the treatment and prevention of further seizures. This is given as a 6-gram bolus over 15–20 minutes followed by continuous infusion at 2 grams per hour. Ten percent of eclamptic women will have a second seizure while receiving IV magnesium. In these women, it is reasonable to give a second bolus of 2 grams IV magnesium sulfate.[12] Blood pressures should be aggressively controlled so as to maintain systolic blood pressure between 140 and 160 mmHg and diastolic blood pressure between 90 and 105 mmHg.[12] Standard doses of IV labetalol and/or hydralazine are the preferred agents in this scenario.[12]

Fetal well-being should be monitored throughout an eclamptic episode. Fetal heart rate tracings may show bradycardia, late decelerations, diminished variability, and tachycardia.[12] These changes are due to maternal hypoxemia, maternal acidosis, and irregular uterine contractions. Often, these fetal findings will resolve spontaneously within 10 minutes after conclusion of seizure activity.[12] The decision to proceed with cesarean delivery should occur after maternal stabilization has occurred and should be based on gestational age, fetal condition, presence of labor, and cervical Bishop score.[12] Cesarean delivery is recommended for those considered remote from delivery after maternal stabilization.[12]

HELLP syndrome (hemolysis, elevated liver enzymes, and low platelet count) is a further element of the preeclampsia spectrum. HELLP occurs in 0.2–0.8% of pregnancies and will coexist with preeclampsia in 70–80% of cases.[21] Hypertension is present in most cases, but is not required by definition and may be subtle or absent in cases as well.[21] Risk of developing HELLP syndrome is higher in patients who have a first-degree relative with a medical history of HELLP.[22] A patient with a history of HELLP has a higher risk of developing HELLP (14–24%) and preeclampsia (22–28%) in subsequent pregnancies.[21,23,24]

Management recommendations for gestational hypertension and preeclampsia without severe features are similar. Once the diagnosis of either gestational hypertension or preeclampsia without severe features has been made fetal surveillance should be performed with an ultrasonographic evaluation of fetal weight and amniotic fluid index as well as non-stress testing. Fetal movement should be assessed daily by the patient. Twice weekly blood pressure monitoring and weekly assessment of platelet counts and liver enzymes should be performed. Bedrest should not be recommended for women falling within this category. Antihypertensive medications should not be initiated in patients who maintain blood pressures below 160/110 mmHg. The optimal timing for delivery of these patients has been debated, but current recommendations are for delivery at 37 0/7 weeks gestation or at time of diagnosis if past 37 0/7 weeks gestation. If the patient is greater than 37 weeks gestation with an unfavorable cervix, induction of labor should be initiated with cervical ripening via prostaglandin therapy.[11,25] Patients within this category without blood pressure greater than 160/110mmHg and without maternal symptoms should not receive intravenous magnesium sulfate for seizure prophylaxis.[9]

Management recommendations for patients with preeclampsia with severe features or HELLP syndrome are more aggressive, calling for closer antenatal surveillance and earlier delivery. Once the diagnosis has been made, management should not be based on the amount of (or change in the amount) proteinuria present. For patients with stable maternal/fetal conditions, close inpatient observation is recommended. The administration of antenatal corticosteroids is recommended for optimal fetal lung maturity prior to 34 0/7 weeks. If patients develop persistently severe hypertension (systolic BP of 160mmHg or greater or diastolic BP of 110mmHg or greater), the use of antihypertensive medications is recommended. For patients at or beyond 34 0/7 weeks or earlier with unstable maternal/fetal conditions delivery is recommended. These patients should receive parenteral magnesium sulfate for seizure prophylaxis and this should be continued intraoperatively if a cesarean section is necessary. Typical dosing is intravenous magnesium sulfate given at a 4–6 gram loading bolus over 20–30 minutes followed by a maintenance dose of 2 grams per hour for at least 24 hours but this may be institution dependent.[5] If HELLP is diagnosed prior to 34 0/7 weeks gestation and maternal/fetal conditions are stable delay of delivery is recommended for a 24–48 hour time period to allow for administration of corticosteroids. For patients with preeclampsia with severe features or HELLP syndrome prior to viability, delivery after maternal stabilization is recommended, expectant management is not appropriate. These patients would benefit from neuraxial anesthesia if platelet count allows and invasive hemodynamic monitoring should not be routinely used.[9]

Women with gestational hypertension have a 16–47% risk of development of gestational hypertension in subsequent pregnancies and 2–7% risk of developing preeclampsia with future pregnancy.[10] For a patient with a history of pregnancy complicated by preeclampsia, the risk of gestational hypertension is 13–53% and preeclampsia is 16% in future pregnancies.[10] Objective risk factors for preeclampsia have been defined as history of preeclampsia, multifetal gestation, chronic hypertension, pre-existing diabetes mellitus, renal disease, and autoimmune disease. A patient is considered to be at increased risk of preeclampsia development if 1 or more of these features are present. Patients identified as having an elevated risk of developing hypertensive disorders in pregnancy benefit from daily low-dose aspirin. Current guidelines recommend that high-risk patients be started on low-dose aspirin (60–150 mg/day) between 12 and 28 weeks of gestation. This has been shown to reduce the occurrence of preeclampsia, preterm birth, and IUGR.[3,26] Moderate risk factors have also been identified and a patient may benefit from daily low-dose aspirin if several of the following features are present: nulliparity, obesity, family history of preeclampsia, sociodemographic characteristics (African American, low socioeconomic status), age >35 years, personal history of SGA fetus, previous adverse pregnancy outcome, or >10-year pregnancy interval.[3] Patients with a history of preeclampsia in previous

Table 35.1 Low-Dose Aspirin and Preeclampsia[3]

Risk Level	Risk Factors	Recommendation
High	History of preeclampsia, multifetal gestation, chronic hypertension, Type I or II diabetes mellitus, renal disease, autoimmune disease	Low-dose aspirin if one or more of these risk factors are present
Moderate	Nulliparty, obesity, family history of preeclampsia in first-degree relative, African American race, low socioeconomic status, advanced maternal age, history of low birthweight or small for gestational age fetus, previous adverse pregnancy outcome, greater than 10-year pregnancy interval	Consider low-dose aspirin if the patient has several of these moderate risk factors

From LeFevre M on behalf of the U.S Preventative Services Task Forces. Low-dose aspirin use for the prevention of morbidity and mortality from preeclampsia: U.S. preventative services task for recommendation statement. *Ann Intern Med.* 2014;161:819–26.

pregnancies may benefit from modifiable lifestyle activities such as weight loss and increased physical activity as well as preconception counseling if subsequent pregnancies are desired.[9]

Chronic Hypertension and Superimposed Preeclampsia

Chronic hypertension is defined as the diagnosis of hypertension with or without antihypertensive treatment prior to conception or before 20 weeks gestational age.[9,27] It is estimated that between 1% and5% of pregnancies in the United States are affected by chronic hypertension.[28,29] Although 75–80% of women with essential hypertension will have uncomplicated pregnancies, these women are at increased risk for exacerbation of hypertension, superimposed preeclampsia, stroke, acute renal failure, pulmonary edema, placental abruption, fetal growth restriction, preterm delivery, maternal death and perinatal death.[27–31]

Studies have demonstrated the risk of superimposed preeclampsia in patients with underlying chronic hypertension to be 23%.[29] There is also a threefold increased risk of stillbirth and 2.5-fold increase in delivering a baby that is small for gestational age.[10] The risk is multifactorial and is increased with black ethnic origin, severity of pre-existing hypertensive disease (worse outcomes if baseline systolic blood pressure is greater than 130 mmHg or diastolic blood pressure is greater than 80mmHg), the duration of chronic hypertension (longer than 4 years since diagnosis), the presence of comorbidities such as obesity, preexisting diabetes mellitus, preexisting renal disease, smoking, the need for antihypertensive medications both prior to and during pregnancy, and a medical history of a previous pregnancy affected by preeclampsia (Box 35.4).[29,32–34]

These patients present special diagnostic and treatment challenges for providers during pregnancy. Occasionally secondary hypertension is diagnosed in pregnancy. Most commonly seen underlying secondary causes of hypertension in this population include pheochromocytoma, primary aldosteronism, Cushings syndrome, and coarctation of the aorta.[10,35] The physiologic decrease in first and second trimesters blood pressure with third trimester increase may be exaggerated in patients with underlying chronic hypertension. Often they are found to be normotensive at early appointments and may be erroneously diagnosed with gestational hypertension later in pregnancy.[10] Health care providers must be able to distinguish those with superimposed preeclampsia without severe features from those with superimposed preeclampsia with severe features as management guidelines differ for these groups. If the only manifestation of disease is blood pressure elevations greater than 160 mmHg systolic or 110 mmHg diastolic this is considered superimposed preeclampsia without severe features.[9] Severe features include any evidence of end-organ damage.

For patients with chronic hypertension and poor pre-pregnancy blood pressure control home blood pressure monitoring is recommended.[9] If these patients were accustomed to regular exercise prior to pregnancy, this should be continued as tolerated throughout the pregnancy. Classic hypertension lifestyle modifications such as salt restriction and weight loss should not be implemented during pregnancy.[9]

Box 35.4 Risk factors for the development of superimposed preeclampsia

African American ethnicity
Severity of preexisting hypertensive disease – worse outcomes if systolic blood pressure greater than 130mmHg or diastolic blood pressure greater than 80mmHg
Duration of chronic hypertension – longer than 4 years since initial diagnosis
Presence of comorbidities – obesity, preexisting diabetes mellitus, preexisting renal disease
Smoking
Need for antihypertensive medication prior to and during pregnancy
Medical history of previous pregnancy affected by preeclampsia

Women with persistent blood pressure elevations of systolic blood pressure greater than 160 mmHg or diastolic blood pressure greater than 105 mmHg antihypertensive medications should be treated with a goal blood pressure value of 120–160 mmHg systolic and 80–105 mmHg diastolic. The recommended antihypertensive agents for use in pregnancy are labetalol, nifedipine, and methyldopa (Table 35.2). Certain antihypertensive agents such as angiotensin converting enzyme inhibitors, angiotensin receptor blockers, renin inhibitors, and mineralocorticoid receptor antagonists should be avoided both in pregnancy and in reproductive aged women.[9]

Patients with chronic hypertension should undergo serial ultrasongraphy to evaluate fetal growth with follow-up umbilical artery Doppler velocimetry assessment if growth restriction is demonstrated. For patients who require antihypertensive medications, antennal testing with non-stress tests should be used in addition to serial ultrasonography.[9] Patients with uncomplicated chronic hypertension should undergo delivery no earlier than 38 0/7 weeks gestational age. If chronic hypertension is complicated by superimposed preeclampsia prior to 34 0/7 weeks corticosteroids should be administered to optimize fetal lung maturity.[9] If the pregnancy is complicated by preeclampsia without severe features, current recommendation is for delivery no earlier than 37 0/7 weeks without the use of parenteral magnesium sulfate.[9] For patients with pregnancy complicated by superimposed preeclampsia delivery at 34 and 0/7 weeks with the use of parenteral magnesium sulfate, therapy is recommended.[9] Delivery prior to 34 and 0/7 weeks gestational age or completion of corticosteroid treatment should be reserved for the setting of uncontrollable severe hypertension, eclampsia, pulmonary edema, abruptio placentae, disseminated intravascular coagulation, and nonreassuring fetal well-being.[9]

Postpartum Hypertension

The incidence and natural history of hypertension in the postpartum period is difficult to definitively describe as most postpartum patients do not undergo blood pressure monitoring prior to their 6-week postpartum office visit. There is conflicting data regarding resolution of gestational hypertension and preeclampsia. Typically in patients with antepartum preeclampsia, blood pressure decreases within 48 hours of delivery but will often increase again 3–6 days post-delivery.[32,36] It has been demonstrated that hypertension and proteinuria resolve within the first postpartum week. For women with persistent hypertension after 6 weeks postpartum, consideration of evaluation for secondary hypertension should be performed. Women with persistent proteinuria after 6 weeks postpartum should also be evaluated for underlying renal disease by renal specialists.[10]

The most common causes for hypertension persisting greater than 48 hours post-delivery are gestational hypertension, preeclampsia, or essential hypertension (preexisting or newly presenting). The differential diagnosis for new onset hypertension in the postpartum period is broad and should include pain, anxiety, volume overload, medication affects (NSAIDs, ergot derivatives, indomethacin, ephedrine), persistence of gestational hypertension/preeclampsia, late onset eclampsia/HELLP syndrome, preexisting hypertension, cerebral vasoconstriction syndrome (associated with thunderclap headaches and various neurologic deficits), TTP, and cerebral venous thrombosis or stroke (Box 35.5).[32,37] Maternal outcomes vary and depend of the severity and etiology of the hypertension, presence of organ dysfunction at presentation, and quality of management. Complications with high rates of elevated mortality include cerebral infarction/hemorrhage, congestive heart failure, pulmonary edema, and renal failure.[32]

All postpartum patients diagnosed with gestational hypertension, preeclampsia with or without severe features, or superimposed preeclampsia should be monitored in the hospital for a 72-hour period postpartum

Table 35.2 Common Oral Antihypertensive Agents in Pregnancy

Drug	Dosage	Comments
Labetatol	200–2,400 mg/day orally in two to three divided doses	Well tolerated; Potential brochoconstrictive effects; Avoid in asthmatics and congestive heart failure patients
Nifedipine	30–120 mg/day orally of a slow release preparation	Do not use sublingal form
Methylopa	0.5–3 g/day orally in two to three divided doses	Childhood safety data up to 7 years of age; May not be effective in control of severe hypertension
Thiazide diuretics	Depends on the agent	Second-line agent
Angiotensin-converting enzyme inhibitors/Angiotensin receptor blockers		Associated with fetal anomalies; contraindicated in pregnancy and preconception period

Hypertension in pregnancy. Report of the American From College of obstetricians and Gynecologists' Task Force on Hypertension in Pregnancy. *Obstet Gynecol.* 2013 Nov;122(5):1122–31.

Box 35.5 Differential diagnosis for the new onset postpartum hypertension

Pain

Anxiety

Volume overload

Medication affects –NSAIDs, ergot derivatives, indomethacin, ephedrine

Persistent gestational hypertension/preeclampsia

Late onset eclampsia/HELLP syndrome

Preexisting hypertension

Cerebral vasoconstriction syndrome

TTP

Central venous thrombosis or stroke

as well as in the outpatient setting 7–10 days after delivery. Risk of eclamptic seizures does exist. Nonsteroidal anti-inflammatory agents are known to often contribute to elevated blood pressure and an alternate analgesic should be considered if hypertension persists more than 1 day postpartum.[9] If a patient presents in the postpartum period with new onset hypertension with neurologic symptoms or otherwise severe features of preeclampsia parenteral administration of magnesium sulfate should be administered. Antihypertensive medications should be given if postpartum blood pressures persistent greater than or equal to 150 mmHg systolic or 100 mmHg diastolic.[9] Further complications such as renal failure, pulmonary edema, heart failure, and further neurologic complications are best managed by a multidisciplinary team in conjunction with obstetric services.

Future Implications

Hypertensive diseases in pregnancy not only have acute maternal and fetal implications but may also be a marker of long-term consequences to come. At this time it is uncertain if preeclampsia is the manifestation of pre-disposition to cardiovascular disease that becomes evident during the physiologic stress of pregnancy or if later cardiovascular disease is a result of a cardiovascular system weakened by pathologic mechanisms that take place during a pregnancy affected by preeclampsia.[10]

Both women and children affected by hypertensive disorders in pregnancy have been found to have twice the risk for developing future cardiovascular sequelae such as heart disease, atherosclerotic disease, myocardial infarction, congestive heart failure, stroke, and venous thromboembolism.[9,27,38,39] The risk of developing future cardiovascular disease is greater if a patient has multiple pregnancies affected by preeclampsia, delivered at less than 37 0/7 weeks gestational age, or had a pregnancy affected by intrauterine growth restriction.[9,39–41] Some studies suggest the risk is at least equal to the risk of cardiovascular disease seen with obesity, diabetes, and smoking.[42,43] There is also long-term psychological effects of preeclampsia that have been demonstrated. Interestingly patients affected by preeclampsia with severe features or HELLP syndrome have a 5-year risk of self-reported depression or anxiety of 32% and a 19% risk of self-reported marital problems or divorce.[23] This finding has been attributed to the psychologic stress of poor neonatal or long-term outcomes related to prematurity as well as the implications this disease spectrum has on future pregnancies.[23]

Current recommendations for patients with a history of preeclampsia resulting in delivery prior to 37 and 0/7 weeks gestational age or with an obstetric history of recurrent preeclampsia state they should undergo yearly assessment of blood pressure, lipids, fasting blood glucose and measurement of body mass index.[9] Although definitive data is lacking, it is recommended that lifestyle modifications should be made as necessary to help maintain healthy body weight, incorporate a daily aerobic exercise routine, well-balanced low-fat diet high in fiber, vegetables, and fruits, and to avoid tobacco so as to generally strive for adequate health and nutrition.[9]

Concluding Remarks

Disorders of hypertension in pregnancy are being continuously studied to provide the most accurate definitions, management strategies, templates for patient discussions regarding pregnancy outcomes and future pregnancy implications, and preventative options. Although the causative mechanism remains unproven, research advancements for a better understanding of underlying placental factors, functional endothelial components, maternal cardiovascular adaptation, and pre-disposition to these disorders remain on the forefront of academic efforts to improve antenatal and postpartum outcomes for mothers and neonates affected by this disease spectrum.

References

1. National High Blood Pressure Education Program Working Group on High Blood Pressure in Pregnancy. Report of the national high blood pressure education program working group on high blood pressure in pregnancy. *Am J Obstet Gynecol* 2000;183:S1–S22.
2. Berg CJ, Callaghan WM, Syverson C, Henderson Z. Pregnancy related mortality in the United States, 1998 to 2005. *Obstet Gynecol* 2010;116:1302–9.
3. LeFevre M on behalf of the U.S Preventitive Services Task Force. Low-dose aspirin use for the prevention of morbidity and mortality from preeclampsia: U.S. preventative services task for recommendation statement. *Ann Intern Med* 2014;161:819–26.
4. Say L et al. Global causes of maternal death: A WHO systematic analysis. *Lancet Global Health* 2014;2(6):e323–33.
5. Sperling J et al. The role of headache in the classification and management of hypertensive disorders in pregnancy. *Obstet Gynecol* 2015;126:297–302.
6. Basso O, Rasmussen S, Weinberg CR, Wilcox AJ, Irgens LM, Skjaerven R. Trends in fetal and infant survival following preeclampsia. *JAMA* 2006;296:1357–62.
7. Waterstone M, Bewley S, Wolfe C. Incidence and predictors of severe obstetrical morbidity: Case–control study. *BMJ* 2001;322:1089–93.
8. Lain KY, Roberts JM. Contemporary concepts of the pathogenesis and management of preeclampsia. *JAMA* 2002;287:3183–6.
9. Hypertension in pregnancy. Report of the American College of Obstetricians and Gynecologists' Task Force on Hypertension in Pregnancy. *Obstet Gynecol* 2013 Nov; 122(5):1122–31.
10. Foo L, Lees CC, McEniery CM, Wilkinson IB. Hypertension in pregnancy: Natural history and treatment options. *Curr Hypertens Rep* (2015)17:36.
11. Sibai, B. Diagnosis and management of gestational hypertension and preeclampsia. *Obstet Gyneol* 2003;102:181–92.
12. Sibai B. Pregnancy and coexisting disease: Hypertension. In *Obstetrics: Normal and Problem Pregnancies*. Ed. Gabbe S, Niebyl J, Simpson JL, Landon M, et al. Philadelphia: Elsevier Saunders, 2012;779–824. Print.
13. Hauth JC, Ewell MG, Levine RL, et al. Pregnancy outcomes in healthy nulliparous women who subsequently developed hypertension: Calcium for preeclampsia prevention study group. *Obstet Gynecol* 2000;95:24.
14. Barton JR, O'Brien JM, Bergauer NK et al. Mild gestational hypertension remote from term: Progression and outcome. *Am J Obstet Gynecol* 2001;184:979.
15. Huppertz B. Placental origins of preeclampsia: Challenging the current hypothesis. *Hypertension* 2008;51(4):970–5.
16. Sibai B, Dekker G, Kupferminc M. Preeclampsia. *Lancet* 2005;365(9461):785–99.
17. Levine RJ, et al. Soluble endoglin and other circulating antiangiogenic factors in preeclampsia. *N Engl J Med* 2006;355(10):992–1005.
18. Levine RJ, et al. Circulating angiogenic factors and the risk of preeclampsia. *N Engl J Med* 2004;350(7):672–83.

19. Bashat AA. Pathophysiology of fetal growth restriction: Implications for diagnosis and surveillance. *Obstet Gynecol Surv* 2004;59:617–27.
20. Laura AM, Pels A, Helewa M, Rey E, von Dadelszen P, On behalf of the Canadian Hypertensive Disorders of Pregnancy (HDP) Working Group. Pregnancy hypertension: an international journal of women's cardiovascular health. *Cardiovascular Health* 2014;4:105–145.
21. Abildgaard U, Heimdal K. Pathogenesis of the syndrome of hemolysis, elevated liver enzymes, and low platelet count (HELLP): A review. *Eur J Obstet Gynecol Reproduc Biol* 2013;166:177-123.
22. Lachmeijer AM, Arngrimsson R, Bastiaans EJ, et al. A genome-wide scan for preeclampsia in the Netherlands. *Eur J Hum Genetics* 2001;10:758–64.
23. Habli M, Eftekhari N, Wiebracht E, et al. Long-term maternal and subsequent pregnancy outcomes 5 years after hemolysis, elevated liver enzymes, and low platelets (HELLP) syndrome. *Am J Obstet Gynecol* 2009;201:385.e1-5.
24. Hupuczi P, Rigo B, Sziller I, Szabo G, Szigeti Z, Papp Z. Follow-up analysis of pregnancies complicated by HELLP syndrome. *Fetal Diag Ther* 2006;21:519–22.
25. Sibai, B. Gestational hypertension – Preeclampsia. *Obstet Gynecol* 2003.
26. Henderson J, Whitlock E, O'Connor E, Senger C, Thompson, J, Rowland, M. Low-dose aspirin for the prevention of morbidity and mortality from preeclampsia: A systematic evidence review for the U.S. preventative services task force. *Ann Intern Med* 2014;160:695–703.
27. Amaral L, Cunningham M, Cornelius D, LaMarca B. Preeclampsia: Long-term consequences for vascular health. *Vasc Health Risk Mgmt* 2015: 11 403–415.
28. Bateman BT, Bansil P, Hernandez-Diaz S, Mhyre JM, Callaghan WM, Kuklina EV. Prevalence, trends, and outcomes of chronic hypertension: A nationwide sample of delivery admission. *Am J Obstet Gynecol* 2012;2006(2);165–9.
29. Lecarpentier E, Tsatsaris V, Goffinet F, Carbol D, Sibai B, et al. Risk factors for superimposed preeclampsia in women with essential chronic hypertension treated before pregnancy. *PLoS One* 2013;8(5):e62140. doi:10.1371/journal.pone.00062140.
30. Gilbert WM, Young AL, Danielsen B. Pregnancy outcomes in women with chronic hypertension: A population-based study. *J Reprod Med* 2007;52:1046–51.
31. Kuklina EV, Ayala C, Callaghan WM. Hypertensive disorders and severe obstetric morbidity in the United States. *Obstet Gynecol* 2009; 113:1299–306.
32. Sibai, B. Postpartum hypertension – Preeclampsia. *Am J Obstet Gynecol* 2012 Jun;206(6):470–5. doi: 10.1016/j.ajog.2011.09.002. Epub 2011 Sep 16.
33. Chappel LC, Enye S, Seed P, Briley AL, Poston L, et al. (2008) Adverse perinatal outcomes and risk factors for preeclampsia in women with chronic hypertension: A prospective study. *Hypertension* 51:1–8.
34. Sibai BM, Lindheimer M, Hauth J, Caritis S, VanDorsten P, et al. Risk factors for preeclampsia, abruptio placentae, and adverse neonatal outcomes among women with chronic hypertension. National Institute of Child Health and Human Development Network of Maternal-Fetal Medicine Units. *N Engl J Med* 1998;339:667–71.
35. Malha L, August P. Secondary Hypertension in pregnancy. *Curr Hypertens Rep* 2015;17;53.
36. Walters BN, Walter T. Hypertension in the puerperium. *Lancet* 1987;2:330.
37. Ghuman N, Ehiener J, Tendler BE, White WB. Hypertension in the postpartum woman: Clinical update for the hypertension specialist. *J Clin Hypertens (Greenwich)* 2009;11:726–33.
38. Kessous R, Shoham-Vardi I, Pariente G, Sergienko R, Sheiner E. Long term maternal atherosclerotic morbidity in women with pre-eclampsia. *Heart* 2015;101(6);526–529.
39. Mongraw-Chaggin ML, Cirillo PM, Cohn BA. Preeclampsia and cardiovascular disease: Prospective evidence from the child health and development studies cohort. *Hypertension* 2010;5:166–71.
40. Funai EF, Paltiel OB, Malaspina D, Friedlander Y, Deutsch L, Harlap S. Risk factors for pre-eclampsia in nulliparous and parous women: The Jerusalem perinatal study. *Paediatr Perinat Epidemiol* 2005;19:59–68.
41. Ray JG, Vermeulem MJ, Schull MJ, Redelmeier DA. Cardiovascular health after maternal placental syndromes (CHAMPS): Population-based retrospective cohort study. *Lancet* 2005;366:1797–803.
42. Roberts JM, Hubel CA. Pregnancy: A screening test for later life cardiovascular disease. *Women Health Issues* 2010;20:304–7.
43. Romundstad PR, Magnussen EB, Smith GD, Vatten LJ. Hypertension in pregnancy and later cardiovascular risk: Common antecedents? *Circulation* 2010;122:579–84.

Cardiovascular Disease in Pregnancy

Cornelia R. Graves

Introduction

In this chapter, the complex issues associated with cardiac disease during pregnancy will be explored. Changes in maternal physiology, which are important to understanding the management of cardiovascular diseases, will be discussed. The need for a coordinated care team consisting of obstetricians, maternal fetal medicine specialists, cardiologist and obstetrical anesthesiologist from the preconception through post-delivery will be emphasized.

Scope of the Problem

Cardiovascular disease is the leading cause of indirect maternal death in the United States; it complicates up to 4% of all pregnancies.[1] Recent data suggests unrecognized or uncontrolled cardiovascular disease has been a leading contributor to rise in maternal mortality in this country over the last 10 years.[2] Intensive care unit (ICU) admissions due to maternal cardiac disease comprise up to 15% of obstetric ICU admissions, but account for up to 50% of maternal deaths.[3] Many advances in the treatment of cardiovascular diseases have changed the landscape of cardiac disease in pregnancy. Prior to 2007, most lesions encountered in pregnancy were acquired lesions. Due to the changes in care of congenital heart disease, many patients who present with cardiac risk factors have been corrected by surgery at birth.[4]

Pregnancy presents unique challenges to providers who care for patients with cardiovascular disease in pregnancy as common complaints of normal pregnancy such as dyspnea, fatigue, palpitations and pedal edema may mimic symptoms of worsening disease making the situation difficult for clinical assessment (Table 36.1).

Maternal Physiology

Pregnancy is associated with a number of cardiovascular and circulatory changes that can significantly impact underlying cardiac disease. Many of these changes begin as early as 5 weeks and peak in the early third trimester. Cardiac output (CO) increases during pregnancy by approximately 50%.[5] The degree of change at a particular moment is acutely influenced by changes in maternal position. For example, CO is higher in the left lateral decubitus position as opposed to the supine position; the supine position can reduce CO by as much as 25–30% due to aorto-caval compression.[6] Stroke volume is also increased. In order to maintain normal blood pressure, systemic vascular resistance decreases and begins to rise in the early third trimester. There is an increase in heart rate by 10–15 beats per minute,[5]

Also present is an increase in blood volume, which is a primarily an increase in plasma volume. Mean corpuscular volume is only increased by 20%. This increase in plasma volume is modulated by sodium retention and changes in renin–angiotensin regulation. These changes cause a physiologic anemia of pregnancy. Pulmonary artery vascular resistance is decreased along with pulmonary colloid osmotic pressure. This decreased is most pronounced in the postpartum period. Pregnancy is a hypercoagulable state and the risk of thrombotic events are higher during pregnancy and in the immediate postpartum period. The postpartum period is also associated with dramatic alterations in hemodynamics during the first 12–24 hours after delivery as the gradual cardiac adaption of pregnancy returns to its pre-pregnancy state. All of these changes represent unique challenges to the clinician but must be understood in order to take appropriate care of this patient population.[7]

The implication of these physiologic changes during pregnancy means that the patient undergoes wide fluctuations in the cardiovascular system during the pregnancy and in the postpartum period which may lead to rapid maternal decompensation. Knowledge of

Table 36.1 Signs and Symptoms of Normal Pregnancy versus Heart Failure

Present in Normal Pregnancy	Suggest Cardiac Pathology
Fatigue	Chest pain
Exertional dyspnea	Severe breathlessness, orthopnea, paroxysmal nocturnal dyspnea (PND), cough
Palpitations	Atrial flutter or fibrillation, supraventricular tachycardia (SVT)
Elevated jugular venous pressure	Systemic hypotension
Sinus tachycardia (10–15%) above normal heart rate	Sinus tachycardia, >15% above normal rate
Full volume pulse	
Third heart sound	Fourth heart sound
Systolic flow murmur	Pulmonary edema
Pedal edema	Pleural effusion

Box 36.1 Hemodynamic adaptations to pregnancy

Cardiac output – increased by 30–50% by end of first trimester. Increase continues throughout gestation. Cardiac output increases in labor by up to 50% with pushing. Epidural anesthesia may blunt this change

Stroke volume – increased by 30%

Circulating blood volume – reaches maximum of 40% to 24 weeks gestation

Heart rate increases by 10–30 beats/ minute

Decreased systemic vascular resistance resulting in a drop in blood pressure until the third trimester when resistance begins to rise

Dilutional anemia secondary to increased plasma volume

Increased coagulation factors

maternal physiology will allow the clinician to anticipate and develop an appropriate care plan for these patients (Box 36.1).

Evaluation of the Heart During Pregnancy

Evaluation of cardiac studies during pregnancy can be difficult for those that are unfamiliar with changes that occur during the pregnancy. The chest radiograph of a pregnant patient may demonstrate apparent cardiomegaly, an enlarged left atrium and increased vascular markings. This is due to the rotation of the cardiac silhouette closer to the left side of the chest and the increase in volume status associated with pregnancy.

Normal echocardiography (ECHO) studies in pregnancy may increase mild tricuspid, mitral or pulmonary regurgitation. A slight increase in left atrial size occurs. Left ventricular end diastolic dimensions may be increased by 6–10%. A small pericardial effusion is not uncommon.

Electrocardiography can demonstrate right axis deviation and a right bundle branch block, Q-waves in lead III and T-wave inversion in leads III, V2 and V3.[8]

Preconception Counseling

Preconception counseling should ideally be performed on every patient with preexisting cardiovascular disease. This counselling should be performed at an institution that has expertise in cardiac disease and high-risk pregnancy care. The goals of preconception counseling should be to minimize the risks, determine whether or not cardiac intervention may be required prior to pregnancy, to identify recurrence and genetic risks and to determine the appropriate center for delivery. Long-term maternal risks and alternative options such as surrogacy and adoption should be addressed. In addition, an evaluation of the patient's current medications and alternatives should be reviewed. Drugs such as angiotensin-converting enzyme (ACE) inhibitors and angiotensin receptor blockers (ARBs) should be discontinued prior to pregnancy due to the potential risk for teratogenicity.

The initial visit should involve a detailed history including pregnancy history, electrocardiogram (ECG) as well has an echocardiogram. Transthoracic ECHO may be helpful in the assessment of valvular function and to determine the degree of shunting. Pulmonary artery pressure is best assessed through cardiac catheterization and should be performed whenever an increase in right-sided pressure is suspected. The performance of stress ECHO testing may be helpful in identifying patients with cardiomyopathy in which pregnancy may present significant risks.[9]

The New York Heart Association Classification is commonly used to identify patients at risk for complications during pregnancy (Box 36.2). Data suggest that 44% of patients may change classification during

Box 36.2 New York heart association classification system

Class I No limitations with physical activity. Ordinary physical activity does not precipitate cardiovascular symptoms such as dyspnea, angina, fatigue or palpitations

Class II Slight limitation of physical activity. Ordinary physical activity will precipitate cardiovascular symptoms. Patients are comfortable at rest.

Class III Less than ordinary physical activity precipitates that markedly limit activity. Patents are comfortable at rest

Class IV Patients are uncomfortable with any physical activity. Symptoms are present at rest

the pregnancy.[10] Patients with Class III and IV disease at the time of conception should the counseled regarding the significant risk of maternal morbidity and mortality. Another classification developed by Clark et al. stratifies risk of maternal mortality based on the cardiac lesion (Table 36.2).[11] The Cardiac Disease in Pregnancy (CARPREG) risk score can also be used to predict the risk of a cardiac event during the pregnancy (Table 36.3),[12] Most recently, the World Health Organization (WHO) proposed a classification for cardiac risk during pregnancy.[13]

Genetic counseling should be performed on all patients affected by congenital heart disease. If the patient is affected by most forms of congenital heart disease the risk of recurrence in her fetus is 3–4%. If there is an affected sibling, the risk of recurrence approaches 10%. Left-sided lesions such as a bicuspid aortic valve and left outflow tract obstructive lesions may have a higher risk of recurrence as well again approaching 10%.[14] Autosomal-dominant disease such as Marfan's syndrome and hypertrophic obstructive cardiomyopathy have a 50% risk of recurrence in offspring. Patients with cono-truncal abnormalities are often associated with the 22q11.2 deletion (DiGeorge) syndrome. If the patient has not been tested previously, genetic testing should be offered to patients with this lesion. Those carrying the deletion have a 50% change of their offspring being affected (Box 36.3).[15]

During the preconception evaluation, the patient should be counseled on whether pregnancy is a feasible option. Some experts suggest that patients with

Table 36.2 Maternal Mortality Associated with Pregnancy

Group I	Group II	Group III
Mortality risk less than 1%	Mortality risk of 5–15%	Mortality risk of 25–50%
Corrected tetralogy of fallot Pulmonic/tricuspid disease Mitral stenosis (NYHA I and II) Patent ductus arteriosus – repaired Ventricular septal defect Atrial septal defect Bioprosthetic valve	**A** Mitral stenosis- NYHA III and IV Previous MI Uncomplicated tetralogy Aortic coarctation – Uncomplicated Aortic stenosis Marfan's normal aortic root **B** Mitral stenosis with atrial fibrillation Mechanical heart valve	Aortic coarctation – complicated Marfan's syndrome with aortic root involvement Cardiomyopathy Pulmonary hypertension

Table 36.3 CARPREG Risk Score: Predictors of Maternal Cardiovascular Events

New York Heart Association (NYHA) functional class>II
Cyanosis (room air saturation <90%)
Prior cardiovascular event
Systolic ventricular ejection fraction <40%
Left heart obstruction

For each CARPREG predictor that is present, a point is assigned.
Risk Estimation of Cardiovascular Complications

Number of predictors	Risk of cardiac event in pregnancy (%)
0	5
1	27
>1	75

Box 36.3 Risk of fetal cardiac abnormality by maternal lesion

Atrial septal defect (ASD) 3–10[3] (4%)
Ventricular septal defect (VSD) 4–22 (7%)
Left outflow obstruction 6–26 (10%)
Right outflow obstruction 4–15 (5%)
Marfan's syndrome 50%
22q11 deletion syndromes 50%
Hypertrophic cardiomyopathy 50%

Marfan syndrome with a dilated aortic root, pulmonary hypertension, severe left heart obstruction and unresolved peripartum cardiomyopathy should be counseled not to become pregnant. Pregnancy is contraindicated in patients with WHO IV status.

Contraceptive counseling including permanent options should be presented to the patient during this session. If pregnancy does occur in this patient population, termination of pregnancy should be offered due to the significant risk of maternal mortality.

Congenital Heart Disease

In the United States, most congenital heart lesions are identified and repaired during the early neonatal period. Most women with repaired congenital heart lesions will have uncomplicated pregnancies although about 30% may have a decrease in functional class. Most of these patients improve post-delivery. Approximately 1% will have a late pregnancy cardiac event with dysrhythmias and heart failure being the most common events.[16] The provider should keep in mind that in under-developed countries, some congenital lesions may go undetected until adulthood. This may increase the risk of complications during pregnancy and delivery.

Congenital Heart Disease – Intracardiac Communications

Atrial septal defects (ASD), ventricular septal defects (VSD) and patent ductus arteriosus (PDA) allow shunting of the blood across the defect. Over time these can lead to ventricular dysfunction and pulmonary hypertension. Left untreated, these shunts will change flow from left–right to right–left across the shunt resulting in Eisenmenger's syndrome. Intracardiac communications are the most common lesion in pregnancy. They may present in young adults as a paradoxical embolism often causing a transient ischemic attack. The risk of venous thromboembolism is ~5%.

Most small lesions are well tolerated in pregnancy and are not associated with complications. Large lesions (greater than 1 cm) may be associated with increased pulmonary pressures. Repaired lesions do not usually present a problem in pregnancy. In unrepaired lesions, prompt treatment of ventricular arrhythmias, hypertension and tachycardia is paramount to avoidance of an increase in the left to right shunt. The mode of delivery should be determined by obstetrical needs. An assisted second stage may be used in those patients for which pushing may increase the risk of arrhythmias.[17,18]

Congenital Heart Disease – Pulmonary Hypertension and Eisenmenger's Syndrome

Pulmonary hypertension still remains one of the most concerning cardiac lesions for both the mother and the fetus. Maternal mortality is approximately 30–50% and the fetal loss rate is also increased due to spontaneous abortion and intrauterine growth restriction. The increased volume load associated with pregnancy along with falling systemic vascular resistance increases the right to left shunt; this exacerbates cyanosis. Acute blood loss may thus, along with other hemodynamic changes that may occur in pregnancy, precipitate cardiovascular collapse. Death may occur during labor and delivery but the risk of maternal death may extend to weeks post-delivery due to thrombus formation or right ventricular failure. Although pulmonary vasodilator therapy has led to improved outcomes, if women with Eisenmenger's syndrome becomes pregnant she should be offered therapeutic termination of pregnancy.[19]

The mode and timing of delivery needs to individualized depending on maternal cardiac status. A multidisciplinary team approach including obstetricians, maternal-fetal medicine specialists, anesthesiologists and cardiologists should be formed. An individualized care conference should be held prior to delivery. Regional anesthesia should be used with caution as hypotension may be fatal. Intra-arterial monitoring as well as central venous pressure monitoring is recommended regardless of mode of delivery. Post-delivery care includes meticulous monitoring in an intensive care setting with anticoagulation to avoid thrombus.

Patients should remain in the hospital for 7–10 days postpartum given the rate for post-delivery complications.[20]

Congenital Heart Disease: Cyanotic Heart Conditions

In the United States, most patients with cyanotic heart disease are repaired in the first few years of life. Unrepaired lesions carry an increased risk of maternal and fetal morbidity. Recent data suggest that fetal outcome is related to the degree of maternal cyanosis.

When oxygen saturation is less than 85%, only 12% of babies were live born.[21]

Tetralogy of Fallot

Tetralogy of fallot (TOF) is comprised of the tetrad of the following findings: ventricular septal defect, overriding aorta, right ventricular septal outflow obstruction and right ventricular hypertrophy. Corrected TOF is usually well tolerated in pregnancy; however, long-term complications are still an issue. Unrepaired TOF is associated with significant cyanosis and is usually not associated with a successful pregnancy. Complications including right ventricular failure, sudden cardiac death and cardiac dysrhythmias can occur. In patients with unrepaired tetralogy of fallot (including those with palliative shunts), pregnancy is not advised due to poor maternal and fetal outcomes.[22] A significant number of patients develop pulmonary regurgitation after repair of TOF; this may lead to RV enlargement and dysfunction, decreased exercise tolerance and arrhythmias. With residual lesions, maternal complications including heart failure exist and there is an increased risk of fetal loss and intrauterine growth restriction.[23] Mortality rates occur at ~1% annually, for 25 years post pregnancy. Management during pregnancy should be geared toward controlling symptoms as they occur.

Transposition of the Great Vessels (Impaired Systemic Right Ventricle)

D-transposition of the great arteries is the most common form of cyanotic congenital heart disease in the neonatal period. Associated lesions include VSD, subpulmonary outflow obstruction and coarctation of the aorta.

In patients with d-transposition, the aorta arises from the right ventricle and the pulmonary artery arises from the left ventricle. Repairs involve redirecting circulation for the deoxygenated blood. This leads to right ventricle becoming the systemic ventricle. As pregnancy progresses, this ventricle may be vulnerable to progressive failure. Although pregnancy can be successful in these patients, a small study noted that in one-third of patients right ventricular dilatation progressed and did not resolve after pregnancy.[24]

Comprehensive cardiac evaluation is recommended prior to pregnancy; however, in patients with repair, pregnancy outcomes appear to be good.[25]

Inherited Lesions

Marfan Syndrome

Marfan syndrome is an autosomal dominant condition in which 80% of patients will have cardiac symptoms. Aortic dilatation and dissection account for the majority of morbidity and mortality in patients with Marfan syndrome, but aortic rupture and dissection can occur in patients with normal aortic root (<1%). Data suggest that the risk of aortic rupture or dissection is approximately 10% if the aortic root is 4 cm or greater. Patients with aortic root measurements greater than 4.5 cm should have repair prior to conception. The hallmark of care in these patients is to avoid hypertension and tachycardia. Some authors suggest beta-blockade during the pregnancy in order to avoid progressive dilatation of the aortic root during pregnancy. Unlike other cardiac lesions, cesarean section is recommended in patients with aortic root dilatation 4 cm or greater.[26]

Bicuspid Aortic Valve and Aortic Stenosis

Severe aortic stenosis is almost always in Western societies related to a bicuspid aortic valve. Severe aortic stenosis (mean gradient 40 mm Hg) should be repaired prior to pregnancy with valvuloplasty when possible. Maintenance of cardiac output is the major issue associated with aortic stenosis. Due to the relative hypervolemia associated with gestation, pregnancy is usually well-tolerated. With severe disease, cardiac output may be relatively fixed and the patient will operate in a narrow therapeutic window. Decreasing preload will result in both poor coronary artery perfusion and cerebral perfusion. Labor delivery and termination of pregnancy may therefore impose the greatest risk of these patients. Hypotension associated with blood loss, the placement of regional anesthesia or significant aorto-caval compression may result in sudden cardiac death. The clinician should be careful to avoid bradycardia or tachycardia when caring for these patients (see Box 36.3 for a discussion on fetal inheritance of maternal cardiac lesions).[27]

Myocardial Infarction

Although coronary artery disease is still rare in women of reproductive age, the incidence of myocardial infarction (MI) during pregnancy has been increasing. As more women postpone childbearing into their forties and sometimes early fifties and with the rising health epidemics of obesity, diabetes and hypertension, chest pain in pregnancy should be fully evaluated. Acute myocardial infarction in pregnancy can be associated with significant maternal morbidity and mortality. Roth et al. reviewed 123 pregnancies with 125 well-documented myocardial infarctions. In that study, most common location for the infarct is the anterior wall, which carried a maternal death rate of 21%. Maternal death most often occurred at the time of the infarct or if the patient delivered within 2 weeks of the event.[28] The diagnosis of MI during pregnancy is performed using the same modalities used for the non-pregnant population. ECG with an elevated troponin or creatine kinase MB fraction (CKMB) establishes the diagnosis.

Once a MI is suspected, treatment includes the administration of morphine, oxygen, sublingual nitroglycerine and chewed aspirin (160–325 mg). Cardiac catheterization with embolic therapy and stent placement are not contraindicated in pregnancy. Expert opinion recommends postponing delivery for 2–3 weeks post-infarction to minimize the additional cardiac demands of labor and delivery. Route of delivery should be individualized as cesarean delivery may be associated with a higher maternal mortality risk.[29]

Peripartum Cardiomyopathy

Peripartum cardiomyopathy (PPCM) is classically defined as the development of cardiac failure in the last month of pregnancy or within 5 months postpartum. Criteria for diagnosis include the absence of an identifiable cause for cardiac failure (such as severe hypertension) and the absence of recognizable heart disease prior to the last month of pregnancy. Additional criteria include left ventricular systolic dysfunction, ejection fraction less than 45%, shortening fraction less than 30% and left ventricular end-diastolic dysfunction dimension of greater than 2.7 cm/m^2 body surface area. This definition excludes women who present early in pregnancy and is meant to exclude those patients who present in heart failure from other causes, including hypertensive heart disease and preeclampsia.[30]

The exact cause of PPCM is unknown. Genetic factors may play a role as recent studies have suggested approximately 5% of patients may carry the same gene as seen in patients with dilated cardiomyopathy. Seventy-five percent of cases are diagnosed in the first month postpartum with 45% of cases presenting in the first week. The incidence of peripartum cardiomyopathy varies, but in the United States it has been suggested that it occurs in 1 in 3,000 cases in pregnancy. PPCM can occur in women of all reproductive ages. Women with underlying medical issues such as hypertension, thyrotoxicosis or undiagnosed cardiac disease may be at increased risk. One case–control study in United States found that when compared to non-African American women, African American women had a 15.7-fold relative risk for the development of PPCM.[31]

Patients often present with complains of shortness of breath, palpitations, orthopnea, fatigue and cough. ECG may show non-specific findings. B-type natriuretic peptide (BNP) will be markedly elevated. Echocardiography is essential for the establishment of the diagnosis. If the patient is hypertensive, the clinician should consider preeclampsia as the primary diagnosis as the disease process may present with pulmonary edema and left ventricular dysfunction.

The goals of therapy are to reduce preload with diuretic therapy, reduce afterload with vasodilator therapy and reduce myocardial oxygen requirements. If these therapies fail to improve contractility, then digoxin or a beta agonist may be considered. Anticoagulation therapy should be considered in patients with significant ventricular dilation or atrial dysrhythmia.

The mode of delivery in still pregnant patients with PPCM should be determined by obstetrical indications. Cesarean section has not been demonstrated to improved outcomes. Regional (epidural) anesthesia is not contraindicated. The clinician may consider an assisted second stage for patients with significant cardiac dysfunction.

Patients with PPCM should be counseled regarding the risk of future pregnancies. Studies have noted that patients who fail to normalize cardiac function within 6 months postpartum carry a mortality risk of 85% in 5 years. Patients with incomplete recovery (ejection fraction<50%) have a high rate of decompensation in a subsequent pregnancy and should be counseled against future conception.

Bioprosthetic and Mechanical Heart Valves

Bioprosthetic heart values do not present a significant change in management as they are not associated with an increased risk of thrombosis during pregnancy. Patients with mechanical prosthetic valves pose a unique challenge as no optimal coagulation agent has been shown to be completely safe in pregnancy. The efficacy of warfarin is well established as if provides the greatest protection against vascular thrombosis When the international normalized ratio (INR) ranges from 2.5 to 3.5 throughout pregnancy, the risk of thrombotic event is 3.9%. However, warfarin is associated with embryopathy at 6–9 weeks gestation and does cross the placenta during the second and third trimester, which can increase the risk of fetal intraventricular hemorrhage. Unfractionated heparin is associated with the highest risk of maternal thromboembolism during pregnancy (33%). This may be due to the difficulty of effective monitoring of the activated partial thromboplastin time (aPTT) or the failure to recognize the increase in renal excretion associated with advancing gestation. Low molecular weight heparin (LMWH) can be used but early use is associated with inadequate dosing leading to maternal value thrombosis and death. LMWH may be used as an alternative to warfarin therapy if dosed twice daily (usually at least 1 mg/kg) during pregnancy with a target anti-factor Xa level of 0.8–1.2 IU/ml at 4 to 6 hours post-dosing monitoring weekly. The use of LMWH should be restricted to patients who can maintain compliance. While prosthetic valve thrombosis is a rare complication in the non-pregnant patient, the risk of during pregnancy may be as high as 10%. Recent data suggest that low-dose thrombolysis in pregnant women with mechanical mitral thrombosis under transesophageal echocardiography did not increase maternal mortality. Perinatal mortality was 20%; these deaths, however, occurred in patients who required repeat treatment.[32]

Concluding Remarks

Although cardiac disease complicates only 4% of all pregnancies in the United States, cardiovascular complications are a leading cause of maternal morbidity and mortality. Pregnancy is associated with a number of changes in the cardiocirculatory system that can have a significant impact on underlying cardiac disease. An understanding of these changes is essential to providing appropriate care to these patients. Patients with underlying cardiovascular disease should be evaluated prior to pregnancy when possible. While labor and delivery may be associated with marked fluctuations in cardiac output, there is no data to suggest that cesarean delivery is safer in most cases. Cesarean section should be reserved for standard obstetrical complications or for those patients in which labor and delivery is relatively contraindicated, i.e. Marfan syndrome with a dilated aortic root.

Meticulous management of the patient with cardiovascular disease requires a team of providers all skilled in taking care of this population. Delivery should occur at centers with resources to support both the mother and her unborn child.

References

1. Berg CJ, Atrash HK, Koonin LM, Tucker M. Pregnancy related mortality in the United States 1991–1997. *Obstet Gynecol* 2003 Feb;101(2);289–296.
2. Berg, CJ, Chang, J, Callaghan WM et al. Pregnancy related mortality in the United States 1991–1997. *Obstet Gynecol* 2005;100(2):289–96.
3. Loverro G, Pansini V, Greco et al. Indications and outcome for intensive care unit admission during puerperium. *Arch Gynecol Obstet* 2001;264(4):195–8.
4. Balint OH, Sui SC, Mason, J et al. Cardiac outcomes after pregnancy in women with congenital heart disease. *Heart* 2010;96:1656–61.
5. Robson SC, Hunter S, Boys RJ, Dunlop W. Serial study of factors influencing changes in cardiac output during human pregnancy. *Am J Physiol* 1989;256:1060.
6. Metacalf J, Ureland K. Maternal cardiovascular adjustments to pregnancy. *Prog Cardiovac Dis* 1974;16:363.
7. Robson SC, Hunter S, Moore M, Dunlop W. Haemodynamic changes during the puerperium: A Doppler and M-mode echocardiographic study. *BJOG* 1987;94:1028–32.
8. Schwartz DB, Schamroth L. The effect of pregnancy on the frontal plane QRS axis. *J Electrocardiol* 1979;12:279–83.
9. Marelli AJ, Mackie, AS, Ionsecu-Itu R, Rhame E, Pilote L. Congenital heart disease in the general population: Changing prevalence and age distribution. *Circulation* 2007;115:163–72.
10. Nishimura RA, Otto Sm, Bonow RO, Carabello BA, Ervin JP III, Guyton RA, O'Gara PT, Ruiz CE, Skubas NJ et al. Guideline for management of patients with valvular heart disease: A report of the American College of Cardiology/American Heart Association Task Force of Practice Guidelines 2014.
11. Clark, SL. Structural cardiac disease in pregnancy. In *Critical Care Obstetrics*, Cotton DB, Phelan JP Clark SL, eds. Oradell: Medical Economics; 1987:92.
12. Siu SC Sermer M, Colman JM, Alvarez AN, Mercier LA, Morton BC et al. Prospective multi-study of pregnancy

outcomes in women with heart disease. *Circulation* 2001;104:515–21.

13. Regitz,-Zagrosek V, Blomstrom Lundquist C, Borghi C, Cifkova R, Ferreira R, Foldard JM, Gibbs JS, et al. ESC Guidelines on management of cardiovascular disease during pregnancy: The Task Force of Management of Cardiovascular Disease during Pregnancy of the European Society of Cardiology(ESC). *Eur Heart J* 2011;32:3145–97.
14. Kerstjens-Federiske W, Su Marchie Sarvaasg, Ruiter J, Van Den Akker P, Temmerman A et al. Left ventricular outflow obstruction: Should cardiac screening be offered to first degree relatives. *Heart* 2011;97:1228–32.
15. Lin AE, Basson CT, Goldmuntz E, Gagoulas PL, McDermott DA, McDonald-McGuinn DM, McPherson E, Morris CA, et al. Adults with genetic syndromes and cardiovascular abnormalities: Clinical history and management. *Genet Med* 2008;10:469–94.
16. Aggarwal N, Suri V, Kaur H, Chopra S, Rohila M, Vijayvergiya R. Retrospective analysis of outcome of pregnancy in women with congenital heart disease: Single centre experience from North India. *Aust N Z J Obstet Gynaecol* 2009;49:376–81.
17. Webb G, Gatzoulis MA. Atrial defects in the adult: Recent progress and overview. *Circulation* 2006;114(15):1645–53.
18. McMahon CJ, Feltes TF, Fraley JK et al. Natural history of growth of secundum atrial septal defects and implications for transcatheter closure. *Heart* 2002;87(3):256–9.
19. Partin C. The evolution of Eisenmenger's eponymic enshrinement. *Am J Cardiol* 2003;92:1187–91.
20. Benza RL, Miller DP, Barst RJ, Badesch DB, Frost AE, McGoon MD. An evaluation of long-term survival from time of diagnosis in pulmonary arterial hypertension from the REVEAL Registry. *Chest* 2012;142:448–56.
21. Presbitero P, Somerville J, Stone F, Atura E, Speigelhalter D, Rabajoli F. Pregnancy and cyanotic congenital heart disease: Outcome of mother and fetus. *Circulation* 1994;89:2673–6.
22. Naguib M, Dob D. A functional understanding of moderate to complex congential heart disease and the impact of pregnancy Part II: Tetralogy of Fallot, Eisenmenge's syndrome and the Fontan operation. *Int J Obtest Anesth* 2010;19:306–12.
23. Gelson E, Gatzoulis M, Steer PJ, Lupton M. Johnson M. Tetralogy of Fallot: Maternal and neonatal outcomes. *BJOG* 2008;115:398–402.
24. Tobler D, Fernandes SM, Wald RM, Landzberg M, Salehian O, Sui SC et al. Pregnancy outcomes in women with transposition of the great arteries and arterial switch operation. *Am J Cardiol* 2010;106:417–20.
25. Metz TD, Jackson GM, Yetman AT. Pregnancy outcomes in women who have undergone an atrial switch repair for congenital d-transposition of the great arteries. *Am J Obstet Gynecol* 2001;205:273.
26. Rossiter J, Renke J, Morales A, Murphy E, Pyertiz R. A prospective longitudinal evaluation of pregnancy in Marfan syndrome. *Am J Obstet Gynecol* 1995;92:1599–606.
27. Gandhi M, Martin SR. Cardiac disease in pregnancy. *Obstet Gynecol Clin N Am* 2015;42:315–33.
28. Roth A, Elkayam U. Acute myocardial infarction associated with pregnancy. *Ann Intern Med* 1996;125:751–62.
29. James A, Jamison M, Biwas M, Brancazio LR, Swamy, G, Myers ER. Acute Myocardial infarction in pregnancy: A United States population-based study. *Circulation* 2005;113:1564–71.
30. Habli M, O'Brien T, Nowack E, Khoury S, Marton JR, Sibai B. Peripartum cardiomyopathy: Prognostic factors for long-term maternal outcome. *Am J Obstet Gynecol* 2008;199(4):415.
31. Isezuo SA, Abubakar, SA. Epdemiologic profile of peripartum cardiomyopathy in a tetriary care hospital. *Ethn Dis* 2007;17:228–33.
32. Hagen I, Ross-Hesselink JW, Ruys T, Merz W, Goland S, Gabriel H, Lelonek M, Trojnarska O et al. Pregnancy in women with a mechanical heart valve. Data of the Euroepan Society of Cardiology Registry of Pregnancy and Cardiac Disease (ROPAC). *Circulation* 2015;132:132–42.

Pulmonary Disease in Pregnancy

Joseph Shumway and Isaac Babarinsa

Introduction

Pulmonary symptoms in pregnancy may indicate intrinsic disease or reflect cardiac and systemic disorders. The relative frequencies of disease are related to geography, regional illness prevalence, population migrations and category of health care facility. Pulmonary disease may be infectious, metabolic, allergic-immunologic, and secondary to systemic or cardiac dysfunction, neoplastic or those that tend to be seen acutely in the course of childbirth.

This chapter excludes the upper respiratory diseases as well as sinusitis.

Scope of the Problem

Infectious, chronic and malignant diseases of the respiratory tract may occur singly or concurrently, but infectious diseases are major contributors to the overall burden of global disease (1). The pregnant patient is not spared from these disorders. Indeed, her unique physiological state in pregnancy may contribute to delayed diagnosis and predispose to rapid deterioration of respiratory health with increasing gestational age or in the course of labor.

There are few published national or regional data relating to the burden of pulmonary disease. Many pulmonary diseases are uncommon in pregnancy, even though they may result in maternal death or severe maternal morbidity. For example, a large Canadian population cohort study (2) found the incidence of amniotic fluid embolism to be 2.5 per 100,000 deliveries. In 2010, chronic respiratory disease, flu and pneumonia were two of the top 10 causes of deaths in women in the United States (3). Remarkably, they were not among the top 10 causes of deaths in women in the reproductive age group (18–44 years) in the same cohort. Respiratory distress syndrome was among the most frequently-diagnosed conditions in severely unwell obstetric patients in the United States (4) when data was compared between different decades of care. Pregnancy rates remained steady between 3% and 4% among patients with cystic fibrosis (CF) in the United States between 1990 and 2014 (5), but in the overall CF-affected population, asthma, allergic bronchopulmonary aspergillosis, massive hemoptysis and pneumothorax occurred in 28.2%, 5%, 1.3% and 0.5%, respectively.

Assessment of Acute and Chronic Respiratory Health

Many respiratory symptoms in pregnancy, except coughing, may be attributable to hormonal, mechanical and biochemical adaptations of pregnancy. Other symptoms may indicate significant cardiac or systemic disease (6). The changing cardiorespiratory profile of advancing pregnancy and the hemodynamic alterations that occur during labor may precariously alter a seemingly stable clinical state in patients with pre-existing pulmonary (and cardiac) disease. Obstetricians should be capable of interpreting the pulmonary parameters described in Box 37.1. For more significant illness, consultation with pulmonary experts and other diagnostic testing such as electrocardiogram, V/Q scan, FEV1, and chest computed tomograph/magnetic resonance imaging (CT/MRI) may be required.

Rapid pulmonary symptom appraisal may be triaged with the following questions: Is it getting worse? Does sitting up relieve the symptom? What medications have you used currently or recently? Has there been had a similar prior illness? Does the patient carry any alert bracelet or card?

A patient with worsened or uncontrolled respiratory dysfunction will eventually develop respiratory failure. See Box 37.2 for clinical findings that indicate increased risk.

Box 37.1 Baseline pulmonary parameters

- Pulse oximetry
  - Abnormal SpO_2 is less than 95% on room air, or a value below 5 units of measurements of pre-existing steady state.
- Arterial blood gases
  - Late in pregnancy, PaO_2 is lower when blood samples are taken in the supine position.
  - A PaO_2 below 8 kPa with normal $PaCO_2$ indicates type I respiratory failure and is commonly suggestive of either an acute pulmonary embolism or pneumonia.
  - For $PaCO_2$ greater than 6.5 kPa prompt ventilatory support is indicated; this is type II respiratory failure.
- Serum electrolytes
  - Serum bicarbonate should range between 18 and 26 mEq/l
  - Potassium below 2 or above 7
  - Calcium above 15 mg/dl
  - Serum pH in pregnancy should demonstrate a mild respiratory alkalosis
- Chest X-ray
  - Maternal irradiation dose for a two-view chest X-ray is 0.1 mSv; fetal dose is 0.002 mGy. These doses are negligible.
- Sputum microscopy and culture.

Box 37.2 Parameters for escalation of care

- Airway obstruction
- Cyanosis
- PaO_2 less than 50 mmHg
- pH less than 7.1 or greater than 7.7
- Respiratory rate greater than 35/min
- Treatment of pneumothorax

Pulmonary Infectious Diseases

Bacterial Pneumonia. The main symptoms of community-acquired bacterial pneumonia (CABP) are dyspnea, fever and cough. It may also include a mild-to-moderate intensity of vague and unilateral chest pain. Tachypnea may be present, but its absence does not exclude pneumonia. Scattered or focal crepitation's (crackles) are invariably audible, especially during deep inspiration. Harsh airway sounds (rales) may also be heard.

Predisposing factors include smoking, asthma, pre-existing pulmonary disorders and HIV. A possible "lethal synergism" has been suggested between the influenza virus and *Streptococcus pneumonia*. There is a possibility that severe bacterial pneumonia is "primed" by a prior influenza infection (7).

Generally, the combinations of clinical, radiological and bacteriologic features are needed to arrive at a diagnosis of community-acquired bacterial pneumonia (CABP). In practice, an initial chest X-ray may not show indicative features. If respiratory symptoms persist after the first 48 hours of treatment, a chest CT scan would yield more information than a repeat chest X-ray (8).

The choice of antibiotic should be consistent with local bacterial prevalence and sensitivity data. Penicillin, Macrolides and Cephalosporin's are first-line choices that should cover most-likely organisms. Dosage may be affected by body mass index (BMI).

Pathogenic organisms of CABP in pregnancy are the same the general population. *Streptococcus pneumonia* is a more frequent cause than *Hemophilus influenza*. Three uncommon but important bacterial causes of CABP are *Pneumocystis carinii* (in patients with high HIV risk) and *Legionella* sp. and *Coxiella burnetti*. Anaerobic organisms are more likely to be associated with post-aspiration CABP.

A combination of β-lactam antibiotics (e.g. Cefotaxime) and a macrolide (e.g. Azithromycin), administered at maximum doses, are useful first-line therapies. *Mycoplasma pneumonia* infection may be typically associated with mild-to-moderate jaundice and associated liver function testing abnormalities. Parenteral antibiotics should be administered 6-8 hourly for at least 48 hours, with consultation indicated if symptoms persist beyond 72 hours. Use of a bedside respiratory spirometer to promote ventilation is clinically useful. The increased frequency of preterm contractions and preterm delivery associated with CABP may be related to pyrexia.

Failure of clinical improvement may indicate a new complication of CABP, infection with an uncommon microbial agent or an initial wrong diagnosis. To put this in context, "pneumonia" was the admitting diagnosis in 10 of a sub-set of 45 pregnant women who were amenable to admission triage and transport, but this diagnosis was not listed among the cause of 95 maternal deaths in the United States (9).

CABP may be complicated by formation of pleural effusion, lung abscess, systemic inflammatory response syndrome and respiratory failure. Thromboprophylactic measures should be instituted for hospitalized pregnant women.

Viral Pneumonias

Influenza

The common influenza virus remains a seasonal affliction. Symptoms may include variable degrees of ill-health, with predominantly upper respiratory viral symptoms including cough, sore throat, chills, fatigue, headache, body aches and fatigue. Fever is not a constant feature.

The known risks for hospital admission are asthma, obesity, Black and ethnic minority, smoking and multiple pregnancies. Pregnancy itself – especially in the third trimester – is a risk factor for critical illness, preterm delivery and death, especially if pneumonia occurs. Of the 788 pregnant women seen in the United States between April and August 2009, 64% were hospitalized, 22.6% were admitted into the intensive care unit (ICU) and 3.8% died (10). The women admitted into the ICU were either obese or had a delay of more than 48 hours before initiating anti-viral drug therapy, or both.

Administration of Oseltamivir (Tamiflu) should not await results of real-time reverse transcriptase polymerase chain reaction (rRT-PCR) or viral culture of swabs taken from the nasal cavity floor. Severely ill patients may require mechanical ventilation or even progression to extra-corporeal membrane oxygenation (ECMO) therapy. ECMO use has been associated with nearly 80% maternal survival; experience was best documented in the 2009 H1N1 influenza epidemic (11). (See Figure 37.1.)

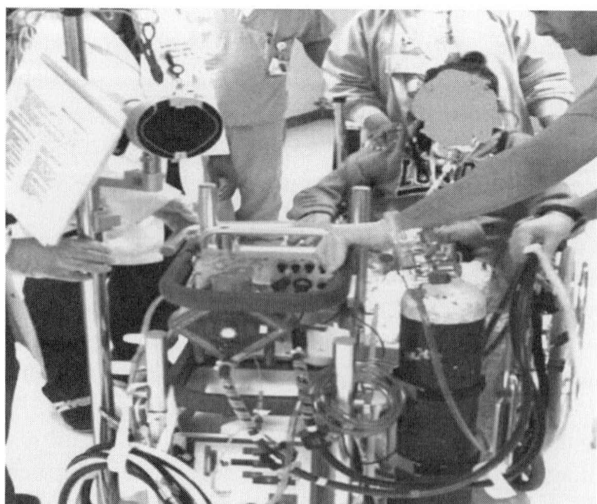

Figure 37.1 Ambulation may occur while on ECMO, following respiratory failure complicating pulmonary tuberculosis. Note the veno-venous circuit connected to the membrane oxygenator. Image provided by Dr Ibrahim Fawzy.

Influenza vaccines should be administered to pregnant women, in view of the increased hazards of influenza during pregnancy.

Middle East Respiratory Syndrome

Infection with the Middle East respiratory syndrome coronavirus presents with a "febrile acute respiratory illness with clinical, radiological or histopathological evidence of pulmonary parenchymal disease e.g. pneumonia or acute respiratory distress syndrome; and direct epidemiologic link with a confirmed case" (www.who.int/csr/disease/coronavirus_infections/MERS_CoV_Update_20_Jan_2014.pdf; Accessed March 1, 2016) (12). Significant illness is rapidly complicated by respiratory and renal failure. Although the origins of the disease are linked to the dromedary camel, most human cases have not had any direct exposure to animals.

Measles

Conjunctivitis, coryza (rhinorrhea) and cough typically follow the prodrome of fever and feeling unwell which is seen in Rubeola (measles) infection. Pneumonia or abnormal liver enzymes indicate moderate to severe disease. The last report of measles in pregnancy in the United States was for a period between 1957 and 1964, but recent Centers for Disease Control and Prevention (CDC) data indicate that futures outbreaks are possible (due to waning herd immunity). This threat would not spare the non-immune pregnant woman (13) who would be at risk for such event.

Chicken Pox

Chickenpox is caused by the varicella zoster virus, a DNA virus of the herpes family. Although most adults have either been immunized or are sero-positive for the virus, a primary infection could be particularly severe in the pregnant woman.

The onset of any significant respiratory symptoms in a pregnant woman with the characteristic rash of chickenpox is a potential indicator of a life-threatening disease (particularly after 24 weeks of gestation). Such women should be initially seen in an isolated area, and universal protective precautions undertaken. Artificial ventilation is often needed, immediate intravenous Acyclovir administration is indicated (13) with concurrent hospitalization.

Pulmonary Tuberculosis

The majority of women with pulmonary tuberculosis (PTB) in pregnancy may not volunteer a "classical" history of chronic cough, hemoptysis or night fever/sweats, but instead may present with unexplained weight loss, poor-progressive weight gain, lethargy and overall feeling of unwell. Hepatosplenomegaly may be demonstrable clinically or on ultrasound examination. Specific radiological findings on the chest X-ray (pulmonary nodules in the upper lung and middle lung fields, cavitation, unilateral pleural effusions and lung scarring) may not be present. Because of these diagnostic difficulties, skin testing is needed. A 20 mm diameter wheal on tuberculin skin testing is consistent with immune reactivity to *Mycobacterium tuberculosis* in patients who cannot easily produce sputum for acid-fast bacilli staining and bacteriology.

Pulmonary TB is classified as a class B1 condition for medical examination of immigrants and refugees into the United States, while "infectious tuberculosis" is in class A category. The latter condition "precludes entry." The typical pregnant woman would therefore be an immigrant or traveler from the Philippines, Mexico, Burma, Vietnam or the Dominican Republic (14). Pulmonary TB is uncommon in developed countries, but it is important to be aware of the risk factors listed in Box 37.3.

Treatment regimens must take into account the current multi-drug resistance present in certain parts of the world. As a minimum, it should include Isoniazid, Ethambutol and Rifampicin. Emerging data reveals that *Mycobacterium tuberculosis* is developing resistance to previous anti-TB medications. Finally, the diagnosis of Pulmonary TB should trigger the need to exclude HIV.

Box 37.3 Indications for TB screening

- Contact with patients who have active, un-treated tuberculosis;
- Congregate communities: shelters for the homeless/refugee sanctuaries/penitentiaries
- Users of "shared" water pipes, especially within migrant communities
- Chronic pulmonary disorders
- HIV positive/those on immune-suppression therapies

Chronic Pulmonary Diseases

Cystic Fibrosis

Cystic fibrosis (CF) is a multi-system disease. The underlying pathophysiology is dysfunction at the subcellular level involving the chloride and sodium pump. The result is formation of viscid mucus, which favors recurrent bacterial colonization and progressive alveolar destruction. Nocturnal desaturation, potentially complicated by sleep apnea, may occur, particularly in the third trimester.

Most women who become pregnant have less severe lung dysfunction than their non-pregnant peers, but the course of pregnancy in CF patients is associated with an overall decline in pulmonary function (10). Respiratory symptoms should be thoroughly investigated and aggressively managed. Assessment for two important organisms, *Burkholderia cepacia* and *Pseudomonas* species, should be performed via sputum bacteriology. Initial treatment of severe illness is with parenteral antibiotics and chest physiotherapy, mucolytics and expectorants.

McMullen et al. provide detailed guideline on the management of cystic fibrosis in pregnancy (15) while Edenborough et al. (16) describe treatment options including respiratory physical therapy (17). Box 37.4

Box 37.4 Optimal clinical care cystic fibrosis

- Control of parallel co-morbidities unique to CF
- Patient education, motivation and counseling
- Biweekly FEV1 assessment.
- Involvement of pulmonary specialty team members
- Review DVT/PE thromboprophylaxis to patient activity level or weight gain
- Perinatal anesthetic consultation
- Individualize the choice of mode of delivery; vaginal route usually preferred
- Ensure that home health assessment and support after hospital delivery are easily accessible

describes optimal clinical care of the respiratory aspects of cystic fibrosis. A successful pregnancy is not felt to be a significant marker of patient well-being for a subsequent pregnancy. All such pregnancies should be planned and considered high risk with comanagement by infectious disease and pulmonary experts.

Box 37.5 lists the frequent comorbidities seen in obstetric patients with CF (18).

Asthma

Asthma symptoms may run a fluctuating course. Fatal asthma events may be associated with an identifiable "trigger" in fewer than half the episodes. The clinical presence sputum neutrophilia and sputum eosinophilia may predict poor control of asthma. Hospitalization rates may be predictable by expiratory peak flow variability. Nocturnal awakenings and severity of episodes are related to overall pulmonary function (19).

Hodder et al. list 46 risk factors for fatal asthma in non-pregnant patients (20). Additionally, alexithymia(or the dysfunction of emotional awareness, social attachments and interpersonal relation) has been associated with near-fatal events or poor asthma control (21). These patients appear to have a profound difficulty in identifying or expressing feelings and body sensations. This group of patients cannot self-manage their disease. For most pregnant asthmatic patients, the overall strategy is to encourage responsible self-management. See Box 37.6 for self-management details.

The management of acute severe asthma in pregnancy is similar to that in non-pregnant women. Tachycardia above 100 indicates imminent severe acute asthma and in pregnancy may represent a more critically perilous state. A recent Cochrane review (22) found no firm conclusions about optimal interventions for managing asthma in pregnancy. The pregnant asthmatic may require induction of labor for obstetric reasons. Prostin (Prostaglandin E2) would appear safe for this purpose, except in a patient who has had a previous "allergic" response to the drug. The use of Prostaglandin F2α (Carboprost) is absolutely contra-indicated.

Box 37.5 Frequent co-morbidities seen in obstetric patients with CF

Anemia
Asthma
Cardiac conduction disorders
Diabetes
Drug abuse
Thrombocytopenia
Thrombophilia
Thyroid disease
Tobacco intake

Box 37.6 Components of asthma self-management plans

- Inhaled short (Salbutamol, Terbutaline) or long-acting β agonists (Formoterol, Salmeterol); inhaler technique must be frequently reviewed
- Inhaled or oral corticosteroids; (for high doses, may need intravenous steroids in labor)
- Mucolytics
- Humidifiers
- Cromoglygate and leukotrienes
- Oxygen therapy
- Abatement of trigger or stimuli (removal of household pets)
- Patient support groups
- Drop-in day care asthma centers
- Family and partner education, information and communication.

Systemic Diseases with Pulmonary Manifestations

Systemic Inflammatory Response Syndrome

The systemic inflammatory response syndrome (SIRS) may occur at any time during pregnancy. A desperately ill pregnant patient may present to the emergency room (ER), or be identified while in labor or after an unremarkable childbirth.

Tachypnea of >20, a serum lactate of >4mmol/L, extremes of temperature (<36° or >38°) and a persistent tachycardia above 100/min suggests the systemic inflammatory response syndrome (SIRS); the severity of the patient's illness is reflected in the degree of tachypnea. Abnormal serum lactate level is a prognostic marker of severe illness, while the titer of Pro-Calcitonin is a guide to the possible needed duration of antibiotic therapy.

Important conditions linked to SIRS are urinary tract infection, pneumonia, upper respiratory tract infection including H1N1, chorio-amnionitis/endometritis, skin and soft tissue infections, especially following cesarean section, and traumatic vaginal deliveries. Group A *Streptococcus* and gram-negative infections are known for sudden onset and rapid deterioration.

One recently proposed clinical tool, the Sepsis in Obstetrics Score (19), was designed specifically for obstetric patients with suspected SIRS. It combines modified selected parameters of the Rapid Emergency Medicine Score (REMS) and of the Acute Physiology and Chronic Health Evaluation (APACHE) score, including respiratory rate, oxygen saturation and lactic acid. A useful risk calculator is accessible online at www.perinatology.com/calculators/spsis%20 Calculator.htmOn

Treatment includes stat doses of intravenous broad spectrum parenteral antibiotics (Cephalosporin and Metronidazole), rapid infusion of a crystalloid solution and vasopressors. Urethral catheterization and central venous monitoring may be indicated. Oxygen therapy may suffice, but some women may require mechanical ventilation. The use of parenteral steroids is controversial.

Goodpasture's Syndrome

Anti-glomerular basement membrane antibody disease (Goodpasture's syndrome) is a systemic vasculitis that affects the microvasculature of the basement membranes of the renal glomeruli and of the pulmonary alveoli. Patients present more frequently with renal insufficiency than with pulmonary features. The main pulmonary symptom is hemorrhage (23). It is diagnosed by finding of a positive anti-glomerular basement membrane autoantibodies in serum.

Anemia requiring blood transfusion or respiratory failure may complicate massive hemoptysis; supportive care is administered but no specific treatment for the pulmonary features is uniformly agreed upon. Supportive care may include plasmapharesis and administration of steroids.

Restrictive Pulmonary Disease

Most women with kyphoscoliosis, congenital myasthenia, spinal muscular dystrophy, bronchiectasis and scleroderma have been diagnosed before pregnancy. Preconception counseling with inclusion of pulmonary risks would be appropriate. After conception, medications that are contraindicated in pregnancy must be stopped or replaced with safer alternatives if possible.

Restrictive pulmonary disease patients lack effective expansion of the lungs. External skeletal or neuromuscular lesions (such as severe kyphosis or myasthenia) or intrinsic gas transfer limitations (such as bronchiectasis) can lead to respiratory failure as a potential consequence. The degree of respiratory reserve, as defined by the forced vital capacity (FVC), may not be predictive of pregnancy outcome. However, patients are expected to experience increasing dyspnea with increasing gestational age. Regularly checked pulse oximetry and spirometry at the beginning of each trimester should be overseen by a multidisciplinary team surveillance.

Twelve patients with restrictive lung diseases, managed through 15 pregnancies were described by Lapinsky et al. (24). Among the five who had kyphoscoliosis or scoliosis, the lowest FVC% predicted was 31%. Another patient with bronchiectasis had the same readings. The lowest FVC% (22%) was in a patient with congenital myasthenia; she required the most intrapartum ventilatory therapy, but had required this antenatally.

Acute Chest Syndrome

Acute chest syndrome (ACS) is among the major causes of death in patients with sickle cell disease (SCD). The precise etiology of ACS remains unclear, but evidence suggests the final common pathway of segmental hypoxia resulting from bone marrow fat embolism, venous thrombosis, pulmonary edema, bacterial pneumonia or and viral pneumonia. Patients may present after normal delivery or operative delivery.

The vaso-occlusive complications of sickle cell disease are not only limited to the long bones. When a patient with sickle cell disease presents with pulmonary dysfunction, ACS should be considered. Cough and fever may not be present. The presence of a wheeze is may indicate bronchoconstriction. Hemoptysis may occur.

Oxygen saturation is often abnormal. The X-ray findings may range from consolidation, hilar infiltrates and pneumothorax or pleural effusion. A positive chest X-ray may define the condition, but a negative one may not exclude it (25) A ventilation-perfusion scan may be indicated if patient appears profoundly unwell and ill out of proportion to the chest X-ray findings.

Initial therapy includes supplementary oxygen, correction of dehydration, administration of analgesics and monitoring of respiratory parameters. A low threshold for prescribing antibiotics empirically exists, but sample cultures should be obtained first. *Streptococcus pneumonia* is a frequent causative infectious agent in patients with SCD due to autosplenectomy. Co-existence of a myocardial dysfunction increases the odds of rapid clinical deterioration, and mechanical ventilation is frequently indicated.

It is good clinical practice to admit these patients for observation. Due consideration should be given to thromboprophylaxis. Consultation with a pulmonologist should be obtained. It is unknown if red blood cell transfusion reduces the duration of ACS, but other co-morbidities may make this therapy necessary. Transfusion-related lung injury is a known complication of blood transfusion in ACS.

Pulmonary Hypertension

Women who have received pre-conceptual counseling for their pulmonary hypertension (PH) have the care advantages of risk assessment and management planning. For newly diagnosed pregnant patients, the demonstration of right ventricular enlargement and accompanying symptoms should narrow the differential diagnosis. Echocardiogram would reveal right ventricular enlargement and function with possible tricuspid regurgitation. Electrocardiogram could show ST-segment depression and T-wave inversion in Leads V1–V4 or prominent R waves in Lead V1. Episodes of intermittent desaturation are not unusual on overnight pulse oximetry. A central line parameter of pulmonary artery systolic pressure of >30 mmHg or a mean pulmonary artery pressure of >20 mmHg is consistent with the diagnosis of PH.

Patients with PH presenting for the first time in pregnancy can only be diagnosed after exhaustive investigation. Differential diagnosis includes exclusion of chronic hemolytic anemias, pulmonary embolism, sleep apnea, prolonged use of appetite-suppressing substances including amphetamines and connective tissue disorders.

Multi-disciplinary care is central to the optimal care of women with PH in pregnancy; such care should include cardiology expertise and or critical care expertise. Low concentration of supplemental oxygen should be considered if PO_2 is <8 kPa and there is no parenchymal lung disease. Nitric oxide therapy, the administration of Prostacyclin analogues, calcium channel blockers, inotropes and phosphodiesterase inhibitors are tailored to individual patient's needs.

Cesarean section may be the safer route of delivery. Triggers of vaso-vagal syncope, such as hyperventilation, Valsalva maneuver and manipulation of the uterine cervix, should be avoided (26).

Most mortality occurs the postpartum period. Complacency must be avoided, thrombo-prophylaxis must be assured and a strict fluid balance must be maintained to optimize clinical outcomes.

Bronchiectasis

Alveolar distension and pulmonary micro-vascular destruction are the long-term outcomes of suppurate pulmonary infections that destroy bronchial epithelial and supportive elastic tissue. This progressive disease commonly worsens during pregnancy. Patients may present with single or repeated episodes of chronic cough, fever, exertional dyspnea or expectoration of offensive-smelling sputum. Halitosis may be present.

Risk factors for bronchiestasis include CF, immune deficiency disorders, congenital pulmonary malformations, history of pulmonary tuberculosis, bronchial malignancy and on rare occasions aspergillosis. An unsuspected inhaled foreign body has been reported. Likewise, some patients may recall childhood or recent pneumonia that was rather difficult to treat.

Examination with chest percussion may not suggest any marked regional differences. Auscultation finding of focal rhonchi and crackles is common. Oxygen saturation readings reflect the extent of oxygenation dysfunction.

Sputum bacteriology, culture and cytology are necessary baseline investigations. Unilateral or segmental lung field hyperluscency with or without emphysema may be seen on chest X-ray. Thickened and dilated bronchograms are identifiable on computed tomography (CT) scan.

The mainstay of treatment is physiotherapy with postural chest percussion and drainage, antibiotic therapy and bronchodilator therapy. Nebulized antibiotics are helpful in severe cases. Inhaled steroids may reduce severity of hypoxia and dyspnea, but respiratory failure is an indication for ICU care. Surgery is rarely needed but could be required for complications such as massive pulmonary hemorrhage (27).

Smoking in Pregnancy

A number of studies about smoking tobacco or marijuana in pregnancy focus on fetal outcomes, as the maternal effects of smoking are unlikely to be reflected during the short time-span of pregnancy.

Between 2000 and 2010, some 10.7% of women in the United States reportedly smoked during pregnancy, and 15% did after delivery. The highest prevalence was in mothers aged 20–24 years (25). In a sample of 350 newly delivered mothers from Lebanon, 8.3% of respondents were water-pipe smokers while 6.3% were "active" cigarette smokers (26).

Exposure of the lungs to inhaled tobacco or other smoke increases the odds to developing chronic bronchitis, impaired broncho-alveolar function, morning sputum production and emphysema. Exercise intolerance is commonly seen in heavy smokers in pregnancy.

Heavy maternal smoking in pregnancy is related to need for chest physiotherapy or respiratory care after administration of a general anesthetic for operative delivery. Deep smoke inhalation followed by a Valsalva maneuver or use of high-resistance inhalation smoking devices (e.g. Hookah) appear to be associated with increased reports of bullous lung disease and baro-trauma, specifically spontaneous pneumothorax and pneumonia-mediastinum (27).

Intrapartum Pulmonary Complications

The active phase of the second stage of labor involves three important phenomena in the mother: Valsalva maneuver (active expulsive efforts against the closed glottis), a 34% increase in cardiac output and reduced end expiratory lung volumes. It is important to identify and effectively manage these changes. Intrapartum pulmonary complications may occur even in previously healthy parturients.

Amniotic Fluid Embolism

The sudden onset of new respiratory symptoms in a laboring woman in (dyspnea, tachypnea, breathlessness, cough and syncope) associated with blood-gas features of respiratory failure should prompt measures to exclude amniotic fluid embolism (AFE), and commence a prompt escalation of care. AFE is also called anaphylactoid reaction of pregnancy and it is more likely in multiparous patients, multiple gestations, induction or augmentation of labor and postdates pregnancies. The crucial clinical symptoms include sudden, unexplained changes in a patient's cardio-respiratory status. There may be dyspnea, chest pain and collapse. Initial features may be suggestive of acute severe asthma in a patient with no similar history.

The US national registry data (28) indicates that AFE is mainly an intrapartum event; only 19% occur delivery at cesarean section, while 11% followed vaginal delivery. More than a third of the patients in the registry had history suggestive of atopy or an allergic experience. The current understanding of the condition involves an immune-based cascade triggered by injection of amniotic fluid into the maternal vascular compartment. Cesarean delivery, maternal age and placental pathology are identified associations (29). Three important differential diagnoses are anaphylaxis, systemic inflammatory response syndrome and pulmonary embolism in that order.

When AFE is suspected, proactive management pathways, based on clinical suspicion alone, should be implemented. High flow oxygen should be commenced by face mask, intravenous access established and urgent pulmonary expert consultation, along with hematology expert consultation, should be obtained. Arterial blood gases and a coagulation profile must be ordered. Chest X-ray would help exclude other possible causes. Electrocardiogram (ECG) may indicate right ventricular strain. Pulmonary support measures along with volume expansion and inotropic support are usually required. The fetal status is indicated if maternal support measures are failing.

Aspiration Pneumonitis

Small quantities of secretions from the oral cavity and upper respiratory tract may be aspirated by up to 50% of healthy adults during sleep (30); these are uneventfully cleared. In labor, gastric stasis, gastro-esophageal sphincter laxity and pH changes may cause the production of significant quantities of such secretions, which may overwhelm and irritate the pulmonary alveoli. The effect is usually immediate, but may be delayed for as long as between 2 and 5 hours.

Sudden respiratory insufficiency in the drowsy, semi-conscious or unconscious parturient should prompt a suspicion of acute aspiration pneumonitis or Mendelsohn's syndrome. Although rare in a patient who is conscious and alert with no gastro-esophageal dysfunction, it can occur in any patient. The use of regional anesthetics for obstetric procedures has also reduced the frequency of aspiration pneumonitis. The preference for use of non-particulate antacids, e.g. sodium citrate as well as the use of H2-receptor blockers (e.g. Ranitidine, proton-pump inhibitors) is helpful. Use of Omeprazole as pre-anesthetic medication has further reduced this condition.

Sudden or repeated coughing, sensation of choking, dyspnea and breathlessness are common signs of aspiration. There may be profuse sweating, a blue hue to the lips and tongue and restlessness. Auscultation of the lung fields may reveal the presence of global or focal crackles and/or wheezing. Arterial blood gases may be normal or abnormal, depending on the volume and pH of the aspirate. A chest X-ray may reveal an air broncho grams; the distribution of lesions may be suggestive patient's position when the aspiration episode occurred.

Initial management includes airway, breathing and maintenance of circulation. High-flow oxygen (10 liters/minute) should be administered by face mask, a parenteral bronchodilator should be administered, a 500 mg dose of corticosteroids administered intravenously, and anesthesiology or pulmonary consultation obtained. If the patient's condition deteriorates, a 0.5 ml of 1:50,000 epinephrine can be administered subcutaneously. Critical care transfer may be needed, bronchoscopic lavage may be indicated.

An audit from Norway (31) identified 11 perioperative obstetric and gynecologic patients with dyspnea, cough, chest tightness, hypoxia, auscultatory and radiographic abnormalities. Five patients reported continued symptoms at 3 months after discharge, but all patients in this cohort were smokers.

Pulmonary Edema

It may initially be difficult to distinguish between AFE aspiration pneumonitis and pulmonary edema (PE) in labor. Unexplained intra-partum coughing, tachypnea, orthopnea and dyspnea may be a result of hypoxemia following interstitial alveolar edema.

PE is generally classified as cardiogenic or non-cardiogenic (32). A recent anesthesiology review, however, regards the problem as two subsets: with hypertension or without hypertension. This clinical distinction allows a focus distinguishing the management of other pulmonary edema from that associated with pre-eclampsia/eclampsia (33). Well-intentioned intravenous fluid therapy or un-restricted infusions in the hypo-albuminemic patient may unfortunately further reduce plasma oncotic pressure and worsen clinical outcomes.

In the setting of pulmonary edema, it is important to stop all infusions immediately, prop up the patient, administer oxygen by face mask and call for help. Auscultation of the chest will reveal crackles at both lung bases. The patient will be hypoxemic and possibly restless and confused. Assessment includes placement of a continuous O_2 saturation monitor, chest X-ray, complete blood count, serum electrolytes, urea, troponin and creatinine. An electrocardiogram may be used to exclude a cardiac event. Transthoracic echocardiogram is useful. If the patient is undelivered, cesarean section (CS) may be seen as part of the resuscitation since it may promote more effective ventilation.

In the presence of severe hypertension and acute pulmonary edema, the choice of agents is limited before delivery. The Task Force on the Management of Cardiovascular Diseases during Pregnancy of the European Society of Cardiology (33) recommends glyceryl trinitrate as the drug of choice in a patient with pulmonary edema complicating preeclampsia/eclampsia. Inhalational glyceryl Trinitrate is used as a one or two metered dose, lasting between 20 and 30 minutes.

Pneumothorax and Subcutaneous Emphysema

Intrapartum spontaneous pneumomediastinum (Hamman's syndrome) is rare. While a sustained or prolonged Valsalva maneuver during the second stage of labor seems a logical explanation, 187 parturients who had the condition did not have a prolonged second stage of labor, had no fetal macrosomia and were all primiparous (34).

It is most important to specifically look for respiratory distress, cyanosis, unilateral chest pain or hyper-resonance of the chest wall to percussion, distant breath or cardiac sounds to auscultation and tracheal deviation. One or more of these may indicate the presence of a tension pneumothorax, which is a medical emergency. Generally, chest X-ray is an adequate initial investigation, but additional imaging may be necessary if the clinical condition worsens or remains static. Bilateral pneumothoraxes may be found. Arterial blood gases are a good indication of severity. Other causes of bullous lung disease must be excluded, particularly unsuspected fungal infections.

In patients with abnormal blood gas results, or those in whom the area of pneumothorax involves more than 25% of one lung, relief is obtained via needle decompression or chest tube placement. Recurrence of the condition in subsequent labors is unpredictable.

Air Embolism

Entry of air through myometrial sinuses, through the right heart to the pulmonary circuit, may cause creation of an intracardiac air column and subsequent bronchospasm, mechanical obstruction and pulmonary edema. The rapidity of events which accompany an air embolism (AE) during labor and cesarean delivery are such that cardio-respiratory arrest may occur before any measure of control is achieved. One sentinel event related to air embolism is exteriorization of the uterus during cesarean section. AE has also been described after normal vaginal delivery, and this rare clinical entity may complicate manual removal of abnormally adherent or retained placenta.

Bradycardia, chest pain and gasping may be consistent with a pre-arrest state. During cesarean section, the anesthesiologist may notice a sudden, unexpected change in cardiopulmonary monitoring parameters. By the time the obstetrician notices profound hypoxia, the patient's neurological prognosis may be grave. Trans-esophageal echocardiography is diagnostic, identifying intra-cardiac air volumes below 0.5 ml.

Even before firm diagnosis, practitioners must utilize standard resuscitation technique including airway, breathing (100% oxygen) and circulation support. External cardiac compression may be required. Placement of a central venous pressure catheter or a pulmonary artery catheter may enhance therapeutic aspiration of the air column (35). The administration of hyperbaric oxygen is the treatment of choice but usually not available urgently.

Pregnancy after Lung Replacement Surgery

Successful pregnancies have followed heart–lung and lung transplants. Most patients described had cystic fibrosis. Patients, partners and family members need to be respectfully counseled about this significant procedure. In a recent Canadian case series, pregnancy was frequently planned even when the risk of death was mentioned to patients in preconception counseling (36). Organ rejection or non-function may occur during or after the pregnancy (36). The real challenge is often in the prompt management of acute pulmonary edema, which may occur without warning. Maternal risks for viral and bacterial pneumonias are increased, which is related to anti-rejection therapy. Denervation of the replacement organ may be associated with gastric atony which worsens the compromised cough reflex and impaired clearance of mucus (37). These issues are important in ventilatory surveillance, anesthetic planning and intrapartum care.

Lung Cancer

Between 1953 and 2013, some 118 women with lung cancer in pregnancy were reported in the English medical literature. Reproductive age women are young, so lung cancer is rarely considered as the cause of vague respiratory symptoms. At gestational ages between 6 and 28 weeks, nine women aged between 24 and 42 years old were diagnosed with lung cancer and found to have metastatic disease (37). None of the women was known to be alive within 5 years of diagnosis.

Concluding Remarks

The proper management of pulmonary disease in pregnancy may have profound effects on patient morbidity and mortality. Preconceptional and prenatal planning may improve the prognosis for patients with known disease but the obstetric care provider must be prepared to care for patients that present with pulmonary crises in labor. Collaborative team management is essential for optimal clinical outcomes.

References

1. Ferkol T, Schraufnagel D. The global burden of respiratory disease. *Ann Am Thoracic Society* 2014 11(3):404–406.
2. Kramer MS, Rouleau J, Bartholomew S, Joseph K for the Maternal Health Study Group of the Canadian Perinatal Surveillance System. Amniotic fluid embolism. Incidence, risk factors, and impact on perinatal outcome. *BJOG* 2012 119:874–879.
3. Women's Health USA 2013. U.S. Department of Health and Human Services, Health Resources and Services Administration, Maternal and Child Health Bureau. *Women's Health USA 2013*. Rockville, MD: U.S. Department of Health and Human Services, 2013.

4. Callaghan WM, Creanga AA, Kuklina EV. Severe maternal morbidity among delivery and postpartum hospitalizations in the United States. *Obstet Gynecol* 2012 120(5):1029–1036.
5. Cystic Fibrosis Foundation Patient Registry. *2014 Annual Data Report*. Bethesda, MD: Cystic Fibrosis Foundation, 2015.
6. ACOG Practice Bulletin No. 100. Clinical Management Guidelines for Obstetrician-Gynecologists. Critical Care in Pregnancy. *Obstet Gynecol* 2009 113(2/1):463–450.
7. Metersky ML, Masterton RC, Lode H et al. Epidemiology, microbiology and treatment considerations for bacterial pneumonia complicating influenza. *Int J Infect Dis* 2012 16:e321–e331.
8. Banker PD, Jain VR, Haramati LB. Impact of chest CT on the clinical management of immunocompetent emergency department patients with chest radiographic findings of pneumonia. *Emerg Radiol* 2007 14(6):383–388.
9. Clark SL, Christmas JT, Frye DR. Maternal mortality in the United States: Predictability and the impact of protocols in fatal postcesarean pulmonary embolism and hypertension-related intracranial hemorrhage. *AMJOG* 2014 211(1):32 e1–e9.
10. Siston AM, Rasmussen SA, Honein MA et al. Pandemic 2009: Influenza A (H1N1) virus illness among pregnant women in the United States. *JAMA* 2010 303 15:1517–1525.
11. Moore SA, Dietl CA, Coleman DM. Extracorporeal life support during pregnancy. *J Thoracic Cardiovasc Surg* 2015 (2015 Dec 22. pii: S0022-5223(15)02521-0. doi: 10.1016/j.jtcvs.2015.12.027. [Epub ahead of print].
12. www.who.int/csr/disease/coronavirus_infections/MERS_CoV_Update_20_Jan_2014.pdf. Accessed March 1, 2016.
13. Rasmussen SA, Jamieson DJ. What the obstetric health care providers need to know about measles and pregnancy. *Obstet Gynecol* 2015 126(1) 163–170.
14. Morbidity Mortality Weekly Report. Disease surveillance among newly arriving refugees and immigrants – Electronic disease notification system, United States 2009. CDC MMWR Summaries 2013 62: 7.
15. McMullen AH, Pasta DJ, Frederick PD et al. Impact of pregnancy on women with cystic fibrosis. *Chest* 2006 129:706–711.
16. Edenborough FP, Borgo G, Knoop C et al. Guidelines for the management of pregnancy in women with cystic fibrosis. *J Cystic Fibrosis* 2008 s2–s32.
17. Flume PA, Robinson KA, O'Sullivan BP et al. Cystic fibrosis pulmonary guidelines: Airway clearance therapies. *Respiratory Care* 2009 54(4):522–537.
18. Patel EM, Swamy GK, Heine RP. Medical and obstetric complications among pregnant women with cystic fibrosis. *Am J Obstet Gynecol* 2015 212:e1–e9.
19. Frey U. Predicting asthma control and exacerbations: Chronic asthma as a complex dynamic model. *Curr Opin Allergy Clin Immunol* 2007 7(3):223–230.
20. Hodder R, Lougheed MD, Rowe BH et al. Management of acute asthma in the emergency department: Nonventilatory management (Review). *Canadian Medical Association Journal* 2010 182(2):E55–E67.
21. Chugg K, Barton C, Antic R et al. The impact of alexithymia on asthma patient management and communication with healthcare providers: A pilot study. *J Asthma* 2009 46(2):126–129.
22. Bain E, Pierides KL, Clifton VL et al. Interventions for managing asthma in pregnancy. *Cochrane Database Syst Rev* 2014 Oct 21:10 CD 010660.
23. Thomson B, Joseph G, Clark WF et al. Maternal, pregnancy and fetal outcomes in de novo anti-glomerular basement membrane antibody disease in pregnancy: A systematic review. *Clin Kidney* 2014 7:450–456.
24. Lapinsky SE, Tram C, Mehta S et al. Restrictive lung disease in pregnancy. *Chest* 2014 145(2):394–398.
25. Bernard AW, Yasin Z, Venkat A. Acute chest syndrome in sickle cell disease. *Hospital Physician* 2007 15–44.
26. Hemnes AR, Kiely DG, Cockrill BA et al. Statement on pregnancy in pulmonary hypertension from pulmonary vascular research institute. *Pulm Circ* 2015 5(3):435–465.
27. Grimme I, Winter R, Kluge S et al. Hypoxic cardiac arrest in pregnancy due to pulmonary haemorrhage. *BMJ Case Reports* 2012 (bcr 2012006741).
28. Clark SL, Hankins GD, Dudley DA et al. Amniotic fluid embolism: Analysis of the national registry. *Am J Obstet Gynecol* 1995 172(1):1158–1167.
29. Abenhaim HA, Azoulay L, Kramer MS, Leduc L. Incidence and risk factors for amniotic fluid embolisms: A population-based study on 3 million births in the United States. *AMJOG* 2008 199(1):49 e1-e8.
30. Marik PE. Aspiration pneumonitis and aspiration pneumonia. *NEJM* 2001 344(9):665–671.
31. Soreide E, Bjornestad E, Steen PA. An audit of perioperative aspiration pneumonitis in gynecological and obstetric patients. *Acta Anesthesiol Scand* 1996 40:14–19.
32. Ware LB, Matthay MA. Acute pulmonary edema. Clinical practice. *NEJM* 2005 353:2788–2796.

33. Regitz-Zagrosek V, Lundqvist CB, Borghi C et al. ESC Guideline on the management of cardiovascular diseases during pregnancy: The Task Force on the Management of Cardiovascular Diseases during Pregnancy of the European Society of Cardiology. *Eur Heart J* 2011 32:3147-3197.

34. Reeder SR. Subcutaneous emphysema, pneumomediastinum, and pneumothorax in labor and delivery. *Am J Obstet Gynecol* 1986 154(3):487–489.

35. Kim CS, Liu J, Kwon J-Y et al. Venous air embolism during surgery, especially cesarean delivery. *J Korean Med Sci* 2008 23:753-761.

36. Shaner J, Coscia LA, Constantinescu S et al. Pregnancy after lung transplant. *Prog Transplant* 2012 22(2):134–140.

37. Boussios S, Han SN, Fruscio R et al. Lung cancer in pregnancy: Report of nine cases from an international collaborative study. *Lung Cancer* 2013 82(3):499–505.

Neurological Disease Complicating Pregnancy

Leah W. Antoniewicz and Karen M. Schneider

Introduction

Neurologic disorders are frequently seen in pregnant patients. Most conditions are chronic and stable, although some improve or worsen during pregnancy. Neurologic disorders may first manifest during pregnancy; it is important for clinicians to distinguish a new disorder from a pregnancy complication. Some disorders have an increased incidence in pregnancy, such as hypertension, Bell's palsy, and some types of stroke. Gestational hypertension (GHTN) is the most common etiology of neurologic conditions. One must also keep in mind that neurologic symptoms can have a psychiatric origin.

Acute neurologic signs and symptoms can be due to intracerebral events (ischemic and hemorrhagic stroke), arteriovenous malformations (AVM), mass effect on the brain (hemorrhage, tumor), meningitis, or other rarer disorders. Computed tomography scan (CT) is generally the first line imaging as it is fast and available. It is the better modality for non-hemorrhagic stroke, subarachnoid hemorrhage, and trauma. Magnetic resonance imaging (MRI) is the better modality for detecting edema, vascular lesions, and other types of intracranial pathology.

This chapter discusses the recognition and treatment of neurologic emergencies, headache syndromes, seizure disorder, multiple sclerosis, myasthenia gravis, and certain neuropathies.

Scope of the Problem

Neurovascular disorders accounted for 10% of maternal deaths in the United States from 1998 through 2005.[1] Therefore, prompt diagnosis and treatment of neurologic emergencies is crucial. These emergencies are often associated with an altered state of consciousness, new-onset seizure, acute headache and/or change in motor or sensory status. Figure 38.1 describes acute onset of neurologic signs and symptoms. Figure 38.2 is an algorithm used for patients with new onset of headache. Figure 38.3 describes the management of pregnant patients with seizure.

Cerebrovascular Disease

Pregnant women have a higher risk of stroke due to physiologic changes and pathophysiologic processes during pregnancy. Half of these events occur postpartum with the other half proximate to delivery. Risk factors include gestational hypertension (most common), gestational diabetes, cesarean section, obstetrical hemorrhage, and postpartum infection.[2] Pre-existing factors are listed in Box 38.1.[3] If a cerebrovascular accident is suspected, the patient should undergo immediate non-contrast CT scan (or MRI if clinically appropriate) and consultation with a critical care specialist and maternal fetal medicine (MFM) specialist. See Box 38.2 for a differential diagnosis of stroke.

Ischemic Stroke

Ischemic stroke is usually associated with headache, hemiplegia, or focal neurologic deficits; occasionally seizures may be associated as well. These events are caused by emboli or thrombi. Up to a third of ischemic strokes are associated with elevated antiphospholipid antibodies and lupus anticoagulant. Embolic strokes usually involve the middle cerebral artery. It can be difficult to differentiate an embolic stroke from an ischemic or hemorrhagic one. If an embolic source can be found after cardiac evaluation, supportive measures and antiplatelet therapy can be started. Full anticoagulation is controversial.

Ischemia caused by thrombi can be arterial (most common) or venous. Often, arterial thrombi cause transient ischemic attacks before stroke, especially if

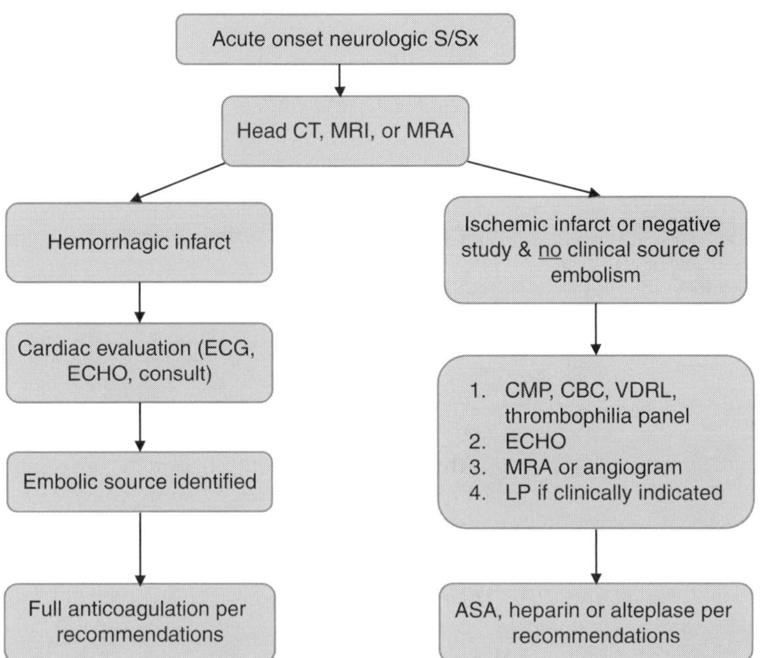

Figure 38.1 Acute onset of neurologic signs and symptoms.

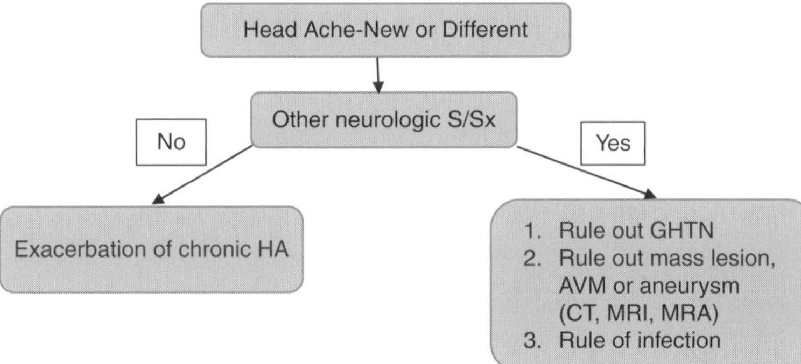

Figure 38.2 New headache algorithm.

the internal carotid artery is atherosclerotic. If hemorrhage is excluded and notable neurologic deficit is present, thrombolytic therapy should ideally be given within a 3-hour window, but can be given up to 4.5 hours after the event. There is a small risk of hemorrhagic conversion (5%).[4] Women should receive antiplatelet therapy for secondary prevention. Venous thrombus of the lateral or superior sagittal sinus usually presents with headache and can commonly be associated with neurologic deficits and seizure. This is often caused by thrombophilia, but can also occur with sepsis and gestational hypertension. Heparin and anticonvulsant medications are the mainstay of therapy, and antibiotics are given if indicated.

Hemorrhagic Stroke

Hemorrhagic stroke can be intracerebral or subarachnoid; this can be differentiated by imaging. Intracerebral bleeds are usually caused by rupture of damaged vessels from chronic hypertension. Thus, in pregnancy, this type of stroke is commonly seen with superimposed GHTN, especially with severe systolic hypertension. This type of stroke can be associated with significant morbidity and mortality so control of blood pressure is very important.

Subarachnoid hemorrhage in pregnancy is very rare and is usually caused by rupture of saccular or berry aneurysms, often at the circle of Willis. The remaining causes (20% of cases) are ruptured AVM,

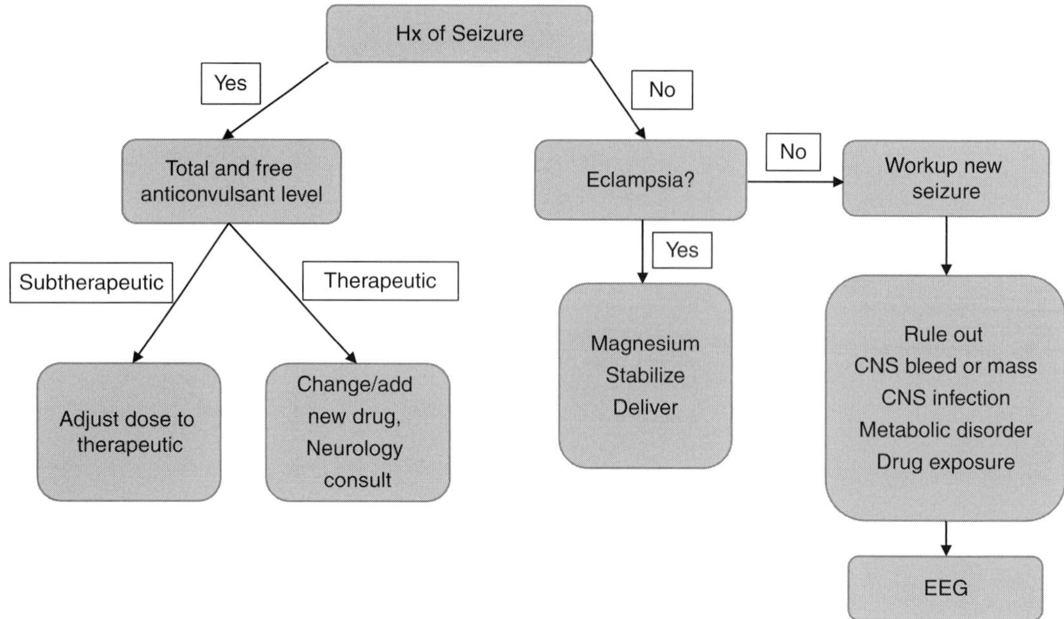

Figure 38.3 Seizure algorithm.

Box 38.1 Preexisting factors which increase risk of cerebrovascular events in pregnancy[3]

Obesity
Diabetes
Hypertension
Smoking
Migraine with aura
Arterial disease
Thrombophilia
Hyperlipidemia
Certain types of heart disease
Substance abuse
Age older than 35
Sickle cell disease
African American race

coagulopathy, angiopathy, venous thrombosis, infection, drug abuse, tumors, or trauma.[5] Aneurysms are more common in patients with Marfan's syndrome or familial polycystic kidney disease. Bleeding from aneurysms tends to occur in older women (>30) and in late pregnancy. The cardinal symptom is a sudden onset of severe headache (referred to as a thunderclap) followed by visual changes, neurologic deficits, and altered consciousness. Treatment is supportive with strict blood pressure control. If the subarachnoid hemorrhage is caused by an aneurysm, repair depends on accessibility of the vessel and other factors.

Box 38.2 Acute stroke differential diagnosis

Hypertensive encephalopathy
Migraine with aura
Seizure with postictal paresis
Posterior reversible encephalopathy syndrome (PRES)
Conversion reaction
Central nervous system tumor or abscess
Head trauma
Systemic infection
Multiple sclerosis
TTP-HUS
Spinal cord disorder (e.g., compressive myelopathy, spinal dural arteriovenous fistula)
Subdural hematoma
Syncope
Toxic-metabolic disturbance (e.g., hypoglycemia, exogenous drug intoxication)
Viral encephalitis (e.g. herpes simplex encephalitis)
Transient global amnesia
Wernicke encephalopathy
Mitochondrial disorder (e.g. mitochondrial encephalopathy with lactic acidosis and stroke-like episodes or MELAS)

Bleeding from an AVM is rare and is not more common in pregnancy. In contrast to bleeding from an aneurysm, AVM bleeding tends to occur in younger patients and occurs equally at all stages of pregnancy. Treatment outside of an acute bleeding episode would depend of many factors, such as symptoms and location. Many recommend treatment if bleeding has occurred by clipping or embolization if possible. Most experts recommend cesarean in the case of an untreated, symptomatic lesion.[5] Early placement of dense regional anesthesia and operative vaginal delivery can be considered in select cases.

Headache

Headache is by far the most common neurological complaint of pregnant women. According to a Centers for Disease Control and Prevention (CDC) study, 20% of women reported a severe headache or migraine within the past 3 months.[6] As previously stated, a new, severe headache or a change in a chronic headache (such as frequency or quality) must be evaluated for an intracranial process or pathology. See Figure 38.2. for further information about evaluation of the patient with headache change.

Gestational hypertension must be ruled out in women of 20 weeks gestation and beyond, as one-third of patients presenting with a complaint of new or changed headache will have preeclampsia. Other headaches that may be worrisome are headaches unrelieved by medication, associated with fever, exertion or in immunocompromised women.

Primary headache types include tension-type headache, migraine, trigeminal autonomic cephalalgias (cluster, etc.), and idiopathic intracranial hypertension (pseudotumor cerebri).

Tension-Type Headache

This is by far the most common headache type experienced. It is usually mild to moderate intensity, bilateral, throbbing, and in the back of the head and neck. It usually responds to over the counter analgesics, rest, massage, heat and ice. Occasionally mild tranquilizers are used.

Migraine

Migraine is the most common headache for which treatment is sought. This is a periodic neurologic disorder with recurrent attacks. It is often unilateral and throbbing or pulsatile and sometimes incapacitating. Associated symptoms may include nausea, vomiting, photophobia, phonophobia, visual disturbances, and even brief neurologic deficits. In pregnancy, the headache frequency usually decreases, but some women experience increased frequency or even have their first migraine episode. Migraine triggers include stress, diet, hormone fluctuations, changes of environment or habits, and sensory stimuli, and many additional activating events.

Three general categories of migraine headache exist: migraine without aura, migraine with aura, and chronic migraine. Migraine without aura is usually unilateral and associated with nausea, vomiting, photophobia, phonophobia, or a combination of these symptoms. Migraine with aura has prodromal symptoms such as visual disturbances or hallucinations.

The actual headache is usually unilateral and can also be associated with the aforementioned symptoms, including brief neurologic deficits. Progression from aura to full migraine can often be averted if abortive therapy is taken. The vast majority of migraine medications are safe in pregnancy. Ergotamines should be avoided completely in pregnancy as they are potent vasoconstrictors and could produce hypertonic uterine contractions.

Prevention of migraines includes non-pharmacologic therapies, such as avoidance of triggers, quality sleep, hydration, regular meals, relaxation, massage, heat/ice, and acupuncture. First-line therapy for acute migraine is 1,000 mg of acetaminophen. Migraines that don't respond to single therapy may respond to a combination of acetaminophen with metoclopramide, or acetaminophen with caffeine and butalbital (Fioricet) with or without codeine. Too frequent use of codeine and/or butalbital can lead to overuse headaches. Meclizine, diphenhydramine, and promethazine are recommended for the initial treatment of nausea and vomiting.

Nonsteroidal anti-inflammatory drugs (NSAIDs) are a second line option; their use is safest in the second trimester. They should be limited to 48 hours of use in the third trimester, and many experts avoid them after 32 weeks of pregnancy for concerns of premature ductus arteriosus closure, oligohydramnios, and platelet inhibition. Opioids are a third-line option. They are habit forming, which could lead to medication overuse, maternal addiction, and neonatal withdrawal. Additionally, they can cause nausea, vomiting, and constipation. They are for acute, short-term use only.

Patients who do not respond to the aforementioned therapies may respond to triptans, a class of serotonin 5-HT-receptor agonists that cause vasoconstriction. Sumatriptan is first-line, and frovatriptan is less desirable because of its longer half-life. Although there is a theoretical risk for uteroplacental vasoconstriction and increased activity, triptan exposure is generally considered safe in pregnancy. Triptans also have the benefits of versatile administration routes (oral, rectal, subcutaneous, intranasal), and they reduce nausea, vomiting, and the need for analgesics. When patients experience migraines that are still refractory and severe, intravenous hydration, opioid, and prochlorperazine can be given. Pretreatment with diphenhydramine will prevent akathisia. Droperidol can also be considered in combination with a triptan, but droperidol can cause extrapyramidal symptoms and arrhythmias. Prednisone or methylprednisolone can be given for intractable cases.

Women who have headaches 15 or more days a month for more than 3 months, and which have the features of migraine headaches on at least eight days per month, should have prophylactic treatment.[7] Low-dose beta- and calcium channel blockers are effective first-line agents. Propranolol, metoprolol, and atenolol can be used, but propranolol has the lowest incidence of intrauterine growth restriction (IUGR). Verapamil is the calcium channel blocker with the best safety and side-effect profile. Low dose selective serotonin reuptake inhibitors (SSRI) or tricyclic antidepressants can be considered in refractory patients, especially those with a history of depression. Certain anticonvulsants, like gabapentin, are an option if no other treatment has worked. Valproate should be avoided, as it is a teratogen and carbamazepine and topimax should be avoided in the first trimester.

Trigeminal Autonomic Cephalalgias

These headaches are characterized by unilateral, brief, usually severely painful attacks with ipsilateral autonomic symptoms. Pain usually reaches full intensity within minutes. Autonomic symptoms include ptosis, miosis, lid swelling, lacrimation, conjunctival injection, rhinorrhea, and nasal congestion. Cluster headaches (a subcategory of trigeminal autonomic cephalalgias) are the most common form and feature severe, brief (15–180 minutes), supraorbital or temporal pain. Headaches will cluster for weeks to months at a time followed by periods of no headaches. Treatment is 100% oxygen and sumatriptan (intranasal or subcutaneous).[5] If prophylaxis is needed, a calcium channel blocker (verapamil) is first-line. These headaches are more common in men and the frequency is not affected by pregnancy.

Idiopathic Intracranial Hypertension (Pseudotumor Cerebri)

This disorder results in increased intracranial pressure, which may be caused by under absorption or over production of cerebrospinal fluid. Headache is the predominant symptom. Visual disturbances are also very common and can even include sight-threatening papilledema. Idiopathic intracranial hypertension is more common in obese patients or those who recently gained weight. Pregnant women tend to develop it in the second trimester.

As part of the diagnosis, lumbar puncture may be performed; opening pressure would be increased. If the patient has headache and papilledema, MRI should be performed to rule out secondary causes of increased pressure. If visual field loss occurs, this can be treated with acetazolamide.[5] In pregnant women repeat lumbar punctures can be considered, and if needed, optic nerve sheath fenestration may be an option. Fortunately, in most pregnant women symptoms completely resolve postpartum.

Postpartum Headache

It is not surprising that headaches are common in the postpartum period. Tension headaches are the most common, followed by migraines. Gestational hypertension should be ruled out. "Danger signs" should prompt imaging and consultation with a neurologist. If the patient had neuraxial anesthesia, postdural puncture headache is a possibility. These post regional anesthesia headaches usually develop within 48 hours, are worse in the prone position, and improve in the supine position.

Most postpartum headaches will resolve within 24 hours. Supportive therapy includes resting supine, opioids, or analgesics that don't affect platelets. Hydration and caffeine have not been shown to be effective.[8] An anesthesiologist or neurologist should be consulted if the patient doesn't improve, as an epidural blood patch may be required.

Medication Overuse Headache

This headache can occur in women who frequently (often daily) use any type of analgesic. The condition can also develop in migraine sufferers. The diagnosis should be suspected in patients with persistent daily headaches, despite therapy. Treatment is simply cessation of the causative agent.

Secondary Headache

There are many processes and disease states that lead to secondary headaches. Sinusitis is a common diagnosis, but many headaches that are diagnosed as sinusitis are actually migraines. A thorough history and physical exam is necessary to establish a diagnosis, and if any "danger signs" are present, imaging should be conducted immediately.

Seizure Disorders

Approximately 1 in 200 pregnancies are affected by seizures; seizure disorders are the second most common neurologic condition seen in pregnant women. Although the vast majority of pregnancies in these patients will have good outcomes, women with epilepsy have higher rates of pregnancy complications. These complications include such as gestational hypertension, preterm labor, cesarean section, longer length of stay, and fetal and maternal mortality.[9] Many antiepileptic drugs (AED) are teratogenic, and abnormal fetal development can occur. Proper preconception and pregnancy management is paramount.

Seizures can be characterized as generalized, involving both sides of the brain, or focal, involving one side of the brain. Generalized seizures involve an abrupt loss of consciousness with or without an aura. The most common seizure types are tonic-clonic and absence. Tonic-clonic seizures former involves tonic, rigid contractions of the body, followed by clonic contractions, complete relaxation, and loss of consciousness. Return to full conscious is gradual and can be prolonged. In contrast, absence seizures feature a brief loss of consciousness without muscle activity.

If a pregnant patient presents with a new seizure after 20 weeks gestation, it is eclampsia until proven otherwise. The patient should be stabilized, particularly her airway, and magnesium should be started while the evaluation is completed. If eclampsia is ruled out or the patient is less than 20 weeks, a new seizure work up should be started. See Figure 38.3 for new seizure workup. Life-threatening causes of seizure are listed in Box 38.3.

Preconception Care of Seizure Disorder Patients

Preconception counseling and optimization can greatly reduce the risk of pregnancy complications when the items listed in Box 38.4 are implemented in the patient care plan.

Patients can be reassured that women who are controlled on their AED and are seizure-free for 1 year have a decreased risk of seizures in pregnancy. Conversely, women who experience at least one convulsion a month will likely have an increase in seizure frequency during pregnancy.[9] Also, emerging evidence shows that women who do not require treatment during pregnancy do not have an increased risk of malformations compared to the general population.[10] Although direct proof of reduced malformations after folate supplementation is lacking, folate supplementation is a reasonable, low-risk intervention in patients on AED's who are trying to conceive. See Box 38.4.

Box 38.3 Life-threatening causes of seizure

- Cerebrovascular accidents
- Infection
- Metabolic derangement
- Drug exposure/withdrawal.

Box 38.4 Preconception plan for seizure disorder patients

- Start folic acid 0.4 mg daily at least 1 month before conception
- Increase folate to 4 mg when she becomes pregnant if taking AED
- If seizure free for 2 or more years, taper AED at least 6 months before conception
- Obtain control with monotherapy if possible at lowest dose possible
- Try changing to a less teratogenic AED if taking valproate
- Stress the importance of medication compliance

Antiepileptic Medication Considerations

Although no anticonvulsant has been shown to be completely safe, uncontrolled seizures are dangerous to the fetus and mother. If a previously well-controlled patient begins to have seizures during pregnancy, the physician should order a blood level of the anticonvulsant if the test is available. Multiple physiologic changes can cause levels to become subtherapeutic. These changes are seen in Box 38.5. Non-compliance with medication because of patient fear for harm to the fetus is not uncommon. Other factors that lower the seizure threshold include sleep deprivation, stress, and pain and hyperventilation during labor.

Unfortunately, studies have only suboptimally defined which AEDs are either superior or inferior to each other with respect to overall teratogenicity. The exception is valproate, which has higher umbilical concentrations and has been linked to poorer neurodevelopment outcomes and neural tube defects. Distal digital hypoplasia is much higher in infants exposed to phenytoin and carbamazepine. Both valproate and carbamazepine should be avoided if there is a family history of neural tube defects. If more than one agent is to be used, combinations of valproate, carbamazepine, and phenobarbital should be avoided. Risk of teratogenicity should not be the sole reason to change a pregnant woman's antiseizure medication for several reasons. First, if the pregnancy is in the organogenesis phase, exposure has already occurred. Second, the fetus will be exposed to more medication due to overlap during the change. Lastly, changing medications can cause seizures.

Box 38.5 **Physiologic changes in pregnancy that may affect anticonvulsant levels**

Blood volume expansion
Delayed gastric emptying
Patient may need to take antacids
Induction of liver enzymes
Placental enzymes
Increased renal clearance
Increased protein binding

Management of Seizure Disorder Patients during Pregnancy

As previously stated, the main therapeutic goal is to prevent seizures by using the lowest possible dose and the lowest number of medications. Free drug levels (if available) and total drug levels should be checked at 5 and 10 weeks gestation and once a trimester thereafter. This is mostly helpful to monitor non-compliance. If levels are sub-therapeutic, they should not necessarily be increased if the patient is seizure free. Protein binding can affect the test results and consultation with a neurologist may be appropriate. If a patient seizes, the dosage should be increased despite therapeutic levels. Folate supplementation should be continued to help prevent malformations. These patients should also undergo routine serum screening for neural tube defects at 14–16 weeks gestation; targeted second trimester ultrasound should be performed at 18–20 weeks to look for malformations. Patients should be offered amniocentesis if the alpha-fetoprotein (AFP) level is elevated and the ultrasound is equivocal or if the AFP is elevated in conjunction with an abnormal ultrasound. In the former scenario, there is a 99% chance of an open neural tube defect if both amniotic fluid AFP and acetylcholinesterase are elevated. In the later scenario, an abnormal karyotype can be ruled out.[11]

Vitamin K supplementation is an inexpensive, low-risk intervention that may help reduce the risk of bleeding in the fetus during the delivery process. Most experts recommend 10–20 mg a day, starting 2–4 weeks before the estimated date of confinement. Babies are also given an intramuscular (IM) injection after birth.

One to two percent of women will seize intrapartum or 24 hours postpartum so it is essential that medications doses are not missed during labor. In the event that a seizure occurs, intravenous lorazepam should be given and the patient and fetus should then be monitored for hypoxia.[11]

Postpartum Management of Seizure Disorder Patients

The new mother needs to be advised of the importance of adequate sleep and compliance with therapy since sleep deprivation lowers the seizure threshold. Additionally, counseling on maternal and infant safety measures in the case of a seizure should be given. Until an adequate sleep pattern is established, the patient should not be alone with the baby while bathing, driving, or other activities that could put her or the baby at risk during a seizure. The baby should be in a safe position for feedings and diaper changes as well. These precautions should certainly continue while the mother is being weaned back to her original dose of medication over the first 2 weeks postpartum.

There is no evidence of long-term deleterious effects of antiseizure medications while breast feeding.[12,13,14] Although all AEDs are excreted in breast milk, the levels in breast milk are considerably lower than from placental transfer. Sedating drugs (benzodiazepines, phenobarbital, primidone) can have side effects in the neonate, however, and breast feeding may need to be interrupted for up to one week ("pump and dump") when these medications are required. Long-acting reversible contraception is an excellent option for breastfeeding women, especially those women on AEDs. Some antiseizure medications induce hepatic enzymes and could make combined oral contraceptives (COCs) less effective. If the patient desires COCs, a higher dose (at least 30 mcg of estradiol) should be prescribed.

Multiple Sclerosis

Multiple sclerosis (MS) is a demyelinating disease, characterized by focal, immune-mediated destruction of myelin sheaths. The disease is associated with a genetic predisposition and likely an additional infectious trigger, such as *Chlamydophila pneumoniae*, human herpesvirus 6, or Epstein–Barr virus.[15] The disease is twice as common in women as in men and usually starts in the twenties and thirties. It is characterized by relapses and remissions. During an exacerbation, progressive neurologic deficits occur, often over several days. These deficits can include unilateral optic neuritis (painful), asymmetric sensory loss, weakness, ataxia, and/or other neurologic symptoms.

MS is not a contraindication for pregnancy, and each patient's care should be considered on a case by case basis. Most patients' MS symptoms improve with pregnancy, likely because it is an immunosuppressive state. Conversely, symptoms generally increase postpartum for up to 3 months. Most studies have not shown any adverse effects on pregnancy outcome with uncomplicated disease. Some women fatigue more easily. Those with bladder dysfunction are at increased risk for urinary tract infections. Women with spinal lesions at or above T6 are at risk for autonomic dysreflexia (massive disordered sympathetic stimulation leading to life-threatening hypertension), which can occur from simply placing a Foley catheter.[15] Some studies have shown an increase in cesarean delivery rates and lower infant birth weights.[16] The rate of induction is also higher.

Treatment of MS during Pregnancy

If possible, discontinuation of disease-modifying therapies is recommended before conception. A wash-out period may be advised as well. Many medications, however, are considered safe for pregnancy although data is limited. These medications include glatiramer acetate, interferons, alemtuzumab, fingolimod, dimethyl fumarate, and natalizumab.[17] Acute and initial attacks are treated with short-term, high-dose intravenous methylprednisolone (daily for 3–5 days, followed by oral for 2 weeks). This is preferred over long-term therapy (especially more than 20 mg a day) because glucocorticoids are not without risk and can cause cleft palate (through the 9th week), maternal and neonatal adrenal suppression, maternal glucose intolerance, and preterm premature rupture of membranes. Pain can be relieved with analgesics, tricyclics, or even antiseizure medications. Baclofen can be used for spasticity. Cholinergics, anticholinergics, and α-blockade can be given for various bladder symptoms.

Postpartum and Lactation

Intravenous immune globulin can prevent postpartum relapses, especially in patients with histories of postpartum exacerbations. This medication is given for 5 days in weeks 1, 6, and 12.[5] Most women choose to forgo disease-modifying therapies while breast feeding, so breast feeding is more common in women with milder disease. Interferon and glatiramer are probably safe during lactation. For patients taking glucocorticoids, it is recommended to pump and discard the milk for the first 4 hours after the dose.

Myasthenia Gravis

This is an autoimmune disorder that causes weakness after repetitive muscle use. It is caused by anti-acetylcholine receptor (AChR) antibodies (80–90%) or muscle-specific tyrosine kinase antibodies (anti-MuSK).[5] Like most autoimmune disorders, it is more common in women and tends to manifest in the twenties to thirties. Mortality is high within the

Box 38.6 Types of myasthenic crises

- Myasthenic crisis – respiratory muscle paralysis, inability to swallow, severe limb weakness
- Refractory crisis – crisis unresponsive to customary therapy
- Cholinergic crisis – nausea, vomiting, diarrhea, abdominal pain, and muscle weakness from excess cholinergic medication

Box 38.7 Basic evaluation of myasthenia gravis patients

- Baseline motor strength
- Baseline respiratory status with pulmonary function tests
- Electrocardiogram (rare instances of focal cardiac necrosis)
- Thyroid function tests (co-morbid autoimmune condition)

first year of diagnosis, so postponement of pregnancy should be encouraged at that time.

Myasthenia gravis (MG) can be ocular or generalized. Ocular MG, as the name suggests, affects the eyelids, and extraocular muscles. Generalized MG often affects the ocular muscles, but also the facial, limb, and bulbar muscles (muscles controlled by the brain stem, like the oropharyngeal and respiratory muscles). The majority of patients present with diplopia or ptosis. Other symptoms can include dysarthria or dysphagia, loss of facial expression, a dropped forward head, proximal limb weakness, or even respiratory compromise.

Respiratory failure constitutes a myasthenic crisis. The three types of crises, all of which can be life-threatening, are listed in Box 38.6.

Management

During pregnancy, patients may have worsening of, improvement of, or no change in disease activity. The physiologic changes associated with pregnancy may require dose adjustments to medications and can affect the course of MG. However, most patients are treated like non-pregnant MG patients. The highest risk of exacerbations is in the first trimester and immediate postpartum period.[19] Evaluation should include the components listed in Box 38.7.

Physical and emotional stress can exacerbate MG, and it is common for patients to experience both during pregnancy. Proper rest and social support is essential. Infections can precipitate exacerbations so it is important that all infections are treated immediately. Similarly, all complaints of cough or shortness of breath need to be evaluated immediately for an exacerbation.

Fetal complications can occur from transplacental passage of AChR and anti-MuSK antibodies. On ultrasound screening, abnormalities can include polyhydramnios (from impaired swallowing), decreased movement, and decreased breathing. Arthrogryposis (joint contractures) multiplex congenital can also be seem. This is a heterogeneous group of disorders characterized by contractures of multiple joints and degeneration of motor neurons. This is probably caused by lack of fetal movement and diaphragmatic excursion. The severity of these findings appears to be inversely proportional to maternal titers.[20] The fetus is at risk during a MG crisis from maternal hypoxia so it should be continuously monitored if viable.

Treatment

Treatment begins with anticholinesterase inhibitors such as pyridostigmine. Hyperemesis and changes in maternal blood volume, renal clearance, and gastric emptying may make dose adjustment necessary. If the patient's symptoms are not controlled, immunosuppressive therapy with glucocorticoids, azathioprine, and cyclosporine can be used.[19] As previously stated, chronic glucocorticoid use carries risk to both the fetus and mother so risk has to be weighed against benefit. Also, while initiating glucocorticoid therapy, MG symptoms may briefly worsen. Use of azathioprine and cyclosporine at high doses carries risk, such as spontaneous abortion, preterm labor, hematologic suppression, and more.

If the patient is refractory to the above therapy, plasmapheresis or high-dose intravenous immune globulin (IVIG) can be used. IVIG can also be used to rapidly improve a patient's status in anticipation of physical stress, like surgery, for example.

Labor in MG Patients

Any pregnant patient with MG should ideally have a consultation with anesthesia in the early third trimester. Regional anesthesia with only local anesthetic is the ideal choice unless she has significant bulbar involvement or respiratory compromise. MG patients are sensitive to narcotics and inhaled anesthetics in that they can cause respiratory depression faster than in other patients. Non-depolarizing muscle relaxants are contraindicated and larger doses of succinylcholine are usually required.

Should the patient be preeclamptic, phenytoin *not* magnesium, should be used for seizure prophylaxis. Hydralazine or methyldopa should be used to control blood pressure as beta and calcium channel blockers should be avoided.

The first stage of labor is not affected by MG, as the uterus is made of smooth muscle. Pain is stressful and can affect an MG patient a great deal. Therefore, an epidural is ideal. The second stage could be affected by fatigue or by decreased proximal strength. Operative vaginal delivery may be necessary, underscoring another reason for epidural pain control. Respiratory status should be monitored at all times. Should the patient need antibiotics, aminoglycosides should be avoided, as they are curariform.

Ten to twenty percent of neonates can develop transient MG symptoms including poor feeding, flaccid tone, poor suckling, feeble cry, and respiratory distress. This is because of transplacental passage of antibodies.[21,22] Mothers taking glucocorticoids and/or anticholinesterase drugs may breast feed. Other immunosuppressive agents should be avoided during breastfeeding until further studies provide more data.

Neuropathies

Neuropathies are common in pregnancy and have a variety of causes, including infection, trauma, and compression. This section will focus on Bell's palsy and Guillain–Barre´ syndrome. For a discussion of traumatic and compression neuropathies, see Chapter 32 on musculoskeletal disorders.

Bell's Palsy

Bell's palsy (BP) is acute paralysis of the facial nerve, often involving all three branches. This results in unilateral weakness of the eye and asymmetric facial expression. Patients may also manifest hyperacusis (a collapsed tolerance to usual environmental sound) and loss of taste. Symptoms and pain develop over 48 hours. Although the exact etiology is unknown, paralysis is the result of nerve inflammation and is often associated with herpes viruses. It is four times more common in pregnancy and most commonly seen in the third trimester or first postpartum week. The disease is associated with gestational hypertension, but otherwise no adverse pregnancy outcomes.[23]

Treatment includes prednisone, and some experts give antiviral medication. The earlier steroids are given, the better the outcome. Supportive treatment includes eye protection to help prevent corneal abrasion (from dryness) and fascial muscle massage.

Although most people with BP will recover completely, only 50% of pregnant women fully recover. Poor prognostic signs include complete paralysis, bilateral palsy, recurrence in a subsequent pregnancy, and a fast rate of nerve function loss.[5]

Guillain-Barré

This syndrome, also known as acute inflammatory demyelinating polyradiculoneuropathy, typically starts within 30 days of an infectious event. It is probably caused by an immune-mediated antibody reaction, which causes demyelination, affecting both sensory and motor nerves. Patients typically have ascending areflexic paralysis. Autonomic dysfunction is common. Respiratory emergencies can occur so patients should be hospitalized as the disease progresses over 1 to 3 weeks. Anesthesia should be consulted for these potential complications, and succinylcholine should be avoided.

The incidence of Guillain–Barré syndrome is not increased in pregnancy. Pregnancy, labor, and delivery are not usually affected.[24] Plasmapheresis or intravenous immunoglobulin are used to treat symptoms, but do not decrease the 5% mortality rate. Seventy-five of patients make a full recovery within a year or less.[25]

Concluding Remarks

Neurologic disorders are common in pregnancy. It is important to recognize emergencies, such as new or severe headaches, seizures, and changes in mental status. Prompt treatment will reduce morbidity and mortality. Gestational hypertension is the most common etiology for new neurologic symptoms. Chronic conditions such as migraines, seizure disorder, multiple sclerosis, and myasthenia gravis can be managed so that there is little or no impact on the pregnancy.

References

1. Berg AT, Scheffer IE. New concepts in classification of the epilepsies: Entering the 21st century. *Epilepsia* 2011;52(6):1058.

2. James AH, Bushnell CD, Jamison MG, Myers ER. Incidence and risk factors for stroke in pregnancy and the puerperium. *Obstet Gynecol* 2005;106:509.
3. Scott CA, Bewley S, Rudd A: Incidence, risk factors, management, and outcomes of stroke in pregnancy. *Obstet Gynecol* 2012;120:318.
4. Van der Worp HB, van Gijn J. Acute ischemic stroke. *N Engl J Med* 2007;357(6):572.
5. Cunningham FG, Leveno, KJ, Bloom, SL, et al. (Eds.). *Williams Obstetrics*, 24th ed. New York: McGraw-Hill, 2010: 1187–1203.
6. Pleis JR, Ward BW, Lucas JW. Summary health statistics for U.S. adults: National Health Interview Survey, 2009. *Vital Health Stat* 2010;10(249):1.
7. Headache Classification Committee of the International Headache Society (IHS). The International Classification of Headache Disorders, 3rd edition (beta version). *Cephalalgia* 2013 Jul;33(9):629–808.
8. Dieterich M, Perkin GD. Post-lumbar puncture headache syndrome. In: *Neurologic Disorders: Course and Treatment*, Brand T, Caplan LR, Dichland J, et al. (Eds). San Diego: Academic Press, 1996: 59.
9. MacDonald SC, Bateman BT, McElrath TF, Hernández-Díaz S. Mortality and morbidity during delivery hospitalization among pregnant women with epilepsy in the United States. *JAMA Neurol* 2015; 72:981.
10. Tomson T, Landmark CJ, Battino D. Antiepileptic drug treatment in pregnancy: Changes in drug disposition and their clinical implications. *Epilepsia* 2013; 54:405.
11. Thomas SV, Ajaykumar B, Sindhu K, et al. Cardiac malformations are increased in infants of mothers with epilepsy. *Pediatr Cardiol* 2008;29:604.
12. Schachter, SC. Management of epilepsy and pregnancy. *UpToDate.* 2016. www.uptodate.com. (Accessed February 25, 2016.)
13. Pennell PB, Gidal BE, Sabers A, et al. Pharmacology of antiepileptic drugs during pregnancy and lactation. *Epilepsy Behav* 2007;11:263.
14. Briggs GG, Freeman RK, Yaffe SJ. *Drugs in Pregnancy and Lactation*, 9th ed. Philadelphia: Lippincott Williams & Wilkins, 2011.
15. Goodin DS. The causal cascade to multiple sclerosis: A model for MS pathogenesis. *PLoS One* 2009;4(2):e4565.
16. Dahl J, Myhr KM, Daltveit AK, et al. Planned vaginal births in women with multiple sclerosis: delivery and birth outcome. *Acta Neurol Scand Suppl* 2006;183:51.
17. Franklin GM, Tremlett H. Multiple sclerosis and pregnancy: What should we be telling our patients? *Neurology* 2009;73:1820.
18. Ciafaloni E, Massey JM. The management of myasthenia gravis in pregnancy. *Semin Neurol* 2004; 24:95.
19. Verspyck E, Mandelbrot L, Dommergues M, et al. Myasthenia gravis with polyhydramnios in the fetus of an asymptomatic mother. *Prenat Diagn* 1993; 13:539.
20. Stafford IP, Dildy GA. Myasthenia gravis and pregnancy. *Clin Obstet Gynecol* 2005;48:48.
21. Morel E, Bach JF, Briard ML, Aubry JP. Neonatal myasthenia gravis. Anti-acetylcholine receptor antibodies in the amniotic fluid. *J Neuroimmunol* 1984;6:313.
22. Shmorgun D, Chan WS, Ray JG. Association between Bell's palsy in pregnancy and pre-eclampsia. *QJM* 2002;95:359.
23. Chan LY, Tsui MH, Leung TN. Guillain–Barré syndrome in pregnancy. *Acta Obstet Gynecol Scand* 2004;83:319.
24. Yuki N, Hartung HP: Guillain–Barré syndrome. *N Engl J Med* 2012; 366:2294.

Renal Diseases in Pregnancy

Moune Jabre Raughley and Gene La Monica

Introduction

Renal disease in pregnancy is rare but carries significant implications both to the fetus and the mother. Obstetricians must have a comprehensive working knowledge of the effects of renal disease on the pregnancy and the pregnancy's effects on the kidneys. This chapter will discuss the normal physiologic renal adaptations to pregnancy and diagnostic evaluation of the renal system. Several individual acute and chronic renal diseases will be described with attention to disease process, general prenatal management and fetal surveillance.

Scope of the Problem

Acute Kidney Disease

Acute kidney injury (AKI), resulting in sudden deterioration of renal function of varying severity, can occur in pregnancy from any of the typical causes as well as unique pregnancy-related etiologies. The extent of AKI can range from mild elevation of serum creatinine to fulminant renal failure requiring dialysis.[1] The incidence of AKI is approximately 1 in 20,000 pregnancies.[2]

Chronic Renal Diseases

Chronic renal diseases have a prevalence of 3% in reproductive-age women.[3] According to US-based population studies, 0.03–0.12% of all pregnancies are complicated by moderate to severe chronic renal disease. This incidence is likely low because many women with moderate to severe disease may be infertile or subfertile due to age or severity of disease. The incidence of mild renal insufficiency in pregnancy is not well known as many women are undiagnosed or the data is not included in reported series. The degree of renal insufficiency may be loosely defined by the creatinine level with mild being a creatinine of 0.9–1.4 mg/dL, moderate 1.4–2.5 mg/dL and severe >2.5 mg/dL.[4]

In general, the prognosis for maternal and fetal outcomes and the severity of the impact that the pregnancy has on the kidney depends on the degree of functional renal impairment prior to pregnancy. The better the prepregnancy renal function, the less likely are poor obstetric outcomes or long-term renal damage. A meta-analysis showed that women with mild renal insufficiency have a very low rate of complications, generally much less than 20%, and that the live birth rate is generally well above 95%. Only 5% of women with mild disease demonstrated irreversible deterioration in kidney function; this was defined as increase in serum creatinine of > 1mg/dL from baseline.[4]

The most common complications of renal disease in pregnancy are chronic hypertension (HTN), preeclampsia (PEC), maternal anemia, intrauterine growth restriction (IUGR), preterm birth and cesarean delivery. According to a small observational study, complications occurred in women with moderate versus severe disease at the following rates: HTN 62% vs. 82%, PEC 58% vs. 64%, maternal anemia 73% vs. 100%, IUGR 35% vs. 43%, preterm birth 30% vs. 86%, live birth rate 88% vs. 64%. Nearly 50% of women with moderate or severe disease had long-term deterioration in their kidney function as a result of pregnancy.[4]

Normal Renal Adaptations to Pregnancy

In pregnancy, the renal system, in concert with the circulatory system, undergoes a dramatic constellation of adaptive changes. The renal plasma flow increases by up to 80% and the glomerular filtration rate (GFR) increases by 50%. This, coupled with physiologic intravascular volume expansion and increased capillary permeability, results in alteration of several laboratory markers (see Table 39.1).[5] Of note, even

Table 39.1 Normal Laboratory Values in Nonpregnant versus Pregnant Women[5,6,33]

Value	Non-Pregnant	Pregnant
Glomerular filtration rate	90–120 mL/min	100–150 mL/min
Creatinine	0.5–0.9 mg/dL (44–80 mmol/L)	0.5 mg/dL
Blood urea nitrogen (BUN)	12 mg/dL	9.0 mg/dL
Uric acid	2.6–5.6 mg/dL	2–3 mg/dL
Serum sodium	136–146 mEq/L	135 mEq/L
Plasma osmolality	275–295 mOsm/kg	270 mOsm/kg
Proteinuria	Up to 150 mg/24 hours	Up to 300 mg mg/24 hours
Serum bicarbonate	22–30 mEq/L	18–20 mEq/L
Serum potassium	3.5–5 mEq/L	3.8 mEq/L

in the absence of hyperglycemia, glycosuria may be present due to a higher filtered glucose load resulting from the increased GFR.[2]

Decrease in systemic vascular resistance and increase in GFR lead to hypertrophy of the kidney thereby increasing the volume by 30%. Progesterone effects on ureteric smooth muscle leads to increased ureteric stasis, capacitance and mild bilateral hydronephrosis. Hydronephrosis is more pronounced on the right side secondary to the dextrorotation of the uterus which impinges more on the right ureter as it travels over the pelvic brim as depicted in Figure 39.1.[5]

Hormonal changes in multiple systems, such as progesterone and relaxin, lead to a decrease in blood pressure (mean value of 105/60 mmHg). The renin–angiotensin–aldosterone system (RAAS) plays a predominant role. Aldosterone levels rise leading to a net gain in fluid balance. Estrogen-mediated increased hepatic angiotensinogen production leads to increased renal angiotensin II production. However, several factors, including refractoriness to angiotensin II, contribute to an overall decrease in blood pressure.[5]

All of the aforementioned changes represent hormonal or mechanical adaptations of the kidney to pregnancy. Other physiologic non-renal adaptations may affect the course of renal disease during pregnancy. Most notably, physiologic modulation of the immune system in pregnancy, aimed at maternal immunologic tolerance of the fetus, can result in variable effects on pre-existing autoimmune diseases in pregnancy.

These adaptive changes reach a peak around the end of the second trimester before beginning to return to pregravid levels. Anatomic changes can take up to 3 months postpartum to return to the prepregnant state.[2]

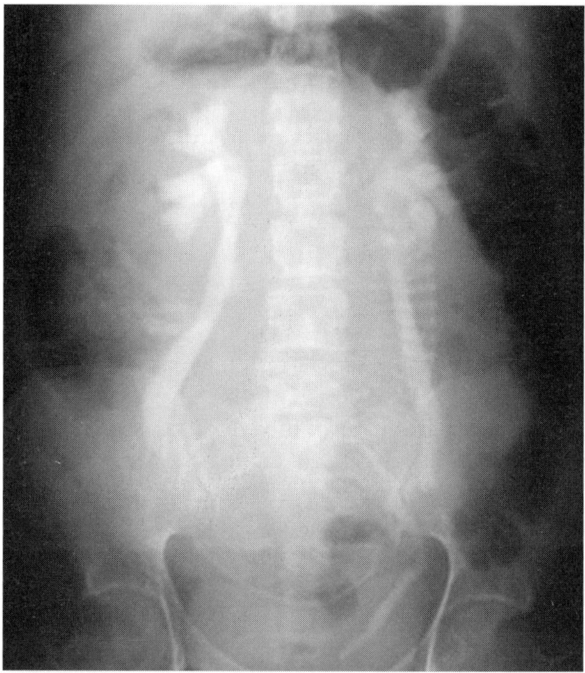

Figure 39.1 Intravenous pyelogram in a woman in the late third trimester showing dilation of the renal collecting system. The hydronephrosis and hydroureter are increased on the right compared to the left due to compression from the dextrorotated uterus.[4]

Diagnostic Evaluation of the Kidney

Acute renal disease incorporates a broad spectrum of clinical manifestations determined by the etiology. Presentation may include but is not limited to a constellation of fever, flank pain/costovertebral angle tenderness, hematuria, vaginal bleeding, pyuria, edema, hypertension/preeclampsia (PEC) thromboembolism, hydronephrosis and sepsis. The presentation of chronic renal diseases varies by disease though many are associated with hypertension, proteinuria, hematuria and nephrotic or nephritic syndrome.[6]

Laboratory Evaluation

Laboratory evaluation for both acute and chronic renal disease should typically include a complete blood count (CBC), a comprehensive metabolic panel (CMP), an assessment of proteinuria and uric acid. The gold standard for measuring proteinuria is 24-hour urine collection for protein and creatinine-clearance. However, this method can be inaccurate due to under collection. It is also cumbersome to collect and delays diagnosis during the collection period. The urine protein to creatinine (P:C) ratio is preferred in nonpregnant patients. There appears to be excellent correlation between the two tests and a P:C ratio of 0.3 is increasingly used in pregnancy to equal 300 mg/day on 24-hour urine collection when a rapid diagnosis is necessary.[7]

Other tests, such as a fractional excretion of sodium (FENa), may also be useful. Baseline labs should be obtained early in pregnancy in all women with known chronic disease. Additional disease-specific labs such as hemoglobin A1C or autoimmune antibody profiles may also be indicated.[6] Kidney biopsy is rarely necessary but when warranted by disease severity, is generally well tolerated and should be performed before the third trimester to minimize risks of bleeding and hematoma formation.[3]

Diagnostic Imaging

Ultrasound (US) is an effective, safe, cost-effective and readily available imaging modality. Its lack of radiation renders ultrasound the preferred first-line diagnostic tool. Magnetic resonance imaging (MRI) should be considered when further imaging is required though availability and cost may be limiting factors. When US and MRI are inconclusive, computed tomography and intravenous pyelogram may be used when a definitive diagnosis is necessary to dictate further management as these modalities expose the fetus to ionizing radiation.[6]

Management by a multidisciplinary team including obstetrics, nephrology, perinatology and nutrition is recommended. Frequency of prenatal visits should be increased with fastidious attention to blood pressure and proteinuria. Although chronic renal insufficiency in the nonpregnant state frequently calls for protein restriction, protein should not be restricted in pregnancy given the increased nutritional demands. A low-sodium diet is however recommended.[6]

Anatomic Abnormalities

Solitary Kidney

Solitary kidney, as a result of congenital absence or prior nephrectomy, may be a rare incidental finding on obstetric ultrasound. The rate of congenital absence is reported to be approximately 1:2,000 people. In those with congenital absence, the prevalence of other concurrent renal anomalies and extrarenal anomalies is high at 32% and 31%, respectively. Given the parallel development of the urologic and genital tracts during embryogenesis, Mullerian tract anomalies are present in 11% of solitary kidney patients.[8]

When no history of active renal disease is present, solitary kidney does not appear to confer additional risk to the pregnancy. Pregnancy appears to be well tolerated with little, if any, long-term effect on renal function. Acute renal failure from ureteric obstruction from the gravid uterus has been reported.[9]

Interestingly, studies on living kidney donors suggest an increased incidence of both preeclampsia and gestational hypertension with odds ratios of 2.4 and 2.5, respectively, compared to non-donors. No differences were noted in the rates of preterm birth or IUGR between donors and non-donors.[10]

Pelvic and Horseshoe Kidney

In the general population, the prevalence of pelvic kidney is approximately 1 in 900 and horseshoe kidney is approximately 1 in 600.[11,12] Both are associated with high rates of other comorbid renal and extrarenal congenital anomalies. Normal physiologic renal adaptation to pregnancy occurs in women with pelvic or horseshoe kidney as there is a normal total mass of renal tissue. These women are usually clinically asymptomatic and unaware of their renal malformation. The diagnosis is often incidental on routine obstetric ultrasound. Figure 39.2 shows a pelvic kidney diagnosed at the time of ultrasound for ectopic pregnancy.

Women may also present in pregnancy with pelvic mass and pain. The anatomic distortion that results from the ectopic location of pelvic and horseshoe kidney causes the ureters to be foreshortened, abnormally placed and susceptible to compression from the growing uterus. This in turn, leads to an increased incidence of urinary tract infections, nephrolithiasis

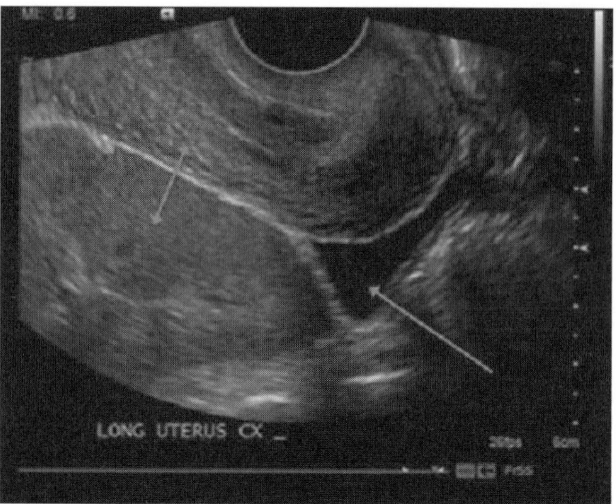

Figure 39.2 Ultrasound of woman with ruptured ectopic pregnancy showing pelvic kidney directly posterior to the empty uterus.[34]

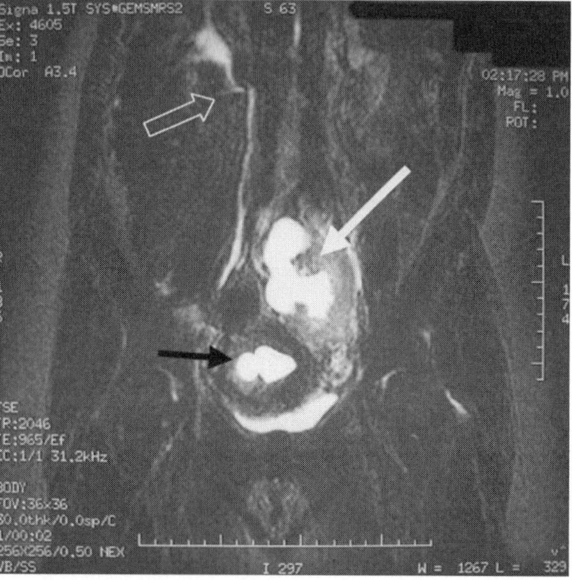

Figure 39.3 Magnetic resonance urogram shows a normal right-sided renal collecting system and ureter (open arrow). There is hydronephrosis of the left pelvic kidney (white arrow). The bicornuate uterus is also shown (black arrow).[35]

and hydronephrosis. Rarely, pelvic kidney can cause obstruction during labor requiring delivery by cesarean[13] Screening urine culture should be performed every trimester and women should be counseled about the signs and symptoms of cystitis and nephrolithiasis. During intrapartum management, labor progress should be monitored for signs of obstructed labor. If cesarean delivery is indicated, the obstetrician must be especially cognizant of potential effects of the altered renal anatomy as well as the possibility of previously undiagnosed Mullerian anomalies. A Mullerian anomaly is seen in Figure 39.3. Further evaluation of the renal tract may be indicated after the postpartum period if the initial diagnosis was made during pregnancy.

Acute Kidney Injury

AKI can be classified according to the mechanism of injury: prerenal or hypovolemic, renal or intrinsic and postrenal or obstructive sources (see Table 39.2).

Table 39.2 Causes of Acute Kidney Injury in Pregnancy[1,2]

Stage	Etiology
Prerenal / hypovolemic	Intravascular hypovolemia / hypoperfusion • Ovarian hyperstimulation syndrome • Hyperemesis gravidarum • Congestive heart failure • Nonsteroidal anti-inflammatory drugs Hemorrhage • Spontaneous abortion • Ectopic pregnancy • Gestational trophoblastic disease • Placenta previa • Placental abruption • Uterine rupture • Postpartum hemorrhage
Renal / intrinsic	Acute tubular necrosis • Hypotension • Sepsis • Disseminated intravascular coagulation Acute interstitial nephritis • Medication toxicity Thrombotic microangiopathy • Preeclampsia /HELLP • Acute fatty liver of pregnancy • Thrombotic thrombocytopenic purpura and hemolytic uremic syndrome Trauma
Postrenal / obstructive	Nephrolithiasis Bilateral ureteral obstruction • Incarcerated uterus • Polyhydramnios • Fibroids • Neoplasm

Injuries may be multimodal if, for example, hemorrhage leads to prerenal azotemia, which, if prolonged, causes acute tubular necrosis as a result of ischemia. This can further complicate the diagnostic process.

Diagnosis of AKI

Early diagnosis of AKI can be challenging in pregnancy as the normal physiologic renal changes can mask injury and delay diagnosis of a reversible etiology such as hypovolemia. A clinical approach to diagnosis of AKI should include accurate assessment of urine output, kidney function tests, proteinuria and serum and urine electrolytes. Oliguria, generally defined as <0.5 mL/kg/h for more than 2 hours, is frequently seen in AKI during pregnancy. Calculation of fractional excretion of sodium (FENa) can help differentiate between prerenal and renal causes. A FENa >1 suggests a prerenal AKI while in intrinsic AKI the FENa is usually <1. Renal insufficiency, serum creatinine >1.1 mg/dL or a doubling of baseline creatinine, may be an indication for delivery depending on etiology.[1]

General Management

Early diagnosis and correction of reversible causes are the mainstay of AKI management. Maintenance of euvolemia, correction of anemia and avoidance of nephrotoxic medications can both prevent and treat AKI. Advanced interventions such as furosemide, renal-dose dopamine and dialysis may be indicated and their effects on timing of delivery should be coordinated between the obstetrician and nephrologist.[1]

Preeclampsia and HELLP Syndrome

Preeclampsia complicates 5% of pregnancies.[14] Generally, establishment of a diagnosis of preeclampsia (PEC) requires a new onset of persistent systolic blood pressure (BP) ≥140 mmHg or diastolic BP ≥90 mmHg after 20 weeks gestation plus proteinuria ≥300 mg/day in a 24-hour urine collection or a urine P:C ratio of ≥0.3.[15] The hemolysis elevated liver enzymes low platelets (HELLP) syndrome is characterized by presence of a microangiopathic hemolytic anemia, elevated liver enzymes twice the upper limit of normal and low platelets below 100,000 mm^3. Hypertension and proteinuria may or may not be present.[2] See Chapter 35 for more information on preeclampsia and hypertensive disorders of pregnancy.

Preeclampsia is associated with systemic endothelial dysfunction and may lead to renal damage through direct and indirect mechanisms. Directly, PEC causes intravascular volume depletion with subsequent decreased GFR, oliguria, elevated serum creatinine and serum uric acid. Indirectly, PEC increases the risk of disseminated intravascular coagulation, placental abruption and postpartum hemorrhage. Coupled with the direct pathophysiologic effects of PEC, these ischemic insults can lead to AKI.[1] Approximately 15% of women with HELLP syndrome develop AKI and between 10 and 46% of those will require dialysis. Renal function usually improves with disease resolution after delivery.[2]

Acute Fatty Liver of Pregnancy

A very rare complication, acute fatty liver of pregnancy (AFLP) is characterized by acute liver failure, coagulopathy and renal dysfunction. It is variably associated with thrombocytopenia, hypoglycemia and hypertension among other findings.[16] The mechanism of renal injury in AFLP may result from a derangement in long-chain fatty acid metabolism.[2] The vast majority of women demonstrate a rapid recovery from renal injury suggesting a largely prerenal component. In a minority of women, however, return to baseline creatinine can be prolonged suggesting superimposed intrinsic renal damage.[16] The critical steps in management include prompt recognition and supportive care for hypoglycemia, anemia/coagulopathy or hepatic encephalopathy when present along with expeditious delivery.[2] Acute fatty liver of pregnancy carries a 10% maternal mortality rate and very high rates of preterm birth, cesarean delivery and fetal demise.[16]

Thrombotic Thrombocytopenic Purpura and Atypical Hemolytic Uremic Syndrome

Thrombotic thrombocytopenic purpura and atypical (non-Shiga toxin) hemolytic uremic syndrome are pregnancy-associated thrombotic microangiopathies characterized by platelet thrombi and fibrin deposition in the microvasculature. They occur at an incidence of 1 in 25,000 women. Presentation may include neurologic symptoms, fever, hemolytic anemia, severe thrombocytopenia and AKI. Pregnancy may be complicated by IUGR, PEC, placental infarct and a maternal mortality rate of 20%. Despite treatment with plasma exchange and plasmapharesis, long-term renal outcome is poor with roughly 75% of women progressing to end-stage renal disease (ESRD).[2]

Nephrolithiasis

The incidence of nephrolithiasis in pregnant women is no different than that in nonpregnant women; however, the underlying risk factors that lead to stone formation differ in pregnancy. Stones complicate 1 in 200–1,500 pregnancies and typically present in the second and third trimester. Hydronephrosis and progesterone-mediated urinary stasis combined with increased excretion of lithogenic factors predispose to stone formation.[17]

As in the nonpregnant population, typical signs and symptoms include flank pain with or without radiation into the groin, abdominal pain, nausea and vomiting, hematuria and costovertebral angle tenderness. Renal and pelvic ultrasound can identify approximately 60% of nephrolithiasis and should be the first-line diagnostic imaging modality.[6,17]

More than 75% of subcentimeter stones pass spontaneously with conservative management consisting of hydration and adequate analgesia.[17] In the presence of obstruction, recalcitrant pain, sepsis or urologic anomalies, urology consultation should be obtained as more advanced therapies are likely indicated.[17]

Asymptomatic Bacteriuria, Acute Cystitis and Pyelonephritis

Physiologic changes to the renal collecting system in pregnancy predispose women to asymptomatic bacteriuria (ASB), which can affect up to 10% of pregnancies. This in turn can lead to acute cystitis and pyelonephritis, which complicate 4% and 2% of pregnancies, respectively. All pregnant women must be screened with a urine culture for ASB in the first trimester. Women with history of recurrent cystitis, diabetes, sickle cell trait/disease, immunosuppression or urinary tract malformations should also be screened in the second and third trimester. The importance of treating pregnant women with ASB must be emphasized since if left untreated, it progresses to pyelonephritis in as many as 40% of pregnancies.

Symptomatic acute cystitis, and most notably pyelonephritis, are associated with significant morbidities such as sepsis, acute tubular necrosis, hemolysis/anemia, acute respiratory distress syndrome (ARDS), hypertension/PEC, preterm delivery, and neonatal sepsis.[18]

Typical causative agents in order of frequency include *Escherichia coli*, *Klebsiella* species, coagulase-negative *Staphylococcus*, *Staphylococcus aureus* and group B *Streptococci* (GBS). Asymptomatic bacteriuria, defined as $\geq 10^5$ colony-forming units on culture from a midstream clean-catch urine specimen, should be treated based on culture speciation and sensitivities. Initiation of empiric treatment for cystitis with oral antibiotics based on clinical presentation and urine dipstick alone is usually adequate though urinary culture and sensitivities should nonetheless be obtained and followed up. Given the potential for severe complications, pyelonephritis should generally be treated with parenteral antibiotics in the inpatient setting until clinically improved. Antibiotics may then be transitioned to oral dosing to complete a 14-day course. Initial evaluation should include a complete blood count (CBC), comprehensive metabolic panel (CMP), urinalysis and culture, renal ultrasound to evaluate for obstruction, stones, hydronephrosis and

Table 39.3 Treatment of Asymptomatic Bacteriuria and Acute Cystitis[18]

Antibiotic	Therapeutic Dosing (7-day course)	Prophylactic Dosing (Remainder of Pregnancy)	FDA Pregnancy Category
Amoxicillin	500 mg po every 8 h	500 mg daily	B
Cephalexin	500 mg po every 6 h	500 mg daily	B
Nitrofurantoin monohydrate macrocrystals	100 mg po every 12 h	100 mg daily	B
Trimethoprim-sulfamethoxazole DS (TMP-SMX DS)	160/80 mg po every 12 h	160/80 mg daily	C[a]

[a] Generally considered safe in second and early third trimester. Neonatal complications may occur if given proximal to delivery.

Table 39.4 Treatment of Pyelonephritis[18]

Antibiotic	Initial IV Treatment	Post-IV Outpatient Treatment (To complete 14-day course)	FDA Pregnancy Category
Ceftriaxone	1–2 g every 24 h	–	B
Ampicillin-sulbactam	1.5 g every 6 h	–	B
Aztreonam[a]	1 g every 8–12 h	–	B
TMP-SMX DS	2 mg/kg every 6 h	160/80 mg po every 12 h	C[b]
Amoxicillin	–	500 mg po every 8 h	B
Amoxicillin-clavulanate	–	875/125 mg every 12 h	B

[a] Alternative for penicillin allergy.

[b] Generally considered safe in second and early third trimester. Neonatal complications may occur if given proximal to delivery.

abscess. Further evaluation should be obtained as indicated for signs of sepsis, pulmonary edema or ARDS. Once treatment is completed for ASB, cystitis or pyelonephritis, a repeat urine culture should be obtained for test of cure. After completing the course of therapeutic antibiotics, women diagnosed with pyelonephritis should continue on prophylactic dosage antibiotics for the remainder of pregnancy.[18] Similarly, women diagnosed with two discrete, urine culture-proven episodes of ASB or cystitis also require antibiotic prophylaxis for the remainder of pregnancy. Table 39.3 shows treatment of asymptomatic bacteriuria and cystitis. Table 39.4 describes treatment of pyelonephritis.

Chronic Kidney Diseases

Antepartum Evaluation, Fetal Surveillance and Postpartum Care in Chronic Kidney Disease

Given that most chronic renal diseases may be complicated by hypertension or PEC, women should have a baseline laboratory evaluation performed either preconceptionally or early in pregnancy. This evaluation should include a CBC and CMP (to assess electrolytes, liver and kidney function) and an evaluation for proteinuria. These tests may be repeated every trimester or more frequently as dictated by severity of disease.

In the absence of IUGR or chronic hypertension, there are no studies establishing clear protocols for increased fetal surveillance in the setting of chronic kidney diseases. Assuming stable disease, the American Congress of Obstetricians and Gynecologists recommends initiating fetal testing at 32 weeks gestation. The frequency of testing has not been well established either but may include nonstress test (NST), biophysical profile (BPP), modified BPP or contraction stress test performed either weekly or twice weekly. Testing may be initiated earlier or more frequently as clinically indicated in unstable or worsening disease.[19] Given the potential for decline into end stage renal disease (ESRD), postpartum care should include close follow up with nephrology and monitoring of blood pressure and renal function.[4]

Chronic Hypertension

Chronic HTN is a common comorbidity of chronic renal disease. Optimizing control is essential to the management of the renal disease. Women with chronic HTN should have the usual baseline laboratory evaluation. Serial ultrasounds for growth should be done every 4–6 weeks starting at 26 weeks or earlier in poorly controlled disease. As previously discussed, antihypertensives that are safe in pregnancy should be used when indicated. See Chapter 34 (Hypertensive Disorders in Pregnancy) for further information.

Renal Transplant

Diseases that lead to renal transplants tend to occur in a younger cohort of women compared to diseases requiring other organ transplantation. As outcomes improve, pregnancy in transplant recipients is seen more frequently. The National Transplantation Pregnancy Registry in the United States recorded 1,356 pregnancies among 857 renal transplant recipients over a 20-year period.[20] Provided a stable immunosuppressive regimen is in place, excellent maternal and fetal outcomes are increasingly common assuming the maternal creatinine remains <1.5mg/dL. Intrauterine growth restriction, PEC, preterm birth and neonatal death rates increase in the presence of maternal hypertension and creatinine >1.5 mg/dL.[2]

Several immunosuppressants such as corticosteroids, azathioprine and calcineurin inhibitors may be safely used in pregnancy, whereas others, such as mycophenolate mofetil, carry a significant risk of teratogenicity. Preconception counseling, pregnancy timing and immunosuppressive management with a multidisciplinary team play an important role in the care of women with renal transplants. Although there are no established protocols for laboratory evaluation in pregnancies with renal transplant, an assessment of the GFR, creatinine and for proteinuria should be performed before conception if possible. Creatinine and proteinuria levels should be rechecked every trimester or as clinically indicated.

Diabetic Nephropathy

Pregestational diabetes complicates 1% of all pregnancies.[21] Of those with type 1 diabetes mellitus, 5–10% have diabetic nephropathy, which is the primary cause of ESRD worldwide.[21,22] Diabetic pregnancies carry an increased risk of hypertensive disorders, IUGR, congenital malformations, preterm birth, intrauterine fetal or neonatal demise and cesarean delivery. The increasing prevalence of pre-gestational diabetes is likely to cause the rates of diabetic nephropathy will continue to rise which may further complicate these pregnancies.

In nondiabetic pregnancies, mild albuminuria is expected due to the increased filtration load. Diabetic nephropathy has been variably defined as having proteinuria in excess of 300–500 mg/dL in 24 hours. Definitions inconsistently include serum creatinine >1.5 mg/dL and presence of hypertension. In the absence of consensus definitions for diabetic nephropathy, the literature demonstrates a general trend where women with mild prepregnancy nephropathy have far less risk of progression of disease post-pregnancy compared to those with moderate to severe disease prior to conception.[21]

Up to 40% of diabetic pregnancies may be complicated by chronic HTN and up to 65% by PEC, which in the setting of pre-existing nephropathy may present a significant diagnostic challenge.[21] Pregnant women with preexisting diabetes therefore should have baseline labs early in pregnancy that include at minimum a CBC, CMP and 24-hour urine collection for protein and creatinine clearance.

Many diabetic patients, even in the absence of chronic HTN, may be treated with renin–angiotensin–aldosterone system (RAAS) blocking agents (ACE-inhibitors and angiotensin receptor blockers), which are known teratogens, and should be discontinued as early as possible upon confirmation of pregnancy or ideally, as part of pre-conception care. Diltiazem may be used for blood pressure control as an alternative. In addition to tight glycemic control, aspirin therapy should be initiated at 12–16 weeks and continued until approximately 34 weeks gestation.[21]

Systemic Lupus Erythematosus and Antiphospholipid Syndrome

Systemic lupus erythematosus (SLE), a multisystem, immune-mediated, connective tissue disease, affects roughly 1–5 in 10,000 women. Lupus nephritis (LN), an immune-complex mediated glomerulonephritis (see Figure 39.4), affects up to 75% of patients with SLE.[23] Lupus may flare in pregnancy and can be difficult to differentiate from PEC.

Antiphospholipid syndrome (APS) is a thrombotic autoimmune disorder characterized by circulating antiphospholipid antibodies. Antiphospholipid syndrome is frequently a feature of SLE but may also occur in isolation. Thrombotic insults leading to vascular lesions

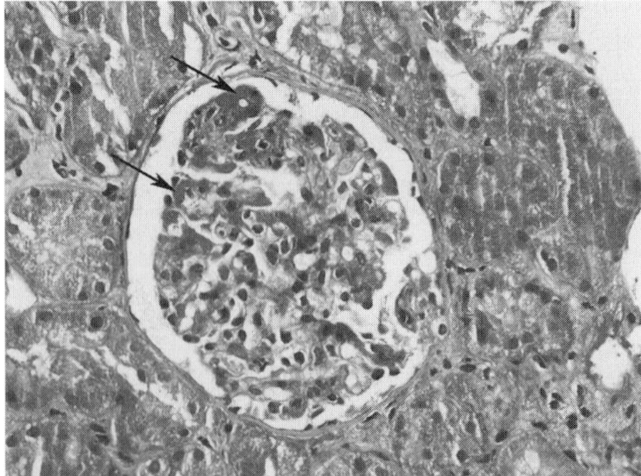

Figure 39.4 Kidney biopsy in a pregnant woman showing diffuse proliferative class IV lupus nephritis (trichrome stain, 400×) with subendothelial deposits (arrows).[25]

in the kidney are the primary cause of renal disease and can lead to APS nephropathy. Antiphospholipid syndrome nephropathy is distinct from lupus nephritis (LN) but seen concurrently in women with systemic lupus erythematosus (SLE). Patients may present suddenly with nephrotic or nephritic syndrome, renal failure, proteinuria, hematuria or hypertension.[24]

When possible, pregnancy should be delayed until autoimmune kidney disease has been in remission for six months and the patient is stable on a regimen of medications that is safe in pregnancy.[25] Pregnancy is not advised if the creatinine is >2.8 mg/dL.[23]

Lupus and APS increase the risk of adverse maternal-fetal outcomes such as spontaneous abortion, IUGR, preterm birth, HTN, PEC, fetal demise and congenital heart block. These risk profiles generally improve when pregnancy occurs in periods of disease quiescence.[23]

Pregnant women with SLE and APS should be managed by a multidisciplinary team with the goal of minimizing flares with pregnancy-safe immunosuppressants, anticoagulation therapy, controlling HTN and appropriate antenatal surveillance. Baseline labs should include CBC, CMP, 24-hour urine collection, anti-Sjogren's syndrome-related antigen A and B antibodies, antiphospholipid antibodies and lupus-like inhibitor.[23]

Dialysis-Dependent Chronic Renal Failure

Pregnant women may require dialysis for similar indications as nonpregnant women. These include severe electrolyte imbalance, metabolic acidosis and volume overload. Fetal complications include a 62% rate of polyhydramnios, 85% rate of preterm delivery (mean gestational age 32 weeks) and 53% rate of cesarean delivery.[4,6] Up to 80% of pregnancies have associated HTN and can develop superimposed PEC. The overall infant survival rate is 40–50% and rate of spontaneous abortion ranges from 12% to 50%.[4]

General management principles include aggressive treatment of anemia, adequate protein and vitamin supplementation and optimal control of blood pressure and volume status.[6] The frequency of dialysis and associated laboratory testing must be individualized and, as it is beyond the scope of the obstetrician, is typically determined by a nephrologist. The obstetrician should pay meticulous attention to maternal blood pressure in order to diagnose and manage PEC early if it develops. Although IUGR is not significantly more common in this population than the general population, fetal growth scans every 3–4 weeks may be reasonable. Continuous fetal monitoring should be done during dialysis sessions (which may be five to six times per week). Consideration should be given to starting testing at 24–28 weeks given that the mean gestational age at delivery is 32 weeks. Additional fetal surveillance for PEC and IUGR should be initiated as indicated and delivery should be timed accordingly.[26]

Chronic Glomerulonephritis

Immunoglobulin A (IgA) nephropathy is the most common of the glomerulonephritidies. Segmental glomerulonephritis, minimal change disease and membranous nephropathy are other chronic glomerulonephritidies that commonly present with nephrotic syndrome. Maternal and fetal outcomes are generally very good when renal function is preserved. There may be an increased incidence of HTN in pregnancy.[6] When renal insufficiency is present, nephrotic syndrome has been associated with an increased incidence of preterm birth, reported as high as 50%, and IUGR at 25%. Pregnancy does not typically adversely impact disease progression although progression to ESRD after pregnancy has been reported.[4,6] General management centers on fluid management, blood pressure control, glucocorticoid treatment and immunosuppression if needed.[25] Early in the course of the pregnancy, involvement of rheumatology and nephrology is recommended. Initial care should include baseline 24-hour urine collection CBC, CMP and serum uric acid. Assuming well-controlled disease, no additional testing is required beyond that for routine obstetric indications.

Renal Malignancy

Although exceedingly rare, renal neoplasms may be diagnosed in pregnancy on routine obstetric ultrasound or in women presenting with flank pain, palpable masses, hematuria and hypertension. Treatment is stage and gestational age dependent with radical nephrectomy being the standard approach. Maternal and fetal outcomes appear to be excellent.[27]

Autosomal Dominant Polycystic Kidney Disease

Autosomal dominant polycystic kidney disease (ADPKD) affects up to 1 in 400 individuals worldwide and is characterized by progressive development of fluid-filled renal cysts. Signs and symptoms include flank pain, hematuria, recurrent cystitis/pyelonephritis or nephrolithiasis. Ultimately ESRD can develop. ADPKD increases risks of hypertension/PEC, preterm birth, urinary tract infections and fetal distress. Pregnancy can significantly worsen renal function and may ultimately lead to ESRD.[28] Antepartum care should focus on the management of concurrent HTN or PEC if present. A urine culture should be done every trimester and for new urinary symptoms. Genetic counseling should be offered to women with ADPKD. Subsets of women with ADPKD develop intracranial aneurysms. Those with a family history of intracranial aneurysm should have a screening brain MRI done preconception with treatment offered before attempting pregnancy.[6]

Medications and Teratogenicity

Many medications frequently used in hypertension and autoimmune or chronic kidney diseases present significant teratogenic risk. RAAS Inhibitors can cause fetal renal tubular dysplasia, anuria-oligohydramnios, pulmonary hypoplasia, fetal hypotension, hypocalvaria, cardiovascular and central nervous system malformations with associated risk of neonatal mortality.[29,30] Surviving infants may have subsequent long-term renal dysfunction. Women on RAAS inhibitors should be counseled to stop these medications before conception. Antihypertensives generally considered safe throughout pregnancy include labetalol, nifedipine, diltiazem, amlodipine, hydralazine and methyldopa. Loop diuretics and clonidine may be used when first-line agents are inadequate.[29]

Alkylating agents such as cyclophosphamide can cause several malformations including imperforate anus, palatal and nasal deformities as well as IUGR later in pregnancy.[31] Immunosuppressants that are safe in pregnancy include corticosteroids, azathioprine and calcineurin inhibitors.[32]

Concluding Remarks

Renal diseases in pregnancy are a complex set of disorders that can present both acutely and chronically. The effects of disease on pregnancy and the effects of pregnancy on the kidney vary in frequency and severity. Most pregnancies with chronic renal disease may be further complicated by HTN and/or PEC. Other examples of obstetric complications include preterm birth and IUGR. General management centers on appropriate selection of medications and avoidance of teratogens and preservation of renal function by controlling blood pressure and fluid status when indicated. Increased fetal testing may be also indicated, which along with timing of delivery, depends on severity of the disease. To optimize maternal and fetal outcomes, pregnant women with renal disease should be cared for by a multidisciplinary team.

References

1. Van Hook JW. Acute kidney injury during pregnancy. *Clin Obstet Gynecol.* 2014;57(4):851–861.
2. Gyamlani G and Geraci SA. Kidney Disease in Pregnancy. *Southern Med J.* 2013; 106(9):519–525.
3. Piccoli G, Daidola G, Attini R, Parisi S, Fassio F, Naretto C, Deagostini M, Castelluccia N, Ferraresi M, Roccatello D, Todros T. Kidney biopsy in pregnancy: Evidence for counseling? A systematic narrative review. *BJOG.* 2013;120:412–427.
4. Ramin SM, Viaeff AC, Yeomans ER, et al. Chronic renal disease in pregnancy. *Obstet Gynecol.* 2006;108:1531–1539.
5. Cheung KL, Lafayette RA. Renal physiology of pregnancy. *Adv Chron Kidney Dis.* 2013; 20(3):209–214.
6. Thadhani RI, Maski MR. Renal disorders. In: RK Creasy, R Resnik, JD Iams, CJ Lockwood, TR Moore, M Greene, editors. *Creasy & Resnik's Maternal-Fetal Medicine: Principles and Practice*, 7th ed. Philadelphia: Elsevier Saunders, 2014.
7. Verdonk K, Niemeijer IC, Hop WCJ, de Rijke YB, Steegers EAP, van den Meiracker AH, Visser W. Variation of urinary protein to creatinine ratio during the day in women with suspected pre-eclampsia. *BJOG* 2014;121(13):1660–1665.
8. Westland R, Schreuder MF, Ket JCF, van Wijk JAE. Unilateral renal agenesis: A systematic review on associated anomalies and renal injury. *Nephrol Dialysis Transplant.* 2013 Jul 10;28(7):1844–1855.
9. Lowes JJ, Mackenzie JC, Abrams PH, Gingell JC. Acute renal failure and acute hydronephrosis in pregnancy: Use of the double-J stent. *J Royal Soc Med.* 1987 Nov 18;80:524–525.
10. Garg AX, Nevis IF, McArthur E, Sontrop JM, Koval JJ, Lam NN, et al. Gestational hypertension and preeclampsia in living kidney donors. *N Engl J Med.* 2015 Jan 8;372(2):124–133.
11. Natsis K, Piagkou M, Skotsimara A, Protogerou V, Tsitouridis I, Skandalakis P. Horseshoe kidney: A review of anatomy and pathology. *Surg Radiol Anat.* 2013 Nov 1;36(6):517–526.

12. Dabiri L, Cheung W. Unilateral Ectopic Right Kidney, an incidental finding during pelvic sonogram. *J Natl Med Assoc.* 2006 Oct;98(10):1710–1712.

13. Zwerbroek W, Brugge Ter HG. Pelvic kidney – A rare cause of obstetrical obstruction. *Eur J Obstet Gynecol Reproduc Biol.* 1995 Jul 7;63:95–96.

14. Wagner S and Craici I. Hypertensive pregnancy disorders and future renal disease. *Curr Hypertens Rep.* 2014;16:484.

15. American College of Obstetricians and Gynecologists Task Force on Hypertension in Pregnancy. Hypertension in Pregnancy. Washington, DC; 2013.

16. Nelson DB, Yost NP, Cunningham FG. Acute fatty liver of pregnancy: Clinical outcomes and expected duration of recovery. *Am J Obstet Gynecol.* 2013;209:456.e1–e7.

17. Semins MJ, Matlaga BR. Kidney stones during pregnancy. *Nat Rev Urol.* 2014;11:163–168.

18. Matuszkiewicz-Rowińska J, Małyszko J, Wieliczko M. Urinary tract infections in pregnancy: Old and new unresolved diagnostic and therapeutic problems. *Arch Med Sci.* 2015; 11(1): 67–77.

19. Antepartum fetal surveillance. Practice Bulletin No. 145. American College of Obstetricians and Gynecologists. *Obstet Gynecol.* 2014;124:182–192.

20. Rickman K, Gohh R. Pregnancy after renal transplantation: A review of registry and single-center practices and outcomes. *Nephrol Dial Transplant.* 2012;27:3428–3434.

21. Leguizamón G, Trigubo D, Pereira JI, et al. Vascular complications in the diabetic pregnancy. *Curr Diab Rep.* 2015;15:22.

22. Piccoli GB, Clari R, Ghiotto S, Castelluccia N, et al. Type 1 diabetes, diabetic nephropathy, and pregnancy: A systematic review and meta-study. *Rev Diabet Stud.* 2013;10(1):6–26.

23. Kattah AG, Garovic VD. Pregnancy and lupus nephritis. *Semin Nephrol.* 2015;35:487–499.

24. Sciascia S, Baldovino S, Schreiber K, et al. Antiphospholipid syndrome and the kidney. *Semin Nephrol.* 2015;35:478–486.

25. Smyth A, Radovic M, Garovic VD. Women, kidney disease and pregnancy. *Adv Chron Kidney Dis.* 2013;20(5):402–410.

26. Chinnappa V, Ankichetty S, Angle P, Halpern SH. Chronic kidney disease in pregnancy. *Int J Obstet Anesth.* 2013;22:223–230.

27. Boussios S, Pavlidis N. Renal cell carcinoma in pregnancy: A rare coexistence. *Clin Transl Oncol.* 2014;16:122–127.

28. Min W, Diping W, Ladan Z, et al. Pregnancy outcomes in autosomal dominant polycystic kidney disease: A case–control study. *J Mat Fet Neonat Med.* 2016;29(5):807–812.

29. Hussain A, Karovitch A, Carson MP. Blood pressure goals and treatment in pregnant patients with chronic kidney disease. *Adv Chron Kidney Dis.* 2015;22(2):165–169.

30. Cooper WO, Hernandez-Diaz S, Arbogast PG, Dudley JA, Dyer S, Gideon PS, et al. Major congenital malformations after first-trimester exposure to ACE Inhibitors. *New Eng J Med.* 2006;354(23):2443–2451.

31. Francis BM, Rogers JM, Sulik KK, Alles AJ, Elstein KH, Zucker RM, et al. Cyclophosphamide teratogenesis: Evidence for compensatory responses to induced cellular toxicity. *Teratology.* 1990;42(5):473–482.

32. Maynard SE and Thadhani R. Pregnancy and the kidney. *J Am Soc Nephrol.* 2009;20:14–22.

33. Kasper DL, Fauci AS, Hauser SL, Longo DL, Jameson JL, Loscalzo J. *Harrison's Principles of Internal Medicine*, 19th ed. New York: McGraw-Hill Medical Publishing Division, 2015.

34. Belotte J, Belotte J, Alexis M, Awonuga A, Aguin TJ. Successful laparoscopic management of ruptured tubal pregnancy with an ipsilateral ectopic pelvic kidney. Case Rep Obstet Gynecol. Published online 2014 July 21. Available at: http://dx.doi.org/10.1155/2014/682737.

35. Kavanagh DO, Fanning N, Heffernan E, Malone DE, Mulvin DM, Quinlan DM. Management of gestational nephrolithiasis in the presence of a bicornuate uterus and pelvic kidney. *Int J Urol.* 2005;12(2):211–213.

Hematologic Diseases Complicating Pregnancy

Natalie Bowersox

Introduction

Pregnancy causes several hematologic changes. Awareness and understanding of these changes are paramount in caring for the pregnant patient during pregnancy, in labor, and the postpartum period. Most disorders can be safely treated during pregnancy. The most common hematologic changes during pregnancy include a physiologic anemia, an elevated white blood cell (WBC) count (leukocytosis), mild decrease in platelets, an increase in procoagulant factors, and a decrease in fibrinolysis.

This chapter will discuss benign hematologic disorders including anemia, thrombocytopenia, thrombophilia, venous thromboembolism, and inherited and acquired bleeding disorders affecting pregnancy and how to treat them.

Scope of the Problem

Anemia is the most common hematologic disorder during pregnancy due to a 40% increase in plasma volume (1). If the anemia is not physiologic and the hemoglobin falls below 11 g/dL, a workup is warranted. The most common cause of anemia in pregnancy is iron deficiency (1). Sickle cell disease is the most common inherited disorder across the world and this affects 300,000 children each year (2). Platelets can be affected by this dilutional effect and thrombocytopenia is seen in 8–10% of pregnancies (1). The most common causes include gestational thrombocytopenia (70%), preeclampsia (21%), and immune thrombocytopenia purpura (ITP; 3%) (3). Pregnancy is a prothrombotic state which results in increased potential clot formation along with both decreased anticoagulant activity and decreased fibrinolysis. These factors can lead to an increase in both venous thromboembolism (VTE) and pulmonary embolus (PE). Inherited disorders are known to cause 50% of cases of VTE, PE, and stroke during pregnancy and include factor V Leiden, Prothrombin G20210, antithrombin deficiency, and protein C and protein S deficiencies (4). Finally, women with inherited bleeding disorders are at an increased risk of bleeding during pregnancy (5).

Physiologic Changes

Plasma volume increases by 10–15% beginning at 6 to 12 weeks gestation and continues to expand until around 30–34 weeks gestation. The largest increases are noted in the second trimester. Overall, this results in a 40–50% increase in volume when compared to non-pregnancy levels. This increase in volume is in response to an underfilled vascular system resulting from systemic vasodilation (1). Plasma volume at term is around 4,700 to 5,200 mL (which is an increase of 1,100 to 1,600 mL during the pregnancy). The volume does decrease immediately postpartum, and then increases again 2 to 5 days later, eventually normalizing at 6 weeks postpartum (6).

Red blood cells (RBC) begin to increase at around 8 to 10 weeks gestation. They rise by about 20–30% by term. This results in an increase of about 250–450 mL. RBC production is increased due to an increase in erythropoietin. In fact, erythropoietin levels increase by 150% at term. Despite this, the increase in plasma volume is greater, and this results in an overall decrease in hemoglobin producing the physiologic anemia seen in pregnancy. The hemoglobin level is lowest in the second trimester and slowly improves as the end of pregnancy approaches (6).

An increase in neutrophil count leads to the leukocytosis seen in pregnancy. The white blood cell (WBC) count starts to increase during the second month, and values around 9,000 to 15,000 are common. The mean WBC count does increase linearly during labor, and values around 10,000 to 16,000 can be seen. The WBC count typically returns to the normal range around

6 days postpartum. Some studies have shown that the percent of bands increases during pregnancy as well (6). Absolute lymphocyte count, including T and B lymphocytes, and the monocyte count do not change during pregnancy. A slight decrease in basophil count occurs and the eosinophil count is slightly elevated. Dohle bodies (which are blue staining cytoplasmic inclusions in granulocytes) are a normal finding in pregnancy.

Platelets are in the normal to slightly decreased range during pregnancy. The value rises after delivery and can stay elevated for 3–4 weeks postpartum. See Table 40.1 for details.

Normal pregnancy is both a hypercoagulable and a prothrombotic state to ultimately protect against excessive bleeding when the placenta separates. Normally, the fibrinolytic system helps to prevent excessive coagulation by removing fibrin and dissolving clots, which allows the blood circulating to move in the vascular beds and helps bleeding to stop quickly following trauma. In pregnancy, the fibrinolytic system's activity will decrease in preparation for labor and delivery. Overall, this leads to a tendency for thrombus formation. Uterine contractions and an increased level of decidual tissue factor assist with this as well. Alternatively, these changes also increase the risk of VTE. There is a return to baseline for these factors by 6–8 weeks postpartum (see Table 40.1 for physiologic hematologic changes in pregnancy). See Box 40.1 for details.

Table 40.1 Physiologic Hematologic Changes in Pregnancy

Factor	Change	Amount
Plasma volume	Increases 40–50%	4700–5200 mL
Red blood cells (RBC)	Increases by 20–30%	250–450 mL
White blood cells (WBC)	Increased	9–15k preg, 10–16k labor
Absolute lymphocyte count	T, B, and monocyte stay same	No change
Platelets	Normal to mildly decreased	No change to slight decrease

Source: References (1, 6).

Box 40.1 Effect of pregnancy on coagulation factors

Protein S, free and total Decreases
Protein C, antithrombin Stable throughout pregnancy
Fibrinogen, factors II, VII, VIII, X, XII, XIII Increases (20–200%)
Von Willebrand's factor Increases
PAI-1, PAI-2 Increases
D-Dimer, plasminogen Increases
Factor V and IX Stable or increase slightly
TAFI (thrombin activatable fibrinolytic inhibitor) Increases

Anemia

Anemia is the most common hematologic disorder during pregnancy. A physiologic or dilutional anemia is associated with a normal pregnancy secondary to a greater plasma expansion relative to the increase in red cell mass. This anemia typically resolves by about 6 weeks postpartum. Interestingly, absence of this dilutional effect is associated with stillbirth. This physiologic anemia makes it difficult to characterize anemia in pregnancy. Anemia should be evaluated with a complete blood count (CBC), peripheral smear, reticulocyte count, serum iron, total iron binding capacity (TIBC), and ferritin level. It is important to keep in mind that 16–29% of pregnant patients become anemic in the third trimester, but fetal requirement are always met (6).

The Centers for Disease Control and Prevention (CDC) defined anemia in pregnancy as hemoglobin levels of less than 11 g/dL (hematocrit less than 33%) in the first and third trimester, and less than 10.5 g/dL (hematocrit less than 32%) in the second trimester (7). The World Health Organization (WHO) defines anemia in pregnancy as hemoglobin less than 11 g/dL or hematocrit less than 33%. WHO defines severe anemia requiring treatment as hemoglobin less than 7 g/dL, and very severe anemia (medical emergency due to the risk of congestive heart failure) as a hemoglobin less than 4 g/dL (8).

Chronic anemia is associated with a myriad of problems and is seen more commonly in developing countries. These problems include increased maternal mortality, increased risk of preterm delivery, spontaneous abortion, low birth weight, and fetal death. Iron deficiency is the most common form of anemia during pregnancy worldwide. Some areas of Africa have reported iron-deficiency anemia rates as high as 75%; this may actually be protective against malaria (9).

In a singleton pregnancy, maternal iron requirements are about 1,000 mg/day. 300 mg is required for the fetus and the placenta, 500 mg for maternal hemoglobin mass, and 200 mg are shed through the gut, urine, and skin. This translates to an increase in daily iron from 18 mg/day to 27 mg/day (1). This demand cannot be met by diet alone for most women. Most women do not have adequate iron stores preconceptually secondary to chronic blood loss from menstruation and/or nutritional deficiencies. Iron can be supplemented either orally (60–120 mg/day of elemental iron) or, in more severe instances, with IV iron infusions, which are safe to use in pregnancy. Pica, the ingestion of substances with no nutrition, is seen more commonly among iron deficient women. Ingestion of starch, ice, clay, and dirt has been reported (9).

Folate deficiency (a megaloblastic anemia) is the second most common cause of anemia. Folate deficiency is rare in the United States and Western countries since food is fortified with folate. Prenatal vitamins also contain folate, which help prevent neural tube defects when give pre-conceptually and in the first weeks of gestation. A woman's body is able to store 5–10 mg of folate. In humans, diet is the only source of folate. Folate is absorbed in the proximal jejunum. Pregnancy requirements are 800 mcg per day, which is two times the non-pregnant requirement of 400 mcg. Anemia from folate deficiency typically presents in the third trimester. Two trials reviewing folate deficiency were not able to show a measurable effect on pregnancy outcome (9).

Vitamin B12 is readily obtained from the diet and stored in the liver. Typically, most people have 2–3 years of storage. Vitamin B12 deficiency (a megaloblastic anemia) is rare in pregnancy as deficiency is typically associated with infertility.

Other causes of anemia should be investigated as well. The microcytic anemias including sickle cell disease (SCD) and B-thalassemia can cause maternal and fetal complications in pregnancy even if the patient is asymptomatic.

SCD is actually a group of conditions that result from an autosomal recessive inheritance of the "sickle" gene (2). This gene produces abnormal hemoglobin due to an amino acid substitution on the beta globin gene, allowing valine to replace glutamic acid at the sixth position forming hemoglobin S rather than hemoglobin A. This causes complex polymers to form red blood cells with abnormal shapes (2). These abnormal red blood cells are more fragile and are held together with weaker bonds, causing a shorter life span of the red blood cells (less than 25 days versus the 120 days of a normal red blood cell). This explains the anemia that is seen in individuals with SCD. Transfusion is recommended if the hemoglobin falls below 6 g/dL (1). The bone marrow cannot keep up with the red cell demands despite an increase in erythropoiesis. According to the World Health Organization, SCD is the most common inherited condition across the world. It has been estimated that over 300,000 children are born each year affected by a hemoglobinopathy (70% of these are due to SCD). Two hundred and fifty million people (4.5% of the population) carry a gene for hemglobinopathy. SCD is found more commonly in individuals whose background is from a tropical area like sub-Saharan Africa, India, and the Caribbean, as well as the Middle East (2). Pregnant women with SCD are considered higher risk and can encounter more medical problems. They should be managed with multidisciplinary team to ensure the best care. SCD is associated with increased infections and thrombotic events as well as increased incidence of eclampsia, intrauterine fetal death, and spontaneous abortion (2). Treatment of SCD should be early and aggressive and is typically accomplished with intravenous hydration, supplemental oxygen, and pain control. Vaso-occlusive crisis, acute chest syndrome, and organ failure can occur and require hospitalization (1).

Finally, aplastic anemia can occur but is rare. This is diagnosed during pregnancy when pancytopenia and diminished bone marrow function are present. This can be treated conservatively with intravenous immunoglobulin (IVIG) and glucocorticoids. There is no evidence that this type of anemia can be transferred to the fetus, but it does tend to recur in subsequent pregnancies.

Thrombocytopenia

Thrombocytopenia is also common during pregnancy. Rates are 8 to 10% (1). Throbocytopenia is typically due to physiologic changes, which lead to an increase in blood volume, platelet activation, and platelet clearance. If the thrombocytopenia is not physiologic, further workup should be completed. The workup should include review of the blood smear, complete blood cell count, reticulocyte count, direct antiglobulin test, liver function tests, thyroid function tests, antiphospholipid antibodies, lupus serology, viral screening, and testing for von Willebrand disease (VWD). Bone marrow biopsies are not usually required (1). The most common causes are gestational thrombocytopenia, immune thrombocytopenia, and preeclampsia (3).

Most cases are due to gestational thrombocytopenia. This is diagnosed in 5% of pregnancies. Typically, patients are asymptomatic. The drop in platelets tends to occur later in the pregnancy (late second or third trimester). In gestational thrombocytopenia, the drop in platelets is less severe, and levels rarely fall below 70,000 (9). Most cases are considered mild with platelet counts of 100,000 to 150,000. There is not a test for this and this is typically a diagnosis of exclusion (3). A return to normal platelet levels follows delivery and there is no association with low fetal platelets.

The second most common diagnosis for thrombocytopenia is ITP. This accounts for 3–4% of cases (10). ITP can be diagnosed any time during the pregnancy, but it typically presents in the first and early second trimester. About a third of cases are diagnosed during pregnancy, while the other two-thirds are found in patients with disease, which presents outside of pregnancy (3). The findings of low platelets (count that drops below 80,000) at the beginning of pregnancy should prompt an evaluation for ITP. Findings on the blood smear usually will show large or normal platelets. Testing for antiplatelet antibodies has not been shown to be beneficial as a sensitive or specific test. Approximately two-thirds of patients do not require treatment. Patients with a history of ITP prior to pregnancy rarely require treatment and they usually need only close observation. Treatment is targeted at severity of the platelet drop, although there is no data to recommend a specific threshold to start treatment. During the first and second trimester, treatment with corticosteroids and/or intravenous immunoglobulin (IVIG) is indicated if the platelet count falls below 30,000, bleeding occurs, or a procedure is planned. In the third trimester, the platelet count may continue to fall and treatment with steroids or IVIG can be indicated. Both of these medications are considered safe during pregnancy, but the risks and benefits must be considered prior to beginning treatment (1). The route of delivery should not be based on the platelet count but on obstetric indications. For pain control, the option of regional anesthesia can still be considered for platelet counts above 80,000–100,000 depending on the comfort level of the anesthesiologist. Patients with thrombocytopenia that does not respond to steroids or IVIG may require splenectomy. This procedure can be performed safely during both the second and third trimester. The first trimester should be avoided due to increased risk of pregnancy loss (11). The use of azathioprine has been described, but no studies have been performed in pregnancy (1). Fetal platelet counts are rarely affected by ITP and newborn platelet counts can be monitored for 5–7 days following delivery for any abnormalities. When the platelet count falls below 50,000 and there are no obstetric complications noted, the diagnosis of ITP can be made (3). See Table 40.2 for details.

Fetal thrombocytopenia caused by neonatal alloimmunization is seen in one to two cases per 1,000 deliveries (10). This develops in utero and can be diagnosed when prenatal ultrasound shows an intracranial hemorrhage.

Preeclampsia is defined as proteinuria and hypertension that presents after 20 weeks gestation. Approximately 20–50% of cases of preeclampsia will be complicated by low platelets. The etiology of this type of thrombocytopenia is not known. The severity of the thrombocytopenia tends to correlate with the severity of preeclampsia. A platelet count of less than 50,000 is considered severe and occurs in less than 5% of pregnancies complicated by preeclampsia. Treatment for preeclampsia is delivery if the gestational age is greater than 34 weeks.

In 10% of women with preeclampsia, hemolysis, elevated liver enzymes, and low platelets (HELLP syndrome) can occur. HELLP syndrome can be diagnosed by the presence of a microangiopathic anemia, elevated lactate dehydrogenase (LDH>600 U/mL), increased aspartate aminotransferase (AST> 70U/mL), and thrombocytopenia (platelet count <100,000/uL) (1). Patients may be asymptomatic, but common symptoms include malaise, right upper quadrant

Table 40.2 Thrombocytopenia

Gestational	ITP
Asymptomatic	Asymptomatic
Diagnosed in third trimester	Occurs at any time, typically first trimester
Less severe, rarely requires treatment	Can be severe, treat if severe, procedure needed, bleeding risk is high Treat with steroids, IVIG If refractory to above, splenectomy
Resolves postpartum	Resolves postpartum, may recur
No fetal effects	Rarely fetal effects

pain, nausea. The right upper quadrant pain is due to obstruction of blood flow in the hepatic sinuses. The treatment for HELLP syndrome is delivery, keeping in mind that patient status may continue to deteriorate for 24–48 hours following delivery. The use of steroids to increase the platelet count has been reported. Twenty percent of cases occur postpartum.

A disorder known as thrombotic thrombocytopenic purpura (TTP) is difficult to distinguish this from HELLP syndrome and can often be diagnosed only after the platelet count remains low for several weeks following delivery. TTP should be treated aggressively as maternal deterioration can rapidly occur. Delivery is indicated and plasma exchange has been used. Maternal complications can include renal failure and neurological damage.

Acute fatty liver of pregnancy (AFLP) is rare and a potentially fatal complication. This occurs in 1/10,000 to 1/15,000 pregnancies. AFLP presents in the third trimester typically between 27 and 40 weeks. The patient presents with symptoms similar to preeclampsia, which include malaise, anorexia, nausea, vomiting, headache, jaundice, and right upper quadrant or epigastric pain. Lab studies may show a CBC with hemoconcentration, normal to low platelets, low fibrinogen, prolonged PT, increased liver function tests including bilirubin, metabolic acidosis with increased creatinine and uric acid, and increased ammonia levels. The standard for diagnosis is liver biopsy but this is rarely done. The goal is timely diagnosis and treatment for the affected mom. Most patients start to improve two the three days after delivery (12).

Thrombosis

Pregnancy is a prothrombotic state and with that comes an increased potential for clots formation (9). Pregnancy requires changes in normal physiology to allow for the hemostatic balance that (1) permits implantation and invasion of spiral arterioles to occur without hemorrhage, (2) results in uteroplacental blood flow maintenance during the third stage of labor, and (3) ultimately causes bleeding to stop once the placenta has separated. This translates to a system that encompasses (a) increased potential to clot, (b) decreased anticoagulant activity, and (c) decreased fibrinolysis. These changes cause the risk of venous thromboembolism (VTE) to increase in pregnancy and can lead to intensified risks of maternal mortality. The VTE risk increases as pregnancy progresses and peaks in the weeks immediately following delivery. According to the MEGA study, a large population-based study, the risk of VTE was increased fivefold during pregnancy and increased to 60-fold for the three months following delivery (13). These increases can be explained by Virchow's triad. Virchow's triad is composed of hypercoagulability, stasis, and endothelial damage. During pregnancy, the increased risk of clotting (hypercoagulable state) is caused by increased clotting factors, impaired breakdown of fibrin, a fall in free protein S, and acquired resistance to activated protein C. Next, venous stasis in the lower extremities is found due to compression of the vena cava and pelvic veins by the enlarging uterus. Finally, endothelial damage is noted during vaginal delivery or cesarean section (1). These factors, in addition to increased venous capacitance, increased insulin resistance, and hyperlipidemia lead to a VTE risk during pregnancy of 1/1,600 births. The majority of VTEs in pregnancy occur on the left side and are ileofemoral due to compression by the gravid uterus on the left iliac vein. The risk for VTE is highest during the first 20 weeks of the pregnancy (and then peaks again postpartum); therefore, those patients who will benefit from prophylaxis should receive medication during the first trimester if possible (4). Prophylactic treatment can be accomplished with either low molecular weight heparin (Enoxaparin, 40 mg subcutaneously once daily for example) or unfractionated heparin (5,000–10,000 units subcutaneously every 12 hours) (4). See Table 40.3 for more details.

Some other risk factors include smoking, prior VTE, obesity, and immobility. Certain conditions during pregnancy can also increase the risk of VTE and include multiple gestations, preeclampsia, bleeding complications, and techniques used in reproductive

Table 40.3 Prophylactic Anticoagulation

Low molecular weight heparin	Enoxaparin, 40 mg SQ daily
	Dalteparin, 5,000 units SQ daily
	Tinzaparin, 4,500 units SQ daily
Unfractionated heparin	UFH, 5,000–7,500 units SQ every 12 hours, first trimester
	UFH, 7,500–10,000 units SQ every 12 hours, second trimester
	UFH, 10,000 units SQ every 12 hours, third trimester

Source: Reference (4)

assistance. Due to the increased maternal mortality associated with VTE, prompt diagnosis and treatment are imperative. Symptoms of deep vein thrombosis (DVT) include swelling, pain and/or redness in an extremity, more commonly a lower extremity (2).

The first line test for diagnosis remains compression duplex ultrasound of the suspected area but this does not diagnose a clot 100% of the time. If index of suspicion is high and duplex ultrasound is negative, magnetic resonance venography, contrast venography, or pulsed Doppler may be used as well. In the non-pregnant patient, measurement of a D-dimer value can help make the diagnosis, but this is not useful in pregnancy as the D-dimer levels are commonly elevated during pregnancy (6).

Pulmonary embolus (PE) can be harder to diagnose during pregnancy as diagnosis requires imaging and thus exposure of the fetus to some radiation. Symptoms of PE include chest pain, shortness of breath, tachycardia, and if severe, hemodynamic instability (2). The preferred test during pregnancy is ventilation/perfusion (V/Q) lung scan as less radiation is used. V/Q scan is preferred over computed tomography pulmonary angiography (CTPA) (1). Prompt diagnosis is critically important, so regardless of the type of testing used it should be done expeditiously.

Heparin is the treatment of choice for VTE and PE. The preferred medication is low-molecular-weight heparin (LMWH) given as twice daily dosing that is weight based. Enoxaparin can be dosed at 1 mg/kg every 12 hours (4). This should be continued until 6 weeks postpartum. LMWH is typically preferred over unfractionated heparin (UFH) because it has fewer side effects and is more efficacious (14). UFH has been linked with heparin-induced thrombocytopenia. The use of anti-Xa levels to adjust dosing of LMWH is controversial as the therapeutic range is not well-defined, and adjustment of dosage to maintain a certain range has not changed outcomes. Patients should be changed to UFH in the final weeks leading up to delivery as PTT levels can be followed and the half-life of UFH is shorter than the half-life of LMWH.

Patients on anticoagulant therapy may benefit from scheduled induction to reduce bleeding risks during delivery and control the timing of the last dose of heparin. If labor begins spontaneously prior to induction, the patient is advised to skip her next dose of heparin. As long as at least 4 hours have passed for the patient on prophylactic heparin, vaginal, or cesarean delivery can occur with only minimal risk of bleeding complications (4). Regional anesthesia can be used if the timing of the last dose of LMWH is greater than 24 hours after a therapeutic dose or 12 hours after a prophylactic dose. Protamine sulfate can be used if rapid reversal of UFH or LMWH is needed to reverse the anticoagulant effects of these medications.

Vitamin K antagonists (such as warfarin) cross the placenta and are teratogenic, and therefore should not be used. If a patient becomes pregnant on a vitamin K antagonist, she should be changed to heparin prior to 6 weeks gestation to avoid damage to the developing embryo (14). Vitamin K antagonists and UFH can be used safely during breastfeeding as only very small amounts have been found in breast milk. Oral thrombin inhibitors and anti-Xa inhibitors are newer and should be avoided in pregnancy as they have not been tested in this patient population (4).

Thrombophilia

Inherited disorders are known to cause 50% of VTE, PE, and stroke cases during pregnancy. Only limited evidence exists to guide practitioners in the screening for and management of thrombophilia disorders during pregnancy. A correlation exists between inherited thrombophilias and VTE, but it is unclear whether they are linked to other adverse events such as uteroplacental issues including fetal loss, preeclampsia, intrauterine growth restriction (IUGR), or abruption. This correlation has led to increased screening for these thrombophilias without a clear or proven link or benefit. According to the American Congress of Obstetrics and Gynecology (ACOG), screening remains controversial and should be done in situations where the results would affect management. This would include "a personal history of venous thromboembolism that was associated with a nonrecurrent risk factor (e.g. fractures, surgery, and prolonged immobilization)," or "A first-degree relative with a history of high-risk thrombophilia." Testing is *not* recommended for patients with recurrent pregnancy loss as it is not clear if treating with anticoagulation actually reduces risks. If testing is indicated, it should be done at least 6 weeks following the thrombotic event and not during a pregnancy. Testing ideally would occur when the individual is *not* on anti-coagulation medication. The exception to this is screening for antiphospholipid antibodies (APA) in the setting of recurrent pregnancy loss (15). Studies have shown that in women with recurrent pregnancy loss, APA syndrome has been linked to 20% of these losses. If untreated 90% of women with APA will experience fetal loss (9).

Factor V Leiden (FVL) is an inherited thrombophilia with a prevalence of 5% in European populations and 3% of African Americans who are not recent immigrants. It is the most common inherited thrombophilia (4). This mutation is not commonly seen in Chinese, Japanese, other Asians, and Black Africans. The mutation found in FVL does not allow FVL to be lysed by activated protein C. Women who are heterozygous for FVL account for about 40% of VTE in pregnancy. For patients with no personal history of VTE or a first degree relative with a previous thrombotic event, however, the risk is about 5–12/1,000 deliveries. This risk does increase to 10% if the patient has a personal history of DVT.

Prothrombin G20210 is the second most commonly diagnosed thrombophilia. This is caused by a point mutation that causes elevated prothrombin levels. This is seen in 3% of European populations and accounts for 17% of VTE that are diagnosed during pregnancy. Patients with a history of VTE in the past who are carriers have a risk of 10% during pregnancy. Patients with no history of VTE who are heterozygous carriers have a risk of less than 1%. Patients with no history of VTE, who are homozygous carriers, have a risk during pregnancy of 2–3%. If a patient is a carrier of both FVL and Prothrombin, her overall hypercoagulable risk is increased. Such a patient would carry a 4–5% risk regardless of personal history (4).

Antithrombin deficiency is rare and is noted to be extremely thrombogenic. About 250 different mutations associated with this disorder are known to decrease gene transcription. This leads to a decreased antigen level and activity, which alters the structure and function and can thus lead to a normal antigen level with decreased antithrombin activity. Antithrombin deficiency affects about 1/2500 people. The non-pregnant patient has a risk of VTE that is increased 25-fold over the general population and the pregnant state further increases this risk. Most patients seen with antithrombin deficiency have a heterozygous condition; patients who are homozygous for this deficiency have little to no antithrombin activity. Homozygous antithrombin deficiency is quite rare (4).

Protein C and protein S deficiency can also be seen. Protein C deficiency is linked to greater than 160 different mutations, which translate to a prevalence of 0.2–0.3% of the population. Patients with a personal or family history have a VTE risk of 2–7% during pregnancy (4). This deficiency can be screened for during pregnancy. Conversely, Protein S deficiency cannot be accurately screened for during pregnancy and testing for this should be done at least 6 weeks postpartum if possible. This deficiency can be due to reduced free protein S antigen levels and activity, which is due to a silenced gene or a gene mutation. Patients with a personal or family history have a VTE risk of 6–7% during pregnancy. Homozygous carriers of both of these can lead to a condition in newborns known as neonatal purpural fulminans, which requires lifetime anticoagulation.

Methylene tetrahydrofolate reductase (MTHFR) mutations have also been studied and were once thought to cause an increased incidence of VTE. It is now known that this mutation alone does not independently increase the risk of VTE. An increase

Table 40.4 Thrombophilia Testing

Thrombophilia	Laboratory Test	Testing During Pregnancy?	Testing During Acute Event?	Testing While on Anti-coagulation?
Factor V Leiden	Activated protein C resistance assay (if abnormal check DNA analysis)	Yes	Yes	No
Prothrombin G20210A mutation	DNA analysis	Yes	Yes	Yes
Protein C deficiency	Protein C activity	Yes	No	No
Protein S deficiency	Functional assay	No[a]	No	No
Antithrombin deficiency	Antithrombin activity	Yes	No	No

[a] If screening needs to be done, free protein S antigen levels of less than 30% in the second trimester, and less than 24% in the third trimester have been set (4).

in homocysteine level is now thought to be a weak risk factor for VTE rather than the modest risk that was presumed in the past. Because of this, evidence appears to be insufficient to recommend screening for this or checking fasting homocysteine levels. An increased level of homocysteine is most commonly due to a homozygous MTHFR mutation. Carriers of homozygous MTHFR C677T and A1298C are seen in 10–16% and 4–6%, respectively (4).

Other more rare thrombophilias include additional mutations on the factor V gene, promoter mutation in the PAI-1 gene, protein Z deficiency, and activity-enhancing mutations in various clotting factor genes. Table 40.4 provides information on thrombophilia testing.

Inherited Bleeding Disorders

Women with inherited bleeding disorders are at an increased risk for bleeding during pregnancy. In the first trimester, bleeding can occur due to a spontaneous miscarriage, implantation bleeding, pregnancy termination, or invasive prenatal diagnostic procedures such as chorionic villus sampling (CVS) or amniocentesis. Bleeding between 24 weeks until just before delivery occurs for about 3–5% of patients with inherited bleeding disorders. This bleeding can be attributed to placental abruption, placenta previa, and vaginal or cervical lesions (5). The care of these patients should involve a multidisciplinary team. Risk for passing on the genetic defect to the fetus depends on the pregnant woman's carrier status and specific disease. Hemophilia A and B, VWD, and factor VII and factor XI deficiency account for 90% of the inherited bleeding disorders.

Hemophilia A and B are X-linked recessive bleeding disorders. Carriers have factor levels that are 50% of normal. In hemophilia A, factor VIII is reduced, while in hemophilia B factor IX is reduced. Baseline factors should be checked at the beginning of the pregnancy, at 28 weeks gestation, and again at 34–36 weeks gestation. Pregnancy will usually lead to normal factor VIII levels, while factor IX is not changed during pregnancy. Invasive testing is the only way to determine if a male fetus is affected when the pregnant woman is a carrier. CVS can be done between 11 and 14 weeks; amniocentesis can be done after 15 weeks (5). The gender of the fetus should be determined to guide delivery planning. Controversy exists regarding route of delivery, but consensus exists that instrumental delivery should be avoided as cranial hemorrhage (cephalohematoma) is a common result of bleeding in affected infants. Many experts report cesarean section as the preferred route of delivery in a patient who is a carrier with a known male fetus (5). Regional anesthesia can be used if factor levels are in a safe range or can be corrected. Intramuscular injections for the newborn should be delayed until the hemophilia testing has been done. Testing should be done on cord blood to avoid bruising or bleeding. The factor levels in the patient must be followed for several days after delivery to ensure that factors do not require replacement. Postpartum hemorrhage risk (rate=22%) is increased both early and late in hemophilia A carriers as factor VIII levels are used up following delivery. Bleeding after delivery should be closely monitored (10).

VWD is an autosomal dominant disorder due to a quantitative or qualitative defect in von Willebrand factor (VWF); three types exist. Women tend to be affected than men given bleeding symptoms such as menorrhagia and postpartum hemorrhage (9). VWF does increase during pregnancy. In normal patients and those with type 1 and 2 VWD, factor VIII levels rise, with the biggest rise noted in the third trimester. Because of these rises, type 1 and type 2 patients will rarely need prophylactic VWF products. This does not hold true for type 3. Type 3 patients will need infusion of plasma-derived VWF containing product at delivery. A typical dose is 40–80 IU/kg and this is followed by 20–40 IU/kg daily for a week. The dose can be tapered over several weeks (10). Patients with type 1 and 2 VWD are at an increased risk of postpartum hemorrhage as factors can fall rapidly at delivery. This risk can be as high as 13–29%. Patients with type 1 VWD should have a factor VIII level checked late in the third trimester and for 1 to 2 weeks postpartum because of this risk. Patients with type 2 can also develop thrombocytopenia late in pregnancy and should have platelet levels monitored for (9).

Disseminated Intravascular Coagulation (DIC)

Several disorders specific to pregnancy can lead to this dangerous bleeding disorder including a dead fetus, placental abruption, and rarely amniotic fluid embolism (AFE) (9). Intrauterine fetal demise can trigger tissue factor release from dead fetal tissue in the maternal circulation, which can trigger DIC. This is not typically seen until the fetus has been expired for 3–4 weeks. If the fetus has been expired for 5 weeks or more, disseminated intravascular coagulation has been reported up to 50% of the time. The severity of DIC associated with placental abruption is related to the degree of placental separation. These patients require rapid recognition followed by volume resuscitation, delivery, and correction of the DIC with blood products. In AFE, DIC is thought to be caused by the deposit of the procoagulant properties of the amniotic fluid into the maternal pulmonary circulation. This leads to a secondary fibrinolytic response. Maternal death due to AFE was noted 86% of the time in 1979, but improved to <30% by 1994 due to better supportive therapy (9).

Concluding Remarks

Pregnancy causes several physiologic changes that directly impact hematologic parameters. This chapter covered the most common disorders and outlined how they are affected by pregnancy and how they affect pregnancy including various anemias, inherited and acquired thrombocytopenias, thrombosis, VTE, PE, thrombophilias, SCD, VWD, and DIC. A thorough understanding of these disorders will allow the care giver to provide excellent care and anticipate any obstacles encountered along the way.

References

1. Townsley DM. Hematologic complications of pregnancy. *Seminars in Hematology* 2013 July;50 (3):221–231.
2. Koh M, Lao ZT, Rhodes E. Managing haematological disorders during pregnancy. *Best Practice & Research Clinical Obstetrics and Gynaecology* 2013;27:855–858.
3. Stasi R. How to approach thrombocytopenia. *American Society of Hematology* 2012;191–197.
4. Lockwood C, Wendel G, Silverman N. ACOG Practice Bulletin No. 138: Inherited thrombophilias in pregnancy. Clinical Management Guidelines for Obstetrician-Gynecologists Practice Bulletin 2014 September. *Obstetrics & Gynecology* 2013 September;122(3):706–716.
5. Kadir RA, Davies J, Winikoff R, Pollard D, Peyvandi F, Garagiola I, et al. Pregnancy complications and obstetric care in women with inherited bleeding disorders. *Haemophilia* 2013 August 30;19(4):1–9.
6. Bauer KA. Hematologic changes in pregnancy. October, 2015; Available at: uptodate.com. Accessed November 13, 2015.
7. Recommendations to Prevent and Control Iron Deficiency in the United States. *CDC MMWR* 1998 April 3;47(RR-3):1–36.
8. World Health Organizations. WHO: Iron deficiency anaemia assessment, prevention and control. A guide for programme managers. 2001; Available at: www.who.nutrition/publications/en/ida/assessments_prevention_control.pdf. Accessed February 29, 2016.
9. Mims M, Prchal J. Chapter 7. Hematology during pregnancy. In: Lichtmann M, Kaushanksy K, editors. *Williams Hematology*, 8th edition; New York: McGraw-Hill, 2010.
10. Karanth L, Kanagasabai S, Abas A. Maternal and foetal outcomes following natural vaginal versus caesarean section (c-section) delivery in women with bleeding disorders and carriers (Review). *The Cochrane Collaboration* 2015;4:2–4.
11. Griffiths J, Sia W, Shapiro AM, Tataryn I, Turner AR. Laparoscopic splenectomy in a pregnant patient with immune thrombocytopenic purpura. *J Obstet Gynaecol Can* 2005;27(8):771–774.
12. Sibai BM. Imitators of severe preeclampsia. *Obstet Gynecol* 2007 April;109(4):956–966.
13. Pomp ER, Lenselink AM, Rosendaal FR, Doggen CJ. Pregnancy, the postpartum period and prothrombotic defects: risk of venous thrombosis in the MEGA study. *J Thromb Haemost* 2008 April;6(4):632–637.
14. Bates SM, Greer IA, Middeldorp S, Veenstra DL, Prabulos AM, Vandvik PO. VTE, thrombophilia, antithrombotic therapy, and pregnancy. Antithrombotic Therapy and Prevention of Thromobosis, 9th edition. American College of Chest Physicians Evidence-Based Clinical Practice Guidelines. *Chest* 2012 February 141(2 Suppl): e691S–736S.
15. Davenport WB, Kutteh WH. Inherited Thrombophilias and adverse pregnancy outcomes. *Obstet Gynecol Clin N Am* 2014;41:133–144.

Gastrointestinal Disorders in Pregnancy

Stephen K. Patrick and Karen M. Schneider

Introduction

Because of anatomic and physiologic changes in the gastrointestinal (GI) tract during pregnancy, GI complaints are common in pregnant women. The majority of women experience some kind of GI disturbance during the course of their pregnancies, most commonly gastroesophageal reflux, constipation, and nausea and vomiting.[1] Other GI disorders including gallbladder disease, irritable bowel syndrome, and infectious diseases are commonly diagnosed and managed by obstetricians. Health care providers must have an understanding of the changes in anatomy and physiology of the GI tract in pregnancy and must be keenly aware of common and unusual GI disorders to evaluate and manage them safely and effectively in the obstetrical patient.

Scope of the Problem

The social and economic impact of gastrointestinal disorders in the United States is tremendous. According to a paper published by Eberhart et al. in *Gastroenterology* in 2009, between 60 and 70 million people in the United States are affected by GI disorders. A determination of the social impact is impossible, but one study from Sander et al. published in the May 2002 edition of *Gastroenterology* states that in the United States in 1998 the "estimated direct costs for all digestive diseases were $85.5 billion." The vast majority of women will complain to their health care providers of one or more of the many benign GI disorders, the most common being nausea, which affects up to 90% of all pregnant women. Vomiting affects over 50% of pregnant women and may simply be caused by pregnancy or may be a symptom of one several more serous GI disorders. Up to 30% of women will present with constipation, over 30% with hemorrhoids, and up to 80% with reflux. Most gastrointestinal disorders in pregnancy only affect the quality of life of the mother; however, others may be life-threatening to the mother and/or the developing fetus. Liver abnormalities such as hepatitis, cholestasis of pregnancy, hepatic dysfunction associated with severe preeclampsia, and fatty liver of pregnancy are certainly less common, but may present with symptoms of one of the common, benign disorders. Therefore, clinicians providing perinatal care must have a thorough understanding of gastrointestinal disorders in pregnancy.

Anatomy and Physiology of the GI Tract

During pregnancy, the enlarging uterus distorts the anatomic positions of the other intraabdominal organs. Relative changes in positions of the stomach, esophagus, small bowel, and colon lead to some of the common GI disturbances and affect preexisting GI disorders. A decrease in overall gastrointestinal motility (with the exception of the stomach) is caused by the elevated progesterone levels associated with pregnancy. Elevated estrogen levels and other hormonal factors may also affect gut motility and increase the transit time of food through the GI tract.[2]

Esophagus: As the pregnant uterus grows, it shifts the esophagus upward until its lower sphincter is pushed into the negative pressure environment of the thoracic cavity. As a result, the pressure in the lower esophagus is decreased and reflux of stomach contents may occur.[3] Esophageal motility is decreased due to slowed peristalsis, an effect of progesterone on the smooth muscle of the esophagus. Additionally, the resting tone of the lower esophageal sphincter is decreased due to the increased progesterone and decreased motilin serum levels associated with pregnancy.[4]

Stomach: The stomach is shifted upward and to the left as the pregnant uterus encroaches on its usual position in the abdominal cavity. Stomach motility is not affected during the course of normal pregnancy, although gastric emptying time is slowed during labor and in patients with hyperemesis gravidarum.[5,6] Studies of gastric acid production and the associated rise or fall in pH during pregnancy have been conflicting. In pregnancy there is an increase in stomach volume and in the production of protective mucus.[7] Because of the alteration in the pressure of the lower esophageal sphincter and the effects of narcotic pain relievers used in the parturient, there is a greater risk of maternal aspiration during labor.

Liver: The liver is pushed upward, posteriorly, and to the right by the enlarging gravid uterus, but its function is not significantly affected by normal pregnancy. The activity levels of the hepatic enzymes lactic dehydrogenase (LDH), aspartate aminotransferase (AST), and alanine aminotransferase (ALT) increase, but remain within the normal non-pregnant ranges during pregnancy. The serum activity of alkaline phosphatase, however, rises significantly in pregnancy due to increases in the placenta and bones. In general, gamma-glutamyl transferase (GGT) activity and serum bilirubin levels – total, free, and conjugated – fall during pregnancy. Total serum bile acid levels do not change during pregnancy and are useful markers in the diagnosis of cholestasis of pregnancy. The serum albumin level begins to fall in the first trimester due to plasma volume expansion.[7]

Gallbladder: The position of the gallbladder shifts with that of the liver as the gravid uterus grows, although this has no significant clinical significance. The motility of the smooth muscle of the wall of the gallbladder is slowed by the increased level of serum progesterone, resulting in biliary stasis. Additionally, an increased amount of cholesterol is produced in bile. Both of these factors increase the risk of formation of cholesterol gallstones.[8]

Pancreas: Not much information is present in the medical literature regarding the changes in the non-endocrine physiology of the pancreas during pregnancy; however, limited data suggests there is an increase in the secretion of pancreatic enzymes and bicarbonate.[9]

Small Bowel: During pregnancy, the small bowel is pushed upward in the abdominal cavity by the growing uterus, although there is no clinical significance in this anatomic shifting. Because of increased serum levels of progesterone and estrogen, there is relaxation of the smooth muscle and a resulting increase in transit time through the small bowel.[10] The increased transit time contributes to GI disorders in pregnancy.

Colon: The colon is affected in several ways during pregnancy. The ascending colon and appendix are progressively pushed upward into the abdominal cavity during pregnancy. The altered position of the appendix may lead to a delay in diagnosing appendicitis in pregnant women. Colonic motility is decreased for several reasons. An increase in the level of serum aldosterone leads to increased water absorption and subsequent decreased transit time in the colon. Progesterone's effect on smooth muscle may play a role in the increased transit time as it does in the gallbladder and small bowel. Finally, the pregnant uterus causes a mass effect particularly on the sigmoid colon; this results in a relative dysfunction in defecation. The mass effect of the uterus also plays a role in the development of hemorrhoids.[11]

Diagnostic Imaging and Procedures of the GI Tract in Pregnancy

When the health care provider orders diagnostic imaging of the GI tract during pregnancy, she or he must be aware of the risks of the imaging procedures to the mother and her developing fetus. In February 2016, the Committee on Obstetric Practice of the American Congress of Obstetricians and Gynecologists (ACOG) published its updated opinion on diagnostic imaging in pregnancy. The imaging techniques of choice for pregnant women are ultrasonography and magnetic resonance imaging (MRI) as they incur no risk to the patient or her developing fetus.[11] Even so, these imaging studies should be ordered only if they significantly impact clinical decision-making while caring for the pregnant patient. Procedures that use x-ray imaging (i.e. computed tomography scans and x-ray imaging) or radioactive contrasts (i.e. radioactive iodine and gadolinium imaging studies) generally do not expose the developing fetus to levels of radiation that cause harm. In the absence of availability of ultrasonography or MRI, other clinically indicated imaging studies involving radiation exposure that will impact clinical decisionmaking should not be withheld from the patient.[12] This includes the use of radioactive contrast media. Diagnostic procedures should not be withheld from the pregnant patient if the procedures are necessary in the diagnosis and treatment of the patient. Endoscopy of both upper and lower GI tract are safe in pregnancy; the major risks to the mother and fetus are associated with the required sedation. Magnetic resonance cholangeopancreatography (MRCP) and endoscopic retrograde cholangeopancreatography (ERCP) are safe when fluoroscopy is used sparingly. Laparoscopic procedures such as appendectomy and cholecystectomy are safe and effective with appropriate maternal and fetal monitoring during the procedure.

Specific Gastrointestinal Disorders

Table 41.1 describes the evaluation and management of acute liver, gallbladder and pancreatic disorders. Table 41.2 reviews laboratory findings in these processes during pregnancy.

Esophageal Disorders

Because of decreased esophageal motility and anatomic changes of the esophagus, new onset and preexisting esophageal disorders are often managed by the prenatal care provider. Except in rare instances, esophageal disorders are not associated with adverse pregnancy outcomes.

Gastroesophageal Reflux Disease

Gastroesophageal reflux disease (GERD) affects up to 80% of pregnant women.[13] The most common symptoms are a burning sensation in the chest, regurgitation of stomach contents, and belching. Only rarely is GERD severe enough in pregnancy to cause problems for the patient or her fetus (see a discussion on esophagitis later). Usually it is an annoyance to the patient and therefore a common compliant to health care providers. The management involves a stepwise approach including lifestyle modifications and pharmacologic therapy.[14] Lifestyle modifications involve elevating the head of the bed, eliminating fatty foods, caffeine, and chocolate from the diet, avoiding eating just before going to bed, and eating frequent but smaller meals. If these measures fail to relieve the symptoms, the patient should be treated medically.

First-line medical therapy is over-the-counter medical treatment. Antacids are safe and effective; the patient should be instructed, however, to avoid bicarbonate-based medications due to the risk of developing maternal and fetal acidosis and maternal fluid retention.[15] The patient should also avoid taking more than the recommended maximum dose of calcium carbonate antacids due to the risk of developing milk-alkali syndrome.[16] If antacids fail, the next options for medical therapy are sucralfate, histamine-2 receptor antagonists and proton pump inhibitors.[14] Sucralfate, a Category B drug, forms a protective layer over the esophageal mucosa relieving the symptoms of GERD. Ranitidine and famotidine are both Category B drugs and are safe and effective H-2 antagonists. Proton pump inhibitors such as lansoprazole, a Category B drug, and omeprazole, a Category C drug, may be considered for treatment. Both H-2 antagonists and proton pump inhibitors (PPIs) reduce the amount of acid produced by the stomach relieving the pain associated with GERD. Patients with intractable GERD may benefit from referral to a gastroenterologist for consultation.

Esophagitis

When a patient presents with unrelenting symptoms of GERD, the health care provider should consider referral the patient to a gastroenterologist for further evaluation. Persistent GERD may lead to erosive esophagitis. Additionally, immunocompromised patients are at risk for *Candida* and CMV esophagitis. Untreated esophagitis may lead to Barrett's esophagus, a risk factor in the development of esophageal cancer. Upper GI endoscopy, which is safe in pregnancy, may be indicated in patients with dysphagia and suspected esophagitis.[17] Treatment of esophagitis is the same as for GERD.

Achalasia

Achalasia is an uncommon disorder of the smooth muscle of the esophagus and the lower esophageal sphincter (LES). The esophagus is dysfunctional and exhibits non-peristaltic contractions, incomplete relaxation of the LES, and increased LES tone resulting in dysphagia and vomiting.[18] Because of the rarity of the disorder, it is not often seen in pregnant women and it is often misdiagnosed as GERD. The decreased motility of the esophagus associated with pregnancy serves to exacerbate this condition

Table 41.1 Evaluation and Management of Acute Liver, Gallbladder, and Pancreatic Disorders

	Acute Viral Hepatitis	Fatty Liver of Pregnancy	Intrahepatic Cholestasis of Pregnancy	Obstructive Cholelithiasis and Acute Cholecystitis	Acute Pancreatitis
Clinical history	Anorexia, nausea, vomiting, low-grade fever, myalgia, right upper quadrant and epigastric pain.	Third trimester, anorexia, nausea, vomiting, malaise, fatigue, headache, and abdominal pain.	Third trimester itching starting with the soles of the feet and the palms of the hands.	Post-prandial right upper quadrant pain, nausea, and vomiting. Fever is present with cholecystitis.	Usually in third trimester, nausea, vomiting, mid epigastric pain referred to the back.
Physical findings	Few findings in acute infection. May have low-grade fever, jaundice, and hepatomegaly depending on the severity of infection.	Febrile, jaundiced, RUQ and epigastric tenderness. May have evidence of preeclampsia/HELLP, encephalopathy, and/or coagulopathy	Physical exam is normal at the onset of symptoms and there is no evidence of a rash. Jaundice may develop later in the course of the disease.	Right upper quadrant tenderness. Murphy's sign is present in cholecystitis. Jaundice may be present.	Fever, tachycardia, abdominal distention, and tenderness.
Imaging	Ultrasonography of the liver and gallbladder to evaluate for gallstones, obstruction, and hepatic lesions.	US, MRI, and CT scanning lack sensitivity and specificity and insufficient for diagnosis. They may help in ruling out other diagnoses.	Not indicated in the evaluation of intrahepatic cholestasis of pregnancy.	Ultrasound of the gallbladder, liver, and ducts. MRCP may be useful if US is inconclusive.	US to evaluate for gallstones. CT or MRI if evidence of pancreatic necrosis.
Lab evaluation	Viral hepatitis panel, liver function studies.	CBC, liver functions, coagulation studies, BUN, creatinine.	Bile acids, cholic/chenodeoxycholic acid ratio, total bilirubin, ALT, AST, PT. PTT, INR.	CBC, liver function panel, amylase, lipase.	CBC, AST, ALT, lipase, amylase, lytes, BUN, LDH, triglycerides, and ABG if dyspneic.
Treatment	Treat based on symptoms and lab abnormalities. Rehydration, antiemetics if indicated.	Early diagnosis, delivery, symptomatic and supportive care.	Ursodeoxycholic acid to control itching and lower bile acids, total bilirubin, and ALT levels. Antihistamines for itching.	Extended spectrum antibiotics for cholecystitis. Cholecystectomy or ERCP for persistent obstruction or failed conservative therapy.	IV hydration, pain control, determine cause, surgical consultation if indicated, calculate Ranson's criteria for survival, fetal monitoring.
Obstetrical implications	Risk of vertical transmission to the fetus.	Increased maternal mortality, multisystem organ failure, IUGR, increased fetal mortality. Immediate delivery.	Maternal risks are low. There is an increased risk of stillbirth. Antenatal testing prior to delivery at 37 weeks.	Uncommon unless acute cholecystitis is associated with sepsis.	Increased maternal mortality, preterm birth, and perinatal demise.

Abbreviations: RUQ – right upper quadrant, US – ultrasound, MRI – magnetic resonance imaging, CT – computed tomography, BUN – blood urea nitrogen, ALT – alanine aminotransferase, AST – aspartate aminotransferase, PT – prothrombin time, PTT – partial thromboplastin time, INR – international normalized ratio, LDH – lactate dehydrogenase, ABG – arterial blood gas.

and may lead to maternal malnutrition and obstetrical complications such as IUGR, preterm labor, and stillbirth. Treatment includes referral to a gastroenterologist, diet modification, and calcium channel blockers to relieve esophageal spasm. In severe cases, total parenteral nutrition, dilation of the esophagus, and/or myotomy of the LES may be required.[19]

Table 41.2 Laboratory Findings in Liver, Gallbladder, and Pancreatic Disorders

	Acute Viral Hepatitis	Fatty Liver of Pregnancy	Intrahepatic Cholestasis of Pregnancy	Obstructive Cholelithiasis and Cholecystitis	Acute Pancreatitis
CBC	May be anemic	Elevated WBC, normal H/H, platelets may be low	Normal	Elevated WBC in cholecystitis.	WBC>12k, elevated Hct
AST and ALT	Extremely elevated	Elevated	Elevated	Mild elevation in cholecystitis. Higher elevation in obstruction.	Usually normal, but elevated in gallstone pancreatitis
LDH	May be elevated but its specificity for liver injury is low	Initially normal, then low as the disease progresses	Normal	Elevated in obstruction.	May be elevated
Electrolytes, BUN, creatinine	Lytes are usually normal unless dehydrated	BUN and creatinine are elevated	Normal	Normal unless there is severe vomiting and dehydration.	Abnormal in severe cases
Bile acids	Elevated	Elevated	Elevated		Normal
Total bilirubin	Elevated in more severe cases	Elevated	Mildly elevated	Elevated with obstruction of hepatic and/or common duct.	Elevated in gallstone pancreatitis
Amylase and lipase	May be elevated in acute severe cases	Elevated in patients with secondary pancreatitis	Normal	Elevated with obstruction of the common duct.	>2–3× normal
Glucose	Hypoglycemia in severe cases	Very low	Normal	Normal	Elevated in severe cases
Coagulation studies	In severe cases INR and PTT are elevated, fibrinogen is low, FSPs are present,	INR and PTT are elevated, fibrinogen is low, FSPs are present,	Normal	Abnormal in prolonged obstruction.	Coagulopathy may be present in severe cases.

Abberviations: CBC – complete bold count, WBC – white blood cell count, H/H – hemoglobiin/hematocrit, Hct – hematocritq.

Hiatal Hernia

The esophagus transits the diaphragm through the esophageal hiatus. When the integrity of the hiatus is compromised, a hiatal hernia may develop allowing the stomach to rise into the thoracic cavity. Although most hiatal hernias are asymptomatic in pregnancy, as the uterus grows and displaces the abdominal contents superiorly, a woman with a previously undiagnosed hernia may develop symptoms. Symptoms mimic those of GERD so the condition is often misdiagnosed. In patients with more severe symptoms of GERD plus chest pain, the diagnosis of hiatal hernia should be considered, and the patient should be referred to a gastroenterologist. Diagnosis is confirmed by endoscopy. Treatment is the same as for GERD; if evidence of incarceration of the abdominal contents through the hernia exists, however, the patient should be referred to a qualified GI surgeon for evaluation.[20]

Mallory–Weiss Tears

Pregnant patients who have intractable vomiting or retching are at risk for tears in the esophageal mucosa, which result in upper GI bleeding. This injury is known as a Mallory–Weiss tear.[21] Patients typically present with acute hematemesis following prolonged vomiting or retching. This condition may occur in patients with hyperemesis gravidarum, gastroenteritis, and other disorders that cause vomiting. Clinicians should have a quick suspicion for the presence of a Mallory–Weiss tear. Management includes stabilization of the patient with intravenous hydration, antiemetics, and evaluation of the underlying cause of the vomiting. Consultation with a gastroenterologist for upper GI endoscopy may be considered. Most patients respond to conservative management; massive bleeding, however, requires aggressive intervention with transfusion and immediate endoscopic or surgical intervention.[22]

Stomach Disorders

Peptic Ulcer Disease

The annual incidence of peptic ulcer disease (PUD) in the United States is around 1.7 per 1,000 population.[23] Pregnancy does not increase the incidence and may have a protective effect.[24] The most common presentation of PUD is a gnawing, postprandial epigastric pain. Duodenal ulcers are a subset of peptic ulcers; their onset of pain is several hours later than other peptic ulcers and they often wake the patient at night. Additional symptoms include heartburn, belching, and bloating. Often patients with PUD report having self-medicated with over-the-counter antacids, H2 antagonists, or PPIs. Risk factors include smoking, chronic use of nonsteroidal anti-inflammatory drugs (NSAIDs), and corticosteroid plus NSAID use. As peptic ulcer disease is associated with *Helicobacter pylori*, evaluation requires *H. pylori* screening. A complete blood count (CBC) is also required to evaluate for potential anemia from a bleeding ulcer. Upper GI endoscopy is the preferred method of diagnosis, but treatment may be initiated based upon symptoms and a positive test for *H. pylori*. In such cases when there is no improvement with treatment, upper GI endoscopy is then indicated. Treatment is with a PPI-based triple therapy; an example therapy is a PPI (i.e. lansoprazole), amoxicillin, and clarithromycin for 7–14 days. After acute treatment, the patient should be maintained on a PPI for up to one year.[25] In the event of treatment failure or recurrence during PPI therapy, the patient should be referred to a gastroenterologist for further evaluation. Misoprostol, a commonly prescribed medication used for the treatment of PUD, is a Category X drug and is absolutely contraindicated for use in pregnant patients with PUD due to its abortifacient and contraction-provoking effects.

Liver Disorders

Viral Hepatitis

Patients with viral hepatitis present with anorexia, nausea, vomiting, low-grade fever, myalgia, jaundice, and right upper quadrant and epigastric pain. The most common cause of jaundice in pregnancy is viral hepatitis; a complete evaluation of the patient, however, is indicated to differentiate gallbladder disease, acute fatty liver of pregnancy, and HELLP syndrome from viral hepatitis. The diagnosis of hepatitis is based upon clinical history, patient risk factors, and physical and laboratory findings. Patients with symptoms should have blood drawn for a viral hepatitis panel, liver function tests, and CBC. Treatment in pregnancy is mainly supportive. Of importance in the obstetrical patient is the concern for vertical transmission of the infecting virus from the mother to the fetus. Vertical transmission of hepatitises A and E is rare as these viruses are transmitted through an oral-fecal route. The hepatitis B virus does not cross the placenta; rather it infects the fetus during delivery or at the time of amniocentesis. The risk of its transmission depends on the viral antigens and antibodies present in the mother. For HBeAg positive mothers, the transmission rate is 70–90%, but the transmission rate drops to 25% for HBeAg negative/HBeAb negative mothers, and 12% for HBeAg negative/anti-HBe positive mothers.[26] For mothers with viremia with hepatitis C the rate of vertical transmission is 4–7%.[27] Hepatitises D and E are rarely transmitted from mother to infant; however, hepatitis G has a vertical transmission rate of 75 to 80%.[28] Regardless of the viral type, the treatment is the same: supportive care. Cesarean delivery is not recommended to reduce the chance of vertical transmission.

Acute Fatty Liver of Pregnancy

Acute fatty liver of pregnancy (AFLP) is one of the liver disorders directly caused by pregnancy. It is a rare condition affecting 1 in 10,000 to 15,000 pregnant women.[29] The cause of the disorder is unknown, but may be related to abnormal metabolism of fatty acids in both the mother and the fetus.[30] The presentation of the patient with AFLP – malaise, anorexia, headache, nausea and vomiting, right upper quadrant pain, fever, and jaundice – is very similar to other liver disorders, including viral hepatitis, HELLP syndrome, and cholestasis of pregnancy. The majority of pregnant women with AFLP present in the third trimester or immediate postpartum period. On physical examination, the patient usually is jaundiced with right upper quadrant or mid epigastric tenderness. Laboratory findings include an elevation of the WBC, ALT, AST, alkaline phosphatase, total and direct bilirubin, INR, PTT, uric acid, BUN, and creatinine. Glucose, fibrinogen, LDH, and platelet count are low.

Some may present with hypertension, multisystem organ failure, and/or coagulopathy; these conditions also seen in patients with preeclampsia and HELLP syndrome. Preeclampsia, HELLP syndrome, and AFLP may be part of a continuum of the same disease process.[31] Patients presenting with preeclampsia and HELLP syndrome usually do not have hypoglycemia and jaundice, two conditions commonly seen in patients with AFLP. Although not necessary to make the diagnosis of AFLP, ultrasound and CT scan may show fatty infiltration of the liver. Patients diagnosed with AFLP require hospital admission, delivery, and intensive supportive care as a delay in delivery may result in the development of multisystem organ failure and maternal and fetal death. The maternal mortality rate is around 18% and the fetal mortality rate is around 23%.[32] In severe cases, patients may develop fulminant, irreversible liver failure requiring liver transplant.

Intrahepatic Cholestasis of Pregnancy

Intrahepatic cholestasis of pregnancy (ICP) is the most common liver disorder caused by pregnancy affecting around 1% of all pregnant women. The cause is likely multifactorial (hormonal, genetic, and environmental), but regardless of the etiology, the end result is an abnormal excretion of bile acids. Because the bile acids are not excreted in a normal manner in AFLP, they accumulate in the skin, causing intense itching.[33] Patients usually present with itching of the palms of the hands and the soles of the feet in the late second or third trimester. The pruritus spreads to the face and trunk as the disease progresses. Physical examination is generally unremarkable, including no evidence of a rash. The patient may exhibit scratch marks as a result of intense itching. Laboratory evaluation to confirm the diagnosis of ICP includes total serum bile acid levels, cholic acid, chenodeoxycholic acid, cholic/chenodeoxycholic acid ratio, total bilirubin, AST, and ALT. The total bile acid levels are elevated, the cholic acid and chenodeoxycholic acid levels are elevated (cholic acid>chenodeoxycholic acid), the cholic/chenodeoxycholic acid ratio is elevated, the total bilirubin, AST, and ALT levels are elevated. The risk of ICP to the mother is solely in the morbidity of the itching. However, for the fetus, there is an increased risk of sudden fetal death, particularly after 36 weeks. The risk of fetal demise is around 11%.[34] Ursodeoxycholic acid is the treatment of choice as it has been proven to improve symptoms and laboratory values.[35] Because of the risk of sudden fetal death, antenatal testing is indicated during medical therapy and delivery is warranted at 37 weeks – sooner if fetal lung maturity is confirmed by amniocentesis. Intrahepatic cholestasis of pregnancy resolves quickly after delivery.

Cirrhosis

Cirrhosis in pregnancy is rare as it causes anovulation and infertility, and it is more commonly diagnosed in women past the reproductive age.[36] Minimal data exists regarding the maternal mortality rate due to cirrhosis, but it has been quoted in the literature as 10.5%.[37] Pregnancy itself does not directly affect cirrhosis, but complications such as esophageal varices, liver failure, ascites and spontaneous bacterial peritonitis, hepatic encephalopathy, splenic artery aneurysm rupture, and postpartum hemorrhage from coagulopathies may complicate the pregnancy.[36] Patients with cirrhosis have an increased risk of spontaneous abortion, preterm labor, maternal and fetal death and should be co-managed with a maternal-fetal medicine specialist and a gastroenterologist.

Pancreatic Disorders

Pancreatitis

The most common cause of pancreatitis in pregnancy is gallstone pancreatitis; less commonly it is caused by alcohol abuse, hyperlipidemia, and hyperparathyroidism.[38] Patients with pancreatitis present with nausea, vomiting, and epigastric pain often referred to the back. Diagnostic evaluation to delineate the underlying cause should include laboratory testing of amylase, lipase, liver functions, lipids, calcium, and electrolytes. Amylase and lipase levels are typically elevated two to three times above normal. Liver functions are abnormal in gallstone pancreatitis; lipids are elevated in pancreatitis caused by hyperlipidemia; calcium is elevated in hyperparathyroidism-related pancreatitis; and electrolyte derangement may occur in any patient diagnosed with pancreatitis. The treatment initially involves identification of the underlying cause along with aggressive electrolyte and fluid replacement. Ultrasound of the liver, gallbladder, and pancreas is indicated to determine the cause of pancreatitis. If gallstones are identified, the common duct should be evaluated for evidence of obstruction. If ultrasound cannot effectively evaluate the common duct, MRCP, ERCP, or even surgery may be indicated. MRCP is diagnostic only whereas ERCP can be used to eliminate the obstruction of the common duct. Both procedures are safe in pregnancy, but measures should be taken to reduce radiation exposure with ERCP. Pregnant women with pancreatitis are at increased risk for preterm delivery, intrauterine growth restriction (IUGR), and fetal demise, so antenatal testing and serial ultrasonography are indicated.

Gallbladder Disorders

Cholelithiasis

As mentioned earlier in this chapter, pregnancy increases the likelihood of gallstone formation. Most women with gallstones are asymptomatic. Some, however, will develop biliary colic, which is characterized by episodic right upper quadrant pain radiating to the back, often occurring after eating. On physical examination, the patient may be jaundiced and have right upper quadrant tenderness and Murphy's sign. Murphy's sign is a physical finding elicited during hands-on or ultrasound examination of the patient's right upper quadrant. If, during inspiration, the patient reports pain as the examiner applies light pressure in the mid-clavicular, subcostal area, Murphy's sign is present. Obstetrical patients presenting with these symptoms and physical findings should be evaluated with ultrasonography of the liver, gallbladder, and bile collecting system. The indicated laboratory testing includes liver function tests, CBC, amylase, and lipase. Patients with intermittent biliary colic may be managed conservatively with narcotics and diet modification. Patients with evidence of obstruction, pancreatitis, or cholangitis require further evaluation with MRCP or ERCP, management of fluids and electrolytes, and possibly antibiotic therapy. In patients who present with recurrent biliary colic in the first and second trimester, consultation with a general surgeon is recommended to consider elective laparoscopic cholecystectomy.[39]

Cholecystitis

Patients with a history of cholelithiasis may develop obstruction and subsequent cholangitis, cholecystitis, or pancreatitis depending on where the obstruction occurs. The clinical presentation is the same as in cholelithiasis plus fever, tachycardia, and diaphoresis. Initial evaluation is the same as for cholelithiasis. Management begins with intravenous hydration, broad spectrum IV antibiotics (i.e. piperacillin/tazobactam or imipenem/cilastatin), antiemetics, narcotic pain relief, and consultations with a gastroenterologist and a general surgeon. Depending on the condition of the patient, MRCP, ERCP, or cholecystectomy may be indicated. Patients with cholecystitis are at risk for preterm delivery so appropriate monitoring should be undertaken during medical and surgical management.

Small Intestine Disorders

Infectious Diarrhea

Infectious diarrhea is the most common cause of diarrhea worldwide. Many different infectious agents are responsible for acute diarrhea. These include viruses such as rotavirus and enterovirus; bacteria such as *Escherichia coli*, *Shigella* spp., *Salmonella* spp., and *Clostridium difficile*; and protozoa such as *Giardia intestinalis*, *Entamoeba histolytica*, and *Cryptosporidium parvum*. Symptoms of infectious diarrheas include nausea, vomiting, abdominal cramping, watery stools, bloody diarrhea, myalgia, and fever. Physical examination is not particularly helpful in determining the cause of the diarrhea. Physical exam will, however, give the health care provider an idea of the patient's hydration status. Since most cases of infectious watery diarrheas are viral and self-limiting, the initial workup should only include an assessment of fluid status, serum electrolytes, and CBC. Treatment should be directed to restore normal hydration, to correct electrolyte imbalances, and to provide symptomatic relief of the diarrhea. Loperamide is commonly used for symptomatic relief.

Patients with bloody diarrhea are evaluated in a fashion similar to watery diarrhea but with the addition of stool microscopy and culture. Microscopy is indicated to look for protozoa, and the culture assess for bacteria.[40] Treatment is the same as for watery diarrhea but should include antimicrobial therapy to cover the most likely infectious agent. Sulfamethoxizole–trimethoprim is a common choice for treatment, but this medication should be avoided if delivery is anticipated due to neonatal risks of jaundice. Metronidazole is a good choice if protozoa are suspected. Risks to the mother and fetus are minimal as long as electrolyte levels are corrected and hydration is maintained.

Irritable Bowel Syndrome

Irritable bowel syndrome (IBS) is one of the most common GI disorders. Patients with IBS present with a constellation of symptoms including abdominal cramps, bloating, and alternating diarrhea, flatulence, and constipation. Unless the patient has more worrisome symptoms such as weight loss, bloody stools, or iron-deficiency anemia, the diagnosis is confirmed by history and a normal physical examination. Patients with a more complicated history should be referred to a gastroenterologist for further evaluation. IBS incurs no significant maternal or fetal morbidity. Treatment is based upon relief of symptoms. The patient with IBS should be instructed to drink more water, take a fiber or polycarbophil compound supplement, and avoid caffeine, legumes, and lactose in the diet.[41,42]

Crohn's Disease

Crohn's disease (CD) is a chronic inflammatory disorder that may affect any part of the GI tract. Patients with CD usually present with a history of the disease. Symptoms include rectal bleeding, fever, weight loss, anorexia, nausea, and vomiting. Physical examination is nonspecific, although mouth or anal lesions may be noted. Laboratory testing is of little value. Diagnostic imaging is limited to MRI and ultrasonography during pregnancy, although these studies are of limited value. Upper and lower GI endoscopy are safe in pregnancy and more likely to render a diagnosis. The disease is characterized by skip ulcerative lesions anywhere along the GI tract.

Dietary modifications and medical therapy are the mainstays of treatment. The most commonly prescribed medications are sulfasalazine, mesalamine, and corticosteroids. These medications are generally considered safe in pregnancy and should not be discontinued so to avoid relapses and complications during pregnancy.[43] Although pregnancy does not affect the course of CD, the disease does have effects on pregnancy. There is an increased risk of spontaneous abortion and preterm birth,[44] and the patient should be assessed for these risks throughout the pregnancy. The pregnant patient with CD should be co-managed with a gastroenterologist during the pregnancy.

Small Bowel Obstruction

Bowel obstruction in pregnancy is rare, but the diagnosis should be considered in any pregnant patient presenting for evaluation of nausea, vomiting, abdominal distention, and absent passage of flatus. The most common cause is abdominal adhesions, so when a patient has a history of abdominal surgery or infection, the diagnosis of obstruction should be entertained in a symptomatic patient. If the health care provider has a high suspicion for bowel obstruction, the patient should undergo the appropriate x-ray, ultrasound, or CT scan imaging and surgical consultation.[45] If bowel obstruction is confirmed, surgery should be considered. Delay in diagnosis and surgical intervention may result in significant maternal and fetal morbidity.

Colon Disorders

Appendicitis

In pregnancy, the position of the appendix changes depending upon the gestational age. As the pregnant uterus grows, the appendix moves upward from its usual anatomic position. Patients with acute appendicitis, one of the most common surgical emergencies diagnosed during pregnancy, present with nausea, vomiting, fever, and first, periumbilical pain followed by right lower quadrant pain. Later in pregnancy, the characteristic finding of tenderness at McBurney's point may shift to a location higher on the right side of the abdomen or the right flank. This makes the diagnosis more challenging.[46]

Prompt diagnosis of appendicitis is required to avoid the risk of appendiceal perforation and maternal sepsis. Appropriate diagnostic imaging should not be withheld during pregnancy if the diagnosis is suspected. Immediate surgical consultation is indicated. Laparoscopic appendectomy is the preferred surgical procedure during pregnancy; this is, however, dependent upon the laparoscopic skills and preference of the surgeon.[47] Regardless of the choice of approach to the appendectomy, maternal and fetal morbidity and mortality are reduced when there is no delay in the decision to perform surgery.

Constipation

Constipation is one of the most common complaints during pregnancy due to increased water absorption, decreased colonic motility, and the pressure effect of the gravid uterus on the sigmoid colon. Patients with uncomplicated constipation of pregnancy may be treated with reassurance, dietary advice (i.e. increase water intake and fiber consumption), and medical therapy for persistent constipation with abdominal discomfort. Medical therapy options include bulk forming agents, stool softeners, lubricant laxatives, osmotic laxatives, and stimulant laxatives.[48] Constipation of pregnancy is not associated with maternal or infant morbidity and mortality. Patients with symptoms beyond the normal constipation of pregnancy should be referred to a gastroenterologist.

Ulcerative Colitis

Ulcerative colitis (UC) is an inflammatory condition of the colon. Patients with this disease characteristically complain of lower abdominal cramping and frequent stools. The stools are often bloody or with mucous discharge. On physical examination, the patient may have fever, tachycardia, and abdominal tenderness. The preferable method of diagnosis is by colonoscopy and mucosal biopsy.

Most pregnant patients with the disease present with a history of UC and may already be on medical treatment. UC is not typically affected by pregnancy; pregnancy may, however, be affected by it. Significantly increased risks of spontaneous abortion and preterm birth have been reported in women with active disease as compared to women with inactive disease at the onset of pregnancy.[49] Treatment with sulfasalazine and corticosteroids have not been shown to affect the already increased spontaneous abortion and preterm birth rates associated with UC. Neonatal outcomes are the same as in healthy women.[49] Women with UC who are considering pregnancy should try to conceive when the disease is in remission, and those who conceive while undergoing medical treatment should continue it throughout the pregnancy. All women with UC should take a folic acid supplement due to malabsorption of this vitamin and because lowered folic acid levels are present in patients taking sulfasalazine.

Anus

Hemorrhoids

Due to the effects of pregnancy on the GI tract, hemorrhoids are a common complaint in pregnant women. Patients with hemorrhoids may complain of constipation, hard stools, blood on the feces or toilet tissue, and anal itching. Hemorrhoids do not affect the fetus, but cause significant consternation in the mother. After ruling out other causes of rectal bleeding, patients may be treated by increasing dietary fiber, prescribing stool softeners, increasing liquid intake, and using anti-hemorrhoidal creams.

Concluding Remarks

Gastrointestinal complaints are common during pregnancy and are usually indicative of one of the many benign discomforts of pregnancy. However, more serious and potentially life-threatening disorders may present with similar symptoms. It is for this reason that health care professionals providing obstetrical care have a thorough understanding of gastrointestinal disorders. Benign conditions may be managed by the perinatal health care provider. However, patients with persistent GI symptoms or preexisting GI disorders should be managed in consultation with an appropriate specialist.

References

1. B. O'Brien, Q. Zhou. Variables related to nausea and vomiting during pregnancy. *Birth*. 1995;22:93–100.
2. A.A. Flick, D.A. Kahn. Chapter 8. Maternal physiology during pregnancy and fetal and early neonatal physiology. In: A.H. DeCherney, L. Nathan, N. Laufer, A.S. Roman, eds. *Current Diagnosis and Treatment: Obstetrics and Gynecology*, 11th ed., New York: McGraw-Hill, 2013.
3. M. Chiloiro, G. Darconza, E. Piccioli, et al. Gastric emptying and orocecal transit time in pregnancy. *J Gastroenterol*. 2001;36:538–543.
4. N.D. Christofides, G.M. Bloom. Decreased plasma motilin concentration in pregnancy. *Br Med J*. 1982;285:1453.
5. E.M. Whitehead, M. Smith, Y. Dean, G. O'Sullivan. An evaluation of gastric emptying times in pregnancy and the puerperium. *Anaesthesia*. 1993;48(1):53–57.
6. B.D. Maes, B. Spitz, Y.F. Ghoos, et al. Gastric emptying in hyperemesis gravidarum and non-dyspeptic pregnancy. *Aliment Pharmacol Ther*. 1999;13:237–243.
7. Y, Bacq. The liver in normal pregnancy. In: *Madame Curie Bioscience Database [Internet]*. Austin, TX: Landes Bioscience; 2000–2013. Available from: http://www.ncbi.nlm.nih.gov/books/NBK6005/.
8. F. Kern Jr, et al. Biliary lipids, bile acids, and gallbladder function in the human female. Effects of pregnancy and the ovulatory cycle. *J Clin Invest*. 1981;68(5):1229–1242.
9. A. Vanagunas, J. Pandolfino. Chapter 30. Gastrointestinal complications in pregnancy. In: J.J. Sciarra, ed. *Gynecology and Obstetrics* (CD ROM), Volumes 1–6, 2004 edition.
10. A. Wald, et al. Effect of pregnancy on gastrointestinal transit. *Dig Dis Sci*. 1982;27(11):1015–1018.
11. A. Vanagunas. Glob. libr. women's med. (ISSN: 1756–2228) 2008; DOI 10.3843/GLOWM.10172.
12. Committee on Obstetric Practice, American College of Obstetricians and Gynecologists. Committee Opinion, Number 656. Guidelines for Diagnostic Imaging During Pregnancy and Lactation. February 2016.

13. Rey E et al. Gastroesophageal reflux symptoms during and after pregnancy: A longitudinal study. *Am J Gastroenterol.* 2007;102:2395–2400.

14. R.A. Ali, L.J. Egan. Gastroesophageal reflux disease in pregnancy. *Best Pract Res Clin Gastroenterol.* 2007;21(5):793–806.

15. U. Mahadevan. Gastrointestinal medications in pregnancy. *Best Pract Res Clin Gastroenterol.* 2007;21(5):849–877.

16. R. Law, C. Maltepe, P. Bozzo, A. Einarson. Treatment of heartburn and acid reflux associated with nausea and vomiting during pregnancy. *Can Fam Phys.* 2010;56(2): 143–144.

17. M.S. Cappell. The safety and efficacy of gastrointestinal endoscopy during pregnancy. *Gastroenterol Clin N Am.* 1998;27(1):37–71.

18. D. Spiliopoulos, M. Spiliopoulos, A. Awala. Esophageal achalasia: An uncommon complication during pregnancy treated conservatively. Case Reports in Obstetrics and Gynecology, vol. 2013, Article ID 639698, 4 pp.

19. W.G. Paterson, R.K. Goyal, F.I. Habib. Esophageal motility disorders. GI Motility online, 2006. doi:10.1038/gimo20. Published May 16, 2006.

20. S. Roman, P.J. Kahrilas. Clinical review: The diagnosis and management of hiatus hernia. *BMJ.* 2014;349:g6154.

21. D.Y. Graham, J.T Schwartz. The spectrum of the Mallory–Weiss tear. *Medicine (Baltimore).* 1978;57(4):307–318.

22. L. Michel, A. Serrano, R.A. Mallory–Weiss syndrome. Evolution of diagnostic and therapeutic patterns over two decades. *Ann Surg.* 1980;192(6), 716–721.

23. J.J.Y. Sung, E.J. Kuipers, H.B. El-Serag. Systematic review: The global incidence and prevalence of peptic ulcer disease. *Aliment Pharmacol Ther.* 2009;29:938–946.

24. M.S. Cappell, et al. Gastric and duodenal ulcers during pregnancy. *Gastroenterol Clin.* 1998;27(1):169–195.

25. W.D. Chey, B.C. Wong. American College of Gastroenterology guideline on the management of *Helicobacter pylori* infection. *Am J Gastroenterol.* 2007;102(8):1808–1825.

26. G. Borgia, M.A. Carleo, G.B. Gaeta, I. Gentile. Hepatitis B in pregnancy. *World J Gastroenterol.* 2012;18(34):4677–4683.

27. E.A. Roberts, L. Yeung. Maternal-infant transmission of hepatitis C virus infection. *Hepatology.* 2002;36(5 suppl 1):S106-S113.

28. R. Wejstål, A. Widell, G. Norkrans. Perinatal transmission of hepatitis G virus (GB virus type C) and hepatitis C virus infections–a comparison. *Clin Infect Dis.* 1999;28(4):816–821.

29. W.J. Watson, J.W. Seeds. Acute fatty liver of pregnancy. *Obstet Gynecol Surv.* 1990;45:585–591.

30. L.L. Bellig. Maternal acute fatty liver of pregnancy and the associated risk for long-chain 3-hydroxyacyl-coenzyme a dehydrogenase (LCHAD) deficiency in infants. *Adv Neonatal Care.* 2004;4(1):26–32.

31. H.H. Ko, E. Yoshida. Acute fatty liver of pregnancy. *Can J Gastroenterol.* 2006;20(1):25–30.

32. B. Sibai, L. Kustermann, J. Velasco. Current understanding of severe preeclampsia, pregnancy-associated hemolytic uremic syndrome, thrombotic thrombocytopenic purpura, hemolysis, elevated liver enzymes, and low platelet syndrome, and postpartum acute renal failure: different clinical syndromes or just different names? *Current Opinion in Nephrology & Hypertension*, 1994 Jul;3(4):436–445.

33. B.A. Mullally, W.F. Hansen. Intrahepatic cholestasis of pregnancy: Review of the literature. *Obstet Gynecol Surv.* 2002;57(1):47–52.

34. N.M. Fisk, G.N. Storey. Fetal outcome in obstetric cholestasis. *Br J Obstet Gynaecol.* 1988;95(11):1137–1143.

35. F. Azzaroli, L. Turco, A. Lisotti, C. Calvanese, G. Mazzella. The pharmacological management of intrahepatic cholestasis of pregnancy. *Curr Clin Pharmacol.* 2011;6(1):12–17.

36. J. Tan, B. Surti, S. Saab. Pregnancy and cirrhosis. *Liver Transpl.* 2008;14:1081–1091.

37. M.M Steven. Pregnancy and liver disease. *Gut.* 1981;22: 592–614.

38. J.J. Eddy, M.D. Gideonsen, J.Y. Song, W.A. Grobman, P. O'Halloran. Pancreatitis in Pregnancy: a 10 year retrospective of 15 Midwest hospitals. *Obstet Gynecol.* 2008;112(5):1075–81.

39. S. Swisher, P. Schmidt, K. Hunt, D. Hiyama, R. Bennison, E. Swisher, J. Thompson. Biliary disease during pregnancy. *Am J Surg.* 1994;168:576–579.

40. A.C. Casburn-Jones, M.J.G. Farthing. Management of infectious diarrhoea. *Gut.* 2004;53(2):296–305.

41. L.J. Brandt, W.D. Chey, A.E. Foxx-Orenstein, L.R. Schiller, P.S. Schoenfeld, B.M. Spiegel, et al. An evidence-based position statement on the management of irritable bowel syndrome. *Am J Gastroenterol.* 2009;104 Suppl 1:S1–35.

42. P.R. Gibson, J. Varney, S. Malakar, J.G. Muir. Food components and irritable bowel syndrome. *Gastroenterology.* 2015;148(6): 1158–1174.e4

43. F.M. Habal, G.R. Greenberg. Safety of 5-aminosalicylic acid (Asacol) in pregnancy. *Am J Gastroenterol.* 1990;85:127.

44. M. Morales, T. Berney, A. Jenny, P. Morel, P. Extermann. Crohn's disease as a risk factor for the outcome of pregnancy. *Hepato-gastroenterology.* 2000;47(36):1595–1598.

45. S. Meyerson, T. Holtz, M. Ehrinpreis, et al. Small bowel obstruction in pregnancy. *Am J Gastroenterol.* 1995;90:299–302.

46. J.B. House, C.L. Bourne, H.M. Seymour, K.L. Brewer. *J Emerg Med.* 2014;46(5):741–744.

47. C. Palanivelu, M. Rangarajan, R. Parthasarathi. Laparoscopic appendectomy in pregnancy: A case series of seven patients. *J Soc Laparoendosc Surg.* 2006;10(3):321–325.

48. M. Trottier, A. Erebara, P. Bozzo. Treating constipation during pregnancy. *Can Family Phys.* 2012;58(8):836–838.

49. O.H. Nielsen, B. Andreasson, S. Bondesen, S. Jarnum. Pregnancy in ulcerative colitis. *Scand J Gastroenterol.* 1983;18(6):735–742.

Selected Endocrine Disorders in Pregnancy

Kenneth K. Chen

Introduction

In this chapter, the complex interactions between the maternal endocrine system and the fetal-placental unit will be explored in detail. These adaptations are extensive and are crucial for pregnancy, delivery and lactation to occur successfully. Disease manifestations can be altered by the pregnancy state and may often be difficult to distinguish from the overlap of symptoms that occur in normal pregnancy. This chapter provides a comprehensive overview of all endocrine disorders as well as normal physiological changes that occur with each endocrine axis during pregnancy.

Scope of the Problem

Endocrine disease is relatively common in pregnancy; thyroid disorders alone affect up to almost 1 in 10 women during pregnancy and in the postpartum period (1). Uncontrolled endocrine disorders in pregnancy, whether poorly controlled preconception or newly diagnosed, are associated with a variety of adverse fetal outcomes and maternal morbidity. Appropriate treatment of preexisting endocrine disorders is an essential part of prenatal care to ensure maternal and fetal well-being.

Thyroid Disease

Thyroid Physiology in Pregnancy

Three major factors alter maternal thyroid physiology in pregnancy. These include significant alterations in iodide physiology, the stimulation of the thyroid by an increase in human chorionic gonadotropin (hCG), and an increase in thyroxine-binding globulin (TBG).

Maternal plasma iodine levels drop in pregnancy due to increased renal clearance as well as an increase in transplacental passage of iodine to the fetus to support fetal thyroid function. To sustain these roles, adequate iodine intake for pregnant and lactating women is estimated at 150–200 mg/day. This is provided to US patients via prenatal vitamins and iodized salt. In world regions with marginal iodine intake and inadequate supplementation, the demands of pregnancy can result in overt iodine deficiency and thyroid enlargement (goiter) as the thyroid gland attempts to produce sufficient thyroid hormone (2).

Structural homology exists between the thyroid-stimulating hormone (TSH) and hCG molecules and their receptors (3). As a result, rising hCG levels during the first trimester cause a transient fall in the TSH level. Conditions that give rise to higher hCG levels (e.g. multiple pregnancies, trophoblastic disease, hyperemesis gravidarum) can result in biochemical derangement, which may otherwise suggest thyrotoxicosis (see more on this condition in the later discussion).

The increase in estrogens produced by the fetal–placental unit stimulates hepatic production of TBG. This increase in TBG results in higher levels of total T4 and T3 but free T4 and free T3 levels remain fairly constant throughout pregnancy (1,4).

Hypothyroidism in Pregnancy

Management of thyroid diseases during pregnancy requires special considerations because pregnancy induces major changes in thyroid function, and maternal thyroid disease can have adverse effects on the pregnancy and the fetus. The avoidance of both maternal and fetal hypothyroidism is of major importance because of potential damage to fetal neural development, an increased incidence of miscarriage, and pre-term delivery (5,6). Universal screening of pregnant women for thyroid disease is not yet supported by adequate studies. Case reports targeted to specific groups of patients who are at increased risk, however, support selected screening (1,7).

Both overt and subclinical hypothyroidism can have adverse impacts on the course of pregnancy or fetal development. Overt hypothyroidism (found in 1% of pregnant women) should be corrected before initiation of pregnancy; preconception levothyroxine (L-T4) dosage should bring the TSH level to <2.5 mU/L (1,7). It is generally recommended that a 25–30% increase in L-T4 dose be prescribed to these women as soon as pregnancy is confirmed in order to reduce the risk of maternal hypothyroidism throughout the first trimester (2,8). Women with subclinical hypothyroidism (serum TSH above the upper reference limit but free T4 [fT4] within the reference limits) should also be treated with T4 replacement as there is some evidence that this is associated with increased rates of pre-term delivery and placental abruption. Also, there is observational evidence demonstrating that women suffering from overt or subclinical hypothyroidism deliver babies with an average intelligence quotient (IQ) score below the mean IQ score of children born to healthy women and women on T4 replacement (9,10). The importance of maternal thyroid hormone replacement is emphasized by the fact that the fetal thyroid does not develop until the second trimester of pregnancy and fetal thyroid hormone production does not become optimal until mid-gestation.

Maintenance of a serum TSH <3.0 mU/L is acceptable in the second and third trimesters of pregnancy. Thyroid function tests can be performed once a trimester and 4–6 weeks after any dose adjustments. Just as it is important to avoid under treatment (with emphasis on fetal neurodevelopment), it is important to avoid overtreatment as this may cause lower birthweights (11). After delivery, the dose of L-T4 therapy can usually be reduced back to the preconception dosage after checking a repeat set of thyroid function tests at the 6-week postpartum visit.

Levothyroxine is safe and appropriate for use in pregnancy. It is advisable to change the treatment for women on other forms of thyroid replacement, such as liothyronine (T3) to T4 as T3 does not cross the placenta. Patients should be advised to take their L-T4 at least 30 minutes before breakfast, and their prenatal vitamins at least 2 hours thereafter. L-T4 is excreted into breast milk, but not at levels sufficient to affect neonatal thyroid function and so breastfeeding can be undertaken as normal.

Hyperthyroidism in Pregnancy

If a suppressed TSH is detected during pregnancy, hyperthyroidism must be distinguished from normal physiology (gestational thyrotoxicosis) and hyperemesis gravidarum because of the potential adverse effects on the mother and fetus. Miscarriage, preterm labor, and fetal growth restriction are some of the adverse outcomes of uncontrolled thyrotoxicosis in pregnancy (12).

Hyperthyroidism in pregnancy is not rare; estimated prevalence is 0.1–0.4% with Graves' disease accounting for 85% of cases and toxic solitary or multiple nodules plus thyroiditis accounting for most of the rest. Hydatidiform molar disease is a very uncommon cause in modern obstetric practice since the advent of dating ultrasounds.

Gestational thyrotoxicosis presents in the mid to late first trimester; hyperemesis is a common symptom. Classical hyperthyroid symptoms are absent or minimal apart from weight loss, which is often the result of malnutrition secondary to vomiting. The suppression in TSH is mediated by rising human chorionic gonadotropin (hCG) levels and therefore gestational thyrotoxicosis will usually self-resolve by mid-gestation at the latest. Approximately 50% of women suffering from hyperemesis have a subnormal TSH and elevated fT4 level. In this setting, the assessment of free triiodothyronine (fT3) level and thyroid stimulating immunoglobulin (TSI) level are helpful as 90% of hyperemesis cases have normal fT3 and most cases of Graves' disease will be TSI positive.

Propylthiouracil (PTU) and methimazole (MMZ) both cross the placenta but can be used in pregnancy. For hyperthyroidism diagnosed during the first trimester, PTU is preferred to MMZ because of the latter's association with congenital abnormalities such as choanal atresia and aplasia cutis. If a woman has been able to control her hyperthyroidism with MMZ prior to pregnancy, however, she should remain on this drug so as to maintain good control. Recent guidelines have recommended switching over therapy from PTU to MMZ at the beginning of the second trimester because of the increased risk of idiosyncratic hepatic reactions with PTU (1,7). Patients should be counseled about the rare but very serious risk of agranulocytosis with both medications. PTU is generally preferred over MMZ in breastfeeding mothers as the passage of MMZ in breast milk is slightly higher. As a clinical response to PTU or MMZ is delayed until the thyroid hormone stored in colloid is used up, β-blockers may be required for a brief period (usually between 2 and 6 weeks) to control the symptoms of thyrotoxicosis.

Therapy should be adjusted to maintain maternal fT4 in the upper non-pregnant reference interval, as overcorrection into the lower reference interval may render the fetus relatively hypothyroid. TSH receptor antibodies can cross the placenta and cause fetal hyperthyroidism in a very small proportion of pregnant women with Graves' disease. If pregnant patients are taking the appropriate dosage of PTU or MMZ, the fetus should be protected from since these medications cross the placenta. Fetal ultrasounds should be performed on a regular basis to assess for fetal tachycardia, hydrops, fetal goiter (see Figure 42.1) and growth restriction. Untreated fetal hyperthyroidism as a result of transplacental passage of antibodies is associated with a mortality rate of up to 15%. After delivery, it is important to continue screening the neonates for neonatal thyrotoxicosis as they will continue to have maternal TSH receptor antibodies for approximately 3 months after birth, but will no longer be receiving any anti-thyroid medications through placental transfer.

Women with well-controlled Graves' disease during pregnancy should be warned about the possibility of postpartum flare-up, which usually occurs between 6 weeks to 6 months postpartum. It is not recommended that radioactive iodine therapy be used during pregnancy and lactation.

Postpartum Thyroiditis

Postpartum, subacute lymphocytic thyroiditis occurs in approximately 8% of all pregnancies (13), usually between 6 weeks and 6 months after delivery, but it can occur up to one year later. The incidence in women with coexistent autoimmune disorders such as type I diabetes mellitus is as high as 25% (14). Women who have positive anti-peroxidase antibodies or those who has had the condition with previous pregnancies have a greater risk of developing postpartum thyroiditis (PPT).

The classic description of PPT includes thyrotoxicosis followed by hypothyroidism. Not all women demonstrate evidence of going through both phases; approximately one-third of patients will manifest both phases, while one-third of patients will have only a thyrotoxic or hypothyroid phase. The thyrotoxic phase tends to occur 1–4 months after delivery of a child, lasts for 1–3 months and is associated with

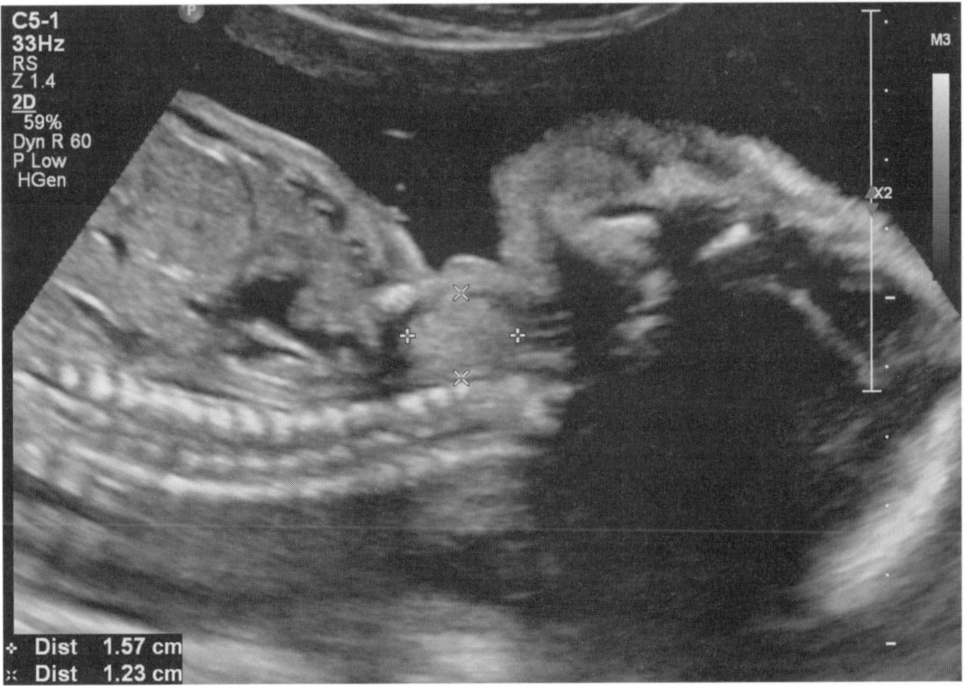

Figure 42.1 A fetal goiter is isolated by the symbols on this ultrasound. Figure courtesy Dr Poonam Charan, Prof. Ricardo Palma Dias, and Dr Elske Posma, Ultrasound Department and Fetal Medicine Unit, Royal Women's Hospital, Melbourne, Australia.

symptoms including anxiety, insomnia, palpitations, fatigue, weight loss, and irritability. Since these symptoms are often attributed to postpartum issues and the stress of having a new baby, the thyrotoxic phase of PPT is often overlooked. However, if the symptoms are brought to the attention of a medical provider, it may be difficult to distinguish the diagnosis between PPT and postpartum flare-up of Graves' disease. If a woman is not breastfeeding, providers may consider an I-131 uptake scan to differentiate between the two differential diagnoses; findings include globally increased uptake for Graves' disease versus globally reduced uptake for PPT.

It is much more common for women to present in the hypothyroid phase, which typically occurs 4–8 months after delivery and may last up to 9–12 months. Typical symptoms include fatigue, weight gain, constipation, dry skin, depression, and poor exercise tolerance. A lot of these women are mistaken for "postpartum depression" in particular. Most women will have return of their thyroid function to normal within 12–18 months of the onset of symptoms. Approximately 20% of those that go into a hypothyroid phase will, however, remain hypothyroid permanently. It is thus very important to continue ongoing monitoring of thyroid function tests so that intervention can occur early.

Thyroid Nodules

The prevalence of thyroid nodules is approximately 4–7% in the general US population. Thyroid nodules are more common in females, and this predisposition exists throughout all age groups. Prevalence increases with age, with spontaneous nodules occurring at a rate of 0.08% per year beginning early in life. Iodine deficiency is another well-documented risk factor. Most solitary thyroid nodules (STN) are benign hyperplastic lesions but 5–20% of these are true malignancies. Previous head and neck radiation exposure is a risk-factor for these malignancies (15).

The effect of pregnancy on the natural history of thyroid cancer is controversial. Some studies have found no apparent effect (16,17), whereas others suggest that there is an increased risk of malignancy in nodules, which develop during pregnancy and that such cancers may be more aggressive (18,19). The intrinsic TSH-like activity of hCG has been postulated to play a role in the progression of cancers found early in gestation (19).

In women of reproductive age, approximately 65% of thyroid malignancies are papillary, 30% are follicular, 3% are medullary, 1% are anaplastic, and 1% are lymphoma or metastases to the thyroid. Diagnosis is made by fine needle aspiration biopsy (FNAB). A diagnosis of medullary or anaplastic carcinoma or lymphoma warrants immediate surgery. Patients with well-differentiated thyroid malignancies could undergo a near total thyroidectomy in the second trimester or following delivery. Adjuvant radioiodine therapy is delayed until the postpartum period; this delay does not seem to alter the prognosis of thyroid carcinoma (20). Patients who have had a history of thyroid cancer should be on thyroid hormone suppression therapy and it is generally recommended to aim for a TSH level of around 0.1 throughout pregnancy.

If a pregnant patient presents with a new onset thyroid nodule, which is rapidly growing, FNAB should be performed immediately. If a thyroid nodule has been there for some time, a thyroid ultrasound could be performed and FNAB can be performed on the lesions that display higher-risk features sonographically (e.g. solid hypoechoic nodules, irregular edges, presence of microcalcifications, concurrent presence of abnormal cervical lymph nodes).

Calcium Metabolism and Parathyroid Disease

Calcium Metabolism

The normal fetal skeleton accumulates approximately 30 g calcium by term, proportional to the fetal weight. The largest proportion (80%) of that accumulation occurs in the third trimester, at a rate of about 250–300 mg/day.

Hyperparathyroidism

Primary hyperparathyroidism is usually diagnosed during pregnancy through routine blood testing following prolonged or extremely severe hyperemesis gravidarum. In some cases, the serendipitous finding of nephrocalcinosis, renal calculi, or excessive calcification of the placenta during fetal ultrasonography provokes diagnosis. Primary hyperparathyroidism is due to the presence of parathyroid adenoma and may occasionally be part of the multiple endocrine neoplasia (MEN-1 or MEN-2a) syndrome. Primary hyperparathyroidism is diagnosed by identifying an elevated serum calcium level together with an elevated parathyroid hormone level. Mild cases may often be overlooked as the serum calcium level may appear normal due to lower albumin levels in pregnancy. Urinary calcium excretion is typically not used as part of the diagnostic evaluation as it is usually increased in normal pregnancy anyhow. Ultrasound is the modality of choice to identify the location of the pituitary adenoma(s) given that radioisotope studies are contraindicated in pregnancy. Maternal hypercalcemia affects the fetus by causing parathyroid suppression.

The incidence of primary hyperparathyroidism in a woman of childbearing age is approximately 1 in 10,000. In pregnancy, hypertension or preeclampsia occurs in up to 25% of cases (21). Maternal mortality may result from pancreatitis or severe acute kidney injury. Significant fetal morbidity with mortality rates of up to 40% occurs when the maternal hypercalcemia is severe (>14 mg/dL). This morbidity is due to the increased risk of stillbirth, IUGR, premature labor, neonatal hypocalcemic tetany, and/or cardiac arrhythmias, which can frequently cause prolonged neonatal intensive care unit (NICU) admissions.

Symptomatic primary hyperparathyroidism is best treated by minimally invasive surgical removal of the parathyroid adenoma during the second trimester after embryogenesis is complete. If surgery is not performed, then it is prudent to keep the patient well hydrated and administration of medications such as calcitonin or bisphosphonates should be considered on a case-by-case basis.

Hypoparathyroidism

Hypoparathyroidism is very rare in pregnancy and may be part of the autoimmune polyglandular syndrome, which is frequently associated with mucocutaneous candidiasis and adrenal insufficiency. It may also be due to surgical removal of all parathyroid glands as part of a total thyroidectomy for thyroid cancer or Graves' disease. Maintenance of normocalcemia involves substantial oral supplementation with calcium and activated vitamin D (calcitriol). The doses of supplementation usually have to be increased particularly in the third trimester as there is high fetal uptake of calcium into the skeleton. It is important to avoid prolonged maternal hypocalcemia as this leads to fetal hypocalcemia, which, in turn, may result in fetal hyperparathyroidism with attendant skeletal demineralization, osteitis fibrosa cystica, or even death (22).

Vitamin D Deficiency

It is well documented that vitamin D has a number of important effects on the mother and fetal–placental unit, via both classical actions (calcium metabolism) and non-classical actions such as promoting insulin action and secretion, immune modulation and fetal lung development.

Currently, it is recommended that all pregnant women should consume 400 IU/day of calcium (23) and high-risk women (those with increased skin pigmentation, reduced exposure to sunlight, those who are immobile or obese) should consume at least 1,000 IU/day in order to reduce maternal complications such as preeclampsia, glucose intolerance, and fetal complications such as low birth weight and childhood allergies (24,25).

It is not current practice to routinely screen all pregnant women for their vitamin D levels. It has, however, been suggested that the following patient groups should have their levels checked early during pregnancy – women with known hypocalcemia, gastrointestinal disease, previous alcohol abuse, previous child with rickets (26). It is well accepted that vitamin D supplementation during pregnancy does not lead to any harm at all (23–25).

Osteoporosis

Transient, focal osteoporosis of the hip is a rare self-limited form of osteoporosis usually found during the third trimester or in the early postpartum period. It is generally unilateral and may present either as pain, limp, or even as an acute fracture. Bone mineral density is diminished at the femoral neck and head, with increased water content in the bone and the marrow. It generally resolves spontaneously within 2–6 months. There is no apparent association with maternal calcium balance. Current theories for this focal condition include femoral venous stasis secondary to compression by the gravid uterus, and fetal pressure on the obturator nerve, which results in reflex sympathetic dystrophy (27).

Fragility fractures during pregnancy and the postpartum period may also be due to preconception low bone density and increased bone turnover state due to pregnancy and lactation. Metabolic conditions such as thyrotoxicosis and primary hyperparathyroidism, malabsorptive disorders such as celiac disease, or chronic therapy with heparin, corticosteroids, or anticonvulsants may all cause secondary osteoporosis.

Pituitary Disease

Pituitary Insufficiency

The differential diagnosis of pituitary insufficiency in the pregnant patient is listed in Box 42.1.

The management of the pregnant woman with preexisting pituitary insufficiency centers on adequate hormonal replacement. In general, thyroid hormone and cortisol requirements increase throughout pregnancy due to increased hepatic production of TBG and cortisol-binding globulin (CBG). It is vital that free T4 (FT4) rather than TSH level is monitored as the latter will always be low in patients with hypopituitarism. Hydrocortisone is generally the preferred glucocorticoid replacement therapy of choice as there is minimal transplacental passage to the fetus. Mineralocorticoid replacement is not required in pituitary insufficiency as the renin–angiotensin–aldosterone axis is intact. Regular obstetrical follow-up with serial ultrasounds to detect IUGR is recommended.

Stress doses of glucocorticoids must be given at the time of labor and delivery; refer to Box 42.2 for recommended doses (28).

Sheehan Syndrome

Sheehan syndrome consists of pituitary necrosis secondary to ischemia occurring within hours of delivery. It is usually secondary to hypotension and shock due to an obstetrical hemorrhage (29). It is uncommon in modern obstetrics, but this diagnosis should be considered in a patient who experiences an obstetrical hemorrhage and then fails either to lactate or who has documented hypoglycemia. Investigation should include levels of FT4, cortisol, and prolactin. Prolactin, in particular, is normally elevated in the immediate postpartum period.

Box 42.1 **Causes of hypopituitarism in the pregnant patient**

Pre-existing before pregnancy

Pituitary adenoma
Vasculitis
Infiltrative disorders (hemochromatosis, sarcoidosis, amyloidosis)
Hypothalamic tumors (craniopharyngiomas, germinoma, meningioma, glioma)
Eosinophilic granuloma (histiocytosis X)
Pituitary apoplexy
Prior surgical or radiotherapy treatment

During pregnancy or postpartum

Lymphocytic hypophysitis/infundibulohypophysitis
Sheehan syndrome (peripartum necrosis)

Box 42.2 **Glucocorticoid stress doses**

1. Hydrocortisone 100 mg IV on call to operating room or at onset of labor
2. Hydrocortisone 100 mg IV q8 h over course of surgery or labor and delivery
3. Hydrocortisone 50 mg IV q8 h day 1 post-operative or postpartum
4. Hydrocortisone 25 mg orally q8 h day 2 post-operative or postpartum
5. Usual pre-admission doses of hydrocortisone orally from day 3 post-operative or postpartum

Lymphocytic Hypophysitis

This condition is autoimmune in nature and is manifested by massive infiltration and destruction of pituitary parenchyma by lymphocytes and plasma cells. It can occur during pregnancy but is particularly prevalent in the postpartum period. It is associated with symptoms of hypopituitarism and/or symptoms relating to an enlarging pituitary gland such as visual field defects and worsening headaches. Treatment is generally conservative and involves identification and correction of any pituitary deficits, particularly that of ACTH secretion (30). There is no evidence that high-dose corticosteroids are of benefit in treating this destructive process. Most patients progress to chronic hypopituitarism.

Prolactinomas

Prolactinomas are the most common pituitary tumors seen in women of reproductive age (31) and are responsible for about one-third of all cases of female infertility (32).

It is uncommon for pregnancy to occur in women with untreated prolactinoma as hyperprolactinemia is associated with infertility. The ability of dopamine agonists to treat hyperprolactinemia restores ovulation in about 90% of patients, many of whom are then able to achieve pregnancy.

Rising estrogen levels during pregnancy have a stimulatory effect on prolactin secretion. This can cause the growth of the adenoma. The risk is much higher for macroadenomas (≥ 10 mm in diameter) compared with microadenomas (< 10 mm in diameter). For this reason, dopamine agonists are always discontinued once pregnancy is confirmed in someone with a microadenoma.

With macroadenomas, dopamine agonists are frequently continued throughout pregnancy in order to prevent tumor growth. Numerous studies have shown that there are no adverse effects on the fetus with the use of bromocriptine. There is much less data on cabergoline. Cabergoline is not favored in pregnancy due to its longer half-life. Some recent studies have linked it to the development of maternal cardiac valve fibrosis (33).

It is recommended that pre-pregnancy baseline visual field testing and MRI imaging of the pituitary be done for women with macroadenomas. These tests should be reviewed on a regular basis throughout gestation for evidence of tumor expansion. This author recommends monthly assessments as well as formal visual field testing every trimester. Magnetic resonance imaging (MRI) of the pituitary is required if tumor enlargement is suspected from the symptoms reported or from any documented changes to the visual fields. There is no role for measuring prolactin levels throughout pregnancy as these levels are known to increase.

In the postpartum period, neonatal suckling has not been shown to stimulate the growth of prolactinomas and so breastfeeding is not discouraged in these women.

Acromegaly

Infertility is common in women with acromegaly, and excess of growth hormone (GH)-associated ovarian dysfunction is often the result of the hyperprolactinemia from pituitary stalk compression; an additional factor is the coexisting polycystic ovary syndrome seen in a number of these patients (34).

Most diagnostic assays are unable to distinguish between pituitary and placental growth hormone, so confirmation of a diagnosis of pituitary growth hormone excess may be delayed until the postpartum period.

Acromegaly can increase the risk of gestational diabetes and gestational hypertension. Associated conditions such as cardiomyopathy and obstructive sleep apnea may manifest for the first time during pregnancy. GH does not cross the placenta, and maternal acromegaly has little direct impact on the fetus. Fetal somatic growth is largely GH-independent, and any macrosomia seen in such pregnancies is likely secondary to maternal glucose intolerance.

Diabetes Insipidus

The development of new onset diabetes insipidus (DI) in the third trimester is usually due to increased vasopressinase activity. This may be caused by either increased placental production or decreased hepatic vasopressinase metabolism due to liver damage from various causes including preeclampsia, acute fatty liver of pregnancy, or HELLP syndrome. This phenomenon is called transient vasopressin-resistant DI of pregnancy.

Preexisting central diabetes insipidus often worsens during pregnancy due to the increased clearance of endogenous vasopressin by increasing levels of vasopressinase. Subclinical central DI can also be unmasked for the first time during pregnancy due to this mechanism.

Vasopressin analogues such as desmopressin (DDAVP) are the treatment of choice for both central DI and transient vasopressin-resistant DI of pregnancy as it is not degraded by vasopressinase.

Thiazide diuretics, also are used for the treatment of nephrogenic diabetes insipidus, are overall considered to be safe during pregnancy. Some case reports of transient oligohydramnios associated with its use do exist (35).

Transient vasopressin-resistant DI of pregnancy tends to resolve within a few days to weeks after delivery. DDAVP transfers minimally into breast milk (36) and is poorly absorbed from the gastrointestinal tract, so its use will not adversely affect an infant's salt/water homeostasis.

Women who have preexisting central DI due to posterior pituitary dysfunction will also have reduced oxytocin production. This has important consequences, as labor may not progress; there is also an increased rate of uterine atony. Conversely, patients on DDAVP therapy who are given oxytocin (Pitocin) for augmentation of labor are at increased risk of developing hyponatremia due to the oxytocin increasing the activity of the vasopressin-2 (V2) receptor.

Adrenal

Adrenal Insufficiency

Primary adrenal insufficiency is most commonly caused by immune-mediated destruction of the adrenal cortex (Addison's disease). Other causes include infection due to tuberculosis (common in the developing world), or hemorrhage affecting both adrenal glands. This diagnosis should always be entertained in patients who have severe lethargy, nausea, and vomiting, which is out of proportion with the normal symptoms of pregnancy. Addisonian hyperpigmentation may be distinguished from chloasma of pregnancy by its presence on mucous membranes and on non-exposed areas. Adrenal antibodies are known to cross the placenta but very rarely result in neonatal disease (37).

Secondary adrenal insufficiency may be caused by pituitary insufficiency or long-term exogenous glucocorticoid therapy which leads to hypothalamic–pituitary–adrenal (HPA) suppression. This is much more common than primary insufficiency. Patients at risk of developing HPA suppression are those who are on a maintenance dosage of prednisone of 5 mg or higher per day, those who have been on courses of prednisone greater than 20 mg per day for at least 3 weeks over the past year, and those who display Cushingoid features.

Normal pregnancy outcomes should be expected as long as the patient takes the appropriate dosages of glucocorticoids and mineralocorticoids; these doses often need to be increased slightly throughout pregnancy as rising progesterone levels act as antagonists to the glucocorticoid and mineralocorticoid receptors. Maternal adrenal insufficiency, which is well treated, has not been known to cause any problems with fetal development.

Hydrocortisone and prednisone are the preferred glucocorticoid replacement agents of choice as their placental passage to the fetus is much lower compared with dexamethasone or betamethasone. Stress doses must always be administered in times of severe hyperemesis or physical stress as well as at the time of labor and delivery; see Box 42.2 for a suggested protocol for stress doses (28).

Pheochromocytoma

This condition, caused by a small catecholamine-secreting tumor, can have profound effects on both mother and fetus. It is important that pheochromocytoma be considered in the differential diagnosis for severe or paroxysmal hypertension in pregnant women particularly in the first half of pregnancy. There is minimal placental transfer of catecholamines (38), but adverse fetal effects are usually a result of catecholamine-induced uteroplacental vasoconstriction and placental insufficiency or even abruption (39). Unrecognized pheochromocytoma is associated with a maternal mortality rate of 50% at induction of anesthesia or during labor (40). The fetal mortality is about 26% in undiagnosed cases and 11% in diagnosed cases.

Fasting plasma metanephrine levels are the most sensitive and specific diagnostic test though it should be noted that baseline levels are slightly increased in pregnancy. Pharmacologic agents such as tricyclic antidepressants, labetalol and methyldopa can cause falsely elevated levels.

Anatomical localization of the tumor is required for definitive treatment once a biochemical diagnosis has been made. In pregnancy, the imaging modality of choice is MRI. Nuclear scanning with metaiodobenzylguanidine (MIBG) is contraindicated in pregnancy. Anatomical localization is also important as a growing, gravid uterus can impact particularly extra-adrenal lesions as they tend to be more influenced by changes in position or by uterine contractions. Physical compression of these lesions can cause hemorrhage into the tumor and/or precipitate a hypertensive crisis.

Medical therapy in the form of alpha-blockade should be initiated once a biochemical diagnosis is made; phenoxybenzamine is considered the agent of choice as it provides long-acting, stable, and non-competitive blockade. Placental transfer of phenoxybenzamine does occur but it is generally considered to be safe (41). Beta-blockade is then instituted after alpha-blockade is achieved to avoid tachyarrhythmias; the dose should be titrated to achieve a maternal heart rate of 80–100 beats per minute. Metoprolol is the preferred agent as other agents such as atenolol have been associated with fetal bradycardia and/or intrauterine fetal growth restriction (42). Hypertensive crises should be treated with phentolamine or nitroprusside. Nitroprusside should be limited due to the risk of fetal cyanide toxicity. It is important to avoid medications that can precipitate a crisis, such as metoclopramide or contrast media.

Surgery in the form of laparoscopic adrenalectomy can be considered once adequate medical therapy and localization of the lesion have been achieved. If the lesion is diagnosed during the first or second trimesters, the best time to operate is during the second trimester. If the lesion is diagnosed during the third trimester, surgery should be delayed until delivery if possible. An elective cesarean section is the delivery method of choice as the process of labor may result in uncontrolled release of catecholamines secondary to pain and uterine contractions.

Primary Hyperaldosteronism

Hypertension with hypokalemia is the classic presentation of hyperaldosteronism although the potassium level may often be normal. This condition is frequently unmasked in the postpartum period as the high progesterone levels during pregnancy antagonize the action of mineralocorticoids on their own receptors.

Both renin and aldosterone levels are increased during pregnancy. Therefore a suppressed renin level may be useful in diagnosing this condition during pregnancy; it should be noted that medications such as beta-blockers and calcium channel blockers (which suppress renin) levels need to be discontinued for at least 2 weeks before formal testing of renin and aldosterone levels.

During pregnancy, it is generally recommended that treatment of hyperaldosteronism with spironolactone be avoided due to its anti-androgenic effects; there is a theoretical risk that ambiguous genitalia might occur in a male fetus. Calcium-channel blockers are regarded to be the most effective antihypertensive agent for this condition as they have some effect in reducing aldosterone synthesis and release. If the hypertension and/or hypokalemia cannot be controlled medically, laparoscopic removal of the affected adrenal gland during the second trimester may be warranted.

Cushing's Syndrome

Cushing's syndrome is not very commonly seen in pregnancy as fertility is generally reduced by altered gonadotrophin secretion in pituitary disease, and increased adrenal androgen secretion in adrenal disease. The clinical features of hypercortisolemia (e.g. weight gain, fatigue, glucose intolerance, and hypertension) greatly overlap with those of pregnancy. More specific features that may suggest hypercortisolemia are red or purple-pigmented striae (compared with pale striae in pregnancy), proximal myopathy, or fractures related to an underlying reduction in bone density.

Complications of maternal hypercortisolemia include a greater incidence of preeclampsia, gestational diabetes mellitus, pre-term delivery, post-operative wound infection, and wound dehiscence. Neonatal adrenal insufficiency can occur as high circulating maternal cortisol levels will typically cause fetal cortisol production to be suppressed in utero (43).

Patients diagnosed with Cushing's syndrome during pregnancy should be considered for surgical treatment (transphenoidal resection of pituitary adenomas or laparoscopic adrenalectomy for adrenal adenomas) before 20 weeks gestation as the fetal outcome is significantly improved (44). Medical treatment can also be considered but is much less effective. Metyrapone has been used, but severe hypertension has been associated with its use. Ketoconazole cannot be used in pregnancy as it is teratogenic in animal studies.

Congenital Adrenal Hyperplasia

Congenital adrenal hyperplasia (CAH) includes a family of monogenic inherited enzymatic defects of adrenal steroid biosynthesis. Manifestations are secondary to an accumulation of precursors proximal to the enzymatic deficiency. The most common form is 21-hydroxylase deficiency; this accounts for more than 90% of cases (45). The presentation can vary, from classic CAH, which presents in the neonatal period with severe virilization and salt wasting, to non-classic (late-onset) CAH, which presents in adulthood with hirsutism and menstrual irregularity. Late-onset CAH can often be difficult to distinguish from polycystic ovarian syndrome clinically. These patients have a reduced fertility rate and usually require assisted reproductive techniques such as ovulation induction to conceive. The spontaneous miscarriage rate is twice that of the normal population and congenital anomalies are more frequent (46).

Once pregnant, fetal risk is dependent on the paternal carrier status given that the mode of inheritance is autosomal recessive. It is recommended that glucocorticoids be commenced before the 9th week of gestation to suppress fetal androgen production only in cases where the father is a carrier of CAH. The glucocorticoid of choice is dexamethasone; dexamethasone readily crosses the placenta because it is not bound to corticosteroid-binding globulin (CBG) and also is not metabolized by placental 11-β hydroxysteroid dehydrogenase. However, as only 1 in 4 female fetuses are affected in a family with CAH, it is important to discontinue therapy as soon as possible in the male fetus and unaffected female fetus to avoid the complications of maternal hypercortisolemia (see description above). Historically, amniocentesis or chorionic villus sampling was required to perform gender determination and direct DNA analysis for the 21-hydroxylase gene CYP21A2, but the recent advent of cell-free fetal DNA has eliminated the risks of these procedures while accurately predicting which one of eight fetuses should stay on dexamethasone therapy throughout the duration of pregnancy (47).

Delivery can be complicated by cephalopelvic disproportion, which can result from maternal android pelvis and can be affected by previous reconstructive surgery (48). Patients with salt wasting are dependent on exogenous glucocorticoid and mineralocorticoid replacement throughout the pregnancy and will require stress dose steroids at the time of labor and delivery (see Box 42.2).

Lipid Disorders

Hypercholesterolemia and hypertriglyceridemia may have significant impacts upon pregnancy. During pregnancy, alterations in maternal lipid metabolism favor fuel production for the developing fetus. In the third trimester, adipose tissue lipolysis increases, elevating the substrates for triglyceride synthesis. Conversely, lipoprotein lipase activity declines, reducing triglyceride clearance (49).

Severe hypertriglyceridemia can occur in patients with hereditary lipoprotein lipase deficiency (49,50). Case reports describe pancreatitis associated with lipid disorders, with maternal mortality rates of up to 20%. Triglyceride levels need to be monitored closely throughout pregnancy and treatment requires drastic dietary fat restrictions as well as medical therapy with fibrates, omega-3-fatty acids and/or niacin. Niacin may cause hepatic toxicity and worsen insulin resistance.

Patients with preexisting hypercholesterolemia on statins (also known as HMG Co-A reductase inhibitors) should discontinue these medications prior to conception as they are known to impair fetal neural lipid synthesis. In cases where patients may have established coronary artery disease, it may be reasonable to resume these medications in the second trimester to reduce the likelihood of coronary events later in pregnancy and/or in the immediate postpartum period.

Concluding Remarks

Endocrine disorders are relatively common in pregnancy. It is important that they are well controlled in order to minimize any adverse outcomes to the mother or fetus. It is also important that the practitioner understands the normal physiological changes that occur with each endocrine axis during pregnancy and to understand the intricate effects of pregnancy on specific hormones in order to appreciate any maternal and/or fetal effects of a particular endocrine condition. Box 42.3 summarizes these effects for easy reference.

Box 42.3 **Effects of pregnancy on specific hormones**

1. Growth hormone (GH) levels rise in pregnancy due to placental production (assays cannot differentiate this from pituitary GH)
2. LH and FSH levels are undetectable during pregnancy due to suppression of high circulating levels of estrogen and progesterone
3. A rise in total T4 and total T3 levels occur due to an increase in thyroxine-binding globulin (TBG) level
4. A progressive rise in serum cortisol levels occur due to an increase in cortisol-binding globulin (CBG) level
5. There is a progressive rise in prolactin level throughout pregnancy due to increasing estrogen levels stimulating pituitary prolactin release
6. There is a reduction in circulating antidiuretic hormone (ADH) in pregnancy due to placental vasopressinase production
7. A sharp rise in renin level occurs throughout the first two trimesters of gestation followed by a plateau in the level (corresponds to aldosterone level & maternal plasma volume level)

References

1. Stagnaro-Green A, Abalovich M, Alexander E, et al. Guidelines of the American Thyroid Association for the diagnosis and management of thyroid disease during pregnancy and postpartum. *Thyroid* 2011; 21: 1081–125.
2. Glinoer D. The regulation of thyroid function in pregnancy: Pathways of endocrine adaptation from physiology to pathology. *Endocr Rev* 1997; 18: 404–433.
3. Yoshimura M, Hershman JM. Thyrotropic action of human chorionic gonadotrophin. *Thyroid* 1995; 5: 425–434.
4. Harada K, Hershman JM, Reed AW, et al. Comparison of thyroid stimulators and thyroid hormone concentrations in the sera of pregnant women. *J Clin Endocrinol Metab* 1979; 48: 793–797.
5. Leung AS, Millar LK, Koonings PP, et al. Perinatal outcome in hypothyroid pregnancies. *Obstet Gynecol* 1993; 81: 349–353.
6. Smallridge RC, Ladenson PW. Hypothyroidism in pregnancy: Consequences to neonatal health. *J Clin Endocrinol Metab* 2001; 86: 2349–2353.
7. De Groot L, Abalovich M, Alexander EK, et al. Management of thyroid dysfunction during pregnancy and postpartum: An Endocrine Society clinical practice guideline. *J Clin Endocrinol Metab* 2012; 97: 2543–2565.
8. Yassa L, Marqusee E, Fawcett R, Alexander EK. Thyroid hormone early adjustment in early pregnancy (the THERAPY) trial. *J Clin Endocrinol Metab* 2010; 95: 3234–3241.
9. Haddow JE, Palomaki GE, Allan WC, et al. Maternal thyroid deficiency during pregnancy and subsequent neuropsychological development of the child. *N Engl J Med* 1999; 341: 549–555.
10. Pop VJ, Kuijpens JL, van Baar Al, et al. Low maternal free thyroxine concentrations during early pregnancy are associated with impaired psychomotor development in infancy. *Clin Endocrinol* 1999; 50: 149–155.
11. Blazer S, Moreh-Waterman Y, Miller-Lotan R, et al. Maternal hypothyroidism may affect fetal growth and neonatal thyroid function. *Obstet Gynecol* 2003; 102: 232–241.
12. Millar LK, Wing DA, Leung AS, et al. Low birth weight and preeclampsia in pregnancies complicated by hyperthyroidism. *Obstet Gynecol* 1994; 84: 946–949.
13. Nicholson WK, Robinson KA, Smallridge RC, et al. Prevalence of postpartum thyroid dysfunction: A quantitative review. *Thyroid* 2006; 16: 573–582.
14. Gerstein HC. Incidence of postpartum thyroid dysfunction in patients with type I diabetes mellitus. *Ann Intern Med* 1993; 118: 419–423.
15. Keh SM, El-Shunnar SK, Palmer T, Ahsan SF. Incidence of malignancy in solitary thyroid nodules. *J Laryngol Otol* 2015; 129 (7): 677–81.
16. Akslen LA, Nilssen S, Kvale G. Reproductive factors and risk of thyroid cancer: A prospective study of 63,090 women from Norway. *Br J Cancer* 1992; 65: 772–774.
17. Herzon FS, Morris DM, Segal MN, et al. Coexistent thyroid cancer and pregnancy. *Arch Otolarynfol Head Neck Surg* 1994; 120: 1191–1193.
18. Rosen IB, Walfish PG. Pregnancy as a predisposing factor in thyroid neoplasia. *Arch Surg* 1986; 121: 1287–1290.
19. Kobayashi K, Tanaka Y, Ishiguro S, Mori T. Rapidly growing thyroid carcinoma during pregnancy. *J Surg Oncol* 1994; 55: 61–64.
20. Moosa M, Mazzaferri EL. Outcome of differentiated thyroid cancer diagnosed on pregnant women. *J Clin Endocrinol Metab* 1997; 82: 2862–2866.
21. Schnatz PF, Thaxton S. Parathyroidectomy in the third trimester of pregnancy. *Obstet Gynecol Surv* 2005; 60:672–682.
22. Mestman JH. Parathyroid disorders of pregnancy. *Semin Perinatol* 1998; 6:485–496.
23. National Institute for Health and Clinical Excellence. *Antenatal Care.* NICE clinical guideline 62. Manchester: NICE; 2008.
24. Hollis BW. Vitamin D requirement during pregnancy and lactation. *J Bone Miner Res* 2007; 22 Suppl 2: V39–V44.
25. Royal College of Obstetricians & Gynecologists. Statement on vitamin D supplementation for pregnant women. www.rcog.org.uk/what-we-do/campaigning and opinions/statement/rcog-statement-vitamin-d-supplementation-pregnant-women (accessed September 12, 2016).
26. Sattar N, Welsh P, Panarelli M, Forouhi NG. Increasing requests for vitamin D measurement: Costly, confusing, and without credibility. *Lancet* 2012; 379: 95–96.
27. Kovacs CS. Calcium and bone metabolism in pregnancy and lactation. *J Clin Endocrinol Metab* 2001; 86: 2344–2348.
28. Chen KK, Powrie RO. Approach to the use of glucocorticoids in pregnancy for non-obstetric indications. In: Powrie RO, Greene MF, Camann W, editors. *de Swiet's Medical Disorders in Obstetric Practice*, 5th edition. Oxford: Wiley-Blackwell, 2010; 736–741.

29. Sheehan HL, Davis JC. Pituitary necrosis. *Br Med Bull* 1968; 24: 59–70.
30. Gillam M, Molitch ME. Lymphocytic hypophysitis. In: Bronstein MD, editor. *Pituitary Tumors in Pregnancy*. Norwell MA: Kluwer Academic, 2001; 131–148.
31. Fernandez A, Karavitaki N, Wass JA. Prevalence of pituitary adenomas: A community based, cross-sectional study in Banbury (Oxfordshire, UK). *Clin Endocrinol (Oxf)* 2010; 72: 377–382.
32. Molitch ME. Disorders of prolactin secretion. *Endocrinol Metab Clin N Am* 2001; 30: 585–610.
33. Zanettini R, Antonini A, Gatto G, et al. Valvular heart disease and the use of dopamine agonists for Parkinson's disease. *N Engl J Med* 2007; 356: 39–46.
34. Nagamani M, Lingold JC, Gomez LG. Hyperthecosis of the ovaries in acromegaly. *Obstet Gynecol* 1980; 56: 258–262.
35. Manikandan K, Raghavan S. Amniotic fluid volume changes in response to frusemide induced maternal fluid shifts. *J Pharmacol Pharmacother* 2014; 5: 153–154.
36. Durr JA. Diabetes insipidus in pregnancy. *Am J Kidney Dis* 1987; 9: 276–283.
37. Gamlen TR, Aynsley-Green A, Irvine WJ, McCallum CJ. Immunological studies in the neonate of a mother with Addison's disease and diabetes mellitus. *Clin Exp Immunol* 1977; 28: 192–195.
38. Dahia PLM, Hayashida CY, Strunz C, et al. Low cord blood levels of catecholamine from a newborn of a pheochromocytoma patient. *Eur J Endocrinol* 1994; 130: 217–219.
39. Combs CA, Easterling TR, Schmucker BC. Hemodynamic observations during paroxysmal hypertension in a pregnancy with pheochromocytoma. *Obstet Gynecol* 1989; 74: 439–441.
40. Lau P, Permezel M, Dawson P, et al. Pheochromocytoma in pregnancy. *Aust N Z J Obstet Gynecol* 1996; 36: 472–476.
41. Santeiro ML, Stromquist C, Wyble L. Phenoxybenzamine placental transfer during the third trimester. *Ann Pharmacother* 1996; 30: 1249–1251.
42. Lydakis C, Lip GY, Beevers M, Beevers DG. Atenolol and fetal growth in pregnancies complicated by hypertension. *Am J Hypertens* 1999; 12: 541–547.
43. Kreines K, DeVaux WD. Neonatal adrenal insufficiency associated with maternal Cushing's syndrome. *Pediatrics* 1971; 47: 516–519.
44. Lindsay JR, Jonklaas J, Oldfield EH, Nieman LK. Cushing's syndrome during pregnancy: Personal experience and review of the literature. *J Clin Endocrinol Metab* 2005; 90: 3077–3083.
45. White PC, Speiser PW. Congenital adrenal hyperplasia due to 21-hydroxylase deficiency. *Endocr Rev* 2000; 21: 245–291.
46. Feldman S, Billaud L, Thalabard J-C, et al. Fertility in women with late-onset adrenal hyperplasia due to 21-hydroxylase deficiency. *J Clin Endocrinol Metab* 1992; 74: 635–639.
47. New MI, Tong YK, Yuen T, et al. Noninvasive prenatal diagnosis of congenital adrenal hyperplasia using cell-free fetal DNA in maternal plasma. *J Clin Endocrinol Metab* 2014; 99: E1022–E1030.
48. Krone N, Wachter I, Stafanidou M, et al. Mothers with congenital adrenal hyperplasia and their children: Outcome of pregnancy, birth and childhood. *Clin Endocrinol* 2001; 55: 523–529.
49. Chiang A-N, Yang M-L, Hung J-H, et al. Alterations of serum lipid levels and their biological relevances during and after pregnancy. *Life Sci* 1995; 56: 2367–2375.
50. Goldberg AS, Hegele RA. Severe hypertriglyceridemia in pregnancy. *J Clin Endocrinol Metab* 2012; 97: 2589–2596.

Diabetes Mellitus in Pregnancy

Mohamad Hamdi

Introduction

Diabetes is a common health problem. When diabetes affects pregnancy, it can lead to serious morbidities and complications. This chapter will discuss the issue of diabetes in pregnancy including scope, classification, diagnosis, complications, and treatment.

Scope of the Problem

Diabetes mellitus is a metabolic disorder characterized by increasing levels of blood glucose as a result of increasing insulin resistance or insulin deficiency. Worldwide, it is estimated that 366 million people are affected with diabetes. the number is expected to increase to 552 million in 2030 (1).

Pregnancy is characterized by an increased prevalence of diabetes secondary to increased diabetogenic hormones including human placental lactogen, insulinase, cortisol and progesterone. This leads to a significant increase in morbidities including risk of birth injury, cesarean delivery, neonatal intensive care unit (NICU) admission and congenital malformations (2,3).

Classification

Diabetes complicating pregnancy can be divided into two broad categories:

1-Pregestational diabetes mellitus: Preexisting diabetes mellitus (type 1 or type 2) in a currently pregnant patient.

2-Gestational diabetes mellitus: Diabetes mellitus first diagnosed during pregnancy.

Pregestational Diabetes

Type 1 Diabetes Mellitus

Type 1 diabetes mellitus is characterized by absolute insulin deficiency secondary to beta cell destruction. In genetically susceptible individuals, an environmental trigger is believed to initiate the beta-cell destruction leading to progressive decline in insulin production and subsequent development of diabetes mellitus.

Type 2 Diabetes Mellitus

Type 2 diabetes mellitus is characterized by increased insulin resistance and impaired pancreatic response to blood glucose levels. Obesity is a major risk factor that predisposes to type 2 diabetes mellitus.

Gestational Diabetes Mellitus

Gestational diabetes mellitus is defined as diabetes first diagnosed during pregnancy. It affects 3–5% of pregnancies (4). It is characterized by a progressive increase in insulin resistance as pregnancy advances. In clinical practice, however, many patients with preexisting diabetes mellitus are first diagnosed during pregnancy and are therefore given the diagnosis of gestational diabetes mellitus even though the undiagnosed condition existed prior to pregnancy. Therefore, testing for persistent diabetes mellitus after pregnancy is important in order to differentiate the two conditions; true gestational diabetes mellitus would, of course, resolve following resolution of pregnancy hormonal changes.

Diabetes complicating pregnancy can also be classified based on associated complications (5). The White's classification is summarized in Table 43.1.

Diagnosis

Pregestational Diabetes

A variety of tests are available to diagnose pregestational diabetes. Both the World Health Organization (WHO) and the American Diabetes Association have published criteria for diagnosis (6,7). These are summarized in Table 43.2. Any one of the thresholds, if abnormal, can be used to make the diagnosis. The diagnostic test chosen should be repeated

Table 43.1 White's Classification of Diabetes in Pregnancy

Gestational Diabetes	
Class A1	Gestational diabetes, diet controlled
Class A2	Gestational diabetes, medication controlled
Pregestational Diabetes	
Class B	Onset at 20 years of age or older or duration less than 10 years
Class C	Onset between age 10 and 19 or duration of 10–19 years
Class D	Onset before age 10 or duration more than 20 years
Class F	Diabetic nephropathy
Class R	Diabetic retinopathy
Class RF	Nephropathy and retinopathy
Class H	Heart disease
Class T	Prior renal transplant

Table 43.2 Diagnostic Criteria for Pregestational Diabetes Mellitus

Time	Value
Fasting plasma glucose	≥ 126 mg/dL
2 hours post 75 g oral glucose challenge test	≥ 200 mg/dL
Glycated hemoglobin (A1C)	≥ 6.5%

on a subsequent day to confirm the diagnosis unless two tests done at the same time were abnormal (8). In patients with overt symptoms of diabetes (such as polyuria, weight loss, thirst), a random glucose level of 200 mg/dL is sufficient for diagnosis.

Gestational Diabetes

The diagnosis of gestational diabetes mellitus is far more controversial. Questions including who, when and how to screen are all debatable.

Historically. pregnant patients are screened with a 50 g one-hour glucose challenge test (GCT). In this test, patients receive a 50 g glucose load followed by a measurement of their blood glucose level one hour later. The test is usually administered between 24 and 28 weeks of gestation. Patients who test above the threshold (either 135 or 140 mg/dL) will receive a diagnostic 3-hour glucose tolerance test (GTT). In a three-hour glucose tolerance test, the patient's blood glucose is measured fasting and then at 1, 2 and 3 hours after a 100 g glucose load. For this test, the presence of two values above the threshold (Table 43.3) on the three-hour test is diagnostic of diabetes (9).

Screening is usually performed between 24 and 28 weeks of gestation, but in patients at high risk for type 2 diabetes, screening earlier in pregnancy is recommended (9). Increased risk factors include patients with gestational diabetes mellitus in a previous pregnancy, obesity, and a history of fetal macrosomia. In the United States, the most common practice is universal screening of all pregnant women. In a study by Danilenko-Dixon et al. (10) that looked at 18,000 patients who received universal screening, only 10% would qualify as low risk enough to be excluded from testing while selective screening will miss around 3% of patients.

The criteria for screening and diagnosis of gestational diabetes were developed more than 50 years ago. They were designed at that time to identify patients at risk of developing type 2 diabetes mellitus after delivery rather than identify patients at risk of perinatal morbidity (11). In 2008, the Hyperglycemia and Adverse Pregnancy Outcomes (HAPO) study (12) was published; it showed that perinatal complications are increased with blood glucose levels below threshold levels diagnostic of diabetes; these risks increase as blood glucose values increase in a continuous fashion. Following the findings of this study, the International Association of Diabetes and Pregnancy Study Groups (IADPSG) developed new guidelines using more stringent thresholds. Universal screening for pregestational diabetes early in pregnancy and screening for gestational diabetes using a 2 hours 75 g oral glucose tolerance test between 24 and 28 weeks are now recommended (13). This approach eliminates the need for a screening and a diagnostic test (50 and 100 g), which makes it easier to administer and more

Table 43.3 Diagnostic Criteria for Gestational Diabetes Mellitus

Time	Carpenter and Coustan (Plasma or Serum)	National Diabetes Data Group (Plasma)
Fasting	95	105
One hour	180	190
Two hours	155	165
Three hours	140	145

Table 43.4 Two-Hour 75 g Oral Glucose Tolerance Test Thresholds

Time	Value
Fasting	≥92 mg/dL
One hour	≥180 mg/ dL
Two hours	≥153

Note: One abnormal value is diagnostic of diabetes.

tolerated by patients. One value above the threshold is diagnostic of diabetes (Table 43.4).

Complications of Diabetes In Pregnancy: Maternal

Retinopathy

Retinopathy is the leading cause of blindness in young adults (14). It is estimated that 4.1 million people are affected with retinopathy in the United States (15,16). It is important to note that retinopathy does not affect patients with gestational diabetes mellitus but rather patients with type 1 and type 2 diabetes.

Retinopathy is classified into two broad categories: non-proliferative and proliferative. Non-proliferative retinopathy is characterized by intraretinal microvascular changes and is subdivided into mild, moderate and severe, while proliferative retinopathy is characterized by retinal surface neovascularization. These changes lead to retinal edema, hemorrhage, scarring and ultimately loss of vision. It is therefore very important to perform a thorough retinal exam by an ophthalmologist to detect any of these abnormalities early in pregnancy for patients with known type 1 or type 2 diabetes.

Pregnancy is a risk factor for worsening retinopathy. Multiple studies have demonstrated an acceleration of retinopathy during pregnancy (15–17). The mechanism of such acceleration is poorly understood. Hormonal, immunologic and hemodynamic changes are all possible contributing factors. The management of diabetic retinopathy should ideally start before pregnancy. Interestingly, tight blood sugar control in early pregnancy has been found in some studies to actually increase the progression of diabetic retinopathy (18). Therefore, control of blood sugar before conception should be the goal.

An ocular exam by an ophthalmologist is important. The American Academy of Ophthalmology recommends eye exams soon after conception and then early in the first trimester followed by re-examination every 3–12 months for patients with no retinopathy or mild to moderate non-proliferative retinopathy and every 1–3 months for severe non-proliferative retinopathy and worse (19). Lasertreatment is safe and should be used in pregnant patients who meet criteria for this intervention.

Hypertension

Hypertension commonly complicates pregnancy; the prevalence of hypertensive disorders is even higher in diabetic patients (20,21) and it affects patients with both pregestational and gestational diabetes. Chronic hypertension, gestational hypertension, preeclampsia and superimposed preeclampsia are all more common in pregnancies complicated by diabetes and therefore contribute to the increased maternal and fetal morbidity associated with diabetes. Prompt identification and treatment of hypertension is important in order to avoid associated complications. Patients generally should have their blood pressure checked early in pregnancy and then every visit afterward. Urine protein should be obtained initially and then urine albumin dipstick should be checked at every visit for diabetic patients. Patients with preexisting hypertension should ideally have their blood pressure optimized using non-teratogenic medications before the onset of pregnancy. Teratogenic antihypertensive medications that must be avoided in pregnancy include ACE inhibitors and angiotensin receptor blockers (22–24).

Nephropathy

The Centers of Disease Control and Prevention (CDC) estimates that 20 million people or 10% of the US adult population suffers from chronic kidney disease (25) with diabetes, which the leading cause of end-stage renal disease. It is estimated that 5–10% of pregnancies complicated by diabetes are affected (26,27). Nephropathy is classified according to the level of albuminuria; levels ≥ 300 mg/24 hours (albumin to creatinine ratio 300 μg/mg) are considered diagnostic. Microalbuminuria, a precursor and strong indicator for development of nephropathy, is defined as albumin excretion of 30–299 mg/24 hours (albumin to creatinine 30–299 μg/mg).

Nephropathy is associated with significant increase in risk of complications; the most commonly increased disease process is preeclampsia (28). Other complications include increasing risks of preterm labor, cesarean section, intrauterine growth restriction and perinatal mortality (26,29). Patients with serum creatinine above 1.4 mg/dL, proteinuria above 3 g/24 hours or severe hypertension have the worst outcome (26,29,30). Many of these outcomes can be improved with early and aggressive intervention and treatment. The diagnosis of preeclampsia can be challenging in patients with nephropathy as many of these patients will have preexisting hypertension, proteinuria or both. A sudden increase in blood pressure or protein is highly suggestive of preeclampsia; therefore, it is important to obtain baseline labs early in pregnancy, which can be used late if preeclampsia is suspected.

The care of patients with nephropathy should be undertaken by a multidisciplinary team experienced in the management of this condition. Management should focus on tight control of blood sugar, aggressive control of blood pressure, early detection of complications, namely preeclampsia as well as extensive monitoring of fetal well-being.

Diabetic Ketoacidosis

Diabetic ketoacidosis (DKA) is a relatively uncommon but very serious and life-threatening complication for both the mother and the fetus. It is much more common in patients with type 1 diabetes mellitus secondary to insulin insufficiency but can still occur in patients with type 2 diabetes. Triggers for DKA include infection, missed insulin dose or undiagnosed diabetes.

DKA occurs as a result of decreased insulin and increased catabolic hormones; this causes increased liver production of glucose and ketones and leads to hyperglycemia, hyperketonemia and acidosis. The increase in hepatic glucose, coupled with poor mobilization into the tissues secondary to lack of insulin, leads these to release ketone bodies.

The pathogenesis of DKA includes hyperglycemia, which leads to profound dieresis with resulting electrolytes imbalance. Subsequent release of stress hormones (catecholamines, cortisol, glucagon) causes a vicious cycle of hyperglycemia, hyperketonemia and electrolyte imbalance, which leads to severe polyuria, polydypsia and ultimately organ dysfunction, lethargy, coma and death.

The patient with DKA usually presents with rapidly worsening polyuria, polydypsia, abdominal pain, nausea and vomiting, hyperventilation, fruity breath, altered mental status or coma. A triggering factor is usually identifiable.

Laboratory assessment of the DKA patient will show hyperglycemia, ketonemia and metabolic acidosis. It is important to note that the degree of hyperglycemia associated with DKA can be much lower in pregnancies complicated by DKA than in the same patients when non-pregnant (31).

The accumulation of acetoacetic acid and betahydroxybutyric acid leads to compensatory hyperventilation, causing reduced CO_2 and consequently loss of bicarbonate. A base deficit of –4 meq/L in the presence of hyperglycemia and ketonemia is therefore diagnostic of DKA (32).

The cornerstone of management of DKA in pregnancy (33) is prompt diagnosis and aggressive and early treatment. Inciting factors such as infections should be identified and eliminated. Blood gases, glucose, ketones and electrolytes should be obtained immediately and then every 1–2 hours to guide the treatment. Aggressive hydration using isotonic sodium chloride should be initiated with a total replacement of 4–6 L in first 12 hours at a rate of 1 L in first hour, 500–1,000 mL/h for 2–4 hours and then 250 mL/h until 80% of fluid deficit is replaced. A 5% dextrose in normal saline should be started when plasma glucose levels reach 250 mg/dL. Insulin is given intravenously at a loading dose: 0.2–0.4 U/kg followed by a maintenance infusion of 2–10 U/h. The infusion (also called insulin drip) can then be titrated based on blood glucose levels.

Serum potassium is particularly important to check and correct due to the close relation of potassium and insulin. In patients with DKA, a total deficit of potassium exists secondary to renal loss from dieresis as well as gastrointestinal loss from vomiting. This hypokalemia can, however, be masked by hemoconcentration as well as displacement of intracellular potassium secondary to insulin deficiency. Therefore, potassium should be infused at a rate of 15–20 meq/L if initially normal or reduced. If elevated, infusion should be withheld until the normal range is achieved. Potassium should then be administered at a rate of 20–30 mEq/L. If the pH is less than 7.1, administer one ampoule of bicarbonate per liter of saline until pH is greater than 7.1.

In viable pregnancies (> 24 weeks gestation), continuous fetal heart rate monitoring should be performed while treating DKA. A fetal heart rate tracing pattern of minimal variability and late decelerations is common; this, however, usually corrects with improvement of maternal status. Emergency delivery should therefore be avoided if it is safe to do so unless fetal distress persists despite correction of maternal condition.

Miscarriage

Diabetes complicating pregnancy has been shown to increase the risk of spontaneous abortion, especially when diabetes is uncontrolled or associated with other comorbidities or complications (34). Preconceptional counseling concerning tight blood sugar control and control of comorbidities is therefore highly important in order to reduce such risk.

Complications of Diabetes in Pregnancy: Fetal and Neonatal

Congenital Malformations

Multiple large studies have demonstrated an increased risk of congenital anomalies in patients with pregestational diabetes. The rate is up to eight times compared to the general population (35–39). The most common anomalies are summarized in Table 43.5. This increased risk is related to the increased glucose levels early in pregnancy during organogenesis. Patients with gestational diabetes who develop increased plasma glucose levels later in pregnancy are therefore spared. The exact mechanism of anomalies is poorly understood but is mostly attributed to abnormal metabolic milieu at the time of organogenesis including hyperglycemia, hypoglycemia, hyperketonemia and increased intracellular free radicals (40,41). Cardiac defects are the most common among all anomalies.

Table 43.5 Congenital Anomalies Associated with Diabetes in Pregnancy

System	Abnormalities
Cardiovascular	Atrial septal defect Ventricular septal defect Transposition of the great vessels Coarctation of the aorta
Nervous	Neural tube defect Microcephaly Anencephaly Hydrocephalus
Gastrointestinal	Duodenal atresia Anorectal atresia Hypoplastic colon
Musculoskeletal	Caudal regression syndrome Talipes Arthrogryposis
Maxillofacial	Orofacial cleft
Urinary	Ureteral duplication Cystic kidney Renal dysgenesis Hydronephrosis

Macrosomia

Contrary to congenital anomalies that are increased only in pregestational diabetes mellitus, increased risks of macrosomia is seen in both pregestational and gestational diabetes. The American Congress of Obstetricians and Gynecologists defines macrosomia as estimated fetal weight above 4000 g. In addition to generalized increase in weight, selective organomegaly occurs in these fetuses. The most common example is increased shoulder width, leading to shoulder dystocia, which is increased three to four times compared to non-diabetic patients (42,43). This leads to increased risk of brachial plexus injury, resulting in permanent impairment in less than 10% of cases (44). Other injuries include facial palsy, fractures and cephalhematoma. In an effort to decrease this risk, ACOG recommends elective cesarean deliveries for diabetic patients with estimated fetal weight equal or above 4,500 g (44). This recommendation is only for diabetic patients.

Respiratory Distress Syndrome

Diabetes in pregnancy, especially with insulin dependent mothers, has been found to significantly increase the risk of respiratory distress syndrome (RDS) in the neonate independent from any other factors (45). RDS results from deficiency in lung surfactant. The exact mechanism of how diabetes causes that is not fully understood but might be related to disrupted synthesis by fetal hyperinsulinemia caused by increased fetal blood glucose.

Hypoglycemia

Hypoglycemia is a common occurrence in newborns of diabetic mothers. Maternal hyperglycemia leads to fetal hyperglycemia and consequently hyperinsulinemia. A sudden drop in plasma glucose following cord clamping can lead to neonatal hypoglycemia, the degree of which is greatly influenced by maternal hyperglycemia late in pregnancy and during the intrapartum period (46). Tight maternal glucose control especially around these times will therefore decrease this risk (47). Most infants of diabetic mothers are asymptomatic and it is therefore imperative for providers to maintain protocols that both check the newborn glucose levels and initiate early feeding to avoid hypoglycemia.

Other Neonatal Complications

Other neonatal complications include hypocalcemia which is presumably secondary to abnormal parathyroid hormone (PTH) production. hyperbilirubinemia, believed to be secondary to polycythemia, frequently seen in infants of diabetic mothers, is another complication as is hypomagnesemia.

Management Strategies

The management of diabetes mellitus complicating pregnancy needs to achieve four goals:

1-Optimizing blood glucose control
2-Ensuring fetal well-being
3-Planning of mode and timing of delivery
4-Postconception testing

Initial Evaluation

In addition to the routine prenatal tests obtained early in pregnancy, the patient with pregestational diabetes should have tests aiming at detecting any existing complications of diabetes as well as establish a baseline to compare any abnormality that might arise during pregnancy to. These investigations are summarized in Table 43.6 (48).

Blood Glucose Control

Optimal blood glucose control is the cornerstone of management of patients with diabetes mellitus in pregnancy and is important to decrease fetal and maternal morbidity and mortality. Both the American College of Obstetricians and Gynecologists and the American Diabetes Association have set target blood glucose levels (49,50). These are summarized in Table 43.7. Patients should be taught how to measure and interpret their glucose reading, what are the warning symptoms of complications and have access to a health care professional to discuss any questions or concerns about their results. Readings should be discussed periodically with their provider and adjustments to treatment made accordingly.

Table 43.6 Initial Evaluation of Patients with Preexisting Diabetes

History	Age of onset Any previously diagnosed complications Diabetes and nutritional education history Current and previous treatment regimens DKA and hypoglycemia episodes and symptom awareness
Physical exam	Height, weight, BMI and blood pressure Dilated eye exam Skin and foot exam
Testing	Routine prenatal tests A1C Lipid profile, liver and kidney function including urine protein Electrocardiogram
Referrals	Ophthalmology for dilated eye exam Dietitian for meal planning and education

Adapted from American Diabetes Association. Initial evaluation and diabetes management planning. *Diabetes Care* 2015;38(Suppl. 1):S17–19.

Table 43.7 Target Blood Glucose Concentrations during Pregnancy

Timing	Blood Glucose Concentration
Fasting	≤ 95 mg/dL
One hour postprandial	≤ 140 mg/dL
Two hours postprandial	≤ 120 mg/dL

Diet and Exercise

It is well known that diet and exercise play a major role in the management of diabetes mellitus in non-pregnant patients by promoting weight loss and increasing end-organ insulin sensitivity. Unfortunately, this is not the case in pregnancy. Most recommendations are based on small studies, expert opinions and extrapolations from non-pregnant patients.

Gestational Diabetes

Patients with gestational diabetes are diagnosed during pregnancy and therefore diet and exercise may be their first line of therapy. The question of how long to try lifestyle changes before introducing another form of therapy was investigated by McFarland and co-workers (51) who conducted a study to determine the length of time required for diet alone to achieve good glycemic control and whether the need for insulin treatment can be predicted at diagnosis of gestational diabetes mellitus. They found that most women who will achieve glycemic control with diet will do that early in the course of the treatment. They also found that women with fasting plasma glucose above 95 mg/dL are unlikely to reach target glucose with diet alone. Therefore the study concluded that dietary therapy should be prescribed for no more than 2 weeks in patients with initial fasting plasma glucose < 95 mg/dL and 1 week in patients with higher values.

All Pregnant Patients with Diabetes

The American College of Obstetricians and Gynecologists, The Royal College of Obstetricians and Gynaecologists and the Society of Obstetricians and Gynaecologists of Canada all recommend some form of exercise in cases of diabetes complicating pregnancy (8,49,52–54). Although historically pregnancy has been a state where weight loss is not recommended, a study by Kiel et al. (55) showed that gestational weight gain for overweight or obese pregnant women less than the currently recommended 15 lb was associated with a significantly lower risk of pregnancy complications; the complications assessed included preeclampsia, cesarean delivery, large for gestational age newborns and small for gestational age newborns. These results were similar for all obesity classes. The authors therefore concluded that limited or no weight gain in obese pregnant women is associated with favorable pregnancy outcomes. Pregnant patients with diabetes should be regularly evaluated by a certified dietician and individualized plans need to be crafted taking into account target sugars, BMI and other existing co-morbidities. Patients with pregestational diabetes usually start pregnancy while on some form of medical therapy in addition to diet and exercise.

Oral Hypoglycemic Agents

Multiple studies have shown that oral hypoglycemic agents can be a viable alternative to insulin for treatment of diabetes in pregnancy. The ease of administration and the lower risk of hypoglycemia and weight gain make these very attractive options to patients. The most commonly used agents in this category are glyburide and metformin.

Glyburide

Glyburide is a second generation sulfonylurea that works by enhancing the release of insulin. Another less important effect is increasing insulin sensitivity. Glyburide reaches peak concentration 2–3 hours after intake with a half-life of 7–10 hours. The starting dose is usually 2.5 mg daily increased by 2.5 mg not less than weekly up to a maximum of 20 mg/day. Side effects are usually mild and include nausea, vomiting, pruritus and uncommonly hypoglycemia. Multiple studies have demonstrated insignificant passage of glyburide to the fetus (56–59). This data alleviated the fear that was historically associated with the use of oral hypoglycemic agents in pregnancy and allowed for a less morbid, more easily administered option for therapy than insulin. One of the most important studies performed to look at the use of glyburide in pregnancy was performed by Langer et al. (59) in which the authors studied 404 pregnant patients randomly assigned to glyburide versus insulin. The primary end point was achievement of the desired level of glycemic control. Secondary end points included maternal and neonatal complications. The study showed similar blood glucose values between both groups with only 4% of the glyburide group requiring insulin. There were no differences regarding neonatal outcomes (large for gestational age, macrosomia, lung complications, NICU admission and fetal anomalies). Glyburide was not detected in the cord serum of any infant in the glyburide group further indicating its safety.

Metformin

Metformin is a biguanide that acts by increasing insulin sensitivity. It is usually started at 500–800 mg per day and gradually increased to a maximum of 2,500 mg per day. The most common side effect is gastrointestinal upset; this can be decreased by gradual increase in dosage. Metformin has been used for a long time in patients with polycystic ovarian syndrome (PCOS) to promote ovulation, promote weight loss and improve metabolic syndrome. Most of the data about its safety is therefore derived from study of PCOS patients who become pregnant while on metformin. In 2008, Rowan et al. published a large study comparing metformin to insulin (60). The authors randomized 751 patients into insulin versus metformin with primary outcomes being neonatal complications. There were no increased perinatal complications in the metformin group compared to insulin.

Other Agents

Acarbose is an oral agent that inhibits alpha glucosidase in the intestines causing a decrease in glucose absorption. It has been shown to be safe and effective but its use is offset by the high rate of gastrointestinal side effects related to unabsorbed glucose. Use of thiazolidinediones, glinides and glucagon-like peptide 1 agonists is not recommended during pregnancy.

Insulin Therapy

When diet, exercise and oral hypoglycemic agents fail to achieve the target glucose levels (usually following 2 weeks of maximum dose therapy), insulin should then be initiated. Pancreatic insulin production follows two patterns. In the fasting state, a basal output of insulin maintains blood glucose within normal range. Following a meal, bolus insulin is released; the amount released depends on the quality and quantity of the meal ingested. Insulin therapeutic plans for diabetes try to mimic these patterns. Insulin does not cross the placenta. When patients use insulin, it is imperative for them to regularly check their blood glucose and be taught to recognize and correct symptoms of hypoglycemia. Patients should have easy access to a health care professional knowledgeable in managing insulin. Table 43.8 summarizes different preparations of insulin as well as their pharmacokinetics.

Insulin is usually administered in two forms, a short or rapid acting before meals and intermediate or more recently long acting for basal action either at bedtime or at breakfast and bedtime. The starting dose of insulin is usually calculated based on the patient's weight (61) and trimester of pregnancy, ranging from 0.7 to 1 U/kg (62) in divided doses. An example of such calculation is presented in Figure 43.1. Patients should check their blood sugar frequently, usually fasting as well as pre- and postprandial and report the readings to their providers. Therapy should be assessed weekly and insulin adjustments made accordingly to achieve target values (63).

Fetal Well-being

As discussed earlier, diabetes complicating pregnancy is associated with multiple complications that can affect fetal well-being and increase morbidity and

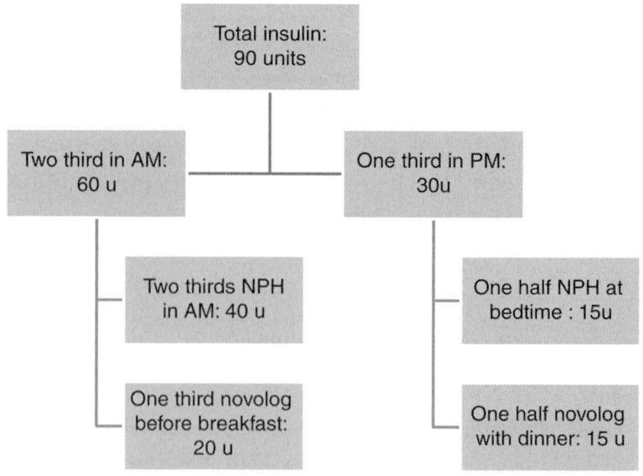

Figure 43.1 Example of insulin dose calculation in a 90 kg patient in the third trimester requiring 90 units of insulin (1 U/kg).

mortality. Therefore, it is important to assess the fetal status periodically especially in pregestational as well as poorly controlled gestational diabetes. Patients with diet controlled gestational diabetes, however, do not need any special testing. Box 43.1 lists recommended fetal well-being assessment based on the American College of Obstetricians and Gynecologists practice bulletin on pregestational and gestational diabetes (33).

Timing and Mode of Delivery

In pregnancies with well-controlled diabetes, there is no indication for early delivery and pregnancy can be allowed to proceed till due date. Earlier delivery is indicated in cases with poor control with amniocentesis for documentation of fetal lung maturity sometimes indicated in cases less than 39 weeks (33,49). Waiting beyond the due date is usually not recommended.

No consensus exists on the optimal regimen to monitor glucose during labor. Most regimen call for checking glucose every 1–2 hours with administration

Table 43.8 Types and Pharmacokinetics of Different Insulin Preparations

Type	Name	Onset	Peak	Duration
Rapid-acting	Lispro (Humalog) Aspart (Novolog)	10–30 minutes	30 minutes to 3 hours	3–5 hours
Short-acting	Regular insulin	30 minutes to 1 hour	2–5 hours	Up to 12 hours
Intermediate-acting	NPH insulin	1.5–4 hours	4–12 hours	Up to 24 hours
Long-acting	Insulin Glargine (Lantus)	4 hours	None	Up to 24 hours

Box 43.1 Fetal assessment in diabetic patients

1-Perform early ultrasound to accurately date the pregnancy and establish viability. This is followed by an anatomy scan at 18–22 weeks to evaluate for any structural anomalies and an echocardiogram if cardiac defects are suspected.

2-Serial growth scans are done to document appropriate growth and detect growth abnormalities every 3–4 weeks.

3-Fetal well-being can be monitored with daily kick count, non-stress test and biophysical profile. These can be initiated between 32 and 34 weeks or earlier if needed. Different institutions have different protocols for monitoring. Twice weekly non-stress testing with weekly biophysical profile is a reasonable regimen.

of rapid acting insulin or dextrose by IV infusion as needed. ACOG recommends keeping blood glucose levels less than 110 mg/dL during labor.

Macrosomia and shoulder dystocia are known complications of pregnancies associated with diabetes. Multiple studies have failed to show any benefit for routine cesarean delivery in cases complicated by macrosomia unless the estimated fetal weight is above 4,500 g (64). It is important to note, however, that ultrasound is not very accurate in estimating the fetal weight in macrosomic fetuses (65).

Management of Gestational Diabetes

Diet and exercise are the mainstay management strategies for gestational diabetes. The input of a nutritionist may be very important. These therapeutic interventions are usually successful when frequent monitoring of blood sugar levels is maintained. Those patients successfully treated with diet and exercise do not require any additional special testing or early delivery. As stated above, if 2 weeks of diet and exercise fail to control the blood sugar, oral agents should be started. If 2–3 weeks of maximum dose fail to provide adequate control, insulin should be started.

Patients who are unable to control their blood sugar levels with these conservative interventions are usually managed similar to patients with pregestational diabetes as far as therapy monitoring, prenatal testing and timing of delivery.

Postpartum Care

Following delivery, women with gestational diabetes mellitus rarely require insulin. It is important to continue checking fasting and 2 hours postprandial glucose in patients who received medications to control their blood glucose and tailor therapy accordingly. It is also important to note that insulin resistance falls rapidly after delivery. This knowledge is crucial in order to avoid therapy induced hypoglycemia. Six to twelve weeks after delivery, a 2-hour 75 g oral glucose tolerance test is recommended to help identify women who either develop type 2 diabetes or may have had undiagnosed diabetes prior to conception (11). The risk of recurrence in subsequent pregnancies is estimated to be around 35% (66) and should be discussed with patients. Patients with gestational diabetes are at increased risk of developing type 2 diabetes later in life (67). Long-term follow-up, preferably every 3 years, is advisable. This can be achieved with either fasting glucose or glucose tolerance testing.

Concluding Remarks

Diabetes is a common and serious comorbidity that can affect pregnancy. Early diagnosis and aggressive treatment can prevent many of the associated complications. Controversy still exists concerning optimal diagnostic test and treatment plan. With proper care, patients can expect favorable pregnancy outcome.

References

1. Imes CC, Burke LE. The obesity epidemic: The United States as a cautionary tale for the rest of the world. *Curr Epidemiol Rep*. 2014;1(2):82–8.
2. Yang J, Cummings EA, O'Connell C, Jangaard K. Fetal and neonatal outcomes of diabetic pregnancies. *Obstet Gynecol*. 2006;108(3 Pt 1):644–50.
3. Knight KM, Pressman EK, Hackney DN, Thornburg LL. Perinatal outcomes in type 2 diabetic patients compared with non-diabetic patients matched by body mass index. *J Matern Fetal Neonatal Med*. 2012;25(6):611–5.
4. Coustan DR. Gestational diabetes. *Diabetes Care*. 1993;16 Suppl 3:8–15.
5. White P. Pregnancy complicating diabetes. *Am J Med*. 1949;7(5):609–16.
6. American Diabetes A. Diagnosis and classification of diabetes mellitus. *Diabetes Care*. 2010;33 Suppl 1:S62–9.

7. Use of Glycated Haemoglobin (HbA1c) in the Diagnosis of Diabetes Mellitus: Abbreviated Report of a WHO Consultation. WHO Guidelines Approved by the Guidelines Review Committee. Geneva, 2011.

8. American Diabetes A. Standards of medical care in diabetes – 2014. *Diabetes Care*. 2014;37 Suppl 1:S14–80.

9. Committee on Practice Bulletins--Obstetrics. Practice Bulletin No. 137: Gestational diabetes mellitus. *Obstet Gynecol.* 2013;122(2 Pt 1):406–16.

10. Danilenko-Dixon DR, Van Winter JT, Nelson RL, Ogburn PL, Jr. Universal versus selective gestational diabetes screening: application of 1997 American Diabetes Association recommendations. *Am J Obstet Gynecol.* 1999;181(4):798–802.

11. Metzger BE, Buchanan TA, Coustan DR, de Leiva A, Dunger DB, Hadden DR, et al. Summary and recommendations of the Fifth International Workshop-Conference on Gestational Diabetes Mellitus. *Diabetes Care*. 2007;30 Suppl 2:S251-60.

12. Lowe LP, Metzger BE, Dyer AR, Lowe J, McCance DR, Lappin TR, et al. Hyperglycemia and Adverse Pregnancy Outcome (HAPO) Study: associations of maternal A1C and glucose with pregnancy outcomes. *Diabetes Care*. 2012;35(3):574–80.

13. International Association of Diabetes, Pregnancy Study Groups Consensus P, Metzger BE, Gabbe SG, Persson B, Buchanan TA, et al. International association of diabetes and pregnancy study groups recommendations on the diagnosis and classification of hyperglycemia in pregnancy. *Diabetes Care.* 2010;33(3):676–82.

14. Klein BE. Overview of epidemiologic studies of diabetic retinopathy. *Ophthal Epidemiol.* 2007;14(4):179–83.

15. Verier-Mine O, Chaturvedi N, Webb D, Fuller JH. Is pregnancy a risk factor for microvascular complications? The EURODIAB Prospective Complications Study. *Diabet Med.* 2005;22(11):1503–9.

16. Chew EY, Mills JL, Metzger BE, Remaley NA, Jovanovic-Peterson L, Knopp RH, et al. Metabolic control and progression of retinopathy. The Diabetes in Early Pregnancy Study. National Institute of Child Health and Human Development Diabetes in Early Pregnancy Study. *Diabetes Care.* 1995;18(5):631–7.

17. Diabetes C, Complications Trial Research G. Effect of pregnancy on microvascular complications in the diabetes control and complications trial. The Diabetes Control and Complications Trial Research Group. *Diabetes Care*. 2000;23(8):1084–91.

18. The Kroc Collaborative Study Group. Diabetic retinopathy after two years of intensified insulin treatment. Follow-up of the Kroc Collaborative Study. *JAMA*. 1988;260(1):37–41.

19. American Academy of Ophthalmology. Diabetic Retinopathy, Preferred Practice Pattern. Updated 2016.

20. Kitzmiller JL, Block JM, Brown FM, Catalano PM, Conway DL, Coustan DR, et al. Managing preexisting diabetes for pregnancy: Summary of evidence and consensus recommendations for care. *Diabetes Care.* 2008;31(5):1060–79.

21. Nielsen LR, Damm P, Mathiesen ER. Improved pregnancy outcome in type 1 diabetic women with microalbuminuria or diabetic nephropathy: Effect of intensified antihypertensive therapy? *Diabetes Care.* 2009;32(1):38–44.

22. Brown MA, Hague WM, Higgins J, Lowe S, McCowan L, Oats J, et al. The detection, investigation and management of hypertension in pregnancy: Full consensus statement. *Aust N Z J Obstet Gynaecol.* 2000;40(2):139–55.

23. Shotan A, Widerhorn J, Hurst A, Elkayam U. Risks of angiotensin-converting enzyme inhibition during pregnancy: Experimental and clinical evidence, potential mechanisms, and recommendations for use. *Am J Med.* 1994;96(5):451–6.

24. Alwan S, Polifka JE, Friedman JM. Angiotensin II receptor antagonist treatment during pregnancy. *Birth Defects Res A Clin Mol Teratol.* 2005;73(2):123–30.

25. CDC. Chronic Kidney disease issue brief. 2015.

26. Landon MB. Diabetic nephropathy and pregnancy. *Clin Obstet Gynecol.* 2007;50(4):998–1006.

27. Carr DB, Koontz GL, Gardella C, Holing EV, Brateng DA, Brown ZA, et al. Diabetic nephropathy in pregnancy: Suboptimal hypertensive control associated with preterm delivery. *Am J Hypertens.* 2006;19(5):513–9.

28. Sibai BM. Risk factors, pregnancy complications, and prevention of hypertensive disorders in women with pregravid diabetes mellitus. *J Matern Fetal Med.* 2000;9(1):62–5.

29. Gabbe SG, Graves CR. Management of diabetes mellitus complicating pregnancy. *Obstet Gynecol.* 2003;102(4):857–68.

30. Miodovnik M, Rosenn BM, Khoury JC, Grigsby JL, Siddiqi TA. Does pregnancy increase the risk for development and progression of diabetic nephropathy? *Am J Obstet Gynecol.* 1996;174(4):1180–9; discussion 9–91.

31. Oliver R, Jagadeesan P, Howard RJ, Nikookam K. Euglycaemic diabetic ketoacidosis in pregnancy: An

unusual presentation. *J Obstet Gynaecol.* 2007;27(3):308.

32. Parker JA, Conway DL. Diabetic ketoacidosis in pregnancy. *Obstet Gynecol Clin North Am.* 2007;34(3):533–43, xii.
33. Bulletins ACoP. ACOG Practice Bulletin. Clinical Management Guidelines for Obstetrician-Gynecologists. Number 60, March 2005. Pregestational diabetes mellitus. *Obstet Gynecol.* 2005;105(3):675–85.
34. Miodovnik M, Lavin JP, Knowles HC, Holroyde J, Stys SJ. Spontaneous abortion among insulin-dependent diabetic women. *Am J Obstet Gynecol.* 1984;150(4):372–6.
35. Jensen DM, Damm P, Moelsted-Pedersen L, Ovesen P, Westergaard JG, Moeller M, et al. Outcomes in type 1 diabetic pregnancies: a nationwide, population-based study. *Diabetes Care.* 2004;27(12):2819–23.
36. Evers IM, de Valk HW, Visser GH. Risk of complications of pregnancy in women with type 1 diabetes: Nationwide prospective study in the Netherlands. *BMJ.* 2004;328(7445):915.
37. Macintosh MC, Fleming KM, Bailey JA, Doyle P, Modder J, Acolet D, et al. Perinatal mortality and congenital anomalies in babies of women with type 1 or type 2 diabetes in England, Wales, and Northern Ireland: Population based study. *BMJ.* 2006;333(7560):177.
38. Diabetes in Pregnancy: Management of Diabetes and Its Complications from Preconception to the Postnatal Period. National Institute for Health and Clinical Excellence: Guidance. London2008.
39. Reece EA, Sivan E, Francis G, Homko CJ. Pregnancy outcomes among women with and without diabetic microvascular disease (White's classes B to FR) versus non-diabetic controls. *Am J Perinatol.* 1998;15(9):549–55.
40. Cousins L. Etiology and prevention of congenital anomalies among infants of overt diabetic women. *Clin Obstet Gynecol.* 1991;34(3):481–93.
41. Lee AT, Reis D, Eriksson UJ. Hyperglycemia-induced embryonic dysmorphogenesis correlates with genomic DNA mutation frequency in vitro and in vivo. *Diabetes.* 1999;48(2):371–6.
42. Acker DB, Sachs BP, Friedman EA. Risk factors for shoulder dystocia. *Obstet Gynecol.* 1985;66(6):762–8.
43. Rouse DJ, Owen J, Goldenberg RL, Cliver SP. The effectiveness and costs of elective cesarean delivery for fetal macrosomia diagnosed by ultrasound. *JAMA.* 1996;276(18):1480–6.
44. American College of Obstetrics and Gynecology Committee on Practice Bulletins-Obstetrics. ACOG Practice Bulletin Number 49, December 2003: Dystocia and augmentation of labor. *Obstet Gynecol.* 2003;102(6):1445–54.
45. Robert MF, Neff RK, Hubbell JP, Taeusch HW, Avery ME. Association between maternal diabetes and the respiratory-distress syndrome in the newborn. *N Engl J Med.* 1976;294(7):357–60.
46. Francois R, Picaud JJ, Ruitton-Ugliengo A, David L, Cartal MJ, Bauer D. The newborn of diabetic mothers. Observations on 154 cases, 1958–1972. *Biol Neonate.* 1974;24(1):1–31.
47. Persson B, Gentz J, Kellum M. Metabolic observations in infants of strictly controlled diabetic mothers. Plasma levels of glucose, FFA, glycerol and B-beta-hydroxybutyrate during the first two hours after birth. *Acta Paediatr Scand.* 1973;62(5):465–73.
48. American Diabetes Association. Initial evaluation and diabetes management planning. *Diabetes Care.* 2015;38 Suppl:S17–9.
49. American College of Obstetricians and Gynecologists Committee on Practice Bulletins--Obstetrics. ACOG Practice Bulletin. Clinical management guidelines for obstetrician-gynecologists. Number 30, September 2001 (replaces Technical Bulletin Number 200, December 1994). Gestational diabetes. *Obstet Gynecol.* 2001;98(3):525–38.
50. American Diabetes Association. Management of diabetes in pregnancy. *Diabetes Care.* 2016;39 Suppl 1:S94–8.
51. McFarland MB, Langer O, Conway DL, Berkus MD. Dietary therapy for gestational diabetes: How long is long enough? *Obstet Gynecol.* 1999;93(6):978–82.
52. Committee on Obstetric P. ACOG committee opinion. Exercise during pregnancy and the postpartum period. Number 267, January 2002. American College of Obstetricians and Gynecologists. *Int J Gynaecol Obstet.* 2002;77(1):79–81.
53. RCOG. Exercise in pregnancy. Statement number 4. 2006.
54. Davies GA, Wolfe LA, Mottola MF, MacKinnon C, Society of Obstetricians and gynecologists of Canada, SOGC Clinical Practice Obstetrics Committee. Joint SOGC/CSEP clinical practice guideline: Exercise in pregnancy and the postpartum period. *Can J Appl Physiol.* 2003;28(3):330–41.
55. Kiel DW, Dodson EA, Artal R, Boehmer TK, Leet TL. Gestational weight gain and pregnancy outcomes in obese women: How much is enough? *Obstet Gynecol.* 2007;110(4):752–8.
56. Elliott BD, Langer O, Schenker S, Johnson RF. Insignificant transfer of glyburide occurs across the human placenta. *Am J Obstet Gynecol.* 1991;165(4 Pt 1): 807–12.

57. Elliott BD, Schenker S, Langer O, Johnson R, Prihoda T. Comparative placental transport of oral hypoglycemic agents in humans: A model of human placental drug transfer. *Am J Obstet Gynecol.* 1994;171(3):653–60.

58. Garcia-Bournissen F, Feig DS, Koren G. Maternal-fetal transport of hypoglycaemic drugs. *Clin Pharmacokinet.* 2003;42(4):303–13.

59. Langer O, Conway DL, Berkus MD, Xenakis EM, Gonzales O. A comparison of glyburide and insulin in women with gestational diabetes mellitus. *N Engl J Med.* 2000;343(16):1134–8.

60. Rowan JA, Hague WM, Gao W, Battin MR, Moore MP, Mi GTI. Metformin versus insulin for the treatment of gestational diabetes. *N Engl J Med.* 2008;358(19):2003–15.

61. Langer O, Anyaegbunam A, Brustman L, Guidetti D, Levy J, Mazze R. Pregestational diabetes: Insulin requirements throughout pregnancy. *Am J Obstet Gynecol.* 1988;159(3):616–21.

62. Jovanovic L. Role of diet and insulin treatment of diabetes in pregnancy. *Clin Obstet Gynecol.* 2000;43(1):46–55.

63. Langer O. Management of gestational diabetes: Pharmacologic treatment options and glycemic control. *Endocrinol Metab Clin North Am.* 2006;35(1):53–78, vi.

64. Sokol RJ, Blackwell SC, American College of Obstetricians and Gynecologists. Committee on Practice Bulletins-Gynecology. ACOG practice bulletin: Shoulder dystocia. Number 40, November 2002. (Replaces practice pattern number 7, October 1997). *Int J Gynaecol Obstet.* 2003;80(1):87–92.

65. Combs CA, Rosenn B, Miodovnik M, Siddiqi TA. Sonographic EFW and macrosomia: Is there an optimum formula to predict diabetic fetal macrosomia? *J Matern Fetal Med.* 2000;9(1):55–61.

66. MacNeill S, Dodds L, Hamilton DC, Armson BA, VandenHof M. Rates and risk factors for recurrence of gestational diabetes. *Diabetes Care.* 2001;24(4):659–62.

67. Kim C, Newton KM, Knopp RH. Gestational diabetes and the incidence of type 2 diabetes: a systematic review. *Diabetes Care.* 2002;25(10):1862–8.

Connective Tissue Disorders and Pregnancy

Joseph E. Peterson

Introduction

This chapter will attempt to guide the clinician in the management of patients with connective tissue disorders prior to conception, throughout the antepartum period to delivery, and in the immediate postpartum period. Criteria and features of the connective tissue disorder diagnoses, unique challenges of management for each, and plans for delivery and follow-up will be introduced. When applicable, we will also discuss the long-term implications for patients who have a connective tissue disorder and have had a past pregnancy and/or wish to become pregnant again.

Connective tissue disorders can be grouped as either (1) auto-immune mediated or (2) hereditary. Either type of connective tissue disorder can be debilitating for patients under normal circumstances. Due to the unique physiologic changes of pregnancy, the impact on patients with connective tissue disorders is worthy of examination prior to conception and also warrants close follow-up during pregnancy and in the immediate postpartum period.

This set of disorders can present diagnostic dilemmas when pregnant patients present with symptoms and signs coincident with both their preexisting disorder as well as disease processes that are unique to pregnancy, such as preeclampsia. Even lacking a pathologic diagnosis, a pregnant patient may undergo changes that can either be confused for or mask underlying connective tissue disease. Also, a preexisting diagnosis for many of the connective tissue disorders puts patients who become pregnant at an increased risk of other complications of pregnancy such as preeclampsia and also increases the need for cesarean delivery.

This interplay of mechanisms, particularly with immune-mediated disorders, will find the pregnancy having direct impact, both positively and negatively, on the manifestations of the disorder. Conversely, it is important for the clinician to know how the disorder can impact both mother and fetus in a planned or current pregnancy.

Scope of the Problem

The immune mediated disorders consist of systemic lupus erythematosus, Sjögren's syndrome, rheumatoid arthritis, and less commonly, scleroderma and poly/dermatomyositis. The preponderance of patients effected by these disorders are females, and of those, the majority are childbearing age [1]. Even those disorders, which are more frequently found in patients in their fourth decade of life and beyond, have potential for increasing impact during pregnancy; recently more women increasingly delay childbearing until later in life. The clinician should have a high index of suspicion for the diagnosis of new cases of these disorders during pregnancy and must also focus on the needs of the pregnant patient with preexisting disease.

Systemic lupus erythematous (SLE) affects between 15 and 50 patients per 100,000 in the United States. It is estimated that 0.15–1.5 million adults in the United States have SLE [1,2]. Sjögren's syndrome is also one of the more common connective tissue disorders, with a prevalence that varies from country to country, from 0.2% to 2.1% of studied populations. However, it is less likely to impact pregnancy due to the later age of onset [3]. Rheumatoid arthritis has an international prevalence and impacts 0.4–1.3% of the population. In the United States, 1.5 million adults are afflicted with this disease [4]. A less common disorder, scleroderma, is found in 24–27 patients per 100,000 [5,6]. Poly/dermatomyositis is considered rare and affects an unknown, but small segment of the population. Estimates place its occurrence in the United States at 0.5–8.4 cases per million population [7].

Hereditary disorders such as Marfan syndrome, Ehlers Danlos syndrome, and osteogenesis imperfecta, though even less common than the

Table 44.1 Hereditary Connective Tissue Disorders with Frequency [8]

Hereditary Connective Tissue Disorders	Prevalence
Marfan syndrome	1 in 3,000–5,000
Ehlers Danlos syndrome	1 in 5,000 (all types)
Osteogenesis Imperfecta	1 in 30,000–60,000

immune-mediated disorders, deserve attention due to their unique and potentially severe maternal and fetal impact. Table 44.1 summarizes the prevalence of these uncommon hereditary disorders.

Immune-Mediated Disorders

Systemic Lupus Erythematosus

SLE is one of the most common rheumatologic connective tissue diseases. SLE, like many of the immune-mediated connective tissue disorders, has strict criteria for diagnosis. These criteria need not be met all at once but may be present in one patient sequentially. In new patients without known SLE, careful history taking and examination for current signs and symptoms, as presented in Table 44.2, is paramount to making the diagnosis.

Unfortunately, many signs and symptoms of SLE can mimic changes inherent to pregnancy, clouding the diagnosis and therefore management of the patient presenting later in pregnancy. For instance, a malar rash or anemia may be present in both SLE and normal pregnancy.

Preconception

If a diagnosis is known or suspected at the time of a pre-conceptual visit, the patient should be encouraged to delay conception until symptoms have been absent for at least 6 months. A shorter time period from symptom onset to pregnancy has been associated with more adverse outcomes [11]. Alternatives to a high-risk pregnancy include surrogacy or adoption. The medication leflunomide has a prolonged presence in a patient's serum; documented absence of leflunomide should be confirmed prior to attempts at conception.

Labs

Baseline preeclampsia labs should be drawn initially and each trimester for later comparison, should signs and symptoms develop later in pregnancy. These labs

Table 44.2 Criteria for Diagnosis of Systemic Lupus Erythematous (adapted from [9,10])

Criteria	Finding
Malar rash	Flat or raised, fixed erythema, sparing the nasolabial folds, on the malar eminences
Discoid rash	Erythematous raised patches, may be accompanied by scaling and scarring
Photosensitivity	Skin rash upon exposure to sunlight, historically reported or observed
Oral ulcers	Physician-observed, painless oral or nasopharyngeal ulcers
Non-erosive arthritis	Tenderness, swelling or effusion in two or more peripheral joints
Pleurites or pericarditis	Pleuritic – historically reported or heard by physician. Pericarditis – on ECG or rub heard
Renal disorder	Persistent proteinuria (>0.5 g/day or 3+ on urine dip) or cellular casts (any type)
Neurologic disorder	Seizures or psychosis with neither medication nor metabolic cause
Hematologic disorder	Hemolytic anemia with reticulocytosis, leukopenia on two occasions, lymphopenia on two occasions, or thrombocytopenia (<100,000/mm^2) without medication-induced cause
Immunologic disorder	Anti-DNA antibody, anti-Sm, anti-phospholipid antibodies, false-positive syphilis test
Positive antinuclear antibody	Detection of antinuclear antibody by immunofluorescence in the absence of medication as causative agent.

include complete blood count (CBC), renal function studies, liver function tests (LFTs) and uric acid. The clinician should also obtain lupus anticoagulant, anticardiolipin IgG and IgM, antiT double-stranded deoxyribonucleic acid (dsDNA) antibodies, and complement levels (CH50, C3, C4), which are specific to SLE. These should be used for tracking the disease during each trimester as well. Testing for anti-Ro/SSA and anti-La/SSB antibodies should also be done due to the significance for the fetus. Of note, the clinician should not initiate therapy based on the findings of these blood tests alone but should make decisions in conjunction with the entire clinical evaluation [12].

Antepartum Management

Patients with SLE should be managed conjointly with maternal-fetal medicine specialists including a multidisciplinary approach including a rheumatologist's evaluation at least once every trimester [13]. Along with the normal ultrasounds for dating and anatomy, routine antepartum monitoring should be performed at least weekly according to American Congress of Obstetrics and Gynecology (ACOG) guidelines beginning at estimated gestational age (EGA) of 30–32 weeks.

Hypertension, proteinuria, thrombocytopenia, and seizures are not features of a normal pregnancy, but their mere presence does not help the clinician trying to distinguish between preeclampsia and a lupus flare or lupus nephritis; all of these are more likely to occur during pregnancy [11]. In these situations, laboratory evaluation may be helpful in distinguishing the diagnosis. Some labs that may be otherwise diagnostic for SLE, however, may not be abnormal in pregnancy. For instance, a normal complement titer does not guarantee an absence of a diagnosis of SLE as complement 3 (C3) and complement 4 (C4) levels may not be abnormal in pregnancies with preeclampsia. The onset of signs and symptoms prior to 20 weeks EGA is more likely, however, to be consistent with lupus nephritis [12]. See Box 44.1 for more features that differentiate between new-onset preeclampsia versus lupus nephritis.

Overall, maternal mortality is increased by 20 times in patients with SLE. These patients are also at increased risk for preterm labor, unplanned cesarean delivery, fetal growth restriction, preeclampsia, thrombosis, infection, thrombocytopenia and need for transfusion [14]. Predictors for adverse outcomes include active disease in the 6 months prior to or during pregnancy, a history of or current lupus nephritis, discontinuation of hydroxychloriquine, concurrent antiphospholipid syndrome, and thrombocytopenia [12].

Box 44.1 Preeclampsia vs lupus nephritis [12]

Lupus nephritis

Proteinuria with sediment (red and white cells and asts)

Low or decreasing complement levels

Less prominently elevated LFTs and/or uric acid

Leukopenia

Preeclampsia

Simple proteinuria without sediment

Normal or increased complement levels

Prominently elevated LFTs and/or uric acid

Normal white blood cell count

In the patient with SLE, there are risks to the fetus other than the obstetrical. Patients with anti-Ro/SSA and anti-La/SSB antibodies have an increased risk for a fetus with complete heart block (CHB) and should have increased monitoring to account for this possibility [15]. Due to this association, if CHB is found in a fetus of a previously undiagnosed patient, the presence of SLE or other auto-immune disease processes with anti-Ro/La antibodies should be considered. Even without progression to CHB, there is also risk to children born of mothers who are positive for anti-Ro/La antibodies of milder manifestations of neonatal lupus syndrome. These outcomes are less severe, with the primary manifestations being transient dermatologic changes, though hematologic derangements (thrombocytopenia, hemolysis) may occur as well [16].

Treatment and Medications

When dealing with connective tissue disorders, appropriate treatments should not be withheld solely due to the pregnant state, but only if the treatment may be toxic to the developing fetus. A patient with SLE who is currently controlled on medications should continue these medications when contemplating pregnancy unless the medications are contraindicated. If the patient becomes pregnant while uncontrolled or has a symptom flare, as with many medications in pregnancy, new dosages should be begun at or titrated to the lowest effective dose [12].

Low-dose aspirin may be used for SLE patients who are at increased risk for preeclampsia for symptom control as well as risk reduction. Hydroxychloroquine should be continued, particularly since cessation is associated with an increased risk of flare. Generally, glucocorticoids are used at the lowest possible dose and with counseling regarding the risk of cleft lip and palate if used in the first trimester. Patients receiving long-term steroid treatment should receive a stress-dose at the time of delivery [17]. Other drugs used during pregnancy for the management of SLE are summarized in Table 44.3.

Postpartum Considerations

Because there is increased risk of lupus flare in the puerperium, reported to be as high as 25–60%, patients should be counseled and encouraged to consult their physician should worsening of disease occur in the postpartum period [12]. Treatments can then be administered without consideration of fetal

Table 44.3 Drugs for Use during Pregnancy in Systemic Lupus Erythematous and Other Immune-Mediated Connective Tissue Disorders (Adapted from [12,17])

Use of Drugs in Pregnancy		
	Drug	**Notes**
Allowed	NSAIDs	Controversial finding of increased first trimester risk of miscarriage. Use in third trimester may cause closure of ductus arterioles and oligohydramnios. Aspirin OK throughout.
	Hydroxychloroquine	Cessation associated with increased risk of flare.
	Glucocorticoids	Increased risk of cleft palate/lip with first trimester use.
	Azathioprine	
	Cyclosporine	
	Tacrolimus	
	Methyldopa, labetalol, nifedipine, hydralazine	Used for hypertensive control in preference to ACE inhibitors and angiotensin II receptor blockers.
Use with caution	Rituximab	May result in fetal B-cell lymphocytopenia
	Belimumab	
Contraindicated	ACE inhibitors and ARBs	Significant fetal risk through all trimesters but may be necessary in scleroderma-related renal crisis
	Cyclophosphamide	Teratogenic
	Mycophenolate mofetil	
	Methotrexate	Teratogenic
	Leflunomide	May remain in patient's serum for up to 2 years after cessation

or neonatal impact unless the patient is breastfeeding. If breastfeeding, consideration needs to directed toward using medications that are safe in lactation. The LactMed database [19] is an important resource for the obstetrician in this regard. Recommendations remain similar to those during pregnancy, including the contraindication for cyclophosphamide and methotrexate.

Sjögren's Syndrome

The characteristic features of Sjögren's syndrome (SS) are dry eyes and mouth, enlarged parotid glands, and in the majority of cases, anti-Ro/La antibodies. There is a large overlap with other connective tissue disorders, in particular SLE, so many of the same recommendations can apply if the patient has a primary rheumatologic disease and the Sjögren's syndrome is secondary. The clinician may have difficulty distinguishing between SS and other autoimmune rheumatologic diseases as there is no single distinguishing diagnostic test.

Preconception

Research and interpretation of pregnancy outcomes are necessarily confounded in those cases where secondary Sjögren's (sSS) exists with other rheumatologic diseases. The evidence is conflicting still even in those with primary Sjögren's syndrome (pSS). Some case–control studies show no difference in outcomes of patients with pSS [20], while others show an increase not only in heart block, as expected from the high rate of anti-Ro/La antibody presence, but also an increase in spontaneous abortions, preterm delivery and cesarean delivery. This increase exists in patients who have preexisting disease as well as those who receive the diagnosis after becoming pregnant [21]. Therefore, the patient with primary Sjögren's, and certainly the patient with secondary Sjögren's, should be counseled that any pregnancy should be classified as high risk. As with SLE, a 6-month symptom and flare-free or symptom-managed interval before pregnancy is recommended [18].

Labs

As mentioned previously, there is no specific lab test to confirm SS. However, for monitoring purposes, in addition to standard prenatal labs, ESR and C reactive protein (CRP) (which may be elevated in those with resultant higher cardiovascular risk), anti-Ro/La antibody titers, anti-nuclear and anti-centromere antibody titers, and liver function tests should be drawn for comparison [22].

Antepartum Management

Since the peak incidence of Sjögren's disease is in the fourth and fifth decades of life [1], a subsequent paucity of cases exist to study. Strong recommendations regarding its management during pregnancy therefore do not exist. It is generally accepted, however, that the pregnant patient with SS should be managed with a multidisciplinary approach and a keen eye for flares and exacerbation of symptoms [18]. No specific recommendations for antepartum fetal surveillance exist. However, similar to SLE, if anti-Ro/SSA and anti-La/SSB antibodies are present in the patient with SS, the fetus is at increased risk for the development of neonatal lupus and of complete heart block. For this reason, if anti-Ro/La antibodies are present, it would be prudent to apply the same principles for increased surveillance as with SLE.

Many signs and symptoms of SS can be difficult to differentiate from the common complaints of pregnancy. These include mild anemia and thrombocytopenia, urinary frequency, or dyspepsia. Fatigue is the most common complaint in SS. It may be difficult if not impossible for the clinician to discern if the fatigue is pathologically increasing due to Sjögren's or simply due to the pregnancy. However, SS affects multiple organ systems; when this results in pathologic symptoms, they should be deemed as worrisome and not attributed solely to pregnancy. These could include persistent cough or throat clearing with globus, evidence of thyroiditis, urinary dysuria and urgency, and vulvovaginal dryness and pruritus with dyspareunia [22].

Treatment and Medication

Rituximab may provide relief from fatigue in the non-pregnant patient [22], but is not recommended in pregnancy [19]. NSAIDs are likely to provide some relief of joint symptoms with the standard precautions regarding use in the first and third trimesters. Lubricating eye drops may be used for the relief of ophthalmologic symptoms. A vaginal lubricant may aid in symptoms related to vaginal dryness. Due to the risk of preterm labor with poor dentition, the patient with SS would do well to maintain her oral hygiene, which can be made difficult without the lubricating qualities of saliva. Pilocarpine and cevimeline (for salivary stimulation) have not been tested in pregnant patients but are considered safe for use in pregnancy [19]. Other medications chosen for symptomatic relief or to address other pathologic exocrine and extraglandular manifestations of SS should be selected in coordination with the patient's rheumatologist.

Postpartum Considerations

There are no specific sequelae unique to SS of concern in the postpartum period other than surveillance for the development of neonatal lupus in the fetus. Breastfeeding considerations need to ensure the patient's medications are safe for breastfeeding.

Rheumatoid Arthritis

The woman with rheumatoid arthritis (RA) can expect to have inflammatory-mediated symptoms, which predominantly manifest in the peripheral joints. The disease exists in both juvenile and adult forms, and it is one of the more likely pre-existing connective tissue disorders to be encountered by the clinician treating pregnant patients. Clear criteria based on a scoring system are available from the American College of Rheumatology [24]. The criteria can be found at www.rheumatology.org/Portals/0/Files/2010%20Rheumatoid%20Arthritis%20Classification_EXCERPT%202010.pdf A simple 1:1 relationship does not exist between signs, symptoms, and score but instead relies on relative weighting of the number, location, and asymmetry of affected joints, presence of rheumatoid factor, abnormalities of CRP or ESR, and duration of symptoms.

Preconception

The pregnant patient who presents with a known diagnosis of RA can be given reassurance that a planned pregnancy is most likely to result in improvement of her symptoms (up to 90% of pregnant women with RA) rather than exacerbation [25]. Discussion of discontinuation of medications for RA can be undertaken at this time, with the understanding that symptoms are likely to improve once pregnancy is achieved. Evidence is unclear about why this disease process tends to improve in pregnancy, but a mismatch in HLA antigens between mother and fetus seems to play a role [26]. She should be counseled that though her symptoms are likely to improve *during* pregnancy, the postpartum period will see not only a return of symptoms within 3–4 months, but in approximately one-third of women, a flare as well [25,27]. As previously stated, if a patient is using leflunomide, pregnancy should not be attempted until the drug is fully eliminated from her system.

Labs

Laboratory values used in diagnosis of RA are not necessary for tracking during pregnancy, though they may aid the clinician in diagnosis if disease is only suspected. Rheumatoid factor, CRP, and ESR are used for initial diagnosis. There is no need for obstetricians to monitor changes of these labs during pregnancy.

Antepartum Management

As with other connective tissue disorders, there is considerable overlap of symptomatology with RA and normal pregnancy including fatigue, anorexia, and nonspecific musculoskeletal symptoms. If extraarticular symptoms and signs are present, such as rheumatoid nodules, vasculitis, or plueritis, the practitioner would, however, need to consider RA exacerbation in the differential diagnosis. Management is focused mainly on relief of these symptoms.

Studies show conflicting results regarding risk for hypertension and miscarriage with RA, but generally, there does not appear to be a significant impact of RA itself on pregnancy outcomes. The fetal and neonatal affects are not predominantly from the disease process but interestingly stem more from the effects of medications used in its management. Patients who have poorly controlled disease and require glucocorticoids for disease suppression are more likely to have small for gestational age infants as well as preterm delivery [28].

As with other connective tissue disorders, the pregnant patient with RA should receive the benefit of a multidisciplinary approach to the management of her pregnancy. There are no specific recommendations for antepartum fetal surveillance or maternal fetal medicine (MFM)consultation, but co-management with a rheumatologist is recommended [18].

Treatment and Medications

As an immune-mediated connective tissue disorder, many of the medications recommended for the treatment of RA are equivalent to those listed in Table 44.3 for use with SLE. The same precautions and stipulations for their use exist when considering treating RA in pregnancy. Due to the likelihood of remission or lessoning of symptoms, aspirin, NSAIDs, and glucocorticoids are the mainstays of treatment in the pregnant patient with more aggressive treatment usually unnecessary. Similar to SLE, NSAIDs should be avoided in the first and third trimesters and glucocorticoids should be maintained at the lowest possible dose necessary. Sulfasalazine also has anti-inflammatory properties and, based on studies involving inflammatory bowel disease, has been deemed safe for use in pregnant patients with RA [17]. Unique to the treatment of RA are penicillamine and gold salts. Penicillamine is rated as class D by the FDA and should not be used during pregnancy. Gold salts should probably be substituted with a well-studied alternative that is more definitively known to be safe since experience with gold salts in pregnancy is quite limited [29].

Modifications to the patient's day-to-day mechanical functioning such as those introduced by physical and occupational therapists may be beneficial to patients in order to teach them how to properly protect the affected joints and mitigate the impact of pain, inflammation, and chronic degradation on activities of daily living.

Postpartum Considerations

Patients can expect a return of symptoms in the postpartum period, usually within the first 3–4 months. It is possible that these symptoms may be severe enough to be classified as a flare.

Pregnancy itself may increase the risk of a patient developing RA at a later point in her life, with the risk being greatest in the immediate postpartum period after a first pregnancy and lasting up to 9 months afterward [30]. Some authors believe breast feeding may be associated with an increased risk of flare as well as development of new disease [30]. Conversely, the largest longitudinal study found that breastfeeding may provide protection from RA in patients without the disease [31]. It is difficult to differentiate between the expected return or flare of RA in the postpartum period when searching for a link to breastfeeding.

As there is significant overlap in the medications used for relief of symptoms in RA and in SLE, consultation with the LactMed database [19] can be helpful in choosing medications for use in the breastfeeding patient with RA. Contraindications exist to the use of cyclophosphamide and other immunomodulary and cytotoxic agents as well as methotrexate, all of which are typically used for the treatment of moderate to severe RA.

Scleroderma

Also known as systemic sclerosis, scleroderma is an uncommon disease in the pregnant patient, primarily due to the average age of onset being from the fourth to sixth decades of life. Beyond the expected skin thickening from overproduction of collagen, typical manifestations include Reynaud's phenomenon and gastroesophageal reflux. Pulmonary involvement is also common, resulting in dyspnea. However, due to the potential for catastrophic complications particularly in those with end-organ involvement [18], vigilance in diagnosis, counseling, management, and monitoring the presence of the disease and its sequelae is important for the obstetrician caring for the patient with scleroderma.

Preconception

Patients should be counseled that the rate of miscarriage appears to be higher in both those patients with preexisting disease as well as those who eventually receive the diagnosis [32]. Pregnancy with scleroderma is considered high risk due to the increased rate of preterm delivery, intrauterine growth restriction, low-birth-weight infants, increased hospital stay, and preeclampsia in those with active disease [33–35]. Although most women with well-controlled or mild disease will have normal outcomes, pregnancy should be delayed in those with recent onset of scleroderma, especially those positive for Scl-70 antibodies (associated with the diffuse form of the disease). Pregnancy avoidance is recommended for those with severe end-organ damage [34]. Renal crisis may present challenges in maintaining both maternal and fetal health. Though a patient with a history of renal crisis is not more at risk for a repeat occurrence during pregnancy, this patient should be encouraged to pursue stabilization of her disease prior to attempting conception as chronic kidney disease is associated with more adverse maternal and fetal outcomes [18]. Patients can expect to see improvement in their Reynaud's but worsening of GERD. Skin changes tend to remain stable throughout the pregnancy, but worsen in the postpartum period [33].

Labs

It is important to know baseline pulmonary and renal function as compromise of these organs comes with higher risk of adverse outcomes. Patients with recent diagnosis/onset of disease should be tested for Scl-70 antibodies as their presence is associated with higher risk of recurrence and worsening of disease [34]. Baseline preeclampsia labs, including LFTs, could prove useful in distinguishing those with new onset renal crisis versus preeclampsia later in the pregnancy.

Antepartum Management

Patients with scleroderma should be concurrently managed with a rheumatologist and maternal fetal medicine sub-specialist [18,34]. No clear recommendation for antenatal testing exists. These patients warrant increased surveillance due to the increased risk for IUGR and preterm delivery.

Gastroesophageal reflux and some dyspnea are common and expected consequences of pregnancy. These concerns, along with edema or arthralgia, may be difficult to distinguish from normal complaints of pregnancy. Worsening dyspnea may, however, indicate underlying cardiac or pulmonary disease. The clinician should promptly work up symptoms or signs suspicious for even mild cardiopulmonary involvement in the pregnant patient with known or suspected scleroderma given the known increased morbidity and mortality associated with pulmonary hypertension.

Pregnant scleroderma patients with rapidly increased thickening of the skin during pregnancy are at risk for renal crisis and accompanying malignant hypertension [36]. As with the nephritis in an SLE flare, differentiating between scleroderma renal crisis and preeclampsia may be difficult. Scleroderma renal crisis does not increase LFTs, however, as is usually seen in preeclampsia, and there is rarely sediment or severe proteinuria with renal crisis. Despite the risk to the developing fetus, rheumatologists recommend that a woman with scleroderma and in renal crisis receive an ACE inhibitor based on its life-saving impact [18,32]. If this course is chosen, the patient should be counseled on the utility of the conservation of maternal life and health weighted with the very real risk of fetal impact throughout all trimesters. Alternately, the patient can be supported with dialysis and fetal monitoring in the intensive care unit [32].

Treatment and Medications

As with other immune-mediated connective tissue disorders, treatment is focused on symptom control, primarily via the control of inflammation and with anti-rheumatic drugs. In this regard, NSAIDs and glucocorticoids are the mainstays of treatment. Patients can receive the same standard treatment for arthralgias and gastroesophageal reflux disease (GERD) used in normal pregnancies. Recommendations for medications used in the treatment of patients with scleroderma with end-organ involvement are similar to those used in SLE and can be utilized with the standard precautions as outlined in Table 44.3.

Postpartum Considerations

After delivery, patients are likely to see return of their Raynaud's, improved GERD, and have potential worsening of the skin changes associated with scleroderma [33]. It is unclear if pregnancy impacts the potential for developing or worsening scleroderma, but those with newly diagnosed disease and Scl-70 antibodies do appear to be more at risk for progression of their disease after a pregnancy [34]. Close follow-up with a rheumatologist is recommended.

Miscellaneous

Polymyositis and Dermatomyositis

Polymyositis and dermatomyositis are characterized by progressive weakness of skeletal muscles. They are differentiated by the presence of a rash on the face, trunk, elbows, knees, and hands in dermatomyositis. Electromyography and muscle biopsy are necessary for the diagnosis. The paucity of data regarding these disease processes in pregnancy prevents formulation of definitive counseling or management plans. In several case series, there appears to be an increased risk of IUGR, preterm delivery, and miscarriage, particularly in those in whom the disease begins or worsens during pregnancy. It would consequently be prudent to manage the patient cooperatively with a rheumatologist and maternal fetal medicine consult. Treatment is based around the same medications and strategies as with other immune-mediated connective tissue disorders and tight control or inactivity of the disease appears to correlate with better maternal and fetal outcomes [18,36,37].

Undifferentiated, Mixed Connective Tissue Disease and Overlap Syndrome

All the entities previously mentioned share many features, both clinically and in laboratory assessment. Though criteria may exist for a definitive diagnosis of each process, these diseases do not always exist in isolation but rather in patients with features that are incomplete for diagnosis. Overlap between diseases may be present or a patient may encompass more than one disease process.

Due to the scarcity of data regarding these undifferentiated, mixed and overlapped diseases and pregnancy, it is not beneficial to attempt to discern specific management strategies for each unique presentation. It would rather behoove the clinician to simply be aware that this potential for overlap may further complicate the interpretation of clinical data in the pregnant patient with connective tissue disorders that are immune-mediated. Because outcomes in these patients appear to be similar to those with SLE, counseling should include the same discussion about the likelihood of a normal pregnancy course with the increased risk for maternal and fetal complications including flare, preeclampsia, preterm delivery, and IUGR. If the patient appears to have mixed features, management should still focus on early diagnosis of worsening disease, symptom relief with the anti-inflammatory, anti-malarial, and anti-rheumatic medications, treatment for end-organ disease, and multidisciplinary consultation [18,36].

Hereditary Connective Tissue Disorders

The hereditary connective tissue disorders are rare. Due to their dramatic impact on collagen and subsequent risk for catastrophic bleeding caused primarily by vascular rupture, it is important to address their implications and management during pregnancy.

Marfan Syndrome

As an autosomal dominant disease, the patient is unlikely to present to the obstetrician lacking a known diagnosis of Marfan syndrome. Aside from the classic phenotypical features characteristic of the disease, patients with Marfan syndrome also have cardiovascular changes that can complicate or become worsened by pregnancy.

Preconception

Patients should be referred to a genetic counselor prior to conception due to the autosomal dominant pattern of inheritance, as the fetus has at least a 50% chance of transmission [38,39]. A screening echocardiogram is recommended, especially for the assessment of the aortic root along with potential valvular involvement. MRI or CT should be used to assess the length of the entire aorta through the arch and descending portions. Those patients with aortic root dilation beyond 4–4.5cm should be counseled on the high risk of rupture and repair is therefore suggested pre-conceptually. Rupture may, however, occur at any dilation [39]. There also appears to be an increased risk for preterm delivery in these patients [40].

Antepartum Management

Early consultation with a geneticist and maternal fetal medicine sub-specialist is recommended for pregnancy planning and monitoring [38]. Since the risks of Marfan syndrome are primarily to the mother, no clear recommendations for fetal surveillance exist. A referral to a cardiologist is encouraged, as well as regularly scheduled echocardiograms every 1–2 months [39].

Measures should also be taken to shorten the second stage of labor and decrease the maternal effort expended. Operative vaginal delivery decreases the risk of undue pressure on the vascular system and decreases risk of aortic rupture for those patients with dilation under 4.5cm. Cesarean delivery should be undertaken in those with dilation >4.5cm. Delivery should take place where immediate access to a cardiothoracic surgeon is available [39].

The pregnant patient with Marfan syndrome is more likely to experience postpartum hemorrhage [40]. The clinician should therefore insure that the resources and medications for management are available in such cases.

Treatment and Medications

In all patients with Marfan syndrome (not only those with noted aortic root dilation), strict blood pressure control (<130 systolic) should be achieved with beta blockers in order to decrease the risk of further dilation and rupture [39].

Prophylactic surgical treatment of aortic root dilation is not usually recommended during pregnancy. However, if the aortic root is found to be >5 cm and rapidly enlarging during pregnancy, discussion should be undertaken regarding the risks of dissection and rupture versus surgery during pregnancy [39]. Successful emergent surgical repair of an aortic dissection may be possible concurrent with delivery in the third trimester if the dissection is not fatal to the patient.

Postpartum Considerations

Patients are at risk for continued aortic root dilation and dissection/rupture after delivery [41]. It would therefore be prudent for patients with Marfan syndrome to be monitored closely in conjunction with a cardiologist. Regular visits and possible imaging during the first 6 weeks postpartum could be considered.

Ehlers Danlos Syndrome

Patients with Ehlers Danlos syndrome (EDS) typically have hyperelasticity and mobility of the skin and joints as well as generally more fragile tissue. Multiple subtypes exist, each with varying degrees of expression of these features; different tissues may be affected. Development of guidelines that apply in all presentations of the disease is therefore not possible. Pregnant patients with EDS are rare, but it is important to recognize the risks associated with the disease during pregnancy regardless of subtype.

Preconception

Due to the varying inheritance patterns associated with each type of the syndrome, consultation with a geneticist is recommended in order to assess risks of transmission to the fetus. A pregnancy in a patient with EDS should be considered high-risk with preterm labor and delivery, uterine rupture, peri-partum hemorrhage, and aortic rupture among the possible complications [42].

Labs

If the diagnosis of subtype is unclear, DNA sequencing may be performed, in order to differentiate and stratify risks of different complications of the syndrome.

Antepartum Management

Early consultation and co-management with a maternal fetal medicine sub-specialist is recommended. A definition of the exact type and therefore unique risks is important in guiding care; genetic input may be required. Prenatal diagnosis of the fetus, with amniocentesis or chorionic villus sampling (CVS) can also aid in management plans [42]. The nature of this disorder creates increased risk over baseline for these procedures. Referral to a cardiologist for an echocardiogram is also recommended due to the risk of vascular complications with all subtypes of the disease [43].

Patients in this high-risk setting with new onset of dyspnea, chest pain, bleeding, or orthostatic intolerance ("drop attacks") should be evaluated immediately to rule out a vascular event [43].

Due to the risk of uterine rupture, early delivery has been recommended, from 32 to 36 weeks, with the mode to be determined in consultation with all invested parties. Poor healing of wounds, whether incisional or unintended lacerations, should be factored in to the decision. Retention sutures are recommended in repairs [42].

Use of anesthesia must be individualized for the patient withEhlers-Danlos syndrome (EDS) as the patient may have musculoskeletal compromise impacting access for regional anesthesia, or cervical spine laxity impeding intubation for general administration. Patients with EDS also show a decreased sensitivity to local anesthetics. The subsequent changes in blood pressure with anesthesia are important to note and monitor, especially as they may pertain to subtypes with increased risk of vascular complications. Spontaneous ventilation if possible, gentle tissue handling and copious padding are necessary in the anesthetized patient to prevent iatrogenic damage to tissues [44].

Treatment and Medications

Though the different subtypes may involve varying manifestations and degrees of symptoms, management of common symptoms and complications largely remains the same, regardless of subtype. Acetaminophen is recommended for pain. While NSAIDs may be used with their typical caveats, their use should be minimal in those with EDS subtypes that include easy bruising. Physical therapy can help guide patients in relief of their symptoms and maximizing their functional ability while preventing injury [43].

Postpartum Considerations

Patients with EDS are more prone to hemorrhage and poor wound healing. It is recommended that those with the vascular subtype of EDS be counseled against future pregnancies due to high risk of morbidity and mortality [44].

Osteogenesis Imperfecta

As the rarest of the three hereditary connective tissue disorders discussed, osteogenesis imperfecta (OI) is unlikely to be encountered by the obstetrician. At least 15 sub-types of OI exist. Types I–IV are the most common, with type 1 making up 30% [45]. However, type II is unlikely to ever be seen or addressed in pregnancy as this type in the fetus usually results in an IUFD. There is little evidence beyond case reports regarding the natural history during pregnancy of a patient with any of the other subtypes of OI, which range in severity from mild to moderate. Knowledge of how the disorder affects the non-pregnant patient does, however, allow some general observations and recommendations to be made for management. Treatment should be tailored to the severity of the individual's disease [42].

Preconception

The majority of common subtypes of OI are autosomal dominant in inheritance; therefore, the patient should receive counseling from a geneticist to ascertain family history, specific gene mutations, and risk of transmission and implications for the fetus. If the patient has severe scoliotic deformities, the patient should be counseled on the physiologic changes of pregnancy related to abdominal and chest cavity volume that may have greater than normal impact, potentially resulting in early delivery due to maternal compromise. Bisphosphonates, commonly used to treat the decreased bone density in OI, should be discontinued prior to planned pregnancy as their impact on the fetus is unknown [46].

Labs

DNA sequencing can determine the maternal diagnosis if it is unclear in milder disease. If the specific subtype and therefore mutation is known, an amniocentesis or CVS can yield cells in which the mutation may be sought, affording fetal diagnosis and improved counseling as well. Baseline preeclamptic labs may be clinically useful as these patients are possibly at increased risk for preeclampsia. calcium, phosphate, vitamin D, parathyroid hormone, CK, and CRP levels should also be checked every trimester [46].

Antepartum Management

Multidisciplinary management should be undertaken with maternal fetal medicine sub-specialists as well as cardiologists and orthopedists as needed based on a patient's individual presentation [46]. If amniocentesis or CVS is not used to confirm transmission to the fetus, ultrasound may yield characteristic findings of marked bowing and shortening of long bones or of multiple bony fractures. The patient may be at increased risk for preeclampsia as well as IUGR, therefore regular fetal growth scans and testing would be warranted particularly if it is unknown whether the disease has been transmitted to the fetus [42,46].

Pregnancy can often be carried to term in patients with OI. Due to the possibility for worsening cardiac or pulmonary complications (if the vascular or bony deformities of the mother are severe), late-preterm to early preterm delivery may, however, be recommended [46].

Operative vaginal delivery is contraindicated in fetuses with OI. Care should be taken to minimize risk of fracture in the mother with OI as even routine obstetrical manipulations may result in fracture. The mode of delivery should be chosen based on the unique features and severity of the individual patient, understanding that the fetus may suffer fractures in utero prior to delivery regardless of mode. If cesarean is chosen, permanent suture is recommended for closure due to the increased risk of herniation of maternal tissues [42]. Malpresentation is common in patients with OI.

Treatment and Medications

Bisphosphonate therapy should be discontinued during pregnancy. Physical therapy and orthopedic surgery are also standard methods of treatment for OI [46].

Postpartum Considerations

It is unknown if pregnancy presents any risk of worsening of the disease state in the postpartum period and beyond [42].

Concluding Remarks

For most connective tissue disorders, a multidisciplinary approach to management is important. The incorporation of maternal-fetal medicine sub-specialists, rheumatologists, cardiologists, and other necessary specialists will offer the patient the best opportunity for early recognition and management of disease progression or of pregnancy compromise.

Although the majority of pregnancies in women with connective tissue disorders will result in normal outcomes, awareness of the unique challenges these disorders may present during pregnancy is paramount in order to recognize and address fetal and maternal impact in the preconceptual, antepartum, and postpartum states.

Initiation or modification of medications is appropriate to obtain therapeutic effect with the lowest possible dose and with the safest medication. Close patient follow-up during the immediate postpartum period is essential with mindfulness directed toward potential disease exacerbation or return as well as increased risks for development of co-morbidities.

References

1. M. Gaubitz. Epidemiology of Connective Tissue Disorders. *Rheumatology.* 2006; 45: iii3–iii4.
2. Systemic lupus erythematosus. www.cdc.gov/arthritis/basics/lupus.htm. Accessed February 15, 2016.
3. R. Patal, and A. Shahane. The epidemiology of Sjogren's syndrome. *Clin Epidemiol.* 2014; 6: 247–55.
4. Rheumatoid arthritis. www.cdc.gov/arthritis/basics/rheumatoid.htm. Accessed February 15, 2016.
5. M. D. Mayes. Scleroderma Epidemiology. *Rheum Dis Clin North Am.* 2003 May; 29(2): 239–54.
6. M. D. Mayes, J. V. Lacey, Jr., and J. Beebe-Dimmer, et al. Prevalence, incidence, survival, and disease characteristics of systemic sclerosis in a large US population. *Arthritis Rheum.* 2003 Aug; 48(8): 2246–55.
7. Polymyositis. http://emedicine.medscape.com/article/335925-overview#a6. Accessed February 15, 2016.
8. F. G. Cunningham, K. J. Leveno, S. L. Bloom, et al. Connective tissue disorders. In: F. G. Cunningham, K. J. Leveno, S. L. Bloom, et al, eds. *Williams Obstetrics,* 24th ed. New York: McGraw-Hill Education, 2014. AccessMedicine. Web. Accessed February 15, 2016.
9. E. M. Tan, A. S. Cohen, J. F. Fries, et al. The 1982 revised criteria for the classification of systemic lupus erythematosus. *Arthritis Rheum.* 1982; 25: 1271–7.
10. M. C. Hochberg. Updating the American College of Rheumatology revised criteria for the classification of systemic lupus erythematosus [letter]. *Arthritis Rheum.* 1997; 40: 1725.
11. L. W. Kwok, L. S. Tam, T. Zhu, et al. Predictors of maternal and fetal outcomes in pregnancies of patients

with systemic lupus erythematosus. *Lupus*. 2011 Jul; 20(8): 829–36.

12. Pregnancy in women with systemic lupus erythematous www.uptodate.com/contents/pregnancy-in-women-with-systemic-lupus-erythematosus. Accessed February 15, 2016.
13. A. Lateef and M. Petri. Managing lupus patients during pregnancy. *Best Pract Res Clin Rheumatol*. 2013 Jun; 27(3): 435–47.
14. M. E. B. Clowse, M. Jamison, E. Myers, and A. H. James. A National Study of the Complications of Lupus in Pregnancy. *Am J Obstet Gynecol*. 2008 August; 199(2): 127.e1–127.e6.
15. J. P. Buyon, R. M. Clancy, and D. M. Friedman. Autoimmune associated congenital heart block: integration of clinical and research clues in the management of the maternal/ foetal dyad at risk. *J Intern Med*. 2009 June; 265(6): 653–62.
16. E. E. Boh. Neonatal lupus erythematosus. *Clin Dermatol*. 2004 Apr–May; 22(2): 125–8.
17. Use of anti-inflammatory and immunosuppressive drugs in rheumatic diseases during pregnancy and lactation. www.uptodate.com/contents/use-of-antiinflammatory-and-immunosuppressive-drugs-in-rheumatic-diseases-during-pregnancy-and-lactation. Accessed February 15, 2016.
18. O. Ateka-Barrutia, and C. Nelson-Piercy. Management of rheumatologic diseases in pregnancy. *Int J Clin Rheumatol*. 2012; 7(5): 541–58.
19. Drugs and lactation database at the United States National Library of Medicine (LactMed). http://toxnet.nlm.nih.gov/newtoxnet/lactmed.htm. Accessed February 15, 2015.
20. H. J. Haga, C. G. Gjesdal, H.S. Koksvik, et al. Pregnancy outcome in patients with primary Sjögren's syndrome. A case–control study. *J Rheumatol*. 2005 Sep; 32(9): 1734–6.
21. S. De Carolis, S. Salvi, A. Botta, et al. The impact of primary Sjogren's syndrome on pregnancy outcome: Our series and review of the literature. *Autoimmun Rev*. 2014 Feb; 13(2): 103–7.
22. Clinical manifestations of Sjogren's syndrome: Extraglandular disease. www.uptodate.com/contents/clinical-manifestations-of-sjogrens-syndrome-extraglandular-disease. Accessed February 15, 2016.
23. S. Dass, S. J. Bowman, E. M. Vital, et al. Reduction of fatigue in Sjogren syndrome with rituximab: Results of a randomised, double-blind, placebo-controlled pilot study. *Ann Rheum Dis* 2008 Nov; 67(11): 1541–4.
24. D. Aletaha, T. Neogi, and A. J. Silman. 2010 Rheumatoid Arthritis Classification Criteria: An American College of Rheumatology/European League Against Rheumatism Collaborative Initiative. *Arthritis Rheum*. 2010 Sept; 62(9): 2569–81.
25. Y. A. de Man, R. J. Dolhain, F. E. van de Geijn FE, et al. Disease activity of rheumatoid arthritis during pregnancy: Results from a nationwide prospective study. *Arthritis Rheum*. 2008 Sept; 59(9):1241–8.
26. J. L. Nelson, K. A. Hughes, A. G. Smith, et al. Maternal–fetal disparity in HLA class II alloantigens and the pregnancy-induced amelioration of rheumatoid arthritis. *N Engl J Med*. 1993 Aug; 329(7): 466–71.
27. J. L. Nelson and M. Østensen Pregnancy and rheumatoid arthritis. *Rheum Dis Clin North Am*. 1997 Feb; 23(1): 195–212.
28. Y. A. de Man, J. M. Hazes, H. H. van der Heide, et al. Association of higher rheumatoid arthritis disease activity during pregnancy with lower birth weight: Results from a national prospective study. *Arthritis Rheum*. 2009; 60: 3196–206.
29. G. G. Briggs, R. K. Freeman, and S. J. Yaffe. *Drugs in Pregnancy and Lactation: A Reference Guide to Fetal and Neonatal Risk*, 10th ed. Philadelphia, PA: Lippincott Williams & Wilkins, 2014. Books@Ovid. Web. Accessed February 15, 2016.
30. Rheumatoid arthritis and pregnancy. www.uptodate.com/contents/rheumatoid-arthritis-and-pregnancy Accessed February 15, 2016.
31. E. W. Karlson, L. A. Mandl, S. E. Hankinson, et al. Do breast-feeding and other reproductive factors influence future risk of rheumatoid arthritis? Results from the Nurses' Health Study. *Arthritis Rheum*. 2004; 50: 3458–67.
32. Scleroderma in pregnancy. www.uptodate.com/scleroderma-in-pregnancy Accessed February 15, 2016.
33. V. D. Steen. Pregnancy in women with systemic sclerosis. *Obstet Gynecol*. 1999 Jul; 94(1): 15–20.
34. M. Taraborelli, V. Ramoni, A. Brucato, et al. Successful pregnancies but a higher risk of preterm births in patients with systemic sclerosis: An Italian Multicenter Study. *Arthritis Rheum*. 2012 Jun; 64(6): 1970–7.
35. E. F. Chakravarty, D. Khanna, and L. Chung. Pregnancy outcomes in systemic sclerosis, primary pulmonary hypertension, and sickle cell disease. *Obstet Gynecol*. 2008; 111: 927–34.
36. Autoimmune connective tissue disease in pregnancy. www.glowm.com/section_view/heading/Autoimmune%20Connective%20Tissue%20Disease%20in%20Pregnancy/item/167. Accessed February 15, 2016.

37. C.A. Silva, S. M. Sultan, and D. A. Isenberg. Pregnancy outcome in adult-onset idiopathic inflammatory myopathy. *Rheumatology.* 2003; Oct; 42(10): 1168–72.

38. American College of Obstetricians and Gynecologists. Identification and referral of maternal genetic conditions in pregnancy. Committee Opinion No. 643. *Obstet Gynecol.* 2015; 126: e49–51.

39. V. Regitz-Zagrosek, C. Blomstrom Lundqvist, C. Borghi, et al. ESC Guidelines on the management of cardiovascular diseases during pregnancy. *Eur Heart J.* 2011; 32: 3147–97.

40. R. A. Curry, E. Gelson, L. Swan, et al. Marfan syndrome and pregnancy; maternal and neonatal outcomes. *BJOG.* 2014; Apr; 121(5): 610–17.

41. R. T. Donnelly, N. M. Pinto, I. Kocolas, et al. The immediate and long-term impact of pregnancy on aortic growth rate and mortality in women with Marfan syndrome. *J Am Coll Cardiol.* 2012; Jul; 60(3): 224–9.

42. S. P. Chetty, B. L. Shaffer, and M. E. Norton. Management of pregnancy in women with genetic disorders, Part 1: Disorders of the connective tissue, muscle, vascular, and skeletal systems. *Obstet Gynecol. Surv.* 2011; Nov; 66(11): 699–709.

43. Overview of the management of Ehlers Danlos syndromes. www.uptodate.com/contents/overview-of-the-management-of-ehlers-danlos-syndromes. Accessed February 15, 2016.

44. Volkov N, Nisenblat V, Ohel G, and Gonen R. Ehlers-Danlos syndrome: Insights on obstetric aspects. *Obstet Gynecol Surv.* 2007 Jan; 62(1): 51–7.

45. Genetics of osteogenesis imperfecta. http://emedicine.medscape.com/article/947588. Accessed March 1, 2016.

46. M. Cozzolino, F. Perelli, and L. Maggio. Management of osteogenesis imperfecta type I in pregnancy; A review of literature applied to clinical practice. *Arch Gynecol Obstet.* 2016 Jan. Epub ahead of print. SpringerLink. Web. Accessed March 2016.

Dermatologic Disorders and Pregnancy

Colleen K. Stockdale and Sarina Martini

Introduction

The focus of this chapter will be on identifying, diagnosing and treating the dermatoses associated with pregnancy. Normal skin changes will also be discussed.

It is essential to distinguish the different dermatoses from one another as they have different outcomes and treatment options. Pregnancy dermatoses are limited to the peripartum period and typically lack long-standing sequelae. One common symptom of pregnancy dermatoses is pruritus.

In 1982, Holmes and Black, first attempted to simplify the dermatoses of pregnancy into three categories: pemphigoid gestationis, polymorphic eruption of pregnancy and pregnancy prurigo.[1] Over the years the classification and nomenclature of these dermatoses have changed as research has evolved. Much remains to be discovered in regards to pathogenesis of most dermatoses of pregnancy.

The pregnancy dermatoses reviewed in this chapter are (1) polymorphic eruption of pregnancy, (2) pemphigoid gestationis, (3) intrahepatic cholestasis of pregnancy and (4) atopic eruption of pregnancy. This categorization reflects the classification described by Ambros-Rudolph et al. in 2006.[2,3]

Scope of the Problem

It is important to distinguish normal physiologic skin, vascular and integumentary changes, which affect 90% or more of women from actual dermatologic disorders, which affect a much smaller proportion of pregnancies. It is difficult to estimate the economic burden of these dermatologic changes, physiologic or pathologic. Dermatoses are rather uncommon, but can be distressing and difficult to control symptoms. The emotional and physical needs of patients to deal with these issues can be tremendous and time-consuming. The identification of pruritic dermatoses is important for maternal and fetal well-being especially since some skin conditions can be associated with significant disease processes. Further study is needed to determine the impact of these dermatologic disorders on the health care system.

Normal Skin Changes in Pregnancy

Physiologic skin changes associated with pregnancy include hyperpigmentation, striae distensae, vascular, eccrine/aprocrine gland activity and shifts in the immune system.[2] These changes are related to shifts in hormones from the ovary, adrenal glands, pituitary, and placenta.[4]

Common areas of hyperpigmentation are the linea alba, nipple and areolae, vulva, axillae, face and neck. Approximately 90% of all pregnant women have increased melanin deposition in epidermal and dermal macrophages leading to darkening of skin.[4] These changes appear to be more prominent in darkly pigmented individuals and can arise at any time during gestation. It is quite common for nevi to darken during gestation and regress after delivery but persistent in up to 30% of women affected.[4]

Melasma or the mask of pregnancy is a pigmentation of the cheeks and nasal bridge. It affects around 50% of women. Ultraviolet light use may further exacerbate this hyperpigmentation. Therefore, use of broad spectrum UV-A and UV-B sunscreens along with limited exposure to sunlight may help to prevent development and worsening hyperpigmentation. This condition may also be seen in oral contraceptive users.

Striae distensae or stretch marks are very common during the later half of gestation. They are permanent, but tend to fade after delivery. Striae appear as light to dark purplish linear lines across the abdomen, breasts, buttocks and upper legs. See Figure 45.1.

Along with skin changes, it is common for women to experience hair growth.[2] Ovarian androgen production

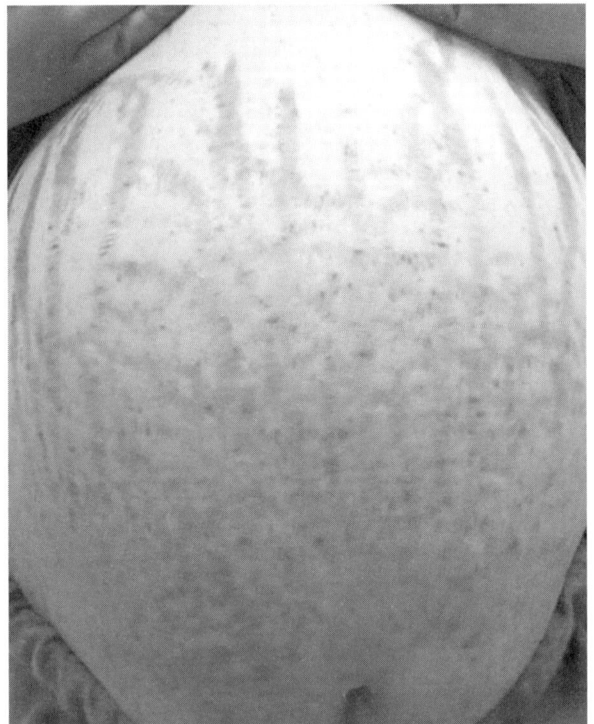

Figure 45.1 Abdominal striae in gravid patient.

has been thought to be the cause of increased growth of body hair in pregnancy. During pregnancy, the hair follicles have prolonged anagen or growth phase and the proportion of hairs entering the telogen or shedding phase declines. At the conclusion of pregnancy, the normal hair cycle resumes; this leads to more hair follicles in the telogen phase. Telogen effluvium is the shedding of these terminal hairs approximately 1–5 months postpartum.[2,4] Normal hair growth is expected to return between 6 and 12 months after delivery.

Vascular changes of the skin commonly seen in pregnancy include spider hemangiomas, hemorrhoids, varicosities of the vulva and lower extremities, palmar erythema, and pregnancy gingivitis and pyogenic granulomas. These changes are related to increased blood flow in the subcutaneous tissues, dilated vasculature and decreases in peripheral vascular resistance.[4] Again, these conditions regress at the conclusion of gestation.

Various changes in skin glands occur. Sebaceous glands have increased activity, which results in worsening acne vulgaris and the development of Montgomery tubercles on the areolae. Montgomery tubercles or glands are small papular projections along the areolas. These changes typically occur in the third trimester and resolve with delivery. The eccrine glands also have increased activity; this leads to hyperhidrosis and dyshidrotic eczema. On the other end of the spectrum, the apocrine glands have decreased activity. This often results in improvement of hidradenitis suppurativa.[2]

The final area of normal physiologic changes in the skin is related to immune system changes. A shift occurs in maternal immune response toward antibody production (T_H2) and away from cell-mediated (T_H1) immunity.[5] This is thought to be advantageous in allowing the "foreign" fetus to develop. This change is postulated as the etiology for increased incidence of autoimmune skin diseases, atopic eczema exacerbations and improvement in psoriasis that are seen in pregnancy.[4]

Dermatologic Disorders Associated with Pregnancy

Polymorphic Eruption of Pregnancy

Polymorphic eruption of pregnancy was previously referred to as pruritic urticarial papules and plaques of pregnancy (PUPPP). This entity was first described by Lawley in 1979.[6] The incidence is approximately 1 in 160 pregnancies. The majority of cases (around 80%) occur in primigravids.[7] This dermatosis typically has a late gestational onset, occurring around the 35th to 39th week.

The polymorphic features include vesicles, target lesions, polycyclic wheals, small bullae, and eczematous changes.[2,8] The key clinical finding of this pruritic eruption is its location. The rash typically begins on the abdomen along the striae with umbilical sparing. The rash can spread to the buttocks and rarely to the extremities. Over time these polymorphic lesions may coalesce. See Figure 45.2. Aroson et al. described three different types of polymorphic eruption of pregnancy based on the visible clinical appearance and location of the lesions.[9] Type I were urticarial papules and plaques, type II were non-urticarial erythema, papules, or vesicles, and type III were a combination of the previous two types. These authors reported in that trimester onset, parity, and direct immunofluorescence findings were not any different between types. Therefore, this separation may not be clinically helpful.

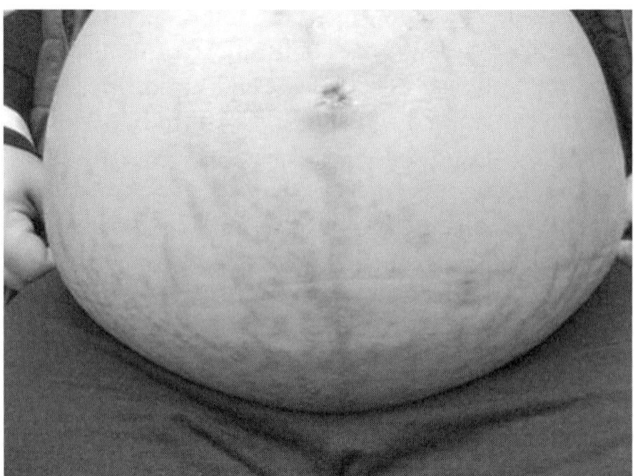

Figure 45.2 Polymorphic eruption of pregnancy in G1P0 at 32 weeks complicated by idiopathic polyhydramnios.

The cause of polymorphic eruption of pregnancy is unknown. One theory is that this condition may be affected by presence of a male fetus. Aractingi et al. compared 10 women diagnosed with polymorphic eruption of pregnancy (PEP) with 26 women who did not have PEP. Six of the ten PEP women were found to have male fetal DNA in their skin samples. None of the control women who were carrying male fetuses were positive for fetal DNA in their skin samples.[10]

Other authors have suggested that this eruption is related to destruction of connective tissue due to distension of the abdominal wall. Support for this theory is the observation that this pathology is usually seen in the later part of primagravid pregnancies. Some researchers, however, have found higher rates of polymorphic eruption of pregnancy among multigestation pregnancies and maternal weight gain.[11,12]

The histopathology of polymorphic eruption of pregnancy is nonspecific and includes epidermal spongiosis, perivascular infiltrate, inflammatory infiltrate along dermis, lymphocytes, histocytes, and eosinophils. Older lesions may show acanthosis, hyperkeratosis, and parakeratosis.[2] Typically, direct immunofluorescence is negative along the basement membrane for complement 3 (C3) or immunoglobulin G (IgG). Some studies have shown positivity for immunoglobulin M (IgM) along the basement membranes.[2,11]

Treatment involves symptomatic relief. Such relief may include topical emollients, topical corticosteroids, and oral antihistamines such as loratidine, certizine, hydroxyzine, or diphenhydramine. In severe symptomatic cases, an oral steroid taper may be used for up to 14 days.

Polymorphic eruption of pregnancy is a self-limited disease and typically the lesions are cleared from maternal skin within 6 weeks of delivery. No associated long-term skin pigmentation or scaring of the skin is associated with this progress. Fetal prognosis is excellent; poor fetal outcomes have *not* been described in the literature.

Pemphigoid Gestationis

Pemphigoid gestationis was previously known as Herpes gestationis. Other terms previously used to name this condition include pemphigus gravidarum, pemphigus pruriginosus, herpes circinatus bullosus, pemphigus hystericus, and dermatitis multiformis gestationis. Holmes and Black renamed the condition pemphigoid gestationis in 1982 because the immunohistochemistry and clinical presentation was most similar to the pemphigoid bullous diseases.[13] Despite the blistering rash that appears similar to herpes viral infections, the term Herpes gestationis has fallen out of favor as viral studies of pemphigoid gestationis have been negative.

This dermatoses presents as an intense pruritic, urticarial eruption on the trunk often involving the umbilicus; 90% of the time lesions start in the periumbilical region and then radiate outwards along the trunk.[14] In the early bullous formation stage, clinicians may find it difficult to distinguish this condition from early polymorphic eruption of pregnancy. Later, as pemphigoid gestationis evolves into tense vesico-bullous lesions, it may be easier to distinguish. See Figure 45.3. Fortunately, this condition can be distinguished by immunohistochemistry as discussed below.

The incidence of pemphigoid gestationis is approximately 1 in 40,000–60,000 pregnancies. It typically occurs in the second and third trimesters, but can be seen in the first trimester and postpartum.[3,13,14] Primary onset of a dermatologic condition after 3 days postpartum is unlikely with this diagnosis.[14] Postpartum flares, however, are common. The flares occur in up to 75% of patients, and they typically occur 24–48 hours after delivery. Resolution of the condition ranges from weeks to several months. Women with pemphigoid gestationis have also experienced recurrences with contraceptive use and with menses. This disease has been described in cases of hydatidiform mole and choriocarcinomas.

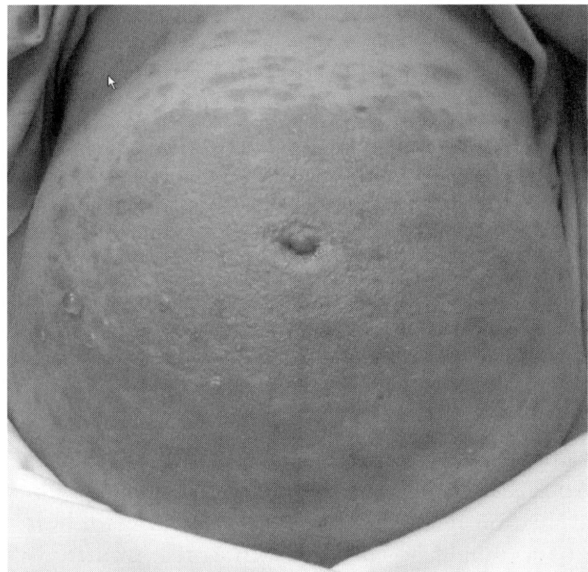

Figure 45.3 Pemphigoid gestationis, which is recurrence for this patient in her second pregnancy.

Unlike, polymorphic eruption of pregnancy, pemphigoid gestationis is associated with fetal effects. Up to 10% of infants born to mothers with pemphigoid gestationis have cutaneous lesions.[13,14] These lesions are self-limited and last around 3 weeks. These lesions are caused by passive transmission of IgG antibodies from mother to fetus. Skin biopsies from infants of affected mothers are typically positive and don't always correlate to clinical manifestations. Some authors have suggested that there is a tendency towards preterm birth and small for gestational age infants.[15]

Jenkins et al. found that approximately 14% of patients studied had an associated autoimmune disorder. The most common autoimmune disorder was Graves' disease. Other patients were noted to have alopecia areata, Hashimoto's thyroiditis, autoimmune thrombocytopenia, and vitiligo.[14]

The pathology of pemphigoid gestationis includes subepidermal blistering, eosinophilic infiltrate in the blister fluid, and edematous upper dermis. The pathologic findings are similar to polymorphic eruption of pregnancy, showing perivascular, lymphohistiocytic infiltrate with eosiniophils. Eosinophils along the basement membrane are seen in almost every case of pemphigoid gestationis. Direct immunofluorescence is the key to diagnosis. A linear deposition of C3, with or without IgG, is present along the basement membrane.[13] Pemphigoid gestationis is associated with human leukocyte antigens (HLA) DR3 and DR4. No clinical associations have been found between HLA type and disease severity, onset, duration, or recurrence. "PG factor" or herpes gestationis factor is an IgG_1 autoantibody directed against the basement membrane in skin.[13]

Women with pemphigoid gestationis have been known to develop bullous pemphigoid later in life. Bullous pemphigoid is an IgG_4 autoantibody to the basement membrane in the skin. Huilaja et al. suggest that the antibody in this disease, which is directed toward collagen XVII components, is related to the poor fetal outcomes associated in this disease. These researchers discovered that collagen XVII is a component in amniotic fluid, which is produced by trophoblastic cell lines. The authors suggest that pemphigoid autoantibodies induce epithelial-stromal microseparation of the placenta, leading to functional failures.[16]

Chi et al., in a small study, found pemphigoid gestationis in the first trimester to be associated with fetal loss. All three women in this study had onset of blisters in the first trimester, along with extensive disease. They received systemic corticosteroids. There was no association found with elevated titer levels and poor fetal outcomes. No association between poor fetal outcomes and corticosteroid use was found.[17]

Treatment of pemphigoid gestationis involves symptomatic relief along with prevention of disease progression and prevention of secondary skin infections. Authors have suggested topical steroids, oral antihistamines, and topical emollients at first signs of the disease.[13,14] Bullous disease typically requires oral corticosteroids such as prednisolone 40 mg daily. Continuation of systemic steroid, at a dose that prevents progression of lesions for 1–2 weeks, along with potential taper and maintenance through pregnancy is the recommended course. The goal should be to use the lowest dose of systemic corticosteroids to control the disease process. It is not uncommon for women to have recurrences in the postpartum period. Such patients may need prolonged therapy. Skin lesions in infants tend to resolve once the maternal autoantibodies are cleared from their systems.

Intrahepatic Cholestasis of Pregnancy

Intrahepatic cholestasis of pregnancy is not a designated dermatosis but has dermatologic sequelae. These sequelae are related to a reversible hormone driven liver disorder.[18–20] The dermatologic changes begin with excoriations secondary to intense pruritis without initial underlying skin lesions. Patients may eventually develop prurigo lesions across the body, most commonly on the extremities, buttocks, and abdomen. The pruritis typically begins on the palms of the hands and soles of the feet in the third trimester of pregnancy. The prevalence varies but has been estimated at 1:1,000–10,000 deliveries.[20] This is particularly higher in the Araucanian population (28%) in Chile and also is increased in Sweden. Overall incidence rates are 0.1–1.5% in Central and North America.[18] A genetic component is present, as 50% of affected women have a family history of the same disease process. A seasonal variation exists, with lower occurrences in the winter in studies conducted in Sweden and Chile.[20] No single cause of this disease is definitively known; intrahepatic cholestasis of pregnancy is likely multifactorial. Postulated contributing factors include elevated hormones, abnormalities in bile acid secretion and metabolism, genetics, and environment components. A recurrence risk of 40–70% is reported. Recurrence may occur not only with future pregnancy but also with oral contraceptive use.

Known fetal risks are associated with intrahepatic cholestasis. It is important to recognize and treat mothers with this condition since pregnancies affected by intrahepatic cholestasis are at risk for premature birth, fetal distress, and stillbirth. The key management component is early diagnosis to avoid these potentially devastating outcomes. Premature birth occurs in 19–60% of pregnancies, whereas intrapartum fetal distress with meconium and/or fetal heart rate abnormalities is seen in 22–30%.[18,21] Stillbirth can affect up to 2% of affected gestations.[22] The poor outcomes are associated with elevated bile acids.

All women with a potential diagnosis of intrahepatic cholestasis should have through evaluation including bile acid levels, transaminases (alanine aminotransferase (ALT), aspart aminotransferase (AST), gamma-glutamyltransferase (GGT), and bilirubin. Bile acids are elevated in ≥90% of women with cholestasis.[22] It should be noted that bile acids are slightly elevated in the normal pregnancy state but they are significantly elevated in intrahepatic cholestasis. Levels above 11 mol/L in the third trimester are considered abnormal.[18] ALT is elevated in 20–60% of patients and GGT is elevated in approximately 30% of patients. Hyperbilirubinemia is found in only 10–20% affected gestations.[18]

The goals of treatment are to reduce fetal risk and also reduce maternal symptoms. Currently the mainstay of management of elevated bile acids in pregnancy is the use of ursodeoxycholic acid.[19,20,22] This is a natural bile acid that stimulates or sequesters bile acids, other hepatotoxic compounds, and progesterone metabolites.[18] The exact mechanism has not been elucidated, but there is a decrease in maternal bile acids. The recommended dose is 15 mg/kg/day to significantly reduce symptoms and improve fetal outcome.

The Society for Maternal Fetal Medicine (SMFM) has recommendations for the screening and care during pregnancy of women with suspected diagnosis of intrahepatic cholestasis. These recommendations include transaminase and direct bilirubin evaluation along with bile acids. Screening for hepatitis C should be considered in at risk women. No current evidence-based recommendations for antenatal testing exist at present as the etiology of intrauterine fetal demise is not understood. Fetal demise typically occurs late in gestation and reassuring antepartum surveillance may not prevent this poor outcome. SMFM advocates delivery between 37 and 38 weeks gestation or sooner if fetal lung maturity is documented.[23]

Most women have resolution of their pruritis within two days of delivery. There is no need to continue ursodeoxycholic acid after delivery.

Intrahepatic cholestasis of pregnancy can be difficult to from between atopic eruptions of pregnancy. The key historical information is the onset of pruritis. Intrahepatic cholestasis typically presents in the third trimester and atopic eruptions tend to occur early in gestation.

Atopic Eruptions of Pregnancy

Atopic eruptions of pregnancy are a group of benign skin changes. This group includes eczema in pregnancy, prurigo of pregnancy, and pruritic folliculitis in pregnancy.[3,24] Atopic eruptions account for 50% or more of the pruritic rashes that develop in pregnancy. These processes typically present in the first half of pregnancy as compared with the previously discussed dermatoses.[3] These pruritic rashes respond well to therapy and are not associated with poor fetal outcome.

It is believed that these atopic atopic eruptions of pregnancy are most commonly due to the t helper cell type 2 (TH2) response. Pregnancy is a state where t helper cell type 1 (TH1) responses are decreased and TH2 responses are enhanced. This is advantageous to the developing fetus, which is antigenically different from the mother host. This may explain why TH1 autoimmune-dominated diseases such as rheumatoid arthritis or multiple sclerosis tend to go into remission during pregnancy and TH2-dominated diseases such as lupus and atopic dermatitis are exacerbated.[24]

Eczema of Pregnancy

In a prospective study conducted in the UK, eczema was the most common dermatosis and was noted in 36% of patients.[24] Women with eczema presented with symptoms in all three trimesters (approximately 24% in first trimester, 44% in second trimester and 32% in third trimester). Twenty-eight percent of women had a personal history of atopic eczema or infantile atopic eczema previous to pregnancy. The remaining women reported a personal or family history of atopy including asthma, eczema, or hay fever. All women had negative indirect immunofluorescent studies. The most common histopathologic skin finding was spongiosis, perivascular mononuclear infiltrate, epidermal hyperkeratosis, and parakeratosis.

Acute pruritic lesions seen in eczema of pregnancy may be erythematous papules and vesicles or extensive areas of weeping with exudates. Chronic features include excoriated papules and plaques, scaling, and lichenification.

Treatment involves symptomatic relief and avoidance of skin irritants. Patients should be instructed to moisturize their skin with emollients and keep the skin hydrated. Patients may bathe, but avoidance of soaps and detergents is essential. Application of emollients after bathing is important. Occasionally a topical corticosteroid may be needed for maintenance. As mentioned above, it is very important with topical corticosteroids to use the lowest potency, which has a positive effect. If oral corticosteroids are needed to decrease eruptions, short burst and tapers are typically effective. Oral antihistamines are also routinely used to help diminish the symptoms of pruritis; these are safe in pregnancy.

One of the more common complications associated with eczema is secondary bacterial infection. When present, therapy should be directed at treatment of *Staphylococcus aureus*. Topical antibiotics may cause further skin sensitization.[24]

Prurigo of Pregnancy

These pruritic lesions are discrete erythematous or skin colored papules. Excoriated surfaces may occur from mechanical trauma such as scratching. The lesions are small papules, typically less than a 0.5 cm, and are located on the extensor surfaces of the extremities and the trunk. Prurigo of pregnancy is a clinical diagnosis and no consistent histological findings are characteristic. Acanthosis and parakeratosis with eosinophilic and/or neutrophilic infiltrate are often present. These lesions can be treated with mild to moderate topical corticosteroids and oral antihistamines.

Pruritic Folliculitis of Pregnancy

This pruritic rash is composed of small, follicular, erythematous papules distributed widely over the trunk. See Figure 45.4. Zoberman and Farmer first described this in six women in 1981.[25] The pathologic analysis from these women showed acute folliculitis and negative direct immunofluorescence. Other authors have classified pruritic folliculitis as an acneiform eruption, which is described as small follicular papules and pustules associated with administration of corticosteroids or progesterones.[26] Conflicting studies have been unable to determine whether this process is associated with elevated androgen levels.[27,28,29]

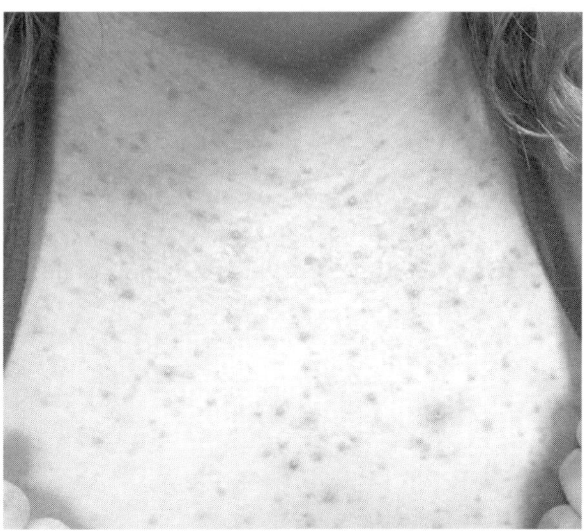

Figure 45.4 Pruritic folliculitis of pregnancy in gravid patient.

Table 45.1 Clinical dermatoses of pregnancy

Dermatoses	Clinical Manifestations	Location	Pathology	Adjunct Labs	Treatment	Fetal Effects
Polymorphic eruption of pregnancy	Pruritic, urticarial rash, erythema, edematous papules	Abdominal onset, umbilical sparing; spreads to trunk, thigh, buttocks	Abdominal distention leading to connective tissue damage and inflammation	–	Topical corticosteroids and oral antihistamines, topical emollients	No concerns
Pemphigoid gestationis	Pruritic urticarial papules and plaques turn into vesicles and then bullae	Begins periumbilical and then spreads outward to abdomen, thighs, palms, and soles	IgG autoantibodies and C3 complement react with basement membranes of skin and placenta, resulting in blister formation and tissue damage	Direct immunofluorescence with linear IgG and C3 along basement membrane	Topical corticosteroid, antihistamines; bullous formation requires oral steroid with taper to maintenance dose	Urticarial to vesicular lesions seen in approximately 10% of newborns; Possible risk for premature birth
Intrahepatic cholestasis of pregnancy	Pruritis without rashes, secondary excoriations, possible jaundice	Palms and soles and then generalized	Complex and multifactorial – hormonal, environmental, genetic-driven liver dysfunction and bile acid metabolism	Elevated serum bile acids and aminotransferases	Ursodeoxycholic acid	Premature birth Intrapartum fetal distress Fetal demise
Atopic eruption of pregnancy	Pruritis, excoriations, eczematous skin	Typically widespread	Reduced Th1 cytokines and increased Th2 cytokine production	–	Topical corticosteroids, oral antihistamines, oral antibiotics if secondary skin infection	No concern

Concluding Remarks

Various pathologic and non-pathologic dermatologic changes are associated with the pregnant woman. Most of these changes are benign and warrant no concern for the fetus and only require symptomatic relief for the patient. It is vitally important that the obstetrician be able to identify and treat intrahepatic cholestasis due to its association with intrauterine fetal demise. It is also important to identify pemphigoid gestationis as this has potential to effect the fetus as well as described earlier. Table 45.1 is a summary of clinical dermatoses of pregnancy.

References

1. R. Holmes, M. Black. The specific dermatoses of pregnancy: A reappraisal with special emphasis on a proposed simplified clinical classification. *Clinical and Experimental Dermatology* 1982; 7: 65–73.
2. C. Ambros-Rudolph, L. Edwards, P. Lynch. *Obstetric and Gynecologic Dermatology*, 3rd ed. Black, M. (ed.), Missouri: Maryland Heights, 2008.
3. C. Ambros-Rudolph, R. Mullegger, S. Vaughan-Jones, H. Keri, M. Black. The specific dermatoses of pregnancy revisited and reclassified: Results of a retrospective two-center study on 505 pregnant patients. *Journal of the American Academy of Dermatology* 2006; 54(3): 395–404.
4. F. Cunningham, K. Leveno, S. Bloom, J. Hauth, D. Rouse, C. Song. Dermatologic Disorders. In: *Williams Obstetrics*, 23rd ed. Twicker, D, Wendel G. (eds). 2010. McGraw Hill, New York.
5. E. Garcia-Gonzalez, R. Ahued-Ahued, E. Aroyo, D. Montes-de-Oca, J. Granados. Immunology of the cutaneous disorders of pregnancy. *International Journal of Dermatology* 1999; 38: 721–729.

6. LC. Parish, JL. Parish. Dermatologic Diseases in Pregnancy. In: Global Library of Women's Medicine.
7. MM. Roth. Pregnancy dermatoses diagnosis, management, and controversies. *American Journal of Clinical Dermatology* 2011; 12(1): 25–41.
8. SV. Jones, C. Ambros-Rudolph, C. Nelson-Piercy. Clinical review: Skin disease in pregnancy. *British Medical Journal*, 2014; 348.
9. I. Aronson, S. Bond, V. Fiedler, S. Vomvouras, D. Gruber, C. Ruiz. Pruritic urticarial papules and plaques of pregnancy: clinical and immunopathologic observations in 57 patients. *Journal of the American Academy of Dermatology* 1998; 39(6): 933–939.
10. S. Aractingi, N. Berkane, P. Bertheau, C. LeGoue, J. Dausset, S. Uzan, E. Carosella. Fetal DNA in skin of polymorphic eruptions of pregnancy. *The Lancet* 1998; 352: 1898–1901.
11. S. Vaughan Jones, S. Hern, C. Nelson-Piercy, P. Seed, M. Black. A prospective study of 200 women with dermatoses of pregnancy correlating clinical findings with hormonal and immunopathological profiles. *British Journal of Dermatology* 1999; 141: 71–81.
12. L. Cohen, E. Capeless, P. Krusinski, M. Maloney. Pruritic urticarial papules and plaques of pregnancy and its relationship to maternal-fetal weight gain and twin pregnancy. *Archives of Dermatology* 1989; 125(11): 1534–1536.
13. R. Jenkins, J. Shornick. Pemphigoid (herpes) gestationis. In: *Obstetric and Gynecologic Dermatology*, 3rd ed, Black, M, Ambros-Rudolph, C, Edwards, L, Lynch P. (eds.). Missouri: Maryland Heights, 2008. pp. 37–47.
14. R. Jenkins, S. Hern, M. Black. Clinical features and management of 87 patients with pemphigoid gestationis. *Clinical and Experimental Dermatology* 1999; 24: 255–259.
15. J. Shornick, M. Black. Fetal risks in herpes gestationis. *Journal of the American Academy of Dermatology* 1992; 26(2): 63–68.
16. L. Huilaja, T. Hurskainen, H. Autio-Harmainen, S. Hofman, R. Sormunen, J. Rasanen, M. Ilves, F. Claus-Werner, L. Bruckner-Tuderman, K. Tasanen. Pemphigoid gestationis autoantigen, transmembrane collagen XVII, promotes the migration of cytotrophoblastic cells of placenta and is a structural component of fetal membranes. *Matrix Biology* 2008; 27(3): 190–200.
17. C. Chi, S. Wang, R. Charles-Holmes, C. Ambros-Rudolph, J. Powell, R. Jenkins, M. Black, F. Wojnaroska. Pemphigoid gestationis: Early onset and blister formation are associated with adverse pregnancy outcomes. *British Journal of Dermatology* 2009; 160: 1222–1228.
18. C. Ambros-Rudolph. Intrahepatic cholestasis of pregnancy. In: *Obstetric and Gynecologic Dermatology*, 3rd ed, Black, M, Ambros-Rudolph, C, Edwards, L, Lynch P. (eds.). Missouri: Maryland Heights, 2008. pp. 57–63.
19. J. Palma, H. Reyes, J. Ribalta, I. Hernandez, L. Sandoval, R. Almuna, J. Liepins, F. Lira, M. Sedano, O. Silva, D. Toha, J. Silva. Deoxycholic acid in the treatment of cholestasis of pregnancy: A randomized, double-blind study controlled with placebo. *Journal of Hepatology* 1997; 27: 1022–1028.
20. H. Reyes. Sex Hormones and biles acids in intrahepatic cholestasis of pregnancy. *Hepatology* 2008; 47: 376–379.
21. A. Riosecco, M. Ivankovic, A. Manzur, F. Hamed, S. Kato, J. Parer, A. Germain. Intrahepatic cholestasis of pregnancy: A retrospective case–control study of perinatal outcome. *American Journal of Obstetrics and Gynecology* 1994; 170(3): 890–895.
22. F. Lammert, H-U. Marschall, A. Glantz, S. Matern. Intrahepatic cholestasis of pregnancy: Molecular pathogenesis, diagnosis and management. *Journal of Hepatology* 2000; 33: 1012–1021.
23. S. Craigo. Understanding intrahepatic cholestasis of pregnancy. Society for Maternal Fetal Medicine Publications and Guidelines 2011. www.smfm.org/publications/96-understanding-intrahepatic-cholestasis-of-pregnancy
24. C. Ambros-Rudolph, S. Jones. Atopic eruption of pregnancy. In: *Obstetric and Gynecologic Dermatology*, 3rd ed, Black, M, Ambros-Rudolph, C, Edwards, L, Lynch P. (eds.). Missouri: Maryland Heights, 2008. pp. 65–72.
25. E. Zoberman, E. Farmer. Pruritic folliculitis of pregnancy. *Archives of Dermatology* 1981; 117(1): 20–22.
26. C. Ambros-Rudolph, M. Black, S. Jones. The popular and pruritic dermatoses of pregnancy. In: *Obstetric and Gynecologic Dermatology*, 3rd ed, Black, M, Ambros-Rudolph, C, Edwards, L, Lynch P. (eds.). Missouri: Maryland Heights, 2008. pp. 76–77.
27. S. Wilkinson, H. Buckler, N. Wilkinson, J. O'Driscoll, M. Roberts. Androgen levels in pruritic folliculitis of pregnancy. *Clinical and Experimental Dermatology* 1995; 20: 234–236.
28. S. Jones, S. Hern, M. Black. Neutrophil folliculitis and serum androgen levels. *Clinical and Experimental Dermatology* 1999; 24(5): 392–395.
29. S. Jones, S. Hern, C. Nelson-Peircy, P. Seed, M. Black. A prospective study of 200 women with dermatoses of pregnancy correlating clinical findings with hormonal and immunopathological profiles. *British Journal of Dermatology* 1999; 141: 71–81.

Selected Infectious Diseases

Marygrace Elson

Introduction

The maternal–fetal dyad presents unique challenges when assessing for and treating infections. Some infections are far more severe in the pregnant woman than in the general adult population. Some infections pose little maternal risk but have potential devastating results for the fetus. TORCH, which includes toxoplasmosis, other (syphilis, varicella zoster, parvovirus B19), rubella, cytomegalovirus, and herpes infections, are some of the most common infections associated with congenital injury. Some infections cannot be eradicated; however, treatment of the mother can prevent vertical transmission to the newborn. Many infections are preventable by vaccination or lifestyle changes to avoid potential exposure.

Scope of the Problem

Maternal infections may cause significant morbidity for both mother and fetus. Vertically transmitted infections may lead to fetal malformations, childhood disabilities, and lifelong consequences for the child and family. Maternal genital infections may increase the risk for miscarriage or preterm delivery or may cause neonatal infection by intrapartum transmission. Prompt diagnosis and treatment may reduce maternal or fetal morbidity. The pre-pregnancy visit is a valuable occasion to identify opportunities for preventive immunization. Prenatal screening may reveal maternal susceptibilities, which can be addressed by immunization either during pregnancy or postpartum. Prenatal visits provide an opportunity for the provider team to discuss possible exposures and suggest preventive measures.

Infectious Diseases That Are More Severe in Pregnancy

It is unclear why some diseases affect pregnant women with more severity than the general population. Decreased cellular (T-cell-mediated) immunity, cytokine changes, and physiologic changes of pregnancy may contribute.

Influenza

Pregnant women account for a disproportionate amount of hospitalizations, intensive care admissions (ICU) admissions, and deaths from influenza compared to the general population. Data from the 2009 influenza A pandemic showed that 509 of 788 influenza cases of pregnant women reported to the Centers for Disease Control and Prevention (CDC) from April to August 2009 were hospitalized. Among the 509 hospitalized, 22.6% were admitted to an ICU. Pregnant women are approximately 1% of the US population, yet accounted for 5% of US deaths from 2009 influenza. Severity of illness was higher for women in the third trimester [1].

Physiologic changes of pregnancy that increase the risk of respiratory failure include elevation of the diaphragm to accommodate the uterus, increased respiratory rate, increased intra-abdominal pressure, decreased chest compliance, and decreased functional residual capacity [2].

Pregnant women with influenza also have an increased risk of premature and cesarean delivery.

Pregnant women suspected to have influenza should be treated immediately with oseltamivir 75 mg bid for 5 days, without waiting for test results. Early treatment with antiviral oseltamivir decreases risk of severe disease, with maximum benefit <48 h. There is a dramatic increase of ICU admission and death if antiviral medication is initiated more than 4 days from onset of symptoms. Chemoprophylaxis can be given to unvaccinated women with known influenza exposure with oseltamivir 75 mg daily for 7–10 days [3]. If pneumonia is diagnosed, the patient should be promptly hospitalized with consideration of broad-spectrum antimicrobial coverage for superinfecting bacteria and low threshold for respiratory support.

The American Congress of Obstetricians and Gynecologists (ACOG) and the CDC recommend vaccination of all pregnant women during influenza season using the intramuscular inactivated vaccine. The intranasal vaccine contains live virus and should not be used in pregnancy.

Hepatitis E

Hepatitis E almost never causes severe complications in the general population, but is a significant cause of fulminant hepatitis failure and mortality in pregnant women, with highest mortality in the third trimester. Endemic areas are India, Southeast Asia, the Middle East, and Africa. Spread is usually fecal–oral route from contaminated drinking water. Presentation is jaundice or hepatic failure and a supporting travel history. Diagnosis is made by serology. Treatment is supportive and often requires ICU admission. Preterm delivery rate is estimated as high as 66% [3]. Mortality rate has been reported as high as 20% [4]. Preventive vaccines are not widely available.

Malaria

Malaria should always be considered in the pregnant woman with fever who has recently traveled to the tropics. The *Anopheles* mosquito carries the parasite. Of the four species of plasmodium causing malaria, *Plasmodium falciparum* is particularly serious in pregnancy and the only species known to sequester in the placenta. This placental sequestration is implicated in the disease process in pregnant women and may be the reason for false-negative testing on rapid diagnostic kits and blood smears. If available, polymerase chain reaction (PCR) assays may overcome the effect of placental sequestration. Pregnancies complicated by *P. falciparum* have increased risk of anemia, spontaneous abortion, stillbirth, preterm delivery, intrauterine growth restriction (IUGR), and neonatal death. *Plasmodium vivax*, the second most common prevalent malarial infection, is associated with low birth weight and anemia [5]. Malaria prophylaxis is a priority for women traveling to or residing in endemic areas, with quinine and chloroquine considered safe in pregnancy. Before providing chemoprophylaxis or treating suspected malaria, consult the CDC website regarding drug resistance patterns [6]: www.cdc.gov/malaria/

Urinary Tract Infection

Pregnant women are more likely to develop ascending urinary tract infection (UTI) and pyelonephritis than nonpregnant women, due to stasis in the urinary tract from progesterone-associated smooth muscle relaxation as well as physical pressure from the pregnant uterus, particularly on the right side, but 75–80% of pyelonephritis is right-sided. Pyelonephritis is associated with preterm labor and delivery. In pregnant women, asymptomatic bacteriuria (>10^5 colony forming units per cc) should be treated due to risk of ascending infection. Clinicians should treat based on local resistance patterns ensuring coverage of the common pathogen *Escherichia coli* [7].

Infectious Diseases That Are More Severe for Fetus than Mother

Cytomegalovirus

Cytomegalovirus (CMV) is the cause of the most frequent congenital infection in America and a leading cause of congenital hearing loss. Both primary and secondary infections occur. After the primary infection, CMV remains latent in host cells. The presence of antibodies to CMV is not completely protective. Secondary infection can occur after reactivation of the latent CMV strain or by reinfection. Humans are the only reservoir. Approximately 50% of children attending day-care centers excrete CMV, and seronegative parents are at risk for acquiring CMV from their children attending day care. Annual seroconversion rates are approximately 10% for parents and uninfected siblings.

Most maternal CMV infections are asymptomatic; however, the mother may have mononucleosis type symptoms. Primary CMV infection is associated with a maternal-to-fetal transmission rate of 30–40% and transmission is highest in the third trimester. Conversely, the risk of severe fetal injury is highest with infection early in pregnancy. Up to 15% of neonates are symptomatic at birth and develop permanent sequelae that involve the central nervous system including developmental delays, seizure activity, and hearing loss. Vertical transmission with a recurrent infection is only 1–2%, with much lower incidence of severe fetal infection.

Fetal ultrasound findings associated with CMV include cerebral ventriculomegaly, hyperechogenic fetal bowel, ascites, intracranial calcifications, and fetal growth restriction. Fetal infection is documented by culture or PCR of amniotic fluid. Elevated IgM suggests new infection, and seroconversion from IgG negative to IgG positive status confirms infection. IgG avidity, which measures how tightly bound the immunoglobulin is to antigen, can help determine if an infection is primary. Recent infections (< 3 months) are less avid while remote infections are more avid (i.e. more tightly bound.) PCR detection in amniotic fluid approaches 100% sensitivity.

There is currently no standard treatment. Ganciclovir and valganciclovir have been used in research protocols. Passive immunization with hyperimmune globulin is also under study. Preventive strategies for CMV include behavior changes for mothers whose children attend day care including frequent hand washing, avoiding sharing food, beverages, towels, and washcloths and avoiding kissing on the mouth. Vaccines are in trials [8].

Toxoplasma gondii

Toxoplasma gondii is a protozoan infection that may be asymptomatic or cause mild viral syndrome symptoms in the mother. The life cycle includes three forms: trophozoite, cyst, and oocyst. Cats are the only host for the oocyst, which is formed in the cat intestine and excreted in the feces. Mammals ingest the oocyst and the trophozoite is then disseminated throughout the body forming cysts in the brain and muscle. Cooking destroys the cyst. Humans are infected by eating undercooked meat containing cysts, or by ingesting oocysts following contact with cat feces or contaminated soil or water.

There is approximately 40% vertical transmission to the fetus with transmission increasing the later in gestation the maternal infection occurs. In contrast, fetal injury is more likely the earlier the fetus is infected. The classic fetal injuries are chorioretinitis, hydrocephalus, and intracranial calcifications.

Maternal diagnosis is by serology, with IgM seropositivity suggestive of acute infection. Fetal ultrasound findings include ventriculomegaly, intracranial calcifications, microcephaly, ascites, hepatosplenomegaly, and growth restriction. Amniotic fluid PCR testing can help in diagnosis. Treatment of the mother reduces the risk for congenital infection. Spiramycin, available through the Food and Drug Administration (FDA,) is recommended to reduce transplacental infection. Fetal infection is usually treated with pyrimethamine, sulfadiazine, and folinic acid. Pregnant women should be counseled to avoid undercooked meat and avoid contact with cat feces to prevent infection. Fruits and vegetables should also be washed [9].

Listeria monocytogenes

Listeria monocytogenes is a bacillus commonly found in soil, which contaminates uncooked meat, raw vegetables, unpasteurized milk, and soft cheese. Approximately 20% of all infections occur in pregnant women, with approximately 20% of these cases resulting in stillbirth or spontaneous abortion. The infection may be subclinical or cause influenza-like symptoms. Infections most commonly occur in the third trimester and are rare earlier in pregnancy.

Listeria has a predilection for the fetal-placental unit. Through hematogenous transmission, the organism forms placental abscesses and causes fetal septicemia. Fetal risks include spontaneous abortion, intrauterine fetal demise/stillbirth, neonatal listeriosis, and meningitis. Standard therapy is ampicillin plus gentamycin. Given the subtleties of presentation, pregnant women should be advised to avoid unpasteurized dairy products and uncooked deli meats [7].

Viral Infections in Pregnancy

Hepatitis

Several different viruses cause viral hepatitis. Symptoms may include jaundice, anorexia, malaise, nausea, and emesis, and right upper quadrant pain. Hepatic transaminases are usually elevated. Most cases are self-limited, but certain types can cause persistent infection and chronic liver disease. Hepatitis viruses A, B, C, and D cause the majority of hepatitis infections in the United States. Hepatitis E is endemic to Asia, Africa, and Mexico. Hepatitis G is a post-transfusion hepatitis (also called GB virus C) similar to hepatitis C [10]. Other viruses causing hepatitis include cytomegalovirus, herpes simplex virus, Epstein–Barr virus, rubella, and yellow fever. Hepatitis A and B can be prevented through vaccination and these vaccines can be given to pregnant patients at risk.

Hepatitis A (HAV) is transmitted by fecal-oral contact. Risks include contaminated food or water, travel outside the United States, illicit drug use, and having a child in day care. HAV does not cause chronic infection but may result in cholestatic hepatitis. Care is supportive. Household contacts should receive HAV immune globulin and HAV vaccine. Infants should receive HAV immune globulin to prevent horizontal transmission after delivery [3].

Hepatitis B (HBV) is transmitted primarily via parenteral exposure, sexual transmission, or perinatal exposure. Approximately 1 million individuals in the United States are chronic carriers. The incidence of acute HBV infection in pregnancy is 1–2 per 1,000, and 5–15 per 1,000 pregnant women have chronic HBV [3]. Incubation is 4 weeks to 6 months following exposure. Of adults who become infected, 85–90% clear their infection. Less than 1% develop fulminant hepatitis with necrosis. Fifteen percent become chronically infected with HBV manifested by detectable levels of HBsAg. Only 15–30% of these with chronic infection will develop liver cirrhosis with risk for hepatocellular carcinoma.

Acute HBV infection is diagnosed by detection of HBsAg and IgM to the core antigen (HBc) or by viral load determination. Pregnant women with known HBV should be vaccinated against hepatitis A to prevent further liver injury. Pregnant women with acute or chronic HBV often benefit from consultation with a hepatologist. Antivirals (Lamivudine, tenofovir, and others) have been used to treat acute and chronic HBV infections in pregnancy.

Similar to HIV, the rate of perinatal transmission correlates with the maternal viral load. Viral load can be measured between 30 and 34 weeks to determine risk of perinatal transmission and determine treatment plan. The risk for maternal–fetal transmission may increase with HBV viral load $> 10^7$ copies/ml. HBV targeted antiviral therapy should be considered to decrease the risk of intrauterine infection in women with viral load $>10^6$ copies/ml. Tenofovir can be considered as a first-line agent. Risk of vertical infection is also associated with maternal HBe antigen positivity. In the United States, all newborns receive HBV vaccine. Infants born to mothers who are HBsAg positive should receive the HBV vaccine series and HBIg. This combination is 85–95% effective at preventing perinatal transmission. Cesarean delivery should not be performed for the sole indication of reduction of vertical HBV transmission [11]. There is no contraindication to breastfeeding.

Hepatitis C (HCV), known as non-A non-B hepatitis prior to the 1980s, is transmitted parenterally and perinatally. The risk of sexual transmission of HCV is substantially lower than HBV. Risk factors include IV drug use and history of transfusion. The blood supply is now screened for HCV and the current major risk factor is IV drug use. More than 50% of individuals affected with HCV are chronic carriers. Universal screening is not yet recommended, but individuals at risk should be tested. The usual therapies of interferon and ribavirin cannot be given in pregnancy, so management is expectant. Perinatal HCV transmission primarily correlates with viral load. Other risk factors for perinatal transmission are maternal IV drug use and HIV co-infection. Pregnant women with HCV should be immunized against HAV and HBV if not immune. There is no contraindication to breastfeeding. There is no effective vaccine against HCV [3].

Hepatitis D (HDV), an incomplete viral particle, uses HBV as a helper virus. Simultaneous HBV infection is required for viral replication. HDV is present worldwide with high prevalence in the Mediterranean basin, Middle East, Central Asia, West Africa, and the Amazon basin. Risk factors include IV drug use and exposure to infected blood products. Patients chronically infected with HBV and HDV have a 70–80% risk of developing cirrhosis and portal hypertension and 25% die of hepatic failure. HBV prophylaxis is effective in preventing perinatal HDV transmission [3].

Hepatitis E is discussed in the section "Infections That Are More Severe in Pregnancy."

Varicella Zoster (Chickenpox)

Primary varicella has a 25-fold risk for complications in adults compared to children, with varicella pneumonia being the most frequent serious complication [5]. Many population studies have suggested higher varicella severity in pregnancy, although more recent studies suggest that mortality may be the same as the general population, with earlier diagnosis and treatment including antivirals. In pregnancy primary varicella has a 10–20% risk of varicella pneumonia and poses risks to the fetus including congenital varicella syndrome. The syndrome is characterized by cutaneous scars, limb hypoplasia, muscle atrophy, malformed digits, psychomotor retardation, microcephaly, cortical atrophy, cataracts, chorioretinitis, and microphthalmia.

Mortality from varicella pneumonia in adults is 5–10%. Pregnant patients with varicella pneumonia may be treated with intravenous acyclovir to reduce the risk of mortality. Varicella zoster immune globulin

(VZIG) or oral acyclovir may reduce risk of severe varicella infection [9]. Immune globulin should be administered to the newborn of a mother who develops active varicella between 5 days before delivery and 2 days postpartum. If possible, delivery should be delayed 5–7 days following the onset of maternal illness to potentially prevent neonatal varicella zoster infection, which has a 20–30% mortality rate. The varicella zoster vaccine (VZV) is 70–80% effective at preventing natural infection [3]. VZV is a live virus vaccine and may not be given in pregnancy.

Parvovirus B 19

Parvovirus B19 (fifth disease) is spread via respiratory droplets, hand to mouth contact, infected blood products, and perinatally. Daycare workers, teachers, and parents are at increased risk of seroconversion. The most common presentation is erythema infectiosum, a "slapped cheek" facial rash and a lacey rash on trunk and extremities. If a pregnant woman is exposed, she should have serologic and DNA testing, with repeat testing in 3 weeks. The presence of IgG antibody indicates prior infection. Pregnant women with confirmed infection are treated supportively, as infection is usually self-limited.

Parvovirus B19 infects red blood cells and their precursors. The effect on the fetal bone marrow can be severe anemia, which leads to high output congestive heart failure and non-immune hydrops. There may also be a direct effect on the fetal myocardium. Serial ultrasounds to evaluate the fetus for hydrops should be performed for 8–10 weeks after maternal illness. Fetal middle cerebral artery (MCA) peak systolic velocity can be helpful to diagnose fetal anemia prior to development of hydrops. If no signs of hydrops occur during this period, no further evaluation is necessary. Fetal mortality from hydrops is approximately 11% when maternal infection occurs in the first 20 weeks of pregnancy. Fetal death is rare when maternal infection occurs after 20 weeks gestation. If hydrops is identified, cordocentesis to evaluate fetal hematocrit for possible intrauterine transfusion is recommended. The majority of fetuses infected with parvovirus B19 have normal long-term development [3].

Measles

Measles, or rubeola, is extremely infectious. With exposure to respiratory droplets, more than 75% of susceptible contacts become infected. The incubation period is 10–14 days. Clinical features are photophobia, fever, Koplik spots (tiny white spots on the buccal mucosa lateral to the molars), and presence of a rash, which begins on the trunk. There may be a productive cough. Diagnosis is by serology or mRNA testing. Pregnant women with measles may require hospitalization and are more likely to develop pneumonia than other adults. Secondary bacterial infections should be promptly treated. There is increased risk of spontaneous abortion and preterm delivery, but low risk of congenital measles infection. Ultrasound findings of congenital measles infection include microcephaly, growth restriction, and oligohydramnios. Vaccination with the two-dose series of the trivalent MMR (measles, mumps, rubella) vaccine prior to pregnancy is the most effective preventive strategy [3].

Rubella

Most rubella infections occur in unvaccinated individuals. The virus is spread by respiratory droplets and incubation period is 12–19 days. Twenty to fifty percent of infections are asymptomatic. The rash begins on the face and neck and spreads to the trunk and extremities, and lasts for approximately 3 days. Serology is used for diagnosis. Although maternal infection is self-limited, congenital rubella is associated with miscarriage and stillbirth. As pregnancy progresses, the risk of congenital rubella syndrome (CRS) decreases, with fetal defects rare beyond 16 weeks gestation. CRS is now rare in the United States. The most common manifestation of CRS is growth restriction. Hearing loss is the most common single defect. Other common defects are cardiac lesions and eye defects [3]. The newborn may have hepatosplenomegaly, thrombocytopenia, and purpuric skin lesions (blueberry muffin lesions). Vaccination with the two dose trivalent MMR vaccine prior to pregnancy is preventive. ACOG recommends routine screening for rubella at the initial prenatal visit, because a significant portion of US women remain susceptible to rubella despite childhood vaccinations [12].

Dengue

Dengue virus (DENV) is transmitted by the bite of infected *Aedes aegyti* mosquitoes. It is a leading cause of febrile illness among travelers returning from Latin America, the Caribbean, and Southeast Asia. Symptoms of infection usually begin 4–7 days after the mosquito bite and typically last 3–10 days.

About 75% of DENV infections are asymptomatic, but around 5% develop severe life-threatening disease. These patients will have persistent vomiting, abdominal pain, peripheral edema, mucosal bleeding, and liver enlargement. Lab findings include leukopenia, thrombocytopenia, hyponatremia, and elevated aminotransferase and alanine aminotransferase. Pregnant women traveling to dengue-endemic regions should observe strict anti-mosquito precautions including use of insect repellant. Dengue is associated with low birth weight, stillbirth, premature birth, and vertical transmission, and the disease may be more severe (or fatal) in pregnant women than the general population. Testing is by PCR. There is no vaccine. Treatment is supportive. Aspirin or NSAIDs should not be given, due to risk of hemorrhage [13].

Zika

Zika virus is transmitted by the same *A. aegyti* mosquitoes that spread dengue virus, and both viruses have the same endemic areas. Sexual transmission has been reported. The incubation period is 3–12 days. Symptoms are non-specific and mild. Aside from avoidance of endemic areas, preventive measures are strict anti-mosquito precautions. Zika during pregnancy has been associated with microcephaly with transmission to the fetus documented in all trimesters. Clinical and epidemiologic information about Zika virus is accumulating. Testing is by PCR. Serial ultrasounds every 3–4 weeks are recommended to assess fetal anatomy and well-being. Consult CDC websites for current information (www.cdc.gov/zika/). There is no vaccine and treatment is supportive. Aspirin or NSAIDs should not be given until dengue infection has been ruled out [14].

West Nile Virus

West Nile virus (WNV) is transmitted by multiple species of mosquitoes. Most infections are subclinical and consist of viral syndrome type symptoms including eye pain. Severe disease is associated with aseptic meningitis, encephalitis, and flaccid paralysis. Treatment is supportive. Overall outcomes in pregnant women are good and outcome is good for the majority of infants. The CDC recommends continuation of breastfeeding. Preventive measures for pregnant women include anti-mosquito precautions [3].

Coxsackie

Coxsackie virus is an enterovirus transmitted by fecal–oral route. It causes hand, food, and mouth disease. Adult illness typically is a self-limited febrile illness needing no treatment. Some studies suggest increased rate of miscarriage with Coxsackie infection in pregnancy [3].

Epstein–Barr Virus

Epstein–Barr virus (EBV) is the cause of infectious mononucleosis. Most adults are seropositive for EBV and primary EBV infection in pregnancy is rare. There is no association with adverse pregnancy outcome [3].

Sexually Transmitted Infections in Pregnancy

The CDC recommends universal prenatal screening for HIV, HBsAg, chlamydia and syphilis, and risk-based screening for HCV and gonorrhea. Universal screening is considered best practice and allows the best outcome for the maternal-fetal dyad, as well as helping diagnose and treat her sexual partner(s).

Chlamydia trachomatis and *Neisseria gonorrhea*

Gonorrhea is less common than chlamydia, with coexisting infection common. Untreated gonorrhea and chlamydia can result in maternal pelvic inflammatory disease, and both are associated with preterm labor, premature rupture of membranes, and low birth weight. In the newborn, both gonorrhea and chlamydia can cause ophthalmia neonatorum. To prevent gonococcal ophthalmia neonatorum, a prophylactic agent (0.5% erythromycin ointment) should be instilled into both eyes of all newborn infants; this procedure is required by law in most states. Neonatal chlamydial infections (including ophthalmia and pneumonia) have occurred less frequently since the institution of widespread prenatal screening and treatment of pregnant women. Nucleic acid amplification techniques (PCR) on urine samples are validated for testing in pregnant women. Chlamydia is usually treated with a single oral 1 g dose of azithromycin, which is safe in pregnancy. Although test of cure is not recommended in non-pregnant patients, a test of cure is advised in pregnant patients. Pregnant women infected with *Neisseria gonorrhoeae* should be treated with dual therapy consisting of ceftriaxone 250 mg in a single intramuscular (IM) dose and azithromycin 1 g orally as a single dose. Partners should be tested and treated. Patients should abstain from intercourse until 7 days after all are treated. Patients who test positive for gonorrhea should always be treated for chlamydia [15].

Pelvic Inflammatory Disease

Pregnant patients with pelvic inflammatory disease generally require inpatient treatment with a CDC recommended regimen of parenteral antimicrobials directed against a polymicrobial infection. Adverse obstetric outcomes are likely [6].

Syphilis

Worldwide, maternal syphilis is a significant cause of spontaneous abortion and stillbirth. Transmission of infection by the spirochete *Treponema pallidum* is by direct sexual contact with ulcerative lesions on skin or mucous membranes. Congenital infection results from transplacental passage of spirochetes. Congenital infection may result in stillbirth, fetal hydrops, or premature labor. The risk of congenital infection is highest in mothers with primary or secondary syphilis in the second half of pregnancy. Fetal ultrasound findings of congenital syphilis include fetal hepatomegaly, ascites, hydrops, and thickened placenta. A positive Venereal Disease Research Laboratory (VDRL) or rapid plasmin reagin (RPR) combined with a positive fluorescent treponemal antibody absorption (FTA) in a woman with no history of syphilis is an indication for treatment.

Pregnant women with syphilis should be treated according to the CDC guidelines for their stage of disease with parenteral penicillin, as should their partner(s). Penicillin allergic patients should undergo desensitization and then treatment with penicillin. The Jarisch–Herxheimer reaction, an acute febrile reaction frequently accompanied by headache, myalgia, and fever, can occur within the first 24 hours following treatment of primary or secondary syphilis and can result in preterm labor [6]. Treponemal tests remain positive for life, with or without treatment. Neonatal syphilis findings include cutaneous lesions on palms and soles, hepatosplenomegaly, jaundice, anemia snuffles, and periostitis. Late neonatal signs include the classic frontal bossing, saddle nose, Hutchinson teeth, eighth nerve deafness, interstitial keratitis, and saber shins [16].

Herpes Simplex

Genital infection with herpes simplex virus (HSV) is common and can result from either HSV 1 or HSV2. Primary and recurrent attacks can be painful. Recurrent infections are usually less severe than primary infection, are associated with fewer lesions and a shorter period of viral shedding. Diagnosis requires viral identification by PCR from lesions, or serologic testing, although serology cannot distinguish between oral and genital HSV infection. Disseminated HSV infection is rare but can occur in pregnancy. Prompt treatment with IV acyclovir is indicated if disseminated HSV is suspected. Congenital HSV infection is rare and includes skin vesicles/scarring, eye disease, microcephaly, or hydranencephaly.

The greatest risk associated with genital HSV exposure is neonatal HSV from intrapartum exposure. Neonatal HSV infection is usually associated with primary maternal infection. Approximately 70% of neonatal HSV infections are caused by HSV 2 and are usually associated with primary maternal infection and approximately 70% of cases are HSV2. Neonatal HSV is treated with IV acyclovir. Women with primary HSV infection during pregnancy should be treated with oral acyclovir, or parenteral for severe infections. Women with active genital herpes or prodromal symptoms at the time of labor should undergo cesarean delivery to reduce the transmission of herpes to the newborn. Some experts recommend cesarean delivery for women with newly acquired genital HSV in the third trimester due to persistent viral titers in genital secretions and lack of maternal type specific antibodies to protect the neonate [17]. Cesarean is not recommended for women with non-genital lesions. After careful examination of the cervix and vagina for coexisting lesions, non-genital lesions may be covered with an occlusive dressing for vaginal birth. Women with a history of genital herpes should be offered prophylactic oral acyclovir or valacyclovir from 36 weeks gestation to reduce recurrence [18].

Trichomonas vaginalis

Infection with *Trichomonas* in pregnancy is associated with premature rupture of membranes, preterm labor, and delivery and low birthweight. It is hypothesized that the host inflammatory response to the infection reduces chorioamniotic membrane strength [19]. Symptomatic women should be treated with metronidazole 2 g orally in a single dose. Partners should also be treated [15].

Bacterial Vaginosis

Although not strictly considered a sexually transmitted infection (STI), women with bacterial vaginosis (BV) are at increased risk for the acquisition of some STIs and complications of pregnancy. Symptomatic pregnant women can be treated with either of the oral or vaginal regimens recommended for nonpregnant women. Although adverse pregnancy outcomes, including premature rupture of membranes, preterm labor, preterm birth, intra-amniotic infection, and postpartum endometritis have been associated with symptomatic BV in some observational studies, data are inconsistent regarding whether treatment of asymptomatic BV among pregnant women who are at low risk for preterm delivery reduces adverse outcomes of pregnancy [15].

Human Papilloma Virus

Human papilloma virus (HPV) is a group of DNA viruses, some of which have a predilection for the genital area. HPV 6 and 11 cause genital warts. Other types, most notably HPV 16 and 18, are associated with the development of lower genital tract dysplasia and cancer. Hormonal effects can cause rapid proliferation and growth of warts during pregnancy. Anogenital warts in pregnancy can be treated with trichloroacetic acid or cryotherapy. Podophyllin and imiquimod should not be used in pregnancy. Vaginal delivery is acceptable unless the wart burden will cause dystocia [3].

Tick-Borne Bacterial Diseases

In pregnancy, symptoms of tick-borne disease may be consistent with preeclampsia or atypical preeclampsia, or may be consistent with the physiologic changes of pregnancy itself. Some of the medications usually utilized for treatment may not be appropriate for pregnancy so the provider must be aware of alternative regimens.

Ticks carry the majority of arthropod-borne bacterial diseases, including those discussed below. Prevention, by wearing insect repellant, keeping skin covered, with pant legs tucked into socks or boots, is the best way to avoid tick-borne disease. If a tick is found attached to a person, it should be detached gently without squeezing the tick, ensuring that the entire tick is removed.

Lyme Disease

Lyme disease is the most common vector-borne disease in the United States. *Borrelia burgdorferi* is the spirochete responsible for infection in the United States and the deer tick is the vector. The presentation and severity of Lyme disease is not affected by pregnancy. Lyme disease is divided into three stages. Stage 1 is an erythema migrans rash near the bite. Stage 2 occurs weeks to months later and consists of neurologic manifestations and less likely cardiac symptoms. Stage 3, or neuroborreliosis, indicates persistent disease and includes chronic arthritis. *B. burgdroferi* rarely crosses the placenta, and there is no evidence for a congenital borreliosis syndrome. Adverse pregnancy outcomes are uncommon and are associated with untreated Lyme disease and infection early in pregnancy. Diagnosis is made clinically because enzyme-linked immunosorbent assay (ELISA) and serology do not become positive until weeks or months after acute infection. Treatment of Lyme disease in pregnancy is the same as for the general population. Oral ampicillin or cefuroxime are efficacious, and erythromycin is an option for penicillin-allergic individuals. Neurologic symptoms require ceftriaxone. Arthritis and joint symptoms require a longer course of treatment. There is no evidence Lyme disease is transmitted in breast milk.

Rocky Mountain Spotted Fever

Rocky Mountain spotted fever (RMSF), the most common fatal tick-borne disease in the United States, is caused by *Rickettsia rickettsiae.* The wood tick and the dog tick are common vectors. RMSF has been identified in the entire continental United States and is more prevalent in the summer. Infected individuals present with fever, malaise, headache, nausea, emesis, and abdominal pain. The rash appears 2–5 days after fever, beginning on the wrists and ankles and spreading to the palms and soles and then limbs and trunk. Delay in diagnosis can lead to a more severe infection, which can mimic preeclampsia, with elevated liver function tests, low platelets, and sometimes proteinuria. RMSF does not appear to be more severe in pregnancy. Diagnosis is by serology or ELISA. Standard treatment for RMSF is usually doxycycline. Chloramphenicol is the drug of choice in pregnancy.

Multiple authors suggest the benefits of tetracycline therapy outweigh the risks if a pregnant patient close to term has a life-threatening infection [20].

Tuberculosis

In the nineteenth and early twentieth century, pregnancy was thought to significantly worsen the outcome of tuberculosis (TB) infection, so much so that termination of pregnancy was recommended. During the second half of the twentieth century larger studies showed that with improved chemotherapy pregnant women have the same prognosis as non-pregnant women [5]. Tuberculosis, caused by *Mycobacterium tuberculosis*, is an important cause of maternal mortality and infant morbidity and mortality around the world, particularly with coexisting HIV infection. The diagnosis of TB in pregnancy can be difficult as many of its symptoms (shortness of breath, fatigue) are common. Any pregnant patient with risk factors for TB who presents with cough, fever, weight loss, or night sweats should be evaluated. Both the World Health Organization and CDC recommend multidrug therapy for several months with protocols utilizing isoniazid, rifampin, ethambutol, and some with pyrazinamide [6].

Vaccine-Preventable Disease

Two vaccines are specifically recommended in pregnancy, seasonal influenza, and adult tetanus, diphtheria, and pertussis (Tdap). These are both inactivated vaccines. Other vaccines are recommended based on patient risk factors and immunization history. These include hepatitis A and B, pneumococcal and meningococcal vaccines. Measles, mumps and rubella (MMR) and varicella zoster virus (VZV) are both live attenuated viral vaccines, which should not be given in pregnancy. Both should be administered to non-immune women immediately postpartum [20].

For pregnant women who must travel in to areas with endemic disease, the CDC website [21] contains up-to-date recommendations for travelers' health: wwwnc.cdc.gov/travel

Concluding Remarks

This chapter has summarized key features of many diseases affecting the maternal–fetal dyad. Maternal infection can cause significant morbidity for both the mother and the fetus. Prompt diagnosis and treatment not only preserves the health of the mother and the fetus, it also may help prevent potentially devastating outcomes.

Recommendations for screening, prevention, and treatment of infectious diseases in pregnancy are constantly evolving. Population epidemiologic data and outcomes data, development of new medications and vaccines, and organisms develop resistance to treatment regimens. The astute clinician will frequently reference the CDC website (www.cdc.gov) in order to obtain the most up-to-date recommendations regarding infectious diseases in pregnancy and provide quality care.

References

1. Siston AM, Rasmussen SA, Honein MA, Fry AM, Seib K, Callaghan WM et al. Pandemic 2009 Influenza A (H1N1) Virus Illness Among Pregnant Women in the United States. *JAMA* 2010;303(15):1517–25.
2. Memoli MJ, Harvey H, Morens DM, Taubengerger JK. Influenza in Pregnancy. *Influenza and Other Respiratory Viruses*. 2012;7(6): 1033–9.
3. Bernstein, HB. Maternal and Perinatal Infection-Viral. In: Gabbe, SG, Niebyl, JR, Simpson, JL, editors. *Obstetrics Normal and Problem Pregnancies*. 6th ed. Philadelphia: Elsevier Saunders; 2012.
4. American College of Obstetricians and Gynecologists. Viral Hepatitis in Pregnancy. ACOG Practice Bulletin No. 86. *Obstet Gynecol* 2007;110:941–55.
5. Sappenfield E, Jamieson DJ, Kourtis, AP. Pregnancy and Susceptibility to Infectious Diseases. *Infect Dis Obstet Gynecol* 2013; Article ID 752852.
6. Adler H, Lambert JS. Clinical Focus: Infections in Pregnancy. *Hosp Pract* 2014;42(2):108–24.
7. Duff P. Maternal and Perinatal Infection – Bacterial. In: In: Gabbe, SG, Niebyl, JR, Simpson, JL, editors. *Obstetrics Normal and Problem Pregnancies*. 6th ed. Philadelphia: Elsevier Saunders; 2012.
8. Soper, D. Congenital Cytomegalovirus Infection: An Obstetrician's Point of View. *Clin Infect Dis* 2013; 57(S4):S171–3.
9. American College of Obstetricians and Gynecologists. Cytomegalovirus, Parvovirus B19, Varicella Zoster and Toxoplasmosis in Pregnancy. ACOG Practice Bulletin No. 151. *Obstet Gynecol* 2015;125:151.
10. Centers for Disease Control and Prevention. Guidelines for Viral Hepatitis Surveillance and Case Management. Atlanta, GA, 2005. www.cdc.gov/hepatitis/pdfs/2005guidlines-surv-casemngmt.pdf (Accessed February 23, 2016.)
11. Society for Maternal-Fetal Medicine, Odom JD, Tita AT, Silverman, NS. Hepatitis B in Pregnancy Screening,

treatment, and prevention of vertical transmission. *Am J Obstet Gynecol* 2016; 214(1):6–14.

12. American Academy of Pediatrics and the American College of Obstetricians and Gynecologists. Perinatal Infections. In *Guidelines for Perinatal Care*. 7th ed. Washington, DC; 2012.
13. Tomashek KM, Sharp TM, Margolis HS. Dengue. Centers for Disease Control and Prevention Yellow Book Chapter 3. wwwnc.cdc.gov/travel/yellowbook/2016/infectious-diseases-related-to-travel/dengue (Accessed February 23, 2016.)
14. Practice Advisory: Interim Guidance for Care of Obstetric Patients During a Zika Virus Outbreak. Society for Maternal-Fetal Medicine and the American College of Obstetricians and Gynecologists. www.smfm.org/publications/220-acog-smfm-joint-practice-advisory-interim-guidance-for-care-of-obstetric-patients-during-a-zika-virus-outbreak (Accessed February 23, 2016.)
15. Centers for Disease Control and Prevention. 2015 Sexually Transmitted Infection Treatment Guidelines. *MMWR* 2015; 64(3): 1–135.
16. Syphilis, congenital. Centers for Disease Control and Prevention. www.cdc.gov/std/stats/congenitalsyphilisdef-rev-jan-2015.pdf (Accessed February 23, 2016.)
17. Brown ZA, Gardella C, Wald A, Morrow RA, Corey L. Genital Herpes Complicating Pregnancy. *Obstet Gynecol* 2005;106:845–56.
18. American College of Obstetricians and Gynecologists. Management of Herpes in Pregnancy. *Prac Bull* No. 82. 2007;109:1489–98.
19. Coleman JS, Gaydos CA, Witter F. Trichomonas vaginalis Vaginitis in Obstetrics and Gynecology Practice: New Concepts and Controversies. *Obstet Gynecol Survey*. 2013;68(1):43–50.
20. Dotters-Katz SK, Kuller J, Heine RP. Arthropod-Borne Bacterial Diseases in Pregnancy. *Obstet Gynecol Survey*. 2013;68(9):635–49.
21. Guidelines for Vaccinating Pregnant Women. Centers for Disease Control and Prevention. http://www.cdc.gov/vaccines/pubs/preg-guide.htm (Accessed February 23, 2016.)

Human Immunodeficiency Virus Infection and Pregnancy

Denise Willers

Introduction

Perinatal human immunodeficiency virus (HIV) transmission has been dramatically reduced in the United States with the employment of increased testing and effective treatment strategies. In 1994, the Pediatric AIDS Clinical Trials Group 076 study reported that use of the antiretroviral zidovudine in the antepartum and intrapartum periods as well as infant oral zidovudine for the first 6 weeks of life could reduce perinatal transmission of HIV from 25% to 8%.[1] While these recommendations still guide treatment, current use of combination antiretroviral therapy (cART) and other interventions now allow for a less than 1% transmission risk.[2–4] Strategies for reduction of HIV transmission in pregnancy are rapidly evolving, especially recommendations for antiretroviral therapy regimens. Additionally, clinical presentations of patients with HIV infection range from straightforward to very complex.

This chapter presents general guidance about testing for HIV during pregnancy and prevention of vertical HIV transmission, from pre-conception care through the post-natal period. Additional resources should be consulted as needed. Recommendations for use of Antiretroviral Drugs in Pregnancy are published by the United States Department of Health and Humans Services and updated regularly; these are accessible at http://aidsinfo.nih.gov/guidelines.[5] The National Perinatal HIV Hotline (1-888-448-8765) can provide guidance for specific patients when experts are not readily available. The hotline can also provide a list of regional experts.

Scope of the Problem

Of the estimated 1.2 million people in the United States living with HIV, 23% are women.[6] Despite the recommendation for universal HIV screening, 12–14% of HIV-infected individuals are unaware of their infection.[6] One-third of new HIV infections can be attributed to sexual contact or IV drug use involving people who are unaware of their HIV infection.[7] An alarming 9,000–10,000 women are infected with HIV annually in the United States. Given that the majority of these infections are a result of heterosexual exposure in women of childbearing age, obstetric providers should be knowledgeable of HIV screening and management during pregnancy.[8]

In the United States, the number of perinatal HIV infections peaked in 1991 at 1,650 and declined to approximately 200 per year by 2002.[9] Despite very effective measures for prevention, 100–150 neonates in the United States continue to be infected annually.[6] For example, in 2010, 6,000–7,000 pregnancies were affected by HIV, and an estimated 162 neonates were perinatally infected. The many barriers that stand between the current rate of HIV vertical transmission and a goal of complete elimination of perinatal HIV transmission are listed in Box 47.1. HIV infection disproportionately affects Black/African American mothers and their infants with a rate of perinatal HIV infection in 2009 of 9.9 infections/100,000 live births in Black infants compared to 0.1/100,000 live births in white infants.[8]

Screening for HIV Infection

Identification of HIV-infected individuals is essential to the prevention of transmission. Since 2006, recommendations have included HIV screening as a part of routine healthcare for people in the United States from ages 13 to 64. Patients with ongoing risk factors should be screened at least annually. Providers are recommended to use opt-out counseling when testing for HIV, in which the patient is tested routinely unless he or she declines.[10]

Universal screening for HIV in pregnancy is well accepted and is a crucial strategy to eliminate perinatal transmission of HIV. Current recommendations include screening all patients for HIV infection at

Box 47.1 Barriers to further reductions in perinatal transmission of HIV

Lack of primary prevention of HIV in girls and women
Lack of adequate contraception and preconception counseling for HIV infected women
Lack of early and adequate prenatal care allowing for detection and treatment of HIV infection
Incident maternal HIV infection during pregnancy
Non-compliance with HIV medication

Box 47.2 Patient factors which indicate repeat HIV testing in the third trimester

A new sexual partner during the pregnancy
Sex with a high-risk or HIV-infected partner
A sexually transmitted infection in the past year
Injection drug use by the patient or her partner

initial presentation for prenatal care, without regard to risk factors and using opt-out counseling. Repeat HIV testing is recommended in the third trimester in women with the personal risk factors seen in Box 47.2.[11] Additionally, universal third trimester testing is recommended in areas with high prevalence of HIV and in centers with at least one diagnosed HIV case per 1,000 pregnant women per year.[10]

In 2014, the Centers for Disease Control and Prevention (CDC) updated the recommendations for laboratory testing for diagnosis of HIV. The CDC currently recommends that specimens sent to the lab are subjected to a fourth-generation combination screen for antibodies to HIV-1 and HIV-2 and a screen for presence of the HIV-1 p24 antigen (HIV 1/2 Ab + p24). Inclusion of a test for the p24 antigen allows detection of HIV infection approximately 15 days after infection occurs, roughly 10 days before antibodies can be detected. See Figure 47.1.

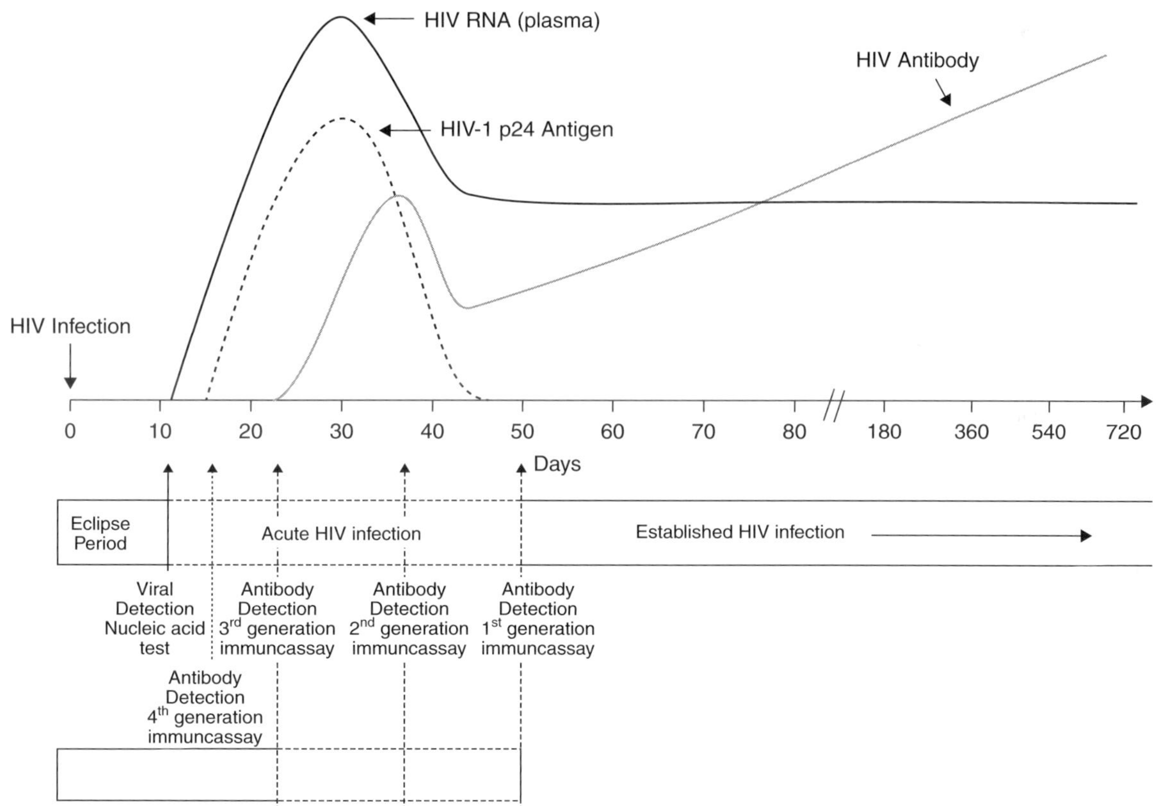

Figure 47.1 Timeline of HIV RNA, HIV-1 p24 Antigen, and HIV antibody levels and the detection timeframe of available HIV tests. From Centers for Disease Control and Prevention and Association of Public Health Laboratories. Laboratory Testing for the Diagnosis of HIV Infection: Updated Recommendations. Available at http://stacks.cdc.gov/view/cdc/23447. Published June 27, 2014.

Non-reactive samples from this initial screening are considered negative unless there is concern for infection within the last three weeks. Reactive samples from this initial test are then analyzed with an immunodifferentiation assay to detect HIV-1 and HIV-2 antibodies. Positivity in this secondary test confirms HIV infection. Samples that are positive on the HIV 1/2 Ab + p24 screen and are non-reactive or indeterminate on the immunodifferentiation assay are then tested for the presence of HIV ribonucleic acid (RNA). This is important to eliminate the possibility of an acute HIV infection that is too early for antibody detection but the p24 antigen is detected.[12] See Figure 47.2.

Any woman presenting in labor without prior HIV testing in her pregnancy or who has any risks for HIV transmission since the last HIV test should be rapidly tested for HIV.[10,11] This testing can be performed in the lab with an HIV 1/2 Ab + p24 test. In some centers, point-of-care testing without the p24 antigen (third generation) is used for initial screening. Point-of-care testing can be completed within 20 minutes and does not require hospital registration. These advantages may outweigh any benefit of inclusion of the p24 antigen test. The immunodifferentiation test can be used to confirm any positive third-generation tests. Additional screening with the HIV 1/2 Ab + p24 or HIV RNA can be performed in patients in whom there is a concern for infection with HIV in the last 3 weeks.[11]

Preconception Care of HIV Infected Patients

The availability of combination anti-retroviral therapy (cART) has allowed HIV-infected women to live longer and healthier lives than ever before. Given that HIV can be transmitted vertically from a pregnant woman to her fetus, it is essential to use effective strategies to prevent this transmission. Such strategies should ideally be initiated before women become pregnant. Providers should thus discuss pregnancy intent and offer contraception or preconception counseling to reproductive aged women. HIV infection should not deter women from becoming pregnant if that is their goal.

Contraception

For HIV-infected women who do not currently desire pregnancy, effective contraception should be encouraged and provided. HIV-infected women can use all available contraceptive options, although known interactions with cART should guide contraceptive choices to provide the most effective therapy. Pharmacokinetic studies have shown a decrease in the levels of estradiol and progestin when combined oral contraceptives, patches, and vaginal rings are used with protease inhibitors boosted with ritonavir.[13–15]. Efavirenz has been shown to decrease progestin levels as well;

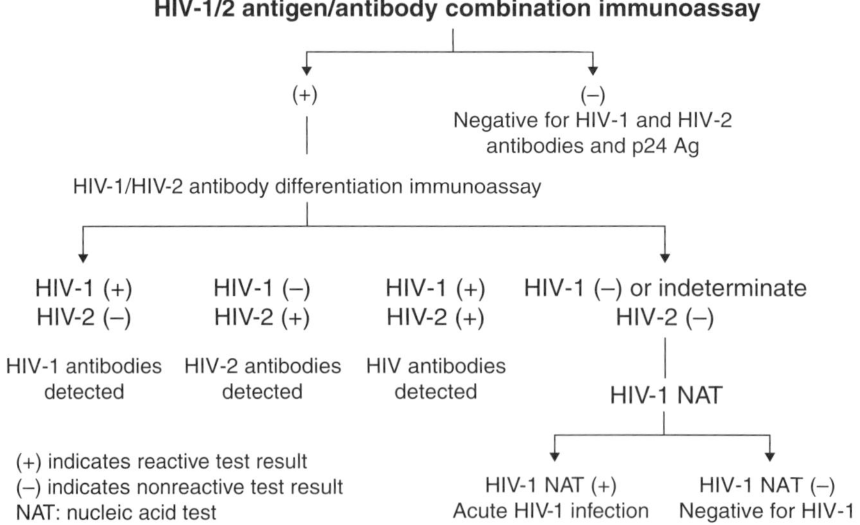

Figure 47.2 Algorithm for screening for HIV in laboratory settings incorporating HIV 1/2 + p24 Ag and the immunodifferentiation assay. From Centers for Disease Control and Prevention and Association of Public Health Laboratories. Laboratory Testing for the Diagnosis of HIV Infection: Updated Recommendations. Available at http://stacks.cdc.gov/view/cdc/23447. Published June 27, 2014.

this decreases effectiveness of progestin containing implantable contraceptives.[16,17] Protease inhibitors boosted with ritonovir are also suspected to decrease the effectiveness of the etonogestrel-implantable contraceptive, although this interaction is less well studied. In contrast, depot medroxyprogesterone has been shown to be effective and can be used without restriction in patients taking cART.[5] Intrauterine devices (IUDs) are considered safe for the prevention of pregnancy in women with HIV and given local action of IUDs, interactions with cART are minimal.[14,18] Sterilization with tubal ligation or vasectomy of the male partner can be considered when fertility is no longer desired. Condom use should be encouraged to protect partners from transmission.

Counseling HIV-Positive Patients

In women planning pregnancy or those declining effective contraception, preconception counseling is indicated. The goals for preconception health care are seen in Box 47.3.[19] HIV-infected women should be further educated concerning the use of antiviral medications to minimize the risk of perinatal HIV infection. Women can be counseled that, if they fully comply with the HIV medication regimen to suppress the HIV RNA to an undetectable level, then the risk of HIV infection of their baby can be less than 1%.[2–4]

Serodiscordant Couples and Conception

Serodiscordant couples, in which one partner is HIV infected and the other is negative, should be counseled about the safest conception options and referred to specialists. Serodiscordant couples, in which the woman is HIV infected, should use self-insemination with the partner's collected semen at the time of ovulation. Syringes can be used for vaginal placement of semen timed with ovulation.[20,21]

In couples in which the man is HIV infected and the woman is HIV negative, insemination from a sperm donor is the only way to eliminate all risk of transmission. If that option is not acceptable to the couple, two low-risk options are available. One option is for the HIV-negative woman to undergo intrauterine insemination or in vitro fertilization with sperm washed using techniques designed to reduce risk of residual HIV virus.[22,23] Alternatively, discordant couples could consider having unprotected intercourse that is limited to the time of the woman's ovulation and the negative partner takes pre-exposure prophylaxis (PrEP) with tenofovir and emtricitabine. This has been shown to have a low risk of transmission when compliance with cART is high.[24]

Any plan for sexual exposure with the HIV-infected partner requires maximal suppression of HIV RNA levels with the use cART and use of PrEP by the HIV-negative partner. The CDC has published guidelines for the use of PrEP.[25] Current recommendations in the United States are for the uninfected partner to take PrEP before and for 28 days following any unprotected sexual activity or semen exposure for pregnancy attempts.[20,21] Testing and treatment of both partners for sexually transmitted infections and evaluation of the female partner for vaginal infections or inflammation is also recommended, as these may increase risk of transmission. HIV-negative patients taking pre-exposure prophylaxis should have renal function monitored and be tested regularly for HIV infection.

Box 47.3 Preconception goals

- Stabilization of medical conditions
- Optimization of social situations
- Treatment of mental health issues
- Evaluation for use of teratogenic medications
- Update immunizations
- Initiation of folic acid
- Reduction of high-risk behaviors
- Screening for sexually transmitted infections
- Screening for genetic disorders that might impact pregnancy

Antepartum Care of HIV-Infected Patients

Risk Factors and Testing

Optimal care for HIV-infected pregnant women includes multidisciplinary care with obstetric care providers who are educated in care of HIV-infected patients and HIV specialty care providers, as well as other medical, mental health, and social services as indicated. Initial evaluation for HIV-infected pregnant women should include review of previous and current HIV RNA levels, CD4 cell counts, and opportunistic infections. Current and prior antiretroviral therapy and genotype testing for medication resistance should also be documented.[5]

Research has universally shown that HIV-1 RNA viral load (total number of HIV particles per mL of blood/serum) during pregnancy and delivery is the most important risk factor for vertical transmission of HIV from mother to offspring.[26–28] The level of HIV-1 RNA at the time of delivery directly correlates with transmission risk.[2,4] The many other factors that additionally contribute to the risk of transmission are seen in Box 47.4.[27–35] When the viral load is undetectable as a result of adherence to cART regimens, however, these factors may contribute minimal additional risk.

Counseling of HIV-Positive Pregnant Women

Patients should be educated about the benefits and goals of treatment of HIV in pregnancy, including the use of cART to lower HIV-1 viral load to undetectable levels as early as possible in pregnancy. Strict adherence to the prescribed drug regimen should be recommended to prevent perinatal HIV transmission and avoid development of drug resistance. Adherence to medication should be assessed at the initial visit and consistently throughout the pregnancy.[5] Counseling must include expected side effects of cART as well as limited long-term data for infants exposed to cART in utero.

Counseling concerning cART should be directive, but non-coercive, and allow patients to make informed decisions about their care.[5] Barriers to medication adherence should be addressed with the patient and support should be provided. Patients should be screened for depression, housing instability, substance use, interpersonal violence, and other complicated social situations, as these contribute to non-adherence to medication.[29] Counseling should deter cigarette smoking, illicit drug use, and unprotected intercourse with multiple partners as these can increase the risk of transmission of HIV to the neonate.[31–35]

Box 47.4 Factors that contribute to risk of perinatal HIV transmission

Acute HIV infection
Low CD-4 counts
Hepatitis B/C coinfection
Sexually transmitted infections
Unprotected vaginal intercourse during pregnancy
Labor
Rupture of membranes
Prolonged rupture of membranes
Vaginal mode of delivery
Chorioamnionitis
Substance use, including smoking

Privacy and protection of health information for HIV-infected patients should be addressed with the patient. The extent of disclosure of HIV status to the patient's partner and other support persons should be queried and assistance with disclosure of status to appropriate persons should be offered. Adherence to prenatal care, HIV care and medications, as well as newborn follow-up and oral zidovudine may be limited if the patient's support persons and infant caregivers are not aware of her HIV status. The patient should be encouraged to limit visitors for prenatal care, delivery, and postpartum care to those who are aware of her status. Clinic and hospital staff should speak to the patient alone about her medical care until her disclosures are known.

Antiviral Therapy

If an HIV-positive woman is not already on antiretroviral therapy, the CDC recommends that such therapy be initiated at time of presentation for prenatal care. If the patient has intractable nausea and vomiting in the first trimester, this medication can be initiated after the nausea improves.[5] Previous recommendations to delay therapy until the end of the first trimester to allow for completion of organogenesis prior to medication exposure are outweighed by evidence that early achievement of undetectable HIV-1 RNA is associated with the lowest rates of vertical transmission.[2] The likelihood of viral suppression by the time of delivery increases when cART is initiated earlier, especially for patients with a high initial HIV viral load.[36] Studies and pregnancy registries show little concern that HIV antiviral medications are teratogenic.[5] Additionally, most pregnancies are not identified before 8 weeks' gestation, when organogenesis is complete. Patients who are currently on cART and whose HIV-1 RNA is below a detectable level should remain on antiviral therapy. Patients who have not achieved viral suppression by 30 weeks may be at increased risk for transmission, therefore suppression by the third trimester is recommended.[5,37]

The data concerning teratogenic risk of antiretroviral medications in pregnancy is incomplete and observational for most medications. Health care providers caring for HIV-infected pregnant women should report all drug exposures to the Antiretroviral Pregnancy Registry at www.APRegistry.com. There were concerns about use of the medication efavirenz, a non-nucleoside reverse transcriptase inhibitor, in the first trimester. This concern was based on primate studies and observational data, which showed an increased risk of central nervous system defects. A meta-analysis evaluating all available studies of efavirenz exposure in the first trimester concluded that the incidence of congenital anomalies, including neural tube defects, was similar to the general population.[38] Current recommendations regarding efavirenz are to avoid use in patients planning pregnancy or not using reliable contraception, and initiate efavirenz after 8 weeks when included in cART regimens during pregnancy. However, given that most pregnancies are not detected prior to 6 weeks when the neural tube closes, patients presenting with pregnancy on efavirenz with a suppressed viral load should be continued on the medication.[5] An ultrasound at 18–20 weeks of pregnancy is recommended for all patients, including those on cART.

If HIV-1 RNA levels are greater than 500 copies/mL, genotypic antiretroviral drug-resistance testing should be performed to guide therapy, although testing may be unsuccessful for HIV-1 RNA levels <1,000 copies/mL. Selection of initial and ongoing regimens for cART in pregnancy should be in conjunction with an HIV specialist when available. The optimal regimen should be based on resistance testing, clinical scenario, prior patient medication regimens, and current guidelines. In addition to minimizing HIV-1 RNA levels, transplacental passage of antiretroviral medications to the fetus is an important mechanism of infant pre-exposure prophylaxis. Nucleoside/nucleotide reverse transcriptase inhibitors (NRTI) cross the placenta and are the backbone for all preferred cART regimens in pregnancy. Preferred regimens include a 2 NRTI backbone with the addition of a protease inhibitor, a non-nucleoside reverse transcriptase inhibitor, or an integrase inhibitor.[5]

Figure 47.3 shows the preferred and alternative regimens for HIV-1 recommended at the time of this publication. Medication recommendations for HIV evolve rapidly and current guidelines can be accessed at aidsinfo.nih.gov and the National Perinatal HIV

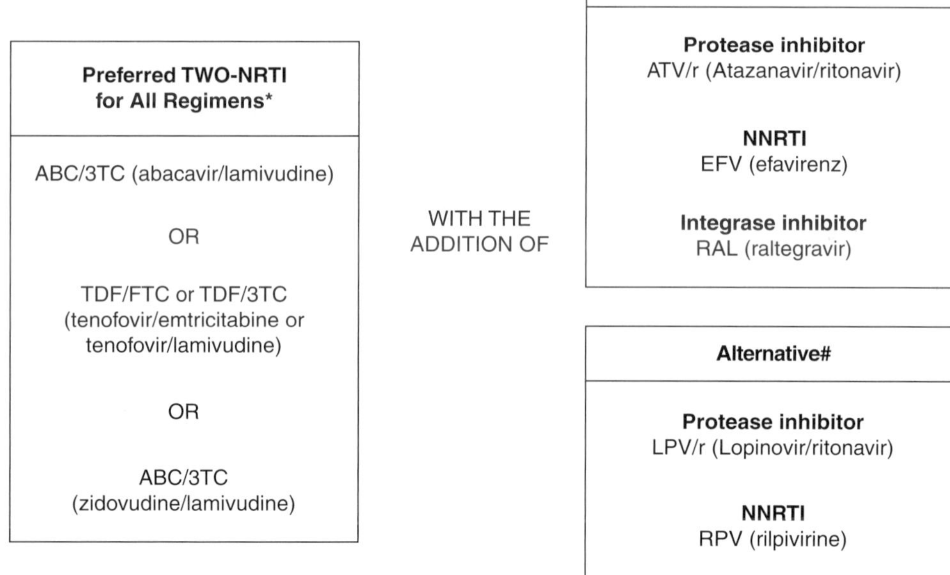

Figure 47.3 Preferred and alternative regimens for HIV-1. Adapted from recommendations for HIV antiviral medication in pregnancy, guidelines updated August 6, 2015.[5] http://aidsinfo.nih.gov/contentfiles/lvguidelines/PerinatalGL.pdf.

* ABC should not be used in patients who test positive for HLA-B*5701. ABC/3TC not recommended with EFV or ATV/r in patients with HIV RNA >100,000 copies per mL. TDF has potential renal toxicity. ZDV/3TC has potential for hematologic toxicities.

\+ ATV/r can cause maternal hyperbilirubinemia. Efavirenz with concern for birth defects in primates. RAL requires twice daily dosing, but has rapid viral load reduction.

\# LPV/r no longer preferred due to nausea, requires twice daily dosing. RPV not recommended with HIV RNA >100,000 copies per mL or CD4<200 cells/mm^3. Do not use with proton pump inhibitors.

Hotline can provide guidance when experts are not readily available.

HIV-2 is endemic to West Africa and makes up a very small portion, approximately 0.01%, of HIV infections in the United States. Improved detection of HIV-2 is, however, provided with the immunodifferentiation assay algorithm compared to previous testing with Western blot. Treatment of HIV-2 in pregnancy should include two NRTI and a protease inhibitor boosted with ritonovir. Infants born to mothers with HIV-2 should receive the standard 6-week zidovudine prophylactic regimen.[5]

HIV-infected patients who are also infected with hepatitis B are treated with medications with action against both viruses. These include tenofovir, emtricitabine, and lamivudine.[5]

Patients with CD-4 counts less than 200 cells/mm^3 should be treated with prophylaxis for *Pneumocystis* pneumonia with trimethoprim/sulfamethoxazole. Trimethoprim has been associated with a small increase in neural tube defects, cardiovascular and urinary tract defects when used in the first trimester. Supplementation of folic acid greater than 400 mcg decreases the rate of these anomalies. Folic acid supplementation may, however, diminish the effectiveness of the prophylaxis and increase the risk of *Pneumocystis* pneumonia. If increased folic acid supplementation is used, it should be limited to the first trimester during organogenesis.[5] Guidance for prevention and treatment for other opportunistic infections in pregnancy are available from the CDC at http://aidsinfo.nih.gov/contentfiles/lvguidelines/adult_oi.pdf.[39]

Laboratory Monitoring/Vaccines

HIV-1 RNA testing should occur at the time of presentation and monthly throughout pregnancy until viral suppression is achieved and then at least every 3 months. HIV-1 RNA testing should be repeated at 34–36 weeks' gestation to guide decisions about delivery plan and optimal treatment of the newborn. CD4 T lymphocyte testing should occur every 3 months and can inform necessity of prophylactic medication against opportunistic infections. Monitoring for complications of antiviral therapy typically includes complete blood count (CBC) and renal and liver function testing, depending on the regimen. Protease inhibitors in cART have been associated with hyperglycemia, but effect on the rate of gestational diabetes in pregnant women is unclear. Standard screening for gestational diabetes at 24–28 weeks is recommended.[5]

Vaccines for influenza (injection only) and tetanus/diphtheria/pertussis are recommended in pregnancy and are safe for patients with HIV. In addition, HIV-infected patients should receive pneumococcal vaccination and hepatitis B vaccination during pregnancy if not current.

Delivery Plan

Decisions about the planned mode of delivery should be made during the antepartum visits. The primary risk factor for transmission at the time of delivery is the HIV-1 RNA level. If the HIV-1 RNA at 34–36 weeks' gestation is > 1,000 copies per mL, then cesarean delivery is associated with a lower risk of vertical transmission compared to vaginal delivery. Planned cesarean in HIV-infected patients with elevated HIV-1 RNA should be performed at 38 weeks to minimize the chance of onset of labor and rupture of membranes. In patients with an HIV-1 RNA level of < 1,000 copies per mL, cesarean delivery is not associated with a lower risk of transmission than vaginal delivery and vaginal delivery is recommended. Patients with a low HIV-1 RNA undergoing cesarean due to obstetric indications should be performed at 39 weeks.[5] Recent adherence to cART should be addressed with the patient by direct questioning about compliance and number of missed doses. Non-adherence to medication in the time since the last HIV-1 RNA test could change the recommendations for delivery method and medications for the patient and her infant.

Situations in which women who are known to be HIV infected but who are not taking cART or those who are newly diagnosed as HIV infected late in pregnancy are often clinical dilemmas. Combination ART should be started as soon as possible. Barriers to adherence for medication continuation should be addressed with the patient. In patients who are nearing 38 weeks gestation, cesarean section should be performed at 38 weeks, or sooner if delivery is indicated. If there is adequate time for suppression of the HIV-1 RNA to a level below 1,000 copies/mL, then HIV-1 RNA can be retested before making decisions about mode of delivery.[36,40] Consultation with infectious disease specialists and/or specialists in the treatment of HIV in pregnancy should occur in these situations. A medication regimen that includes the integrase inhibitor, raltegravir, may be recommended as raltegravir leads to faster viral decay than other antiretroviral medications, with a 2 log reduction in HIV-1 RNA during the first 2 weeks of use and potential decreased transmission to the neonate. Elevation of transaminases have been reported with use of raltegravir in late pregnancy.[5]

Intrapartum Care

Treatment

Intravenous zidovudine (a nucleoside reverse transcriptase inhibitor) during labor and delivery and for at least 3 hours before cesarean section has been a component of perinatal HIV prevention since 1994, when the initial recommendations were established.[1] For patients whose HIV-1 RNA level is >1,000 copies/mL, cesarean delivery and IV zidovudine are recommended, 2 mg/kg IV load over 1 hour, and then 1 mg/kg until delivery. IV zidovudine is not required for patients who are on antiviral therapy and have an HIV-1 RNA <1,000 copies/mL, as there is no evidence that it leads to further reduction in perinatal transmission.[41–43] If there are concerns about adherence or tolerance of oral antiviral medication since the 36-week HIV-1 RNA test, use of IV zidovudine in labor is still recommended. Clinicians my elect to continue to use IV zidovudine in labor regardless of HIV RNA as it is well tolerated.[5] It is recommended that patients who are on cART continue their oral medications on schedule as much as possible to prevent increases in HIV-1 RNA and development of resistant virus.[5]

Vaginal Delivery

Patients who are candidates for vaginal delivery (HIV-1 RNA < 1,000 copies/mL and good adherence to cART) can be allowed to continue their pregnancies until labor occurs, reserving induction of labor for obstetric indications. Lack of adherence should prompt consideration of repeat testing for HIV-1 RNA level if the result can be available when needed. Depending on the patient's clinic scenario, cesarean delivery should be considered if adherence to medication has been poor and there is concern for an elevated HIV-1 RNA.[5]

Management of labor in HIV-infected patients should be guided by goals of (1) decreasing time of rupture of membranes and (2) limiting exposure of the infant to maternal blood. In patients who present with rupture of membranes without labor and who are candidates for vaginal delivery, interventions to decrease the interval to delivery should be considered. These possible interventions include administration of prostaglandins and oxytocin. Data are limited on effects of prolonged rupture of membranes on HIV transmission in patients with HIV-1 RNA levels <1,000 copies/mL, but the available data suggest that there is minimal risk of transmission.[43] Rupture of membranes to expedite delivery (if other methods are not effective) or to prevent splashing, could be considered. Data are limited on use of fetal scalp electrode, operative delivery with forceps or vacuum, and episiotomy; these should be avoided unless there are clear obstetric indications. Delayed cord clamping has not been studied in HIV-infected patients, although there is no indication to limit this practice if indicated.[5]

Cesarean Delivery

HIV-infected patients who are having planned cesarean sections due to HIV-1 RNA >1,000 copies/mL should be scheduled for delivery at 38 weeks gestation. Intravenous (IV) zidovudine should be administered for 3 hours before surgery to ensure adequate levels of zidovudine in the cord blood, and cART therapy should be continued as much as possible, even if oral intake is otherwise limited. Perioperative antibiotics should be administered similarly to other patients undergoing cesarean.[5]

HIV infected patients with HIV-1 RNA < 1,000 copies/mL undergoing cesarean for obstetric indications should be scheduled for 39 weeks.[5]

In patients with planned cesarean section who present in labor or with rupture of membranes, it is unclear whether cesarean section further decreases the risk of perinatal transmission of HIV. Decisions on whether to proceed with vaginal delivery or perform a cesarean section should be individualized with consideration given to the probable time to patient delivery and risk of transmission.[5]

Preterm Labor

Patients presenting with preterm labor and premature rupture of membranes should generally be managed in accordance with obstetric guidelines, including administration of antenatal steroids when indicated. The risk of HIV transmission must be weighed against the known risks of prematurity. Patients who are not taking cART should be started on cART to lower viral levels as quickly as possible.[5]

Postpartum

Postpartum hemorrhage

Methergine (ergot alkaloid) used for postpartum uterine atony can interact with protease inhibitors and other CYP3A4 enzyme inhibitors in cART and lead to excessive vasoconstriction. Thus, other options for postpartum atony should be used and Methergine should be avoided. If other options are not effective, then Methergine can be used in a low dose for a short period of time. Other HIV medications that induce CYP3A4 enzyme activity (nevirapine, efavirenz, etravirine) can lower the effectiveness of Methergine.[5]

Treating the Infant

Post-exposure prophylaxis for infants exposed to HIV at delivery is a key component for the prevention of perinatal transmission of HIV. Oral zidovudine is the standard therapy recommended for infants exposed to HIV. Dosing should be weight based, adjusted for gestational age, and usually continued for 6 weeks. This should be initiated as soon as possible after delivery. Full-term infants who are born to mothers on cART who had a suppressed HIV-1 RNA at the time of delivery are candidates for a 4-week regimen of oral zidovudine; this regimen is considered to be equivalent to 6 weeks in this population.[5]

Infants whose mothers received suboptimal or no antenatal cART or had elevated HIV-1 RNA at delivery are at higher risk of perinatal infection with HIV and may benefit from three doses of nevirapine in addition to oral zidovudine. The first dose is given as soon as possible after birth, the second dose 48 hours later, and the third dose 96 hours after the second dose.[5] Pediatric infectious disease specialists should be consulted for HIV-exposed infants, especially in these complicated cases or if maternal genotype predicts resistance to zidovudine.

HIV-exposed infants should be started on prophylaxis for *Pneumocystis* pneumonia with trimethoprim-sulfamethoxazole at 4–6 weeks, unless HIV nucleic acid amplification testing can presumptively exclude HIV infection (negative HIV-1 DNA/RNA at > 14 days and > 4 weeks).[5]

Exposure to maternal cART during pregnancy can contribute to anemia and neutropenia at birth. CBC testing should be done prior to initiation of zidovudine therapy for infants exposed to HIV. Repeat CBC is recommended at the end of zidovudine therapy.[5]

Nucleoside reverse transcriptase inhibitors such as zidovudine are associated with mitochondrial dysfunction, although the incidence in exposed infants is unclear. This diagnosis should be considered in uninfected infants and children with a history of nucleoside reverse transcriptase inhibitor (NRTI) exposure, who present with severe clinical findings, especially neurologic findings.[5]

No data exist to guide newborn management in terms of timing of circumcision, eye ointment application, or vitamin K injection; bathing the infant before these therapies, however, could be considered. Care of HIV exposed newborns should balance the need for expedited antiretroviral prophylaxis and bathing with the importance of bonding between mother and newborn within the first hours of life.[5]

Counseling of mothers and fathers or other caregivers concerning care of the HIV-exposed infant should include an assessment for any barriers to compliance with the recommended medication and follow-up. Ideally, the infant medication needed for the entire 4–6 weeks of therapy should be provided to the mother at discharge, or availability at the pharmacy should be confirmed. Follow-up with a general pediatrician and a specialist in pediatric infectious disease should be arranged.[5]

Breastfeeding

Even with viral suppression, breast milk can contain HIV and lead to infection of the infant. Thus, HIV-infected women should be counseled not to breastfeed in the United States, where formula feeding is considered safe and acceptable.[5] This recommendation may be different in underdeveloped countries based on safety, availability, and acceptability of infant formula. Additionally, pre-mastication (chewing of food prior to feeding to the child) should be avoided because of reports of HIV infection of infants from this practice.[43]

Infant Testing

HIV antibodies cross the placenta and their presence in the infant up to 18 months or beyond is indicative of maternal, not infant infection. Instead, HIV-1 nucleic amplification testing (DNA or RNA) is used for detection of infant infection. This testing is usually done at birth, 14–21 days of life, 1–2 months, and 4–6 months. HIV infection in the infant can be excluded with negative testing at 1 month and 4 months of age or after.[5]

Maternal Follow-up

Current HIV management guidelines recommend use of cART for all HIV-infected individuals regardless of HIV RNA level or CD4 levels.[5] After delivery, patients should be continued on their cART regimens and infectious disease, as well as gynecologic follow-up, should be arranged. Contraception recommendations should focus on effective methods including long-acting methods of contraception and sterilization when desired.

Concluding Remarks

Elimination of perinatal transmission of HIV is an obtainable goal. Obstetric providers should be familiar with the recommendations for optimal testing for HIV in pregnancy and treatment when HIV infections are identified. Multidisciplinary care including physicians, nurses, case managers, mental health specialists, and social services can provide recommendations and support to patients to promote treatment adherence and minimize risk of vertical transmission of HIV.

References

1. Connor EM, Sperling RS, Gelber R, et. al. Reduction of maternal-infant transmission of human immunodeficiency virus type 1 with zidovudine treatment. Pediatric AIDS Clinical Trials Group Protocol 076 Study Group. *N Engl J Med.* 1994;331(18):1173–1180.
2. Townsend CL, Byrne L, Cortina-Borja M, et al. Earlier initiation of ART and further decline in mother-to-child HIV transmission rates, 2000–2011. *AIDS.* 2014;28(7):1049–1057.
3. Forbes JC, Alimenti AM, Singer J, et al. A national review of vertical HIV transmission. *AIDS.* 2012;26(6):757–763.
4. Ioannidis JP, Contopoulos-Ioannidis DG. Maternal viral load and the risk of perinatal transmission of HIV-1. *N Engl J Med.* 1999 Nov 25;341(22):1698–1700.
5. Panel on treatment of HIV-infected pregnant women and prevention of perinatal transmission. Recommendations for use of antiretroviral drugs in pregnant HIV-1-infected women for maternal health and interventions to reduce perinatal HIV transmission in the United States. Available at http://aidsinfo.nih.gov/contentfiles/ lvguidelines/ PerinatalGL.pdf. Accessed March 19, 2016.
6. Centers for Disease Control and Prevention. Monitoring selected national HIV prevention and care objectives by using HIV surveillance data – United States and 6 dependent areas, 2012. HIV Surveillance Supplemental Report 2014;19(3). www.cdc.gov/hiv/ library/repors/ surveillance/. Published November 2014. Accessed February 27, 2016.
7. Skarbinski J, Rosenberg E, Paz-Bailey G, et al. Human immunodeficiency virus transmission at each step of the care continuum in the United States. *JAMA Intern Med.* 2015;175:588–596.
8. Centers for Disease Control and Prevention. HIV Among Women, Infants, and Children. Available at www.cdc.gov/hiv/group/gender/pregnantwomen/. Page updated June 15, 2015. Accessed March 19, 2016.
9. Centers for Disease Control and Prevention. Reduction in perinatal transmission of HIV infection – United States, 1985–2005. *MMWR* 2006;55:592–597.
10. Branson BM, Handsfield HH, Lampe MA, et al. Revised recommendations for HIV testing of adults, adolescents, and pregnant women in health-care settings. *MMWR* Sept 22, 2006;55(RR14);1–17.
11. ACOG Committee Opinion No 635. Prenatal and perinatal human immunodeficiency virus testing: expanded recommendations. American College of Obtetricians and Gynecologists. *Obstet Gynecol.* 2015 Jun;125(6):1544–1547.
12. Centers for Disease Control and Prevention and Association of Public Health Laboratories. Laboratory Testing for the Diagnosis of HIV Infection: Updated Recommendations. Available at http://stacks.cdc.gov/ view/cdc/23447. Published June 27, 2014. Accessed February 20, 2016.
13. Vogler MA, Patterson K, Kamemoto L, et al. Contraceptive efficacy of oral and transdermal hormones when co-administered with protease inhibitors in HIV-1-infected women: pharmacokinetic results of ACTG trial A5188. *J Acquire Immune Defic Syndr.* 2010;55(4):437–82.
14. Stringer EM, Kaseba C, Levy J, et al. A randomized trial of the intrauterine contraceptive device vs hormonal contraception in women who are infected with the human immunodeficiency virus. *Am J Obstet Gynecol* 2007;197:144.e1–144.e8.
15. Robinson JA, Jamshidi R, Burke AE. Contraception for the HIV-positive woman: a review of interactions between hormonal contraception and antiretroviral therapy. *Infect Dis Obstet Gynecol.* 2012;2012:890160. doi:10.1155/2012/890160. Available at www.hindawi .com/journals/idog/2012/890160/
16. Landolt NK, Phanuphak N, Ubolyam S, et al. Significant decrease of ethinylestradiol with nevirapine, and of etonogestrel with efavirenz in HIV-positive women. *J Acquir Immune Defic Syndr.*

2014;66(2):e50–e52. Available at www.ncbi.nlm.nih.gov/pubmed/24608892.

17. Perry SH, Swamy P, Preidis GA, Mwanyumba A, Motsa N, Sarero HN. Implementing the Jadelle implant for women living with HIV in a resource-limited setting in sub-Saharan Africa: concerns for drug interactions leading to unintended pregnancies. *AIDS.* 2014. Available at www.ncbi.nlm.nih.gov/pubmed/24401645.
18. Morrison CS, Sekadde-Kigondu C, Sinei SK, Weiner, DH, Kwok C, Kokonya D. Is the intrauterine device appropriate contraception for HIV-1-infected women?. *BJOG.* 2001;108: 784–790.
19. ACOG Committee Opinion No 313. The importance of preconception care in the continuum of women's healthcare. American College of Obstetricians and Gynecologists. *Obstet Gynecol.* 2005 Sep;106(3):665–666.
20. Lampe MA, Smith DK, Anderson GJE, et al. Achieving safe conception in HIV-discordant couples: the potential role of oral preexposure prophylaxis (PrEP) in the United States. *Am J Obstet Gynecol* 2011;204:488.e1–8.
21. Matthews L, Smit J, Cu-Uvin S, Cohan D. Antiretrovirals and safer conception for HIV-serodiscordant couples. *Curr Opin HIV AIDS.* 2012, 7:569–578.
22. Ethics Committee of the American Society for Reproductive M. Human immunodeficiency virus and infertility treatment. *Fertil Steril.* 2010;94(1):11–15.
23. Semprini AE, Macaluso M, Hollander L, et al. Safe conception for HIV-discordant couples: Insemination with processed semen from the HIV-infected partner. *Am J Obstet Gynecol.* 2013 May;208(5):402.e1–9.
24. Vernazza PL, Graf I, Sonnenberg-Schwan U, et al. Preexposure prophylaxis and timed intercourse for HIV-discordant couples willing to conceive a child. *AIDS.* 2011;25(16):2005–2008.
25. CDC. Preexposure prophylaxis for the prevention of HIV infection in the United States-2014. www.cdc.gov/hiv/pdf/prepguidelines2014.pdf. Accessed March 19, 2016.
26. Garcia PM, Kalish LA, Pitt J, et al. Maternal levels of plasma human immunodeficiency virus type 1 RNA and the risk of perinatal transmission. Women and Infants Transmission Study Group. *N Engl J Med.* 1999;341(6):394–402.
27. Cooper ER, Charurat M, Mofenson L, et al. Combination antiretroviral strategies for the treatment of pregnant HIV-1-infected women and prevention of perinatal HIV-1 transmission. *J Acquir Immune Defic Syndr.* 2002;29:484–494.
28. Jourdain G, Mary JY, Coeur SL, Ngo-Giang-Huong N, Yuthavisuthi P, Limtrakul A, et al. Risk factors for in utero or intrapartum mother-to-child transmission of human immunodeficiency virus type 1 in Thailand. *J Infect Dis.* 2007;196(11):1629–1636.
29. Whitmore SK, Taylor AW, Espinoza L, Shouse RL, Lampe MA, Nesheim S. Correlates of mother-to-child transmission of HIV in the United States and Puerto Rico. *Pediatrics.* 2012;129;e74–e81.
30. Drake AL, Wagner A, Richardson B, John-Stewart G. Incident HIV during pregnancy and postpartum and risk of mother-to-child HIV transmission: A systematic review and meta-analysis. *PLoS Med* Feb 2014;11(2):e1001608. doi:10.1371/journal.pmed.1001608.
31. Burns DN, Landesman S, Muenz LR, et al. Cigarette smoking, premature rupture of membranes and vertical transmission of HIV-1 among women with low CD4 levels. *J Acquir Immune Defic Syndr Hum Retrovirol.* 1994;7(7):718–726.
32. Turner BJ, Hauck WW, Fanning TR, Markson LE. Cigarette smoking and maternal–child HIV transmission. *J Acquir Immune Defic Syndr Hum Retrovirol.* 1997;14(4):327–337.
33. Rodriguez EM, Mofenson LM, Chang BH, et al. Association of maternal drug use during pregnancy with maternal HIV culture positivity and perinatal HIV transmission. *AIDS.* 1996;10(3):273–282.
34. Bulterys M, Landesman S, Burns DN, et al. Sexual behavior and injection drug use during pregnancy and vertical transmission of HIV-1. *J Acquir Immune Defic Syndr Human Retrovirol.* 1997;15(1):76–82.
35. Matheson PB, Thomas PA, Abrams EJ, et al. New York City Perinatal HIV Transmission Collaborative Study Group. Heterosexual behavior during pregnancy and perinatal transmission of HIV-1. *AIDS.* 1996;10(11):1249–1256.
36. Read PJ, Mandalia S, Khan P, et al. When should HAART be initiated in pregnancy to achieve an undetectable HIV viral load by delivery? *AIDS.* 2012;26(9):1095–1103.
37. Tubiana R, Le Chenadec J, Rouzioux C, et al. Factors associated with mother-to-child transmission of HIV-1 despite a maternal viral load <500 copies/ml at delivery: A case–control study nested in the French perinatal cohort (EPF-ANRS CO1). *Clin Infect Dis.* 2010;50(4):585–596.
38. Ford N, Mofenson L, Shubber Z, et al. Safety of efavirenz in the first trimester of pregnancy: An updated systematic review and meta-analysis. *AIDS.* 2014;28 Suppl 2:S123–S131.
39. Panel on Opportunistic Infections in HIV-Infected Adults and Adolescents. Guidelines for the prevention and treatment of opportunistic infections in HIV-infected adults and adolescents: recommendations from the Centers for Disease Control and Prevention, the National

Institutes of Health, and the HIV Medicine Association of the Infectious Diseases Society of America. Available at http://aidsinfo.nih.gov/contentfiles/lvguidelines/adult_oi.pdf. Accessed March 19, 2016.

40. Aziz N, Sokoloff A, Kornak J, et al. Time to viral load suppression in antiretroviral-naive and -experienced HIV infected pregnant women on highly active antiretroviral therapy: Implications for pregnant women presenting late in gestation. *BJOG* 2013;120(12):1534–1547.

41. Wong VV. Is peripartum zidovudine absolutely necessary for patients with a viral load less than 1,000 copies/ml? *J Obstet Gynaecol.* 2011;31(8):740–742.

42. Briand N, Warszawski J, Mandelbrot L, et al. Is intrapartum intravenous zidovudine for prevention of mother-to-child HIV-1 transmission still useful in the combination antiretroviral therapy era? *Clin Infect Dis.* 2013;57(6):903–914.

43. Cotter AM, Brookfield KF, Duthely LM, Gonzalez Quintero VH, Potter JE, O'Sullivan MJ. Duration of membrane rupture and risk of perinatal transmission of HIV-1 in the era of combination antiretroviral therapy. *Am J Obstet Gynecol.* 2012;207(6):482 e481–485.

Psychiatric Diseases in Pregnancy and the Postpartum Period

M. Camille Hoffman and Gareen Hamalian

Introduction

Psychiatric illness during pregnancy is common and has implications for pregnancy outcomes and lifelong maternal and child health.[1] Psychiatric illnesses may be diagnosed prior to pregnancy, during pregnancy, or during the postpartum period. Like many other medical issues encountered during pregnancy, they may worsen, improve, or remain unchanged as pregnancy progresses. However, unlike some other medical issues, psychiatric disorders are unlikely to spontaneously resolve following delivery.[2] Women with known histories of psychiatric illnesses such as bipolar disorder and postpartum psychosis should be followed closely during pregnancy but also during the postpartum period as incidences of relapse, need for inpatient admission, and their risk for self-harm or harm to their newborns is disproportionately high for their small overall prevalence.[3,4]

Scope of the Problem

The prevalence of perinatal (pregnancy and postpartum) depression is 15–20% for the general population and up to twice as high in more vulnerable populations. This makes psychiatric disease the most common and most recurrent complication of pregnancy.[5] Anxiety disorders affect at least 4–5% of perinatal patients,[6] bipolar disorder affects 1–2% of patients,[7] posttraumatic stress disorder (PTSD) affects 2–15% of patients,[8] obsessive-compulsive disorders affect 2–2.5% of patients,[9] and postpartum psychosis affects 1–2/1,000 patients.[5] Although depression is the most frequently diagnosed psychiatric illness, these other important psychiatric disorders should be considered during pregnancy and the postpartum period.

The Role of the Ob-Gyn in Screening for and Treating Psychiatric Illness during Pregnancy and the Postpartum Period

The American Congress of Obstetricians and Gynecologists (ACOG) advises screening for depressive disorders in pregnancy and the postpartum period.

Additionally, a safety initiative, through the Council on Patient Safety in Women in the United States Preventive Services Task Force (USPSTF) also issued a guideline in 2016 that advises screening of all adults, including during pregnancy and postpartum, for mood disorders.[10]

The recommendation for screening by perinatal care providers has therefore been well established in the past few years. The most commonly used screening tools are the Edinburgh Postnatal Depression Scale (EPDS) and the Patient Health Questionnaire 9 (PHQ9).

EDPS may be used both antepartum and postpartum. This survey is available in many languages. Both 3-question and 10-question versions are available.[5] PHQ9 is commonly used in non-pregnant populations. In pregnant populations, it may result in more false-positive scores as there is overlap with normal pregnancy physiology and symptomatology. It may, however, be used to make a major depressive disorder diagnosis and to monitor changes in symptomatology. A 2-question version also exists.

Baby Blues

Baby blues is a common and transient experience that occurs in up to 85% of new mothers. The baby blues often begin immediately after childbirth when women are predisposed to mood swings and emotional

Box 48.1 Risk factors for baby blues

Lack of support
High-risk or difficult pregnancy
Difficult or traumatic birth
Maternal health comorbidities
Health issues in the baby
Neonatal intensive care unit (NICU) admission
History of prior pregnancy loss
Newborn characteristics such as excessive crying and irritability

fluctuations. Mood may vacillate between crying for no apparent reason and then being very happy the next moment. Baby blues can only last for a few hours to less than 2 weeks. Baby blues should not be diagnosed after 14 days postpartum. If a new mother is more than 14 days postpartum and is still highly emotional, especially if she is down or depressed, further consideration and screening for perinatal depression is necessary.

Lack of sleep in the immediate postpartum period is a major contributor to emotional volatility. Other risk factors for baby blues are seen in Box 48.1. The majority of postpartum women experience mood lability, anxiety, sleep disruption, changes in appetite, irritability, dysphoric mood, and tearfulness. While baby blues is a risk factor for postpartum depression, this depression is an independent diagnosis separate from, and longer lasting than, baby blues.

Treatment of Baby Blues

Baby blues resolves naturally the majority of the time. Patients may be referred to resources such as support groups. Additionally, support can be bolstered through education regarding sleep hygiene and encouragement of new mothers to ask for and accept help from others. Addressing infant behavioral dysregulation, including feeding issues, breastfeeding challenges and concerns, and infant crying may help to alleviate baby blues.

Perinatal Depression

Perinatal depression is a depressive episode, characterized by the same diagnostic criteria as a major depressive episode, which occurs during pregnancy or within 6 weeks of birth. By some definitions, perinatal depression may be diagnosed within a year of giving birth.[2,5]

Perinatal depression most often occurs within the first 3 months postpartum. It may also, however, begin during pregnancy, improve toward the end of pregnancy, and then recur with more severe symptomatology postpartum. It is important to consider that perinatal depression may occur with other changes in the first year postpartum such as weaning or when the menstrual cycle resumes.

Unlike baby blues, depression may last for up to a year or longer depending on a woman's past psychiatric history, interventions used for treatment, and the circumstances of her pregnancy.

Risk factors for perinatal depression are seen in Box 48.2. Depression may be diagnosed as late as 9 to 12 months postpartum. The psychology of perinatal depression, as described in the DSM 5, is described in Box 48.3. Box 48.4 is a description of DSM-5 criteria for peripartum onset of major depression.[5]

Box 48.2 Risk factors for depression

Lack of support
Interpersonal violence
Medical comorbidities including obesity
Difficulties with
- Pregnancy
- Birth
- Postpartum period

Difficulties with infant feeding
History of a prior pregnancy loss or
History of trauma

Box 48.3 DSM 5 description of perinatal depression

Half of postpartum major depressive episodes actually begin prior to delivery. Women with peripartum major depressive episodes often have severe anxiety and even panic attacks. Mood and anxiety symptoms during pregnancy as well as the "baby blues" increase the risk for a postpartum major depressive episode.

Peripartum-onset mood episodes can present either with or without psychotic features. Infanticide is most often associated with postpartum psychotic episodes that are characterized by hallucinations to kill the infant or delusions that the infant is possessed, but psychotic symptoms can also occur in severe postpartum mood episodes without such specific delusions or hallucinations.

Box 48.4 DSM-5 criteria for peripartum onset of major depression

Major depression

At least five symptoms present for at least 2 weeks, for most of the day, nearly every day

A symptom must be

- Depressed mood
- Markedly diminished interest or pleasure in all or most activities

Other symptoms

- Substantial weight loss when not dieting or weight gain, or increase or decrease in appetite
- Insomnia or hypersomnia
- Psychomotor agitation or retardation
- Fatigue or loss of energy
- Feeling of worthlessness or excessive or inappropriate guilt
- Diminished ability to think or concentrate or indecisiveness
- Recurrent thoughts of death or suicidal ideation (with or without a specific plan)
- Symptoms cause clinically significant distress or impairment in social, occupations, or other important areas of functionality
- Symptoms not due to direct physiological effects of a substance or other medical condition
- The occurrence of a major depressive episode is not better explained by schizoaffective disorder or other psychotic disorders and there has never been a manic or hypomanic episode.

With peripartum onset

Onset of mood symptoms happens during pregnancy or in the 4 weeks after delivery.

Depressive episode with insufficient symptoms

Depressed affect and at least one other of the aforementioned symptoms associated with clinically significant distress or impairment persisting for at least 2 weeks.

Treatment for perinatal depression should entail therapies and treatments that are realistic for patient compliance given her life circumstances. Treatments should address lifestyle issues that are beneficial or detrimental to maternal–child mental health and consider pharmacotherapy in moderate to severe cases.[5]

Psychotherapy treatment options include cognitive behavioral therapy, individual or group therapy, dyadic therapy (therapy for mother and baby), and psychotherapy.[11] Lifestyle changes include avoidance of depressants such as alcohol and illicit drugs, and exercise according to ACOG guidelines (30 minutes five or more times per week). The complementary and alternative therapies include bright morning light therapy,[12] acupuncture,[13] yoga, and meditation,[14] omega-3 fatty acids,[15,16] folic acid,[17] and vitamin D,[18] transcranial magnetic stimulation.[19] Other resources include numerous online support groups, psychoeducation, and anticipatory guidance, which may be provided by the inpatient obstetric team or prenatal/postnatal care team.

Caregivers must educate these patients about self-care and encourage them to engage in social and community support groups. Providers should encourage appropriate sleep hygiene; patients should ask for, and accept, help from others with nighttime feeding and daytime performance of maternal activities of daily living and self-care. Treatment may also involve addressing the behavior of the infant and how the behavior may exacerbate maternal emotional complications and symptomatology.

Pharmacotherapy includes restarting any antidepressant medication, which has been successfully used in the past. If a woman is antidepressant naïve, sertraline is the selective serotonin reuptake inhibitor (SSRI) with the largest body of data supporting its safety for use in pregnancy and the postpartum period. If the mother is postpartum and breastfeeding, and has not previously been on an SSRI, medications considered as first-line include Sertraline (Zoloft) 50–200mg, Fluoxetine (Prozac) 20–60mg, Citalopram (Celexa) 20–40mg, and Escitalopram (Lexapro) 10–20mg. The goal of any SSRI treatment is augmentation of the dose in response to symptoms, more frequently than outside of pregnancy and the postpartum period, until remission of symptoms occurs. Providers must ensure the prescribed medication is delivered in an optimal dose and avoid suboptimal dosage.

It is important to consider the risks of untreated maternal psychiatric illness when considering the benefits of pharmacotherapy since exposure to psychiatric illness is a risk for both mother and infant. Postpartum depression is associated with a series of developmental and behavioral issues for the child.

Perinatal Anxiety

Perinatal anxiety encompasses a range of anxiety disorders that may include generalized anxiety, panic disorders, social anxiety, and post-traumatic stress disorder that occur during pregnancy and/or the postpartum period. Anxiety most commonly occurs immediately after delivery until six weeks postpartum. It may, however, begin during pregnancy, after the baby weans, when the mother resumes her menstrual cycle, or in relation to some other trigger. Prenatal anxiety may last from weeks to months to years.[20]

Risk factors for perinatal anxiety include the major life changes associated with motherhood, lack of support, pregnancy, or postpartum difficulties that may include maternal medical comorbidities, birth difficulties, and breastfeeding difficulties. Additionally, prior pregnancy loss, sleep interruption, and the temperament of the baby may also be risk factors for perinatal anxiety.

The psychology behind perinatal anxiety involves the generalized anxiety, which occurs in 6–8% of women in the first 6 months after delivery. A subgroup, 0.5–3%, of women, experience generalized anxiety in the first 6–10 weeks postpartum. Generalized anxiety is characterized by the components listed in Box 48.5.[9]

Guidelines recommend screening using three of the questions from the EDPS the scale ("blamed self unnecessarily when things go wrong," "anxious or worried for no good reason," "felt scared or panicky for no good reason") to screen for problematic perinatal anxiety. The recommended anxiety subscale cutoff score is 6. (It should be noted that EDPS was not designed to measure anxiety solely.) The Perinatal Anxiety Screening Scale (PASS) (a 31-item self-administered screen) was developed and validated to help screen for perinatal anxiety.[21]

Box 48.5 Components of generalized anxiety

- Fear
- Anxiety
- Panic attacks
- Shortness of breath
- Hyperventilation
- Tachycardia
- Dizziness
- Chest pain
- Abdominal pain
- Fear of detachment from the newborn
- Fear of "losing my mind"
- Fear of death
- Feelings of impending doom
- Intrusive thoughts of accidentally or unintentionally harming or killing the newborn
- Intrusive thoughts of accidentally or unintentionally harming or killing oneself

Therapy for anxiety disorders involves similar principles as management for depression. Psychotherapy may be considered along with complementary and alternative therapies such as meditation, mindfulness, deep breathing exercises, yoga, B vitamins, diet and exercise, and avoidance of stimulants.[14]

If the patient has previously been on an SSRI or other non-habit forming medication for anxiety, that medication should be resumed.

If mother's anxiety has been predominately managed with benzodiazepines, a serious conversation regarding the addictive qualities of benzodiazepines and neonatal respiratory suppression as well as withdrawal must occur. Benzodiazepines are not the mainstay of anxiety management and, thus, should not be dispensed routinely by obstetric care providers without psychiatric consultation.

Use of SSRIs for treatment of anxiety often require higher doses than those required to achieve remission with depression. Treatment dosage that achieves remission is the goal.[20]

Bipolar Disorder

The usual age of onset for bipolar disorder is late teens to early adulthood. Risk factors for bipolar disorder are seen in Box 48.6. Patients with bipolar disorder often discontinue their medications when they become pregnant and therefore have a very high rate of relapse. Women with bipolar disorder are more likely to experience relapse and psychiatric admission during pregnancy or the postpartum period compared with any other psychiatric diagnosis. Pregnancy is a vulnerable period for symptom onset or recurrence. Those diagnosed with bipolar disorder are at

Box 48.6 Risk factors for bipolar disorder

- Major life events such as traumatic experiences or death of loved one
- Substance abuse
- Sleep deprivation
- Use of anti-depressant medication
- Advanced paternal age (associated with increased genetic mutations during spermatogenesis)
- Genetics
- Family history of bipolar or depression

high risk for postpartum episodes, including psychosis and mania.[22,23] The diagnosis of bipolar disorder is sometimes made in patients experiencing a first onset of psychosis or mania in the postpartum period.[3]

Bipolar disorder is a mood disorder characterized by mania, hypomania, and depression. Mania is a distinct period of abnormally and persistently elevated, expansive, or irritable mood. Abnormally and persistently increased activity or energy, lasting at least 1 week is present most of the day on nearly every day. During this period, three or more of the following must be present (four if the mood is only irritable): (a) inflated self-esteem, (b) decreased need for sleep, (c) increased talkativeness or pressure to keep talking, (d) flight of ideas or feeling thoughts are racing, (e) distractibility, (f) increase in goal-directed activity, (g) psychomotor agitation, or (h) excessive involvement in activities that have a high potential for painful consequences. Marked impairment in social or occupational functions are present or require hospitalization. The episode must not be attributable to the physiological effects of a substance.[24]

The Mood Disorder Questionnaire has been most studied for screening bipolar disorder. This has been validated for the postpartum period but not during pregnancy.[25,26] Since the most common presentation of bipolar disorder during the perinatal period is a depressive episode, screening for perinatal depression with only instruments like the Edinburgh Postnatal Depression Scale (EPDS) may result in misdiagnosis and or the ongoing under-diagnosis of bipolar disorder.[22]

Over 20% of women who screen positive for depressive symptoms on the EPDS screened positive for bipolar on the MDQ.[22,27] Universal screening for bipolar disorder in pregnancy is not currently recommended by the American College of Obstetricians and Gynecologists but it is prudent to screen women who are found to be depressed or who have risk factors for bipolar disorder such as family history, history of depression, mania, or psychosis. Ideally screening should be done at the initial presentation but should always be done before starting an antidepressant.

Treatment of bipolar disorder ideally involves cooperative management by the patient's obstetrician and psychiatrist. In patients with a known diagnosis of bipolar disorder, treatment is most successful when pregnancy is planned and clinicians can work with the patient to map out management. Since half of pregnancies are unplanned and women with bipolar disorder usually do not experience symptom improvement during pregnancy, it is important that clinicians understand the options and risks associated with pharmacotherapy during pregnancy.

Box 48.7 Pharmacotherapy for bipolar disorder in pregnancy

- Use treatment modalities that have been successful in the past
- Continue effective medications unless significant clinical concerns exist
- Use minimum effective dose
- Use monotherapy when possible.

Women with bipolar disorder have high rates of relapse due to sudden discontinuation of medications during pregnancy. Those with a history of recurrent, severe mood episodes are at risk for impulsivity, poor self-care and suicidality. Clinicians should therefore advise patients and their support networks against rapid discontinuation of medications especially if treatment has helped stabilize a patient's mood currently or in the past. Close clinical follow-up is important even when patients remain on their medications since a large number of women who remain compliant during pregnancy also experience relapse.[3]

The basic principles of pharmacotherapy for bipolar disorder in pregnancy are seen in Box 48.7. Comprehensive counseling should emphasize the importance of sleep, postpartum prophylaxis, risks and benefits of breastfeeding, and social support structure.

Estimation of relapse risk is a useful part of the decision-making process as clinicians and patients collaborate on a risk-benefit analysis looking at benefits of prophylaxis versus the risks of fetal medication exposure. Research is limited in regard to relapse risk but a recent meta-analysis demonstrated that patients with bipolar disorder are at high risk for postpartum relapse with an overall relapse risk of 37%.[3] Prophylactic pharmacotherapy for bipolar disorder is highly effective for relapse prevention making continuation of prophylactic medication during pregnancy critical for mood stability after delivery.

Posttraumatic Stress Disorder (PTSD)

Posttraumatic stress disorder (PTSD) is characterized by distressing anxiety symptoms that are experienced after a traumatic event or events. PTSD may be present prior to pregnancy or may occur in relation to an event that occurs during pregnancy or birth. PTSD

Box 48.8 Risk factors for PTSD

Lack of partner support
Interpersonal violence
Depressive symptomatology
Physical problems and or pain prior to or resulting from birth experience
High health risk behaviors
Prior pregnancy loss
History of childhood trauma

may result from a traumatic birth, although there is often some other event – either conscious or subconscious – that predisposes to PTSD following a traumatic birth. Birth may also serve as a trigger for PTSD if a history of prior trauma exists.[28]

PTSD may last from one month to much longer periods of time. It may also recur due to a birth trigger. PTSD occurs in 2–15% of women in pregnancy and 2–9% of women following childbirth.[8] Risk factors for PTSD are seen in Box 48.8.

PTSD is thought to result from a change in cognition, mood, and the arousal response that is associated with a traumatic event. The patient will attempt to avoid stimuli associated with a traumatic event and often go to great links to do so. PTSD is also a major risk factor for depression. Formal postnatal debriefing for PTSD prevention is not supported by evidence at this time; however, women may benefit from an opportunity to discuss the delivery process.[5]

Treatment depends on individual circumstances, but is often a combination of medication and trauma-focused cognitive behavioral therapy. First-line pharmacological treatment for PTSD includes selective serotonin reuptake inhibitors (SSRIs).[29] They are considered an appropriate choice although not studied specifically for PTSD. SSRIs have been studied in the treatment of depression and anxiety in pregnancy. Current research has explored the labor and delivery experience as a possible trigger for women with preexisting trauma histories.[30]

Obsessive-Compulsive Disorder

Obsessive-compulsive disorder (OCD) occurs when a woman experiences intrusive repetitive thoughts that are frightening, sometimes nonsensical, and may include rituals such as counting, hand washing, cleaning, or other compulsions. OCD may occur with or without depression. Postpartum OCD starts 1–3 weeks to 3 months after delivery but occasionally begins after weaning or after the menstrual cycle resumes. OCD may also occur during pregnancy. Risk factors for OCD are seen in Boxes 48.8 and 48.9.

When diagnosed in the perinatal period, obsessional thinking and compulsive behaviors often focus on the baby or the pregnancy with themes ranging from contamination to fears about fetal death. Compulsive behaviors may include the patient's repeat requests for ultrasounds to check for fetal well-being or repeated washing or changing of the baby to avoid contamination. Patients with OCD often have insight into their obsessions but when severe the symptoms can resemble fixed delusional thinking.

OCD may occur in up to 4% of women. The psychopathology of OCD includes disturbing repetitive thoughts, which may include harming the baby, adapting to compulsive behavior in order to prevent the baby from being harmed, a constant state of hypervigilance, obsessional thoughts about harming the baby, and overriding thoughts about impending doom to the baby or patient herself.

Interestingly, intrusive thoughts occur in up to 80% of pregnant and postpartum women.[31] Hypervigilance associated with motherhood and infancy differs from a formal diagnosis of OCD, or anxiety disorders; however, the nuances are best determined by a mental health professional.

Treatment for OCD includes anticipatory guidance on the frequency of intrusive thoughts and ruminations.[31,32] OCD is challenging to treat and most patients do not achieve full remission. The treatment of OCD in pregnancy and the postpartum period is the same as general OCD with adaptations appropriate to the patient's circumstances. Treatment is usually a combination of pharmacotherapy and cognitive-behavioral therapy. Selective serotonin reuptake inhibitors are recommended for first-line use at higher doses than are commonly used for depression.[33] For refractory cases, atypical antipsychotic medication can be used

Box 48.9 Risk factors for obsessive-compulsive disorder

Family history of OCD or other anxiety disorders
Depressive symptoms and anxiety
Prior pregnancy loss or infant loss
A baby with excessive crying, feeding difficulty, irritability, or sleep issues

for augmentation. If concern exists regarding harm to the baby or patient, safety should be the primary goal and immediate referral to a mental health professional must occur.

Postpartum Psychosis

Postpartum psychosis is a rare disorder that affects an estimated 1–2 per 1,000 newly delivered women. Postpartum psychosis is rare and serious. It is characterized by the sudden onset of psychosis following childbirth or during the postpartum period. It usually involves delusions, poor insight about the illness, lack of awareness of the symptomatology, auditory visual or olfactory hallucinations, and occasional delusions that result in self-harm or harm of the newborn. Postpartum psychosis typically presents more rapidly after birth then depression, anxiety, or PTSD. Its onset is usually between two and 12 weeks postpartum and women with a history of bipolar disorder have a much higher risk of postpartum psychosis, as well as manic episodes, in the first few weeks postpartum.

In postpartum psychosis, the patient's mood fluctuates rapidly. Women may become more confused, have marked cognitive impairment, bizarre behavior, experience insomnia, visual or auditory hallucinations, or other unusual types of hallucinations that include tactile or olfactory. Women may also have moments of lucidity interspersed with the psychosis.

Women with a history of bipolar disorder or postpartum psychosis should be monitored very carefully, especially if they are sleep deprived for 48 hours or more intrapartum or postpartum. Risk factors for postpartum psychosis are seen in Box 48.10. [23] Autoimmune encephalitis has also been identified in a small group of women with postpartum psychosis and may be considered in the differential for a patient with no prior history of psychiatric disorder or risk factors for psychosis

Postpartum psychosis may include delusions about infanticide, homicide, or suicide all of which must be addressed immediately. Women with postpartum psychosis require immediate psychiatric help and usually require hospitalization to protect themselves, their children, and other close relatives. Medication is nearly universally indicated and atypical antipsychotic medications have a reasonable reproductive safety profile.[34]

If immediate patient treatment is needed prior to the arrival of a psychiatric consultant, it is appropriate to initiate treatment with a short-acting benzodiazepine and an atypical antipsychotic such as quetiapine or an older antipsychotic such as haloperidol.

Box 48.10 **Risk factors for postpartum psychosis**

- Diagnosis of bipolar disorder
- History of postpartum psychosis or other psychosis (80% of women with a history of postpartum psychosis will relapse without intervention)
- Family history of postpartum psychosis
- Sleep deprivation
- Discontinuance of mood stabilizers in women with bipolar disorder,
- Prior pregnancy or neonatal loss
- Dysregulated infant
- Primiparity

Once a woman has a postpartum episode with psychotic features, the risk of recurrence with each subsequent delivery is between 30% and 50%.[3,4,23] If a woman has a history of psychosis, in particular in relation to bipolar disorder, preventative treatment with a mood stabilizer is strongly encouraged in subsequent pregnancies. If a woman with this history does not want to start medication in the first or second trimester, starting medication in the third trimester or prior to discharge home postpartum is even more strongly encouraged.

Postpartum psychosis must be differentiated from delirium occurring in the postpartum period. This is distinguished by a fluctuating level of awareness or attention and may be related to underlying organ failure, sepsis, hypovolemia, or other obstetric event. The postpartum period is unique with respect to the degree of neuroendocrine alterations and psychosocial adjustments, the potential impact of breastfeeding on treatment planning and the long-term implications of a history of postpartum mood disorder on subsequent family planning.

For women with a history of isolated postpartum psychosis, the initiation of prophylaxis immediately after delivery appears to be highly effective for relapse prevention and eliminates the risk of in utero medication exposure. Women have multiple contacts with health services during pregnancy, which provide a compelling opportunity for prevention of postpartum psychotic episodes.[3]

A discussion about sleep hygiene and sleep support (including assistance from the partner or other family members or friends) and a discussion around other activities of daily living should be part of anticipatory guidance for all women predisposed to psychiatric disorders during pregnancy or the postpartum period. In particular, this discussion and guidance should occur early in pregnancy in women with this rare but very serious history.

Specific Treatment Options for the Psychiatric Care of Pregnant and Postpartum Women

Box 48.11 describes basic principles concerning psychopharmacotherapy in pregnancy. Further discussion of specific options has been done later in the chapter.

Box 48.11 Psychopharmacotherapy in pregnancy

- A primary factor in initiating or resuming pharmacotherapy during pregnancy is what has and has not worked for a woman in the past and to which medication(s) and dose(s) she responded to remission (fully functional recovery status). Also consider this in the context of the side effect burden.
- Selective serotonin reuptake inhibitor (SSRI) antidepressants are the most frequently used drugs for the pharmacological treatment of major depressive disorder due to their low toxicity, particularly in overdose situations, and their overall safety record. SSRIs are among the most comprehensively studied group of medications taken by pregnant women.
- The serotonin–norepinephrine reuptake inhibitors (SNRI) have been included with the group of SSRI medications as well as separately for pregnancy exposure studies. They have not been as extensively studied as SSRIs.
- Tricyclic antidepressants (TCA) and mirtazapine are less well studied than SSRIs. They may be most useful for women who are not responsive to SSRI, have prohibitive side effects, or who also need medication for neuropathic pain and/or sleep. There are also reports of TCAs being used with success to treat hyperemesis gravidarum in women who have failed more conventional regimens.[35,36]
- Optimize the dose of a single drug before considering additional drug treatments.
- Always inquire about alcohol, cigarettes and other drug use, environmental exposures, and over-the-counter and prescribed medication intake.
- While the concept of reducing the dose or discontinuing an antidepressant before the birth is appealing, no clear advantages for the newborn have been demonstrated that offset the very high risk of recurrence postpartum.

Adapted from Wisner and Shaefer, Psychotropic drugs. In: *Drugs during Pregnancy and Lactation*, Schaefer Paul WJ and Miller PRK (eds.). Cambridge, MA: Elsevier, pp. 294–327.

Lithium

The efficacy of lithium in pregnancy and the postpartum periods is well established. Lithium crosses the placenta. There is an association between lithium exposure and Ebstein's anomaly (small absolute risk) but no established causal relationship. It is recommended that women treated with lithium have a high-resolution ultrasound and fetal echocardiography at 16–18 weeks gestation.[22] Lithium dosage must be adjusted over the course of pregnancy. Increases of both total amount and number of daily doses is common. Levels should be checked more frequently at the end of pregnancy (monthly from the 20th week of gestation and then weekly 4 weeks before delivery) as well as immediately prior to delivery due to potential for lithium toxicity.[37] When emesis or dehydration occur, the lithium dose must be reduced or discontinued and serum levels checked more frequently. If lithium is discontinued during or before labor, it should be restarted immediately after the mother is medically stable. Infants must be monitored for at least the first 48 hours post-delivery.[37]

Lamotrigine

Lamotrigine is approved for the treatment of bipolar depression and maintenance therapy but is not first line for an acute manic episode or postpartum psychosis. It has a favorable reproductive risk profile and is the preferred option for women of childbearing age. Therapeutic dose monitoring is a challenge given limited research.[38] Clinicians should note the significant increase in lamotrigine clearance during pregnancy and make monthly serum levels and dose adjustments as necessary. The dose should also be lowered postpartum.[39]

Mood Stabilizers and Antiepileptics

Other mood stabilizers or antiepileptic drugs such as valproic acid and carbamazepine are used for the treatment of bipolar disorder. Valproic acid has been associated with increased rates of congenital malformations, including neural tube defects and cardiac or craniofacial defects, and, outside of embryogenesis, progressive neurodevelopmental delays. Valproic acid should be avoided during pregnancy. Carbamazepine is also typically avoided in pregnancy due to teratogenic and postnatal developmental effects.

Antipsychotics

Antipsychotics are also used as mood stabilizers and for treatment of postpartum psychosis. The choice of medication depends on specific clinical situations. If a woman has a history of positive therapeutic response to an antipsychotic medication without significant side effects, that medication should be considered first. Use of one medication at therapeutic dose is ideal. Metabolism of antipsychotic medications can change during pregnancy so clinicians must monitor the patient and adjust doses in response to symptoms. Of note, first-generation antipsychotics may help reduce morning sickness due to antinausea effects. With atypical antipsychotics, particularly olanzapine, weight gain, hyperglycemia, and glucose intolerance are potential side effects with significant adverse consequences in pregnancy. Certain antipsychotics such as risperidone increase prolactin levels.

Electroconvulsive Therapy

Electroconvulsive therapy (ECT) is another treatment option for unipolar and bipolar depression during pregnancy or the postpartum period for women who require more acute treatment, especially if they are catatonic, cannot tolerate medications, or are at high risk for self-harm or violence.[22,40]

Concluding Remarks

Perinatal mental illness is common and has multigenerational effects that may include significant maternal morbidity and mortality risks. Caregivers should lead informed discussions early in the prenatal course with review of clinically feasible treatment. The partner and family should be involved if clinically appropriate. The patient must be connected with mental health services before delivery.

Box 48.12 Registries and resources that are useful for perinatal clinicians

A number of registries exist to inform clinicians about the risks of antiepileptic drugs in pregnancy. Women taking anticonvulsants or antipsychotics during pregnancy may be enrolled in the following registries:

1. North American Antiepileptic Drug (AED) Pregnancy Registry: www.massgeneral.org/aed/
2. Europe and other continents: EURAP Registry (International Registry of Antiepileptic Drugs and Pregnancy): www.eurapinternational.org/about/join
3. National Pregnancy Registry for Atypical Antipsychotics (unexposed women may also enroll as controls): http://womensmentalhealth.org/clinical-and-researchprograms/pregnancyregistry/atypicalantipsychotic/
4. https://reprotox.org (requires individual or group subscription)
5. http://mothertobaby.org (free)

Patients must be monitored closely, with adjustment of medication doses across pregnancy and postpartum to maintain therapeutic levels and avoid toxicity. Patients should avoid sleep deprivation. Psychosocial stressors must be addressed. If the patient is stable and chooses to breastfeed, we recommend that someone else feed the baby at night to minimize the risk of relapse associated with postpartum insomnia.

Pharmacotherapy in pregnancy is associated with a constant evolution of standards. A list of useful resources and registries is presented in Box 48.12.

References

1. Stein AP, Goodman, SH, Rapa, E, Rahman A, McCallum M, Howard LM. Pariante C.M. Effects of perinatal mental disorders on the fetus and child. *Lancet*. 2014; 384: 1800–19.
2. Meltzer-Brody S and Jones I. Optimizing the treatment of mood disorders in the perinatal period. *Dialogues Clin Neurosci*. 2015; 17: 207–18.
3. Wesseloo R, Kamperman AM, Munk-Olsen T, Pop VJ, Kushner SA and Bergink V. Risk of postpartum relapse in bipolar disorder and postpartum psychosis: A systematic review and meta-analysis. *Am J Psychiatr*. 2016; 173: 117–27.
4. Bergink V, Bouvy PF, Vervoort JS, Koorengevel KM, Steegers EA and Kushner SA. Prevention of

postpartum psychosis and mania in women at high risk. *Am J Psychiatr*. 2012; 169: 609–15.

5. Howard LMM, Dennis, C, Rochat T, Stein A and Milgrom J. Non-psychotic mental disorders in the perinatal period. *Lancet*. 2014; 384: 1775–88.
6. Goodman JH, Chenausky KL and Freeman MP. Anxiety disorders during pregnancy: a systematic review. *J Clin Psychiatr*. 2014; 75: e1153-84.
7. Hoffman MCR, Karban LV, Durfee MJ, Mazzoni, SE. Maternal and child delivery charges, postpartum charges, and utilization of care among women with bipolar disorder: A cohort study; in review.
8. Yonkers KA, Smith MV, Forray A, et al. Pregnant women with posttraumatic stress disorder and risk of preterm birth. *JAMA Psychiatr*. 2014; 71: 897–904.
9. Miller ES, Hoxha D, Wisner KL and Gossett DR. The impact of perinatal depression on the evolution of anxiety and obsessive-compulsive symptoms. *Arch Women Mental Health*. 2015; 18: 457–61.
10. Siu AL, Force USPST, Bibbins-Domingo K, et al. Screening for depression in adults: US Preventive Services Task Force Recommendation Statement. *JAMA*. 2016; 315: 380–7.
11. Dennis CL. Psychosocial interventions for the treatment of perinatal depression. *Best Prac Res Clin Obstet Gynaecol*. 2014; 28: 97–111.
12. Wirz-Justice A, Bader A, Frisch U, et al. A randomized, double-blind, placebo-controlled study of light therapy for antepartum depression. *J Clin Psychiatr*. 2011; 72: 986–93.
13. Manber R, Schnyer RN, Lyell D, et al. Acupuncture for depression during pregnancy: A randomized controlled trial. *Obstet Gynecol*. 2010; 115: 511–20.
14. Battle CL, Uebelacker LA, Magee SR, Sutton KA and Miller IW. Potential for prenatal yoga to serve as an intervention to treat depression during pregnancy. *Women Health Issues*. 2015; 25: 134–41.
15. da Rocha CM and Kac G. High dietary ratio of omega-6 to omega-3 polyunsaturated acids during pregnancy and prevalence of post-partum depression. *Matern Child Nutr*. 2012; 8: 36–48.
16. Kaviani M, Saniee L, Azima S, Sharif F and Sayadi M. The effect of omega-3 fatty acid supplementation on maternal depression during pregnancy: A double blind randomized controlled clinical trial. *Int J Community Nurs Midwifery*. 2014; 2: 142–7.
17. Chong MF, Wong JX, Colega M, et al. Relationships of maternal folate and vitamin B12 status during pregnancy with perinatal depression: The GUSTO study. *J Psychiatr Res*. 2014; 55: 110–6.
18. Huang JY, Arnold D, Qiu CF, Miller RS, Williams MA and Enquobahrie DA. Association of serum vitamin D with symptoms of depression and anxiety in early pregnancy. *J Women Health*. 2014; 23: 588–95.
19. Kim DR, Sockol L, Barber JP, et al. A survey of patient acceptability of repetitive transcranial magnetic stimulation (TMS) during pregnancy. *J Affect Disord*. 2011; 129: 385–90.
20. Marchesi C, Ossola P, Amerio A, Daniel BD, Tonna M and De Panfilis C. Clinical management of perinatal anxiety disorders: A systematic review. *J Affect Disord*. 2016; 190: 543–50.
21. Somerville S, Byrne SL, Dedman K, et al. Detecting the severity of perinatal anxiety with the Perinatal Anxiety Screening Scale (PASS). *J Affect Disord*. 2015; 186: 18–25.
22. Khan SJ, Fersh ME, Ernst C, Klipstein K, Albertini ES and Lusskin SI. Bipolar disorder in pregnancy and postpartum: Principles of management. *Curr Psychiatry Rep*. 2016; 18: 13.
23. Jones I, Chandra PS, Dazzan P and Howard LM. Bipolar disorder, affective psychosis, and schizophrenia in pregnancy and the post-partum period. *Lancet*. 2014; 384: 1789–99.
24. Amerio A, Odone A, Tonna M, Stubbs B and Ghaemi SN. Bipolar disorder and its comorbidities between Feinstein and the Diagnostic and Statistical Manual of Mental Disorders. *Aust N Z J Psychiatry*. 2015; 49: 1073.
25. Clark CT, Sit DK, Driscoll K, et al. Does screening with the MDQ and EPDS improve identification of bipolar disorder in an obstetrical sample? *Depression Anxiety*. 2015; 32: 518–26.
26. Chessick CA and Dimidjian S. Screening for bipolar disorder during pregnancy and the postpartum period. *Arch Women Mental Health*. 2010; 13: 233–48.
27. Merrill L, Mittal L, Nicoloro J, Caiozzo C, Maciejewski PK and Miller LJ. Screening for bipolar disorder during pregnancy. *Arch Women Mental Health*. 2015; 18: 579–83.
28. Smith MV, Poschman K, Cavaleri MA, Howell HB and Yonkers KA. Symptoms of posttraumatic stress disorder in a community sample of low-income pregnant women. *Am J Psychiatr*. 2006; 163: 881–4.
29. Goodman DJ, Milliken CU, Theiler RN, Nordstrom BR and Akerman SC. A multidisciplinary approach to the treatment of co-occurring opioid use disorder and posttraumatic stress disorder in pregnancy: A case report. *J Dual Diagn*. 2015; 11: 248–57.
30. Beck CT. Birth trauma and its sequelae. *J Trauma Dissoc*. 2009; 10: 189–203.
31. Miller ES, Chu C, Gollan J and Gossett DR. Obsessive-compulsive symptoms during the postpartum period. A prospective cohort. *J Reprod Med*. 2013; 58: 115–22.

32. Miller ES, Hoxha D, Wisner KL and Gossett DR. Obsessions and compulsions in postpartum women without obsessive compulsive disorder. *J Women Health*. 2015; 24: 825–30.

33. Hudak R and Wisner KL. Diagnosis and treatment of postpartum obsessions and compulsions that involve infant harm. *Am J Psychiatr*. 2012; 169: 360–3.

34. Cohen LS, Viguera AC, McInerney KA, et al. Reproductive safety of second-generation antipsychotics: Current data from the Massachusetts General Hospital National Pregnancy Registry for Atypical Antipsychotics. *Am J Psychiatr*. 2016; 173: 263–70.

35. Schwarzer V, Heep A, Gembruch U and Rohde A. Treatment resistant hyperemesis gravidarum in a patient with type 1 diabetes mellitus: Neonatal withdrawal symptoms after successful antiemetic therapy with mirtazapine. *Arch Gynecol Obstet* 2008; 277: 67–9.

36. Guclu S, Gol M, Dogan E and Saygili U. Mirtazapine use in resistant hyperemesis gravidarum: Report of three cases and review of the literature. *Arch Gynecol Obstet* 2005; 272: 298–300.

37. Bergink V and Kushner SA. Lithium during pregnancy. *Am J Psychiatr*. 2014; 171: 712–5.

38. Clark CT, Klein AM, Perel JM, Helsel J and Wisner KL. Lamotrigine dosing for pregnant patients with bipolar disorder. *Am J Psychiatr*. 2013; 170: 1240–7.

39. Deligiannidis KM, Byatt N and Freeman MP. Pharmacotherapy for mood disorders in pregnancy: A review of pharmacokinetic changes and clinical recommendations for therapeutic drug monitoring. *J Clin Psychopharmacol*. 2014; 34: 244–55.

40. Ray-Griffith SL, Coker JL, Rabie N, Eads LA, Golden KJ and Stowe ZN. Pregnancy and electroconvulsive therapy: A multidisciplinary approach. *Journal of ECT*. 2016 Jun;32(2):104–12.

Substance Use in Women and Pregnancy

Natalie E. Roche and Damali Campbell Oparaji

Introduction

Substance abuse disorders in women are prevalent across all socioeconomic classes and occur in women of all ethnic backgrounds. Approximately 8% of people in the United States have some substance use disorder (1).

Women with substance use disorders need the same general health care as women without these disorders. Particular attention is needed toward issues of testing for sexually transmitted infections as well as pregnancy prevention and enhanced prenatal care. This population may lack regular health screening secondary to their substance use disorders and comorbid psychiatric disorders (2).

Scope of the Problem

The care of pregnant women with substance abuse disorders must be tailored to the needs of the individual patient. The prenatal, intrapartum and postpartum care of the woman with a substance use disorder is more challenging because of the additional areas that need to be addressed for successful patient outcomes.

Pregnant women with substance use are generally considered to be at increased risk due to higher rates of miscarriage and stillbirth and pregnancy complications including preterm labor, late or inadequate prenatal care (3). Many psychosocial issues faced by this population are seen in Box 49.1.

Obstetrical Care for Women with Substance Use Disorders

The medical aspects of prenatal care are generally quite similar to high-risk prenatal care. More time, efforts, and resources are needed to address substance use and dependence in addition to management of high-risk pregnancy. The prenatal care of these patients usually requires the use of the ancillary resources seen in Box 49.2.

Screening for substance abuse at the annual screening visit, at preconception visits and during prenatal care is recommended for all patients. It may be difficult for practitioners to realize the volume of patients who face these problems. According to the Substance Abuse and Mental Health Services Administration (SAMHSA) among 15- to 44-year-olds, a total of 11.4% of women were current users of illicit drugs. For the same years 2012–2013, a total of 5.4% of pregnant women were current illicit drug users (4). The prenatal care of these patients will also usually require enhanced prenatal surveillance including additional ultrasound screening for fetal growth.

Prenatal care providers may feel ill equipped to diagnose, treat or refer patients with substance abuse problems. Providers may also have difficulty interfacing with child protective services who may become involved with their substance abusing patients. Ob/Gyn physicians do, however, have unique opportunities to identify women who use tobacco, alcohol and other drugs, to offer guidance and treatment to women with substance use disorders and to educate women about the dangers of substance use and abuse (5).

Neurobiology of Addiction

Addiction has been seen in the past as a failure of will power and a moral deficiency. Current science categorizes addiction as a chronic disease of the brain. Substances that have addiction potential include tobacco, alcohol, cannabis, cocaine and other stimulants, opiates, and sedatives. The greatest potential for addiction after exposure is by the substance tobacco followed by heroin, cocaine and alcohol (6).

Addiction causes a desensitization of the pleasure reward circuitry in the brain. Chronic substance use will dampen pleasure and inhibit motivation upsetting emotional balance. Addicted patients have increased

Box 49.1 Psychosocial issues faced by substance abuse patients

Shame and fear of exposure
Diagnosed or undiagnosed psychiatric illness
Housing issues
Parenting Issues
Domestic violence
Involvement with criminal justice system
Unemployment

Box 49.2 Ancillary resources needed in the care of prenatal substance abuse patients

Social workers
Nutritionists
Financial counselors
Legal counseling services
Substance abuse counseling services
Mental health or psychiatric services providers
Antenatal neonatology consultations
Division of Child Protective Services consultation
Anesthesia consultations.

response to stress, which causes increased craving for drugs. Failure to satiate drug cravings causes negative emotions. Chronic drug use also negatively affects executive functions such as self-regulation, decision making and control of inhibitions; this potentiates relapse. Research has demonstrated the role of genetics, environment and developmental stage on risk of drug addiction and the success of recovery once addicted (7).

Addiction can be divided into three stages. The first stage is binge and intoxication where the reward center in the brain is activated by the release of dopamine. The second stage is withdrawal where normal rewards are replaced by motivation to use drugs, which cause a more potent release of dopamine. Chronic drug use causes smaller release of dopamine over time (downregulation), making the brain's reward system less sensitive to all rewards. The third stage of addiction is preoccupation and anticipation. The downregulation of dopamine in the reward circuitry of the brain also has a negative effect on the frontal cortex. The result is damage to executive functioning of the brain with negative effects on decision making, monitoring of error, self-regulation and ability to select and initiate actions (7). Stages of addictions are listed in Box 49.3.

Box 49.3 Figure stages of addiction

Binge/intoxication (goal euphoria, the good high avoidance of bad feelings)
Withdrawal (bad feelings, decreased energy, decreased excitement)
Preoccupation/anticipation (craving for drug, preoccupation with plans to obtain drug)

Specific Substance of Abuse

Alcohol

Background/Epidemiology

Alcohol use is common in many cultures. Harm is caused when the volume, pattern (binging), quality and or timing (during pregnancy) of the alcohol use presents a problem. Populations with greater wealth have higher alcohol consumption with greater episodic heavy drinking. Ten percent of the world population older than 15 years of age are categorized as heavy drinkers. More males are alcohol users and females are more likely to abstain from use (8,9).

Alcohol abuse can cause many diseases including alcoholic liver disease, acute alcohol poisoning and cancers. Alcohol abuse is also associated with violence, injuries, acquisition of sexually transmitted infections and unplanned pregnancy.

Of pregnant women in the United States, 10.2% reported alcohol use in the past 30 days and 3.1% of pregnant women report an episode of binge drinking. The pregnant women who reported binge drinking had more episodes of binge drinking (4.6% versus 3.1%) compared to non-pregnant women (10).

There is no level of alcohol use that is safe during pregnancy. It is recommended that all pregnant women abstain from all alcohol use. Alcohol is teratogenic and causes damage to the central nervous system, face, and fetal growth with resulting behavioral and intellectual deficits, facial abnormalities, and developmental problems. Abnormalities of the heart and kidneys along with restricted growth in the fetus have been reported. Fetal alcohol syndrome and fetal alcohol spectrum disorders are preventable if women abstain from alcohol use during pregnancy. It is estimated that the prevalence of fetal alcohol syndrome is 2–7/1,000 and fetal alcohol syndrome disorders is up to 20–50/1,000 (11). Alcohol use during pregnancy can also cause miscarriage, stillbirth, prematurity, and increases in the risk of sudden infant death syndrome (SIDS) (12).

Screening

The Centers for disease Control and Prevention (CDC) and ACOG recommend screening all pregnant women for alcohol use regardless of age, ethnicity, race or socioeconomic status (13).

Screening tools such as tolerane, annoyance, cut down, eye opener (T-ACE), car, relax, alone, family, friends, trouble (CRAFFT), cut down, annoyed, guilty, eye-opener (CAGE) and tolerance, worried, eye-opener, amnesia, k-cut down (TWEAK) are available and can help identify problem drinking in reproductive aged women. Any alcohol use during pregnancy is a trigger for intervention with a goal toward all alcohol cessation. See Box 49.4.

Diagnosis

Any alcohol use during pregnancy requires intervention with the goal to stop all alcohol use. The diagnosis of Diagnostic and Statistical Manual of Mental Disorders, fifth edition (DSM-5) for alcohol use disorder follows the chronic disease model. As with other chronic abuse disorders the diagnosis includes increased use over time, tendency for remission and relapse, expansion of time devoted to use or recovery from alcohol use, failure to perform in life activities at school work or home, neglect of other life activities, use of alcohol despite physical risk, presence of craving, use despite alcohol-related problems, use of alcohol despite knowledge of alcohol use disorder and physical dependence (14).

Treatment

Motivational interviewing to establish willingness to change is the first step in treatment (14).

A variety of pharmacological treatments are available for alcohol abuse including benzodiapines, disulfiram, naltrexone and acamprosate. All are category C medications during pregnancy; insufficient studies of these medications in pregnancy and breast feeding are available (15). For each medication, the risk benefits analysis has to be applied taking into consideration the known teratogenic effect of alcohol. The side effects of disulfiram, which blocks the metabolism of acetaldehyde to acetate, would be difficult for most pregnant women to tolerate. Naltrexone is an opiate agonist that blocks some of the euphoric effects of alcohol. Naltrexone is embryocidal at 30–60 times the usual dose in animal models and there are no adequate studies during pregnancy. Use of naltrexone in breastfeeding is contraindicated because the drug is present in breast milk. Acamproste has been associated with teratogenicity in animal models.

Box 49.4 Screening tools for substance abuse disorders

DAST-10 (drug abuse screening test)
CAGE
CRAFFT (available for use without restriction)
T-ACE
TWEAK

Tobacco

Epidemiology

The total percentage of adult smokers in the United States declined to 16.8% of the population in 2014. Despite the continued decrease in the percentage of adult smokers, tobacco remains the number one cause of preventable disease and death in this country (16).

Significant adverse health consequences are associated with smoking. Significant disease and death caused by second hand smoke exposure in the nonsmoking population are also concerning. Most smokers (70%) report a desire to quit. Few smokers are successful in their attempts to quit with success rates for smoking cessation at 4–7% per year. Most smoking attempts are undertaken without ongoing treatment (17).

Women have lower smoking rates than men but experience adverse effects on reproduction in addition to the adverse effects found in all patients (see Boxes 49.5a and 49.5b). Nicotine freely enters the placenta after absorption into the blood stream. Nicotine is found in the placenta and the umbilical cord blood of newborn infants. The negative effects of smoking on reproduction include intrauterine growth restriction (IUGR), disorders of the placenta (abruption and previa), low birth weight, premature rupture of membranes, perinatal mortality and ectopic pregnancy (18). See Boxes 49.5a and 49.5b.

Screening

The US Preventive Services Task Force recommends that all clinicians screen every pregnant patient for tobacco use. Standardized tobacco use screening tools are available such as the five A's of smoking (19).

Box 49.5a Adverse effects associated with tobacco use

Cancers
Cataracts
Heart disease (coronary artery disease, peripheral vascular disease, abdominal aortic aneuyrsm
Lung disease (chronic obstructive pulmonary disease (COPD), bronchitis, emphysemapneumonia)
Periodontal disease
Osteoporosis
Stroke

Box 49.5b Adverse effects on pregnancy associated with tobacco use

Abnormal placentation (placenta previa, placental abruption)
Decreased maternal thyroid function
Cleft lip and cleft palate
Ectopic pregnancy
Intrauterine growth restriction (IUGR)
Low birth weight
Increased perinatal mortality (stillbirth)
Preterm premature rupture of membranes
Reduced fertility

ACOG Committee on Health Care for Underserved Women; American Society of Addiction Medicine. ACOG Committee Opinion No. 524: Opioid abuse, dependence, and addiction in pregnancy. *Obstet Gynecol.* 2012 May;119(5):1070–6. doi: 10.1097/AOG.0b013e318256496e.

Diagnosis

Tobacco use disorder should be addressed using the chronic disease model. This model reflects the chronic nature of the problem and the tendency to experience remission and relapse. The diagnostic criteria in the DSM-5 reflect a pattern of increasing use, unsuccessful attempts to quit or cut down use, craving, disruption at work home or school because of smoking, use despite medical problems associated with smoking, smoking in settings that are hazardous, social problems caused by tobacco use, increasing time and energy spent supporting tobacco use, and the development of tolerance and withdrawal (20).

Treatment

Current treatment for tobacco use disorders as recommended by the US Public Health Service Guidelines includes counseling and the use of Food and Drug Administration (FDA)-approved medications for tobacco cessation. These medications include nicotine replacement, bupropion and varenicline, either alone or in combination. The exceptions to this recommendation include patients who are pregnant and breastfeeding (21).

Treatment recommendations for pregnant and breastfeeding patients are enhanced with counseling using motivational interviewing and close follow-up. The motivational interviewing model includes the four A's listed in Box 49.6.

The US Preventive Services Task Force clinical guidelines found inadequate data to determine safety and efficacy of FDA-approved medications for the treatment of nicotine dependence during pregnancy (22). Clinicians need to make individualized patient specific treatment plans based on assessment of risks and benefits prior to prescribing FDA-approved medications for the treatment of nicotine dependence during pregnancy. See Box 49.7.

Patients and prescribers should be aware that varenicline and bupropion are present in breast milk and that there is insufficient data to evaluate safety and effectiveness during lactation. The benefits of breastfeeding are significant and there is little nicotine in breast milk so nicotine replacement can be considered if risk–benefit analysis supports its use (23). The

Box 49.6 Four A's of smoking cessation

Advise to quit
Assess willingness to stop smoking
Assist patients who have a willingness to quit
Arrange follow-up to track success with smoking cessation or changes in willingness to quit (22)

Box 49.7 FDA-approved medications for smoking cessation

Over-the-counter nicotine replacement
Nicotine gum, nicotine lozenges = category C in pregnancy and breastfeeding
Nicotine patch = category D in pregnancy and breastfeeding
Prescription nicotine replacement
Nicotine nasal spray, nicotine oral inhaler = category D in pregnancy and breastfeeding

breastfeeding mother must not smoke while using nicotine patches since the use of tobacco with nicotine replacement presents a risk of increasing nicotine exposure to the infant. Accidental exposure by children to nicotine replacement can cause severe illness or death (24).

Risk of Relapse

Half of the patients who quit smoking during pregnancy will experience a relapse within 1 year after delivery (25). Careful attention therefore must be paid to former smokers in the postpartum period to advise on the risk of relapse and the dangers of relapse. Patients may be unaware of the risk they present to their children when they smoke. The risks to children include asthma attacks, ear infections, respiratory infections and increased risk of sudden infant death (SIDS). Children are also susceptible to nicotine poisoning. The ingestion of a single cigarette by a child can lead to severe illness and 0.1 mg/kg of nicotine is a lethal does for a child. Family members are also at risk from second hand smoke with increased risk of coronary heart disease, lung cancer and stroke (26).

Tobacco and Other Substances

Tobacco use disorder is likely to be present when there is another substance abuse disorder such as alcohol and or drug abuse. It has been commonly thought that tobacco use disorder is best left untreated in the face of other substance abuse disorders to focus on treatment of the other disorders. There is no evidence to support this belief. Evidence supports treatment of smoking disorders in polysubstance abuse to decrease the risks associated with smoking and to promote longer term recovery from alcohol and drug use (27).

Opiates

Epidemiology

An estimated 15.5 million people are opioid dependent globally; the prevalence is higher in men than women (28). Deaths from drug overdose have steadily risen over the past two decades and have become the leading cause of injury death in the United States. Abuse of prescription drugs – especially opioid analgesic prescription drugs such as hydrocodone, oxycodone, morphine and methadone used to treat both acute and chronic pain – have increasingly been implicated in drug overdose deaths over the last decade (29).

> **Box 49.8 Opiates**
>
> Naturally occurring: derived from the poppy plant – examples include morphine, codeine
>
> Synthetic: examples include fentanyl, heroin, hydrocodone, hydromorphone, meperidine, methadone and oxycodone

The prevalence of opiate use in pregnant women ranges from 1% to 21%. The higher percentage reflects use in an at-risk population. While heroin is the most commonly abused illicit opiate, there is a growing group of women who misuse prescription opiates (30).

Opioid use results in dopamine release with a euphoria rush of intensely pleasurable feelings (euphoria). The opioid use leads to decreased physical pain, decreased emotional pain, decrease in anxiety and cough suppression. Under the influence of opiates, most patients feel calm and euphoric. After the effect of the drug wears off, people experience withdrawal symptoms, including drug craving, anorexia, nausea, abdominal cramping and increased sensitivity to pain.

Opioids range in strength from weak to powerful, are naturally occurring or synthetic and function in a range from pure agonists to pure antagonists. See Box 49.8. The use of opioids is primarily for its agonistic effects. Routes of use of these drugs are intravenous, intramuscular, subcutaneous and intranasal. Opiates are lipid soluble and rapidly crossing the blood–brain barrier subsequently binding to opioid receptors. There are several opioid receptors (mu, kappa and delta). Heroin has a high affinity for the mu receptor. Onset of action and duration depend of the quantity, purity and route of administration.

Opioid receptors are found in every part of the body. High concentrations of the receptor are present in the brain, gastrointestinal tract (GI) tract and spinal cord.

Over time and repeated exposure, tolerance develops. Tolerance is the need for increasing amounts of the substance to achieve the same euphoric feelings or "high." Repeated exposure leads to long-lasting changes in the brain. See Table 49.1.

During pregnancy, opioid use may lead to increased risk of miscarriage, intrauterine growth restriction (IUGR) and after-birth neonatal abstinence syndrome (31).

Table 49.1 Effects of opiod abuse

Short-Term Effects of Opioid Use	Long-Term Effects of Opioid Use
Euphoria – intense pleasure	Physiologic withdrawal
Somnolence	Risks of intravenous use (infectious)
Altered mentation	Hijack pleasure center of the brain
Cardiorespiratory arrest (overdose)	Risk of high-risk sexual behaviors

Box 49.9 Screening tools for opioid and substance abuse disorder

COWS (Clinical Opiate Withdrawal Scale) (33)
DAST-10 (Drug abuse screening test) (34)
CAGE – AID (CAGE adapted to include drugs) (35)
4P'plus screen (copyrighted)
CRAFFT (available for use without restriction)

Screening

Less than one-third of clinicians carefully screen for drug use (32). The consensus panel that developed the clinical guidelines for the use of buprenorphine in the treatment of opioid addiction recommends that all patients be periodically screened for substance use and substance-related problems, not just those who are from a high-risk population. Screening should not be limited to patients with risk factors for substance abuse. This recommendation for universal screening is supported by ACOG, because substance misuse occurs in all racial groups and socioeconomic classes and neighborhoods.

The screening tools available for opioid and substance use disorder are listed in Box 49.9.

Physician barriers to screening may include lack of training, lack of resources to address positive screens and lack of awareness of pervasiveness of the problem throughout society. Providers may have a fear of upsetting and losing patients diagnosed with a substance use disorder. Providers may experience discomfort in discussing prescription drug abuse and skepticism about whether treatment is effective. Any busy clinician may legitimately worry about time investment needed for counseling and referrals for patients who screen positive for substance abuse.

Laboratory testing to confirm or screen for substance abuse is usually done through urine tests because the renal system is the major route of drug excretion. The urine testing is generally inexpensive and rapid. Providers need permission for drug testing. A strategy for incorporation of drug testing into routine prenatal care is to inform patients of that urine drug screens are a part of the routine prenatal lab panel along with complete blood count (CBC), HIV, hepatitis and syphilis. Patients are offered the right of refusal for drug testing and all routine prenatal labs. Random drug checks without permission may be considered unethical and maybe illegal in some locations. Depending on the state the physician may have an obligation to inform the local police or child protective services of positive screens; this can be damaging to the physician–patient relationship.

In our current opioid epidemic, drug overdose is a leading cause of accidental death exceeding motor vehicle accidents (36).

Opioid-dependent women are particularly at risk for death from overdose in the postpartum period where relapse risk is higher. A variety of factors may play a role in increasing postpartum patients' vulnerability. Women may experience mood changes and disorders in the postpartum period; their primary motivation for abstinence is gone with delivery of the infant. Patient education about the risks of relapse and close follow-up are recommended in the postpartum period.

Diagnosis

Opioid use disorder should be approached using the chronic disease model. This model reflects the chronic nature of the problem and the tendency to experience remission and relapse. Diagnostic criteria are seen in Box 49.10.

Treatment

Treatment for opioid addiction starts with an individual who acknowledges her substance abuse problem or reports a desire for help. See Box 49.11. For pregnant women, the mainstay of treatment is medication assistance therapy. Pregnant women are typically highly motivated to seek treatment to help their unborn children. Abrupt withdrawal from opioids is not recommended in pregnancy because abrupt opioid withdrawal can precipitate preterm labor and fetal distress.

Methadone maintenance has been traditionally recommended for these women. In the past several

Box 49.10 Diagnostic criteria for opioid use disorder following a 12-month interval of use/abuse

- Use results in failure to fulfill major obligations
- Recurrent use despite physically hazardous situations
- Recurrent use leading to legal problems
- Continue use despite persistent or recurrent social or personal problems

Box 49.11 Treatment: Behavioral change

Precontemplation
Contemplation
Action
Intervention
Relapse

years, buprenorphine has emerged as a promising therapy for pregnant women. The use of buprenorphine in pregnancy has been shown to improve neonatal outcomes, decreasing the mean dose of morphine needed to wean opiate-dependent infants, decrease in length of hospital stay for management of withdrawal symptoms and decrease mean duration of neonatal abstinence syndrome treatment (37). Withdrawal without medication is associated with high relapse rates (38).

Methadone

Medication assistance programs with methadone were initially started in the 1960s. Federal regulations mandate that only designated centers may dispense and provide methadone along with individual and/ or group counseling. Patients are generally started on a dose of 10 or 20 mg daily and are titrated up 5–10 mg every few days (2–3 days) until they no longer experience withdrawal symptoms. Initially, daily treatment and psychosocial therapy are recommended to address all of the needs of the patient. Daily attendance at methadone clinics may be difficult for some patients.

Daily maintenance doses vary, sometimes going up to and beyond 100 mg daily. Physiologic changes in pregnancy may require an increase in the methadone dose for some women in the second or third trimester. Increase in dose and/or split dosing will usually resolve withdrawal symptoms caused by physiologic increases in blood volume and glomerular filtration rate (GFR), which occur normally in pregnancy.

Buprenorphine

Buprenorphine is a partial opioid agonist and has been available for use since 2002. Clinicians must receive a special waiver to prescribe buprenorphine, which requires that they undergo specialized training and credentialing. A drug addiction treatment act of 2000 (DATA 2000) waiver allows office based prescriptions to be written for medication assistance treatment. Practicing Ob/Gyn physicians are eligible for additional training and DATA 2000 waivers. Buprenorphine is favored by some authors because it has a decreased risk of respiratory depression, decreased sedation, fewer drug interactions and more mild withdrawal symptoms for some patients and has improved safety from overdose. In addition, it may be preferred over methadone because of the decreased outpatient visit schedule; daily visits are not required. Johnson et al. report evidence of less severe neonatal abstinence syndrome (39).

The landmark Maternal Opioid Treatment: Human Experimental Research (MOTHER) study has established the safety and efficacy for the use of buprenorphine as an alternative to methadone. Buprenorphine has been shown to actually lessen the risk of death from overdose.

Buprenorphine is available in a variety of forms and doses: solution, film, patch, tablet and implant. Initiation (usually combination product buprenorphine/naloxone) should begin after induction of a mild to moderate withdrawal. Several protocols exist for transitioning a patient from opiate use to buprenorphine. Potential exists for abuse. Diversion of buprenorphine is also a possibility, but as a partial antagonist, overdose risk is minimized.

Naloxone is an opioid antagonist. This drug blocks the opioid receptor. If the person has already taken the illicit drug, using this medication will precipitate withdrawal and its subsequent symptoms. Naltrexone, the tablet form of naloxone, is used in maintenance treatment of opiate detoxified persons. Naltrexone works by blocking opioid receptors to prevent the illicit use of opiates by preventing the euphoria from the illicit opiate use. One formulation of buprenorphine (trade name Suboxone®) includes both buprenorphine and naltrexone.

Patients who become pregnant while on buprenorphine are generally advised to continue the same dosage but to transition to the singe agent product (buprenorphine only) as opposed to the buprenorphine plus naloxone formulation.

A lack of long-term data exists for infants and children exposed for buprenorphine during pregnancy. High dropout rate due to dissatisfaction with the drug and risk of hepatic dysfunction are concerns.

Buprenorphine Implant

Four implants containing buprenorphine are FDA approved for insertion under the skin of the upper arm in a physician's office; implants remain in the arm for 6 months. The target population for buprenorphine implants are stable patients in recovery treatment, who are able to be maintained on a dose of 8 mg or less daily and who wish to avoid taking daily medication. It is recommended that implant users still see their providers once a month. After the 6-month end period, a certified physician must remove the implants and new implants can be inserted to continue treatment. Providers must be specifically credentialed to prescribe, insert and remove the buprenorphine implants.

Buprenorphine implant is not recommended in pregnancy since animal studies show an increase in adverse reactions; no human studies are available (40).

Community Resources

One of the ways to combat the recent crisis of opioid overdose death is to have wider availability of the medication naloxone. The opioid receptor antagonist reverses opioid overdose and restores normal respiration. Making naloxone available to first responders (fire, police, EMTs) and even lay people can minimize response times for treating opioid overdose and prevent overdose deaths.

Cannabinoids

Marijuana

According to office of national drug control policy, marijuana is the most commonly used illicit drug in the United States. The percentage of Americans who reported using marijuana has doubled in the last decade. Recent marijuana use rose from 4.1% to 9.5% of the US adult population while the prevalence of marijuana use disorder rose from 1.5% to 2.9% in studies conducted by National Institute on Alcohol Abuse and Alcoholism (NIAAA), part of the National Institutes of Health.

Approximately 30% of people who used marijuana met criteria for marijuana use disorder during 2012–2013, as defined by DSM-5. Symptoms of marijuana use disorder include taking the drug over a longer period than was intended by the user; persistent desire to cut down or control use with efforts to do so; failure to fulfill major role obligations at work, school or home as result of marijuana use; presence of tolerance and/or withdrawal.

The most psychoactive component in marijuana is 9 delta-tetrahydrocannabinol (THC) although there are over 60 cannabinoids found in natural marijuana plants (41). THC is lipophilic and accumulates in fatty tissues. This likely accounts for its lengthy elimination process and prolonged detection in drug screens even after discontinued use. THC acts on the brain to cause effects seen in Box 49.12.

THC is metabolized by the liver. Onset of action and duration of effects varies based on route of administration and potency of the product. Onset of action can vary from 30 minutes (from smoking) to 90 minutes (edible forms), and duration of effects typically varies from 3–5 hours.

The marijuana plant contains chemicals that may help to treat a range of illness or symptoms. As of 2016, researchers have not conducted enough clinical trials to satisfy FDA criteria for the use of marijuana plant as an approved medicine. The most widely

Box 49.12 Effects of THC

- Altered senses, sense of time
- Changes in mood
- Impaired body movement, difficulty with thinking and problem solving
- Impaired memory
- Hallucinations
- Paranoia
- Worsening symptoms in patients with schizophrenia (NIH)
- Long-term marijuana can affect brain development, which is particularly harmful in teenagers whose brain is still undergoing maturation and development. Marijuana may reduce thinking, memory and learning functions. These effects are determined by quantity and length of marijuana use, but the effect can be long-lasting and even permanent.

known use of medical marijuana is to treat nausea and as an appetite stimulant. There is more and more interest in use of chemical compounds derived from the marijuana plant for THC and cannabidiol delta tetra-hydrocannabinal (CBD) to treat symptoms of cancer, multiple sclerosis (MS), chronic pain, epilepsy and Parkinson's disease in patients who have not been successfully treated with traditional medical therapies.

Four states (Alaska, Oregon, Colorado and Washington) and the District of Columbia have laws allowing the use of marijuana for recreational use. An additional 19 states have laws permitting the use of marijuana for medical use. All of these states allow adults older than 21 or over to legally possess a small amount of marijuana. The amount allowable varies from state to state and all places except Washington state allow for individuals to cultivate varying numbers of plants. Despite the legality in these territories, federal laws still do not consider marijuana to be legal and federal law supersedes state law. Methods of marijuana consumption are listed in Box 49.13.

Synthetic Cannabinoids

Synthetic cannabinoids have been synthetically produced to mimic the natural compounds. They have significant toxicity and have been utilized recreationally in many areas. These substances are largely unregulated because manufacturers label them as not for human consumption, thereby bypassing FDA regulation.

Synthetic cannabinoids are usually smoked but can be vaped, ingested and snorted. They are less expensive, widely available, not detected by most routine drug screening and often blended with other substances.

The adverse reactions found with synthetic cannabinoids are more severe and can be deadly. Some of the clinical manifestations noted after exposure to synthetic cannabinoids are listed in Box 49.14. There is no consistency in these substances matched under the same name and it is possible that some packages may contain different components with different potencies.

Screening

THC can be identified with standard urine drug screen testing. Drug testing for synthetic cannabinoids is ineffective.

Effects in Pregnancy and Newborn

Marijuana is the illicit drug most commonly used during pregnancy and most women believe that it is relatively safe in pregnancy (42).

Effects of THC on users include central nervous system (CNS) depression but can also cause cardiovascular, respiratory as well as learning and social behavioral problems. Notably THC causes slower reaction times, changes in memory and attention, hypotension, tachycardia, bronchitis, sinusitis and pharyngitis.

Studies have conflicting results regarding the association of congenital anomalies, decrease in birth weight, increased risk of preterm birth or long-term infant child neurodevelopmental sequela with marijuana use. Multiple confounders are noted in many studies of marijuana users including tobacco use, lack or preconception folic acid, lack of early prenatal care and polysubstance use. This lack of evidence presents challenges for providers who counsel against use of this drug. Consensus exists that women should be encouraged at preconception and prenatally to discontinue marijuana use.

Box 49.13 Marijuana ingestion methods

Smoking: Handrolled joints, blunts (emptied cigars that have been partly or completely refilled with marijuana). Pipes or water pipes aka bongs.

Inhaling vapors: This allows users to pull the active ingredients from the marijuana vapors but not the smoke.

Edibles food: Users can mix marijuana in brownies, cookies or candy or brew as a tea.

Marijuana extracts: THC resins – these are extracted from the plant and use in a variety of products hash oil, honey oil or wax. Meant to deliver a large amount of THC to use of these extracts have sent some users to the emergency room.

Box 49.14 Clinical manifestations of synthetic cannabinoids

Agitation, coma, toxic psychosis, seizures, hallucination
Bradycardia, tachycardia, other cardiovascular effects
Rhabdomyolysis
Respiratory depression
Acute kidney injury

Treatment

No pharmacotherapies have proven to be effective treatment for cannabis dependence. Emergency room or detoxification facilities can provide a safe place for stabilization of patients with the severe symptoms (may occur with synthetic cannabinoid exposure). It is imperative that the individuals to have ongoing treatment in the form of counseling and education to adapt a drug-free lifestyle. Cognitive behavioral therapy and incentive vouchers showed up to 3 months of efficacy in promoting abstinence (43).

Stimulants

Stimulants include the class of drugs that make people more alert, increase attention and raise blood pressure. Stimulants come in a variety of forms, including amphetamines, methamphetamines, and cocaine. Prescription medications for attention deficit disorder (ADHA) are also members of the stimulant class and improper use of these medications (diversion or use outside of doctor's prescribing orders) can lead to a wide range of side effects such as hostility, irregular heartbeat, heart failure, and seizures.

According to SAMHSA national survey on drug use and health, 1.5 million people used cocaine in 2014.

The stimulants are highly addictive drugs. Cocaine is derived from the leaves of the coca plant and has limited medical use. As a drug of abuse, it looks like a white powder but very often mixed with various substances to weaken its potency and increase profits. It can be used orally, vaginally, rectally, snorted, smoked (crack cocaine), liquefied by heat and injected into the bloodstream. Cocaine causes excessive release of dopamine and prevention of dopamine reuptake. The result is a massive flood of dopamine that disrupts the normal brain communications and results in a high. Cocaine also enhances norepinephrine and serotonin activity.

Short-term effects of cocaine are extreme euphoria, increase in arousal, alertness and a sense of self-confidence and well-being. Physical effects include increase in body temperature, blood pressure and heart rate, along with constriction of blood vessels, decreased appetite, dilated pupils and restlessness. At its extreme, cocaine can lead hypertensive emergencies, cardiac arrhythmias, seizures and stroke. Long-term effects include nosebleeds, severe bowel decay and increased risk of contracting infectious bloodborne diseases, malnutrition, restlessness, and paranoia with auditory hallucinations.

Methamphetamines are an extremely addictive form of stimulant drug that is chemically similar to amphetamines. They are taken orally, smoked snorted or dissolved in alcohol or water, or injected. Smoking and injecting the drug delivers the drug very quickly to the brain where it produces an intense euphoria. Also known as meth, crystal, chalk and ice, methamphetamines can also be prescribed to treat attention deficit hyperactivity disorder (ADHD). Illicit methamphetamines are produced in homemade labs using over-the-counter ingredients such as pseudoephedrine found commonly in many cold medicines. Long-term effects of methamphetamine use in addition to those described for cocaine include extreme weight loss, severe dental problems (known as meth mouth) and skin sores caused by scratching.

Bath salts (synthetically made and chemically related to cathiones, a stimulant found in the khat plant). Khat is a shrub grown in in East Africa and southern Arabia and people sometimes chew its leaves for their mild stimulant effect, but synthetic varieties are much stronger in potency. These synthetic varieties can be swallowed, snorted, smoked or injected. They are marketed under a variety of street names such as Flakka, bloom, cloud nine, lunar wave, vanilla sky, white lightning, scarface. In addition to the lower anxiety, decreased depression and decreased inhibition, the effects of Bath salts can also produce paranoia, hallucinations, increased sociability and sex drive, panic attacks, agitation and violent behavior. Patients can suffer from dehydration, skeletal muscle breakdown and kidney damage.

Methylenedioxy methamphetamine (MDMA) is a synthetic drug that chemically resembles both stimulants and hallucinogens. Commonly called ecstasy or Molly, it alters mood and perception, and produces feeling of pleasure, increased energy emotional warmth, and a distorted sense of time. It is usually found in a capsule or tablet though some swallow it in liquid form or snort the powder. In addition to causing an increase in dopamine activity, it also increases norepinephrine and serotonin levels in the brain.

The durations of these effects depend on the potency of the drug as well as the method of usage.

Use of these drugs can lead to impaired judgement and risky sexual behaviors. Intravenous use increases the risk for HIV infection, hepatitis, and other bloodborne pathogens. Chronic heavy use has been associated with paranoid ideations, irritability and increased risk of violence.

Screening

Multiple screening tools are available for drug/stimulant use. High sensitivity and specificity have been shown even in pregnancy using CAGE and the two question two item conjoint screen (TICS) (44,45).

Stimulant use disorder should be addressed using the chronic disease model. This model reflects the chronic nature of the problem and the tendency for persons to experience remission and relapse.

Pregnant women who use cocaine or other stimulants are at increased risk for vaginal bleeding, spontaneous miscarriage, growth problems in their fetuses, preterm labor and birth, abruption and intrauterine fetal death. Although all these effects have not been universally confirmed by all studies, it should be noted that many confounders such as multiple drug use, tobacco smoking and other high-risk behaviors are often present.

Initial adverse effects on newborns include autonomic instability, decreased head circumference and low birth weight, hypertonia, tremors and an increased risk of SIDS (46).

Behavioral therapy is the mainstay of treatment for stimulant addiction as currently there are no FDA medications approved to treat stimulant use disorder. The treatment goal is to help the patient resist urges for compulsive stimulant use through group and individual therapy.

Other Drugs of Abuse

Hallucinogens

Hallucinogens are a group of drugs that cause hallucinations (sensations and images that are not real), disconnection and other alterations of perception, thought and feeling.

This group includes mushrooms (psilocybin), the cactus peyote (mescaline), LSD (D-lysergic acid diethylamide) and ayahuasca (dimethyltryptamine (DMT)) tea, dextromethorphan, ketamine, phencyclidine (PCP) and the plant *Salvia divinorum* (salvia). The hallucinogens can be smoked, absorbed by mouth or snorted.

The common pathway for the effects of hallucinogens are interference with serotonin and glutamate. The drug starts to work 20–90 minutes after use and can last for 6–12 hours. The physical findings with use are increased heart rate and nausea. The symptoms include intensified feelings and sensations and alteration in the sense of time.

Long-term effects are flashbacks and persistent psychosis. Deaths have been reported with use of large doses.

The effect of hallucinogens on the developing fetus are unknown.

Some hallucinogens such as PCP have addictive potential with withdrawal symptoms (craving, headaches and sweating). Other hallucinogens such as LSD produce tolerance but are not addictive.

There is no approved medication for the treatment of addiction to hallucinogens. The treatment is inpatient and outpatient behavioral therapy (47). Abstinence from use of hallucinogens is recommended during pregnancy.

Inhalants

Inhalants are volatile substances that have psychoactive properties when inhaled. These substances include volatile solvents, aerosols, gases and nitrites. Examples of substances abused as inhalants include spray paint, glue, cleaning fluids, whipped cream aerosols, nitrous oxide and amyl nitrites. This class of drugs of abuse are generally used more commonly by children and teenagers, but amyl nitrites are substances in this category more commonly used by adults for sexual enhancement.

The effects of the drugs are similar to alcohol with CNS depression. The symptoms are slurred speech, impaired coordination, and feelings of euphoria, dizziness, hallucinations, decreased inhibitions, headache and drowsiness. The chemical content of certain drugs can cause liver, kidney and bone marrow damage and hearing loss.

Repeated use can cause addiction and deaths have been reported rarely from respiratory depression and cardiac arrhythmia.

There is inadequate data to determine risk to the fetus from use of this category of drugs of abuse.

No approved medication for treatment of addiction to inhalants has been identified. Treatment is individual or group therapy (48). Abstinence from use of inhalants is recommended during pregnancy.

Breastfeeding by Patients with Substance Abuse Disorders

Women should be encouraged to breastfeed as it affords newborns and their mothers numerous health and psychological benefits. Many of the major medical societies, public health organizations and local government health departments have put resources toward the renewed support of breastfeeding.

Women with substance use disorder are often given conflicting information regarding to their ability to breastfeed. This population of women often have lower rates of breastfeeding initiation. All substances are found in breastmilk to some small degree. Active polysubstance abuse and HIV are contraindications to breastfeeding. Women who use cocaine, other stimulants, heroin, and synthetic marijuana should be advised to bottle-feed while actively using these drugs (49).

Conversely, women who are on maintenance therapy for opioid dependence with methadone or buprenorphine should be encouraged to breastfeed. Reduced medication needs for breastfed infants with neonatal abstinence syndrome (NAS) have been demonstrated.

Smoking cessation should be encouraged, and mothers should be warned to minimize nicotine intake and to avoid smoking around their infants. The benefits of breastfeeding outweigh any small exposure to nicotine in breastmilk.

Women who drink alcohol should be evaluated for the amount of consumption. Occasional users (one drink or less daily) should be counseled about timing of the drink, which is best after a feed to minimize the amount of alcohol in breastmilk. The consumption of more than one drink a day while breastfeeding should be discouraged.

Women who use marijuana should be encouraged to eliminate its use. THC is found in breastmilk and its effects on the infant are still largely unknown.

Concluding Remarks

Drug dependence is a chronic relapsing disease. Tobacco, alcohol, and illegal substance use is present in all races, socioeconomic groups, and communities. All women should be screened annually, with special attention at preconception visits and initial encounters when seeking prenatal care.

Treatment does work but relapse is part of the illness and should be anticipated. Drug enforcement policies that deter women from seeking prenatal care are contrary to the welfare of the mother and fetus (50).

References

1. Hedden S KJ, Lipari R, Medley G, Tice P. Behavioral Health Trends in the United States: Results from the 2014 National Survey on Drug Use and Health. Center for Behavioral Health Statistics and Quality. (2015). Behavioral health trends in the United States: Results from 2014 National Survey on Drug Use and Health 2015. HHS Publication No. SMA15-4927, NSDUH Series H-50. https://www.samhsa.gov/data/sites/default/files/NSDUH-FRR1-2014/NSDUH-FRR1-2014.pdf, accessed April 30, 2017
2. National Institute on Drug Abuse. Sex and Gender Differences in Substance Use 2015 [cited July 25, 2016]. Available from: www.drugabuse.gov/publications/research-reports/substance-use-in-women/sex-gender-differences-in-substance-use.
3. National Institute on Drug Abuse AAS. Substance Use While Pregnant and Breastfeeding 2015 [cited July 25, 2016]. Available from: www.drugabuse.gov/publications/research-reports/substance-use-in-women/substance-use-while-pregnant-breastfeeding.
4. DrugWarFacts.org GTF. Pregnancy & Substance Use 2013 [cited July 25, 2016]. Available from: www.samhsa.gov/data/NSDUH/2013SummNatFindDetTables/Index.aspx.
5. Chez RE Illicit Drug Abuse and Dependence in Women: ACOG – American College of Obstetricians and Gynecologists. http://www.acog.org/About-ACOG/ACOG-Departments/Tobacco--Alcohol--and-Substance-Abuse/Substance-Abuse/Illicit-Drug-Abuse-and-Dependence-in-Women
6. Anthony JC, Warner LA, Kessler RC. Comparitive Epidemiology of Dependence on Tobacco, Alcohol, Controlled Substances and Inhalants: Basic Finding from the National Comorbidity Survey. *Exp Clin Psychopharmacol.* 1994;2(3):244–68.
7. Volkow ND, Koob GF, McLellan AT. Neurobiologic advances from the brain disease model of addiction. *New Engl J Med.* 2016;374(4):363–71.
8. World Health Organization Alcohol 2015 [cited July 29, 2016]. Available from: www.who.int/substance_abuse/facts/alcohol/en/.
9. Opinion A-C. At-risk drinking and alcohol dependence: obstetric and gynecologic implications. *Obstet Gynecol.* August 2011;118(2 Pt 1):383–8.
10. Control Computational fluid dynamics. MMWR. [cited August 1, 2016]. 1042–6. Available from: www.cdc.gov.
11. Natinoal Institute on Alcohol abuse and Alcoholism NIAAA Overview-alcohol-consumption/alcohol-facts-and-statistics [cited August 1, 2016]. Available from: www.niaah.nih.gov/alcohol-health/overview-alcohol-consumption/alcohol-facts-and-statistics.

12. Available from: www.cdc.gov/ncbddd/fasd/alcohol-screening.html
13. ACOG. Alcohol abuse and other substance use disorders: ethical issues in obstetric and gynecologic practice. ACOG Opinion No. 633. *Obstet Gynecol.* 2015 Jun;125(6):1529-37. doi: 10.1097/01.AOG.0000466371.86393.9b.
14. Association AP. Diagnostic and Statistical Manual of Mental Disorders. 2013;5th Edition(DSM-5).
15. Hale T, Rowe HE. *Medications and Mothers Milk.* 2012;15th edition. New York: Springer Publishing.
16. Control CfD. MMWR. 64(44).
17. Guidelines USDoHaHS-CP. Treating Tobacco Use & Dependence: 2008 Update. 2008. https://www.ncbi.nlm.nih.gov/books/NBK63952/?report=printable (accessed May 15, 2017).
18. ACOG Committee on Health Care for Underdeserved Women; ACOG Committee on Obstetric Practice. Smoking cessation during pregnancy. *Obstet Gynecol.* 2005 Oct;106(4):883–88.
19. Fagerstrom Test for Nicotine Dependence [cited July 8, 2016].
20. Portico Network. Tobacco Use Disorder: Assessment and Diagnosis. 2014.
21. Prochaska JJE. The past, present and future. *Annu Rev Med.* 2016;67:467–86.
22. USPST Force. The Guide to Clinical Preventive Service. 2014.
23. NIH, LacMed, https://toxnet.nlm.nih.gov/newtoxnet/lactmed.htm
24. Mattison D. *Clinical Pharmacology during Pregnancy.* Cambridge, MA: Academic Press, 2013:217–47.
25. Coleman. Trends in smoking before, during, and after pregnancy in ten states. *Am J Prevent Med.* 2003;24:29–35.
26. Control CfD. Health Effects of Second Hand Smoke.
27. Available from: pubs.niaaa.nih.gov/publications/arh293/208–212.htm.
28. Degenhardt L, Charlson F, Mathers B, Hall WD, Flaxman AD, Johns N, Vos T. The global epidemiology and burden of opioid dependence: results from the global burden of disease 2010 study. *Addiction.* 2014;109(8):1320–33.
29. United States Department of Human Services. Opiod Abuse in the U.S. and HHS Actions to Address Opioid-Drug Related Overdoses and Deaths 2015 [cited 2016].
30. Keegan J, Parva M, Finnegan M, Gerson A, Belden M. Addiction in pregnancy. *J Addict Dis.* 2010;29(2):175–91.
31. ACOG Committee on Health Care for Underserved Women; American Society of Addiction Medicine. Opioid Abuse, Dependence and Addiction in Pregnancy. *Obstet Gynecol.* 2012 May;119(5):1070–6.
32. The National Center on Addiction and DrugAbuse. Five Year National Study Reveals: Addiction Treatment Neglected by U.S. Medical System 2012. 1–7. Available from: www.centeronaddiction.org/newsroom/press-releases/addiction-medicine-report-1.
33. Wesson DR. The Clinical Opiate Withdrawal Scale (COWS). *J Psychoac Drugs.* 2003;35(2):253–9.
34. Skinner HA. The drug abuse screening test. *Addict Behav.* 1982;7(4):363–71.
35. Brown RL. Conjoint Screening Questionnaires for alcohol and other drug abuse: Criterion validity in a primary care practice. *Wis Med J.* 1995;94(3):135–40.
36. McCarthy M. Drug overdose has become leading cause of death from injury in US. *BMJ.* 2015 Jun 22;350:h3328. doi: 10.1136/bmj.h3328.
37. Jones HE, Kaltenbach K, Heil SH, Stine SM, Coyle MG, Arria AM, O'Grady KE, Selby P, Martin PR, Fischer G. Neonatal abstinence syndrome after methadone or buprenorphine exposure. *N Engl J Med.* 2010;363(24):2320–31.
38. Jones HE. Methadone maintenance vs. methadone taper during pregnancy: maternal and neonatal outcomes. *Am J Addict.* 2008;7(5):372–86.
39. Johnson RE, Jones HE, Fischer G. Use of bupurenorphine in pregnancy: patient management and effects on the neonate. *Drug Alcohol Depend.* 2003;70(2 Suppl):S87–101.
40. [cited August 23, 2016]. Available from: https://braeburnpharmaceuticals.com.
41. CH A. Pharmacology and effects of cannabis: A brief review. *Br J Psychiatry.* 2001;178:101–6.
42. American College of Obstetricians and Gynecologists Committee on Obstetric Practice.. Marijuana u.se during pregnancy and lactation. *Obstet Gynecol.* 2015 Jul;126(1):234–238. doi: 10.1097/01.AOG.0000467192.89321.a6.
43. Budney AJ, Moore BA, Rocha HL, Higgins ST. Clinical trial of abstinence-based vouchers and cognitive-behavioral therapy for cannabis dependence. *J Consult Clin Psychol.* 2006;74(2):307–16.
44. Midanik LT, Zahnd EG, Klein D. Alcohol and drug CAGE screeners for pregnancy, low-income women: The California Perinatal Needs Assessment. *Alcohol Clin Exp Res.* 1998;22(1):121–5.
45. Brown RL, Leonard T, Saunders LA, Papasouliotis O. A two-item conjoint screen for alcohol and other drug problems. *J Am Board Fam Pract.* 2001;14(2):95–106.
46. Kuczkowski K. The effects of drug abuse on pregnancy. *Curr Opin Obstet Gynecol.* 2007;19(6):578–85.

47. [cited August 1, 2016]. Stimulants Available from: www.drugabuse.gov.

48. [cited August 1, 2016]. Inhalants Available from: www.drugabuse.gov.

49. Briggs G, Freeman RK. *Drugs in Pregnancy and Lactation: A Reference Guide to Fetal and Neonatal Risk*, 10th edition. Philadelphia: Walters Klewer Health, 2014.

50. Committee opinion no. 633 Alcohol Abuse and Other Substance Use Disorders: Ethical Issues in Obstetric and Gynecologic Practice. 2015;633(June):1–9.

Cancer in Pregnancy

Scott D. Richard and Clinton A. Veselis

Introduction

Cancer treatment in pregnancy presents a multifaceted challenge to both the provider and patient. The need for expedient, evidence-based treatments must be often balanced against ethical dilemmas, the potential for teratogenicity, and relative lack of research data. Ultimately, a frank discussion between provider and patient about treatment and pregnancy goals must be had.

Further complicating the diagnosis of cancer in pregnancy are physiologic changes that occur in normally pregnancy that may delay the initial diagnosis of malignancy. Most pregnant women have increased contact with the health care system during their pregnancy, so obstetricians are offered an ideal opportunity to deliver timely diagnosis and potential treatment to these women.

Scope of the Problem

Cancer is one of the leading causes of non-accidental death in women between the ages of 15 and 34 years old in the United States [1]. Unfortunately, newly diagnosed malignancy occurs at a rate of approximately 1 in 1,000 pregnant women [2]. Among the most common malignancies to be diagnosed in this age group are malignant melanoma, breast cancer, leukemia, cervical cancer, central nervous system (CNS) tumors, and non-Hodgkin lymphoma [2]. As the average age for women's first birth continues to rise, it is thought that the incidence of malignancy in pregnancy will also continue to rise [3].

In pregnancy, cancer can be categorized based on time of diagnosis during pregnancy. Falling into one of three broad categories: the antenatal period, time of delivery, or within 1-year of delivery. In one California-based study, the majority of newly diagnosed cases are found within 1 year after delivery (50%) [4].

Breast Cancer in Pregnancy

Epidemiology

Breast cancer is the most common malignancy diagnosed in pregnant and postpartum women. Currently it is expected that 1 in 3,000 pregnant women will be diagnosed with breast cancer. It is expected that this rate will rise as modern women delay childbearing. Average age at diagnosis is between 32 and 38 years.

Pathology appears to be similar between age-matched pregnant and non-pregnant women, but hormone receptor assays are frequently negative in pregnant women diagnosed with breast cancer. One theory is that high serum estrogen levels during pregnancy competitively bind to assays typically used to detect hormone receptor status. When more sensitive assays were employed, Elledge et al. were able to show similar receptor positivity in pregnant and non-pregnant women [5].

Diagnosis

Unfortunately, diagnosis of breast cancer in pregnant women is made difficult by the natural engorgement of breasts. Discrete masses are more difficult to identify, and diagnosis may be delayed from 5 to 15 months [6–9]. This delay has led to a later stage at diagnosis for women who are pregnant when compared to age-matched controls [10]. In order to combat this issue, it is recommended that women who are pregnant continue to practice self-breast exams similar to ones that those who practice self-examination utilize when they are not pregnant. Additionally, the American Congress of Obstetrics and Gynecology (ACOG) recommends that, as part of the routine prenatal examination, women should undergo a comprehensive breast examination.

If a breast mass is identified during pregnancy, then ultrasound and mammography can be utilized to characterize the lesion. With proper shielding, mammograms should pose little risk to the fetus, but it is recommended that mammograms only be utilized to evaluate dominant masses and to locate occult carcinomas [11]. Suspicious lesions should be biopsied, and the pathologist should be made aware of the patient's pregnant status to avoid any misinterpretation of pregnancy-related changes to the breast [12]. A negative mammogram, especially in this population age, does not specifically eliminate a cancer risk; up to 25% of mammograms in patients with cancer in this age group can be negative in the presence of cancer [11]. Needle biopsy, although uncomfortable, poses little risk to the mother or fetus.

Radiographic examinations to determine stage should be modified, or used sparingly, in the presence of a pregnant patient. Timing of the exposure to radiation is of particular importance. During the first trimester, even 0.1 Gray (Gy) of radiation can cause congenital malformations and increase the risk of carcinogenesis or even mental retardation [13]. Chest x-rays with proper shielding are considered safe, but should only be used to determine treatment decisions [7,14]. Average dose of radiation from a chest x-ray is 0.00008 Gy [15]. When bone metastasis is a concern, a bone scan can be utilized; expected dose of radiation for a bone scan is 0.001 Gy [11]. For evaluation of possible liver metastasis, ultrasound is recommended [11].

Treatment

Early Stage Breast Cancer (Stages I and II)

The mainstay of treatment for early stage breast cancer is surgery, even in pregnant women. In order to avoid scatter radiation to the fetus, therapeutic radiation should be avoided [16]. Modified radical mastectomy is therefore the treatment of choice. Some studies have looked at breast conservation surgery in pregnancy with postpartum radiation therapy; the authors have tried to establish predictive risk models to delaying radiation until after pregnancy [7,9,17].

When adjuvant chemotherapy is indicated, timing of the chemotherapy administration is important. Chemotherapy given after the first trimester is generally not associated with fetal malformation, but may lead to premature labor and fetal wastage. Data of the long-term fetal effects of chemotherapy is limited [7,9,18–21]. Due to the high risk of teratogenicity, chemotherapy should never be given in the first trimester. Knowledge of the use of adjuvant hormonal therapy is limited [22].

Late Stage Breast Cancer (Stages III and IV)

Five-year survival for women who are pregnant with stage III and IV breast cancer is around 10% [6,9]. Chemotherapy can be given after the first trimester, and as already mentioned, radiation therapy should not be given due to risk of fetal scatter. Therapeutic abortion has unfortunately not been shown to improve survival [6,7,9,10,13].

Lactation and Breast Cancer

Suppression of lactation does not improve survival, however, if surgery is planned, then lactation should be avoided/suppressed in order to decrease vascularity and blood loss during surgery. If chemotherapy is employed during treatment, then lactation should be avoided since many anti-neoplastic agents can be expressed in breast milk at high levels.

Cervical Cancer in Pregnancy

Epidemiology

Cervical cancer occurs at approximately 13,000 new cases per year, with an estimated 4,100 deaths per year [2,23]. Of women in the age group 20–39 years old, cervical cancer represents the second leading cause of cancer related death in the United States [24]. For all patients with cervical cancer, however, only 1% are pregnant at diagnosis [25]. Abnormal cytology following Papanicolaou (Pap) smear may be found in approximately 5% of pregnancies [26]. Pregnant women have increased health care surveillance as part of regular prenatal visits. Many patients who would otherwise go without care gain access to the health care system when pregnant. This may contribute to the higher incidence of pregnant versus nonpregnant women who are diagnosed with early stage cervical disease [25].

Diagnosis

As in non-pregnant patients, Pap smears for pregnant patients are evaluated using the Bethesda system. Most commonly and in pregnancy, when indicated by American Society for Colposcopy and Cervical Pathology (ASCCP) guidelines, abnormal cervical lesions should be further evaluated by colposcopy to exclude invasive disease. The normal evolution of the cervix in pregnancy actually aids in colposcopic evaluation as the squamo-columnar junction (SCJ) everts. Biopsies should only be taken of the most obviously abnormal areas and endocervical curettage (ECC) should be avoided [27]. Following satisfactory colposcopic evaluation, the diagnostic accuracy is reported as high as 95–99%. The most common complication reported is bleeding from the biopsy site [28]. If colposcopy is deemed inadequate, unlike in non-pregnant patients, follow-up with repeat colposcopy in 6–12 weeks is recommended, as further time may allow the SCJ to evert for adequate evaluation [29]. When there is a concern for malignancy, it is imperative that an experienced clinician evaluate.

Rates of progression of disease are similar to that of non-pregnant patients. One study reports that the rate of progression from dysplasia to a higher-grade lesion postpartum is only 7% [30]. Given the data available, and following adequate colposcopic evaluation, conservative management of cervical intraepithelial neoplasia (CIN) may be reasonable if invasive cancer has been excluded [27]. Rates of regression of abnormal lesions, however, are significantly higher in pregnant patients with nearly 70% of CIN 2 and CIN 3 resolving by 6 months postpartum [31].

Cervical conization and loop electrosurgical excision procedure (LEEP) should be avoided as much as possible in pregnant patients. When performed in pregnancy, there are reported similar complication rates, which include bleeding, infection, preterm premature rupture of membranes, cramping, spontaneous abortion, preterm labor, and pregnancy loss [32]. However, if a LEEP or cone biopsy must be performed to exclude malignancy, the safest time in early pregnancy is generally considered to be the second trimester between 14 and 20 weeks. Later in pregnancy, following documented fetal maturity, these procedures are also considered acceptable.

Treatment

When a cervical biopsy is concerning for microinvasive disease, further tissue is necessary for accurate diagnosis. The primary way to confirm a diagnosis is with a cervical cone biopsy. In accordance with the International Federation of Gynecology and Obstetrics (FIGO) clinical staging classification of cervical cancer, women with stage, IA1 or less, lesions may safely be monitored intermittently during pregnancy, until definitive management can be performed in the postpartum period. Although there is a lack of data for management outcomes for women with adenocarcinoma in situ it is currently managed the same as with microinvasive squamous cell carcinoma via cervical conization [33].

For early, stage I disease, surgical outcomes tend to be excellent. Several small studies suggest that a delay in treatment of stage I disease has similar outcomes as immediate treatment. For example, Sood et al. report that of the 11 women who delayed treatment for an average of 16 weeks, no negative outcomes as a result of delayed treatment in pregnancy were revealed [34].

In patients with stage I disease in early gestation, surgical management with radical hysterectomy, with fetus in situ, is the treat strategy of choice and may be performed up to 20 weeks gestation [35]. If treatment is delayed to allow for delivery in the third trimester, ideally cesarean section is route of delivery to avoid delivery through a cervical lesion and lessen risk of metastasis to the vagina, followed by a radical cesarean hysterectomy [36].

The mainstay for advanced cervical cancer is radiation in combination with a platinum-based chemotherapeutic agent [37]. Radiation therapy should be reserved for patients with advanced disease who are not going to carry the fetus to term, as there is a dose-dependent negative effect on the fetus. Spontaneous abortion has been reported in most cases of therapeutic radiation [38]. Delaying therapy to allow for fetal viability has not been elucidated [34].

Ovarian Cancer in Pregnancy

Epidemiology

Approximately 10% women in the United States at some point in their lifetimes will undergo surgery for an ovarian mass. Of these masses, 20% will harbor malignancy [39]. For pregnant patients, adnexal masses are a relatively common, and for the most part benign, finding. Approximately 70%, of these adnexal masses resolve on their own by the end of the first trimester [40]. Approximately 1–3% of these adnexal masses, however, may turn out to harbor malignancy [41].

Pregnant women with an adnexal mass are most likely to present with symptoms of ovarian torsion [42]. For these patients, it is also important to bilaterally inspect the ovaries at the time of surgery as up to 10–15% of dysgerminomas occur bilaterally. Benign cystic teratomas are the most common neoplasm to be uncovered in pregnancy [40,41]. As masses grow larger than 8 cm, clinicians must become suspicious for complications such as torsion, obstruction of labor, and pain [43]. The incidence of other ovarian tumors such as endodermal sinus tumors, and sex cord stromal tumors are relatively rare in women of reproductive age. These tumors are typically managed in the same manner as non-pregnant patients.

Diagnosis

The majority of suspicious ovarian masses are diagnosed during routine ultrasound for fetal anatomy/growth or during a suspect torsion.

Treatment

For masses that are not rapidly enlarging, are simple cysts, and are less than 8 cm, observation may be recommended [39]. If surgery is determined to be necessary by both maternal-fetal-medicine and gynecologic oncology experts, the recommended time to perform surgery is between 16 and 20 weeks. At this time, the pregnancy is well established and most physiologic cysts have regressed. If cesarean section is the route of delivery, this provides an ideal time for providers to further inspect and stage any pathology.

The majority of ovarian cancers are stage I when diagnosed during pregnancy. Chemotherapy can usually be delayed until after delivery of the fetus for epithelial ovarian tumors. Although rare, germ cell tumors can occur. In these cases, chemotherapy should be undertaken as soon after delivery as possible, or after the first trimester if necessary [6,44].

Hematologic Malignancies and Pregnancy

Epidemiology

Approximately 18% of patients with malignant disease during pregnancy have a hematologic malignancy. The majority of these are a Hodgkin's lymphoma. Currently it is expected that 1 in 6,000 pregnancies will be affected by a hematologic malignancy. Leukemia is relatively rare in this patient population, but presents a very difficult challenge for patient and physician [45].

Diagnosis

Patients with hematologic malignancies often present with hyper-metabolic symptoms such as fatigue, night sweats, nausea/emesis, weight loss. These symptoms can often be mistaken for changes that occur in early pregnancy [46]. Swollen and suspicious lymph nodes can safely be biopsied at any gestational age. In the case of leukemia, bone marrow biopsy can also safely be performed at any gestational age [47].

Positron emission tomography-computed tomography (PET-CT) is contraindicated in pregnancy. The radiographic marker used in this type of evaluation has been shown to cross the placenta and can irradiate the fetus directly [48]. Abdominal-pelvic CT is also contraindicated [49]. In order to stage hematologic malignancies, recommendations are to utilize abdominal ultrasound or non-gadolinium magnetic resonance imaging (MRI) [50].

Treatment

Lymphoma

When lymphoma is diagnosed during the first trimester, consideration should be given to termination. Chemotherapeutic agents should be avoided, but if the patient desires to continue the pregnancy, then delay until the second trimester for chemotherapy is possible. Patients with low-grade or indolent disease can have treatment delayed until after delivery [45].

Leukemia

Treatment for leukemia should be instigated as soon as possible after diagnosis, regardless of gestational age. It is recommended that women in the first trimester undergo termination of the pregnancy. Maternal complications during anti-neoplastic therapy can be high due to extreme pancytopenia and immunosuppression [51].

Concluding Remarks

Many treatment options exist for women diagnosed with cancer during pregnancy. Early referral to a gynecologic oncologist, as well as a maternal fetal medicine specialist, will help the general obstetrician navigate the unique challenges that a cancer diagnosis will have on the patient, her pregnancy, and the fetus. It is important also to realize that a new cancer diagnosis will bring with it a flood of emotional and psychological strain. When deciding how to proceed with a pregnancy, discussions about the effects treatment will have on the fetus and the patient's survival are important. When discussions involve timing of delivery, additional support will be required for the patient and her family. Access to counselors who specialize in cancer support immediately after diagnosis greatly helps patients greatly assess their options, and provides them with much needed psychological support.

References

[1] Antonelli NM, Dotters DJ, Katz VL, Kuller JA. Cancer in pregnancy: A review of the literature. Part I. *Obstet Gynecol Surv*. 1996;51:125–34.

[2] Siegel R, Ward E, Brawley O, Jemal A. Cancer statistics, 2011. *CA: Cancer J Clin*. 2011;61:212–36.

[3] Matthews TJ, Hamilton BE. First births to older women continue to rise. *NCHS Data Brief*. 2014:1–8.

[4] Smith LH, Danielsen B, Allen ME, Cress R. Cancer associated with obstetric delivery: Results of linkage with the California cancer registry. *Am J Obstet Gynecol*. 2003;189:1128–35.

[5] Elledge RM, Ciocca DR, Langone G, et al. Estrogen receptor, progesterone receptor, and HER-2/neu protein in breast cancers from pregnant patients. *Cancer*. 1993; 71(8):2499–506.

[6] Hoover HC Jr. Breast cancer during pregnancy and lactation. *Surg Clin North Am*. 1996; 70(5):1151–63.

[7] Gwyn K, Theriault R. Breast cancer during pregnancy. *Oncology*. 2001; 15(1):39–51.

[8] Moore HC, Foster RS Jr. Breast cancer and pregnancy. *Semin Oncol*. 2000; 27(6): 646–53.

[9] Rugo HS. Management of breast cancer diagnosed during pregnancy. *Curr Treat Options Oncol*. 2003; 4(2):165–73.

[10] Clark RM, Chua T. Breast cancer and pregnancy: The ultimate challenge. *Clin Oncol (R Coll Radiol)*. 1989; 1(1):11–18.

[11] Yang WT, Dryden MJ, Gwyn K, et al. Imaging of breast cancer diagnosed and treated with chemotherapy during pregnancy. *Radiology*. 2006; 239(1):52–60.

[12] Middleton LP, Amin M, Gwyn K, et al. Breast carcinoma in pregnant women: Assessment of clinicopathologic an immunhistochemical features. *Cancer*. 2003; 98(5): 1055–60.

[13] Barnavon Y, Wallack MK. Management of the pregnant patient with carcinoma of the breast. *Surg Gynecol Obstet*. 1990; 171(4):347–52.

[14] Nicklas AH, Baker ME. Imaging strategies in the pregnant cancer patient. *Semin Oncol*. 2000; 27(6):623–32.

[15] Gallengerg MM, Loprinzi CL. Breast cancer and pregnancy. *Semin Oncol*. 1989; 16(5):369–76.

[16] Kal HB, Struikmans H. Radiotherapy during pregnancy: Fact and fiction. *Lancet Oncol*. 2005; 6(5):328–33.

[17] Nettleton J, Long J, Kuban D, et al. Breast cancer during pregnancy: Quantifying the risk of treatment delay. *Obstet Gynecol*. 1996; 87(3):414–18.

[18] Kuerer HM, Gwyn K, Ames FC, et al. Conservative surgery and chemotherapy for breast carcinoma during pregnancy. *Surgery*. 2002; 131(1):108–10.

[19] Giacalone PL. Laffargue F, Benos P. Chemotherapy for breast carcinoma during pregnancy: A French national survey. *Cancer*. 1999; 86(11):2266–72.

[20] Cardonick E, Iacobucci A. Use of chemotherapy during human pregnancy. *Lancet Oncol*. 2004; 5(5):283–91.

[21] Berry DL, Theriault RL, Holmes FA, et al. Management of breast cancer during pregnancy using a standardized protocol. *J Clin Oncol*. 1999; 17(3):855–61.

[22] Issacs RJ, Hunter W, Clark K. Tamoxifen as a systemic treatment of advanced breast cancer during pregnancy – Case report and literature review. *Gynecol Oncol*. 2001; 80(3): 405–8.

[23] Howlader N, Noone AM, Krapcho M, Miller D, Bishop K, Altekruse SF, et al. SEER Cancer Statistics Review, 1975–2013. SEER web site 2016.

[24] Siegel RL, Miller KD, Jemal A. Cancer statistics, 2016. *CA: Cancer J Clin*. 2016;66:7–30.

[25] Duggan B, Muderspach LI, Roman LD, Curtin JP, d'Ablaing G 3rd, Morrow CP. Cervical cancer in pregnancy: Reporting on planned delay in therapy. *Obstet Gynecol*. 1993;82:598–602.

[26] Campion MJ. TV S. colposcopy in pregnancy. *Obstet Gynecol Clin North Am*. 1993;20:153–63.

[27] Wright Jr TC, Massad LS, Dunton CJ, Spitzer M, Wilkinson EJ, Solomon D. 2006 consensus guidelines for the management of women with abnormal cervical cancer screening tests. *Am J Obstet Gynecol*. 2007;197:346–55.

[28] Economos K, Perez Veridiano N, Delke I, Collado M, Tancer M. Abnormal cervical cytology in pregnancy: A 17-year experience. *Obstet Gynecol*. 1993;81:915–8.

[29] ACOG Practice Bulletin #66: Management of Abnormal Cervical. *Obstet Gynecol*. 2005;106:645–64.

[30] Woodrow N, Permezel M, Butter-field L, Rome R, Tan J, Quinn M. Abnormal cervical cytology in pregnancy: Experience of 811 cases. *Aus N Z J Obstet Gynaecol*. 1998;38:161–5.

[31] Yost NP, Santoso JT, McIntire DD, Iliya FA. Postpartum regression rates of antepartum cervical

intraepithelial neoplasia II and III lesions. *Obstet Gynecol.* 1999;93:359–62.

[32] Robinson WR, Webb S, Tirpack J, Degefu S, O'Quinn AG. Management of cervical intraepithelial neoplasia during pregnancy with LOOP excision. *Gynecol Oncol.* 1997;64:153–5.

[33] Lacour RA, Garner EIO, Molpus KL, Ashfaq R, Schorge JO. Management of cervical adenocarcinoma in situ during pregnancy. *Am J Obstet Gynecol.* 2005;192:1449–51.

[34] Sood AK, Sorosky JI, Krogman S, Anderson B, Benda J, Buller RE. Surgical management of cervical cancer complicating pregnancy: A case–control study. *Gynecol Oncol.* 1996;63:294–8.

[35] Monk B, Montz F. Invasive cervical cancer complicating intrauterine pregnancy: Treatment with radical hysterectomy. *Obstet Gynecol.* 1992;80:199–203.

[36] Baloglu A, Uysal D, Aslan N, Yigit S. Advanced stage of cervical carcinoma undiagnosed during antenatal period in term pregnancy and concomitant metastasis on episiotomy scar during delivery: A case report and review of the literature. *Int J Gynecol Cancer.* 2007;17:1155–9.

[37] Morris M, Eifel PJ, Lu J, Grigsby PW, Levenback C, Stevens RE, et al. Pelvic radiation with concurrent chemotherapy compared with pelvic and para-aortic radiation for high-risk cervical cancer. *N Engl J Med.* 1999;340:1137–43.

[38] Kal HB, Struikmans H. Radiotherapy during pregnancy: Fact and fiction. *Lancet Oncol.* 2005;6:328–33.

[39] ACOG Practice Bulletin No. 83: Management of Adnexal Masses. *Obstet Gynecol.* 2007;110:201–14.

[40] Leiserowitz GS, Xing G, Cress R, Brahmbhatt B, Dalrymple JL, Smith LH. Adnexal masses in pregnancy: How often are they malignant? *Gynecol Oncol.* 2006;101:315–21.

[41] Whitecar P, Turner S, Higby K. Adnexal masses in pregnancy: A review of 130 cases undergoing surgical management. *Am J Obstet Gynecol.* 1999;181:19–24.

[42] Schmeler KM, Mayo-Smith WW, Peipert JF, Weitzen S, Manuel MD, Gordinier ME. Adnexal masses in pregnancy: Surgery compared with observation. *Obstet Gynecol.* 2005;105:1098–103.

[43] Hess LW, Peaceman A, O'Brien WF, Winkel CA, Cruikshank DP, Morrison JC. Adnexal mass occurring with intrauterine pregnancy: Report of fifty-four patients requiring laparotomy for definitive management. *Am J Obstet Gynecol.* 1988;158:1029–34.

[44] Boulay R, Podczaski E. Ovarian cancer complicating pregnancy. *Obstet Gynecol Clin N Am.* 1998; 25:385–399.

[45] Pereg D, Koren G, Lishner M. The treatment of Hodgkin's and non-Hodgkin's lymphoma in pregnancy. *Haemotologica.* 2002; 92:1230–37.

[46] Amit O, Barzilai M, Avivi I. Management of hematologic malignancies: Special considerations in pregnant women. *Drugs.* 2015; 75:1725–38.

[47] Rovera F, Frattini F, Coglitore A, et al. Breast cancer in pregnancy. *Breast J.* 2010; 16(Suppl 1):S22–5.

[48] Colletti PM. PET-CT in the pregnant patient. *Am Coll Radiol.* 2012. http://www.imagewisely.org/~/media/ImageWisely-Files/NucMed/PETCT-in-the-Pregnant-Patient.pdf (accessed May 15, 2017).

[49] Brent RL. The effect of embryonic and fetal exposure to x-ray, microwaves, and ultrasound: Counseling the pregnant and non-pregnant patient about these risks. *Semin Oncol.* 1989; 16(5): 347–68.

[50] Austin LM, Frush DP. Compendium of national guidelines for imaging the pregnant patient. *Am J Roentgenol.* 2011; 197(4):W737–46.

[51] Shapira T, Pereg D, Lishner M. How I treat acute and chronic leukemia in pregnancy. *Blood Rev.* 2008; 22:247–59.

Thromboembolic Complications of Pregnancy

Zachary C. Kuhlmann

Introduction

Venous thromboembolism (VTE) during pregnancy is a life-threatening event for the patients who are diagnosed with this condition. Management of VTE and deep vein thrombosis is sometimes different in pregnant patients as compared to non-pregnant patients. This chapter discusses the epidemiology, physiology, risk factors, diagnosis and treatment of VTE in pregnancy. Special considerations at the time of delivery for patients on anti-coagulant therapy and thromboprophylaxis are also described.

Scope of the Problem

Pregnancy increases a woman's risk of having a thrombotic event. Although the overall rate is low, the risk of having VTE during pregnancy or the postpartum period is estimated to be between 1–2/1,000 pregnancies (1,2). It is estimated that up to 80% of thrombotic events during pregnancy are deep venous thrombosis (DVT) and that pulmonary emboli account for much of the remaining thrombotic events (1,2). The risk of a DVT is approximately fivefold higher in pregnant women and between 20- and 60-fold higher in the postpartum period (1,2). These numbers represent 500,000 patients each year who are diagnosed with VTE (3). Thromboembolic events are one of the most common causes of maternal deaths in the United States. This fact differs from underdeveloped nations where hemorrhage is the most common cause of maternal death (4,5).

Physiology

Rudolph Virchow, a nineteenth-century physician, described a triad of physiologic changes that increase the risk of venous thromboembolism (VTE). The triad includes (1) venous stasis, (2) hypercoagulable state, and (3) endothelial damage (6).

Pregnancy affects all three of Virchow's famous triad for thrombus formation. Increased levels of progesterone can lead to vasodilation, which contributes to venous stasis. The gravid uterus also compresses the iliac vein, which likely increases venous stasis and risk of thrombosis (7,8). This compression also is likely the reason there is an increased number of left sided DVT's in pregnant women when compared with DVTs found in non-pregnant individuals (7,8).

Many physiologic changes result in the hypercoagulable state of pregnancy. Estrogen, factors V, VII, VIII, IX, X, XII, Von Willebrand factor, and fibrinogen all increase during normal pregnancy. There is also an increase in plasminogen activator inhibitor. All of these changes result in an increased ability of clot formation (7,8).

Endothelial homeostasis is critical to the avoidance of thrombosis formation. Pregnancy likely disrupts this homeostasis at the level of the placenta. This finding is related to decidual reactions, which are often influenced by hormonal changes of pregnancy (7–9). The compression of the left iliac vein by the right iliac artery likely contributes to endothelial injury during pregnancy (10). Also, the trauma associated with delivery, whether vaginal or cesarean delivery, subjects the endothelium to damage (10).

Risk Factors

Many factors have been identified that increase the risk for thrombosis. Those risk factors can be stratified into three broad categories: (1) factors that are generally shared among the general population, (2) inherited thrombophilias and (3) acquired thrombophilias.

General risk factors for VTE include history of previous VTE, immobilization, malignancy, elevated body mass index, surgery, orthopedic trauma, smoking and hemoglobinopathies (2,8). In pregnancy, the single most important risk factor remains a history of prior VTE; 15–25% of VTEs are recurrent events (1,11,12). Pregnancy-specific risk factors include preeclampsia, antepartum or postpartum hemorrhage, and postpartum infection. The risk of VTE seems to be higher in the postpartum period than during pregnancy itself (11–13).

Simply stated, thrombophilia is a disorder of the hemopoietic system that increases the tendency for occurrence of thrombosis (14). It is estimated that thrombophilia can be identified in up to 50% of individuals diagnosed with VTE during pregnancy (5,11,12). Thrombophilias can be divided into two groups: inherited and acquired.

Inherited thrombophilias include factor V Leiden, prothrombin G20210A, protein C deficiency, protein S deficiency, antithrombin deficiency, and methylenetetrahydrofolate reductase (MTFHR) mutation (9,11,12). Factor V Leiden mutation is the most common inherited thrombophilia; it is present in 5–8% of the population from European ancestry (12). The mutation results in activated protein C resistance and is the most common inherited thrombophilia. Individuals who are heterozygous for the mutation carry a slightly increased risk of VTE during pregnancy of 5–12/1,000 (12). Individuals who are homozygous for the mutation can have up to a 17% risk of VTE if there is a history of VTE in the past or an affected first degree relative (12).

Prothrombin G20210A mutation is the second most common inherited thrombophilia. The mutation is only found in about 3% of the population from European descent and results in an increased amount of prothrombin, thus increasing the risk of thrombosis. Again, an individual who is homozygous has an increased risk of VTE (12).

Deficiencies in either protein C or protein S can result in an increased risk for VTE. In both conditions, over 100 mutations exist and the phenotypic presentation can vary greatly (9,12).

Anti-thrombin deficiency is rare, but extremely potent (9,12). Many mutations exist in the antithrombin gene and, if present, can carry a risk of up to 8% of VTE in the non-pregnant individual and up to 40% in pregnancy when accompanied by a personal or family history of VTE (9,12). Stillbirth rates also appear to be increased with antithrombin deficiency (9).

Homozygous mutations in the MTFHR gene result in hyperhomocysteinemia. The clinical significance of hyperhomocystenemia is unclear, as it is currently thought this condition portrays no increased risk of VTE. The MTFHR mutations themselves also do not carry increased risk of VTE (9,12).

Antiphospholipid syndrome (APLS) is an acquired thrombophilia. The condition is an autoimmune disease where the antibodies bind to negatively charged phospholipids on the cell (15,16).

The diagnosis of APLS is both a laboratory and clinical diagnosis and at least one clinical criteria and one laboratory criteria must be present to make the diagnosis. The clinical criteria for APLS diagnosis include vascular thrombosis or pregnancy morbidity. Examples of pregnancy morbidities that would qualify to make the diagnosis of APLS include fetal death after 10 weeks in a fetus that is morphologically normal, preeclampsia or eclampsia requiring delivery prior to 34 weeks gestation, or three or more consecutive spontaneous abortions that cannot be otherwise explained (15,16). For the laboratory evaluation of APLS, clinical antibodies must be obtained. These include B2 glycoprotein 1, lupus anticoagulant and anticardiolipin antibodies (15,16). These laboratory tests must be confirmed 12 weeks after an initial positive result.

Diagnosis

The timing of diagnosis for VTE is crucial to the outcome of the patient. A delayed diagnosis with a DVT may result in the development of a PE or even death. Clinical suspicion of a VTE should prompt immediate evaluation.

DVTs commonly present with leg swelling and pain/tenderness (1,2). This can create a clinical quandary in some cases since many normal pregnant patients also complain of leg swelling and pain/discomfort. An objective measurement of the lower extremity such as calf circumference, when compared to the contralateral counterpart may aid in the diagnosis (1,2). When performing leg measurements, it is important to verify the same area of the calf was measured on both legs. Typically, a difference of 2 cm or more warrants further investigation (1,2,13).

If a DVT is suspected, the next step after examination is compression ultrasound of the lower extremity. Both the sensitivity and specificity of compression ultrasound for the detection of DVT is > 90% each respectively (1,2). In addition to the sensitivity and specificity, the compression ultrasound is noninvasive and has no radiation (1,2). If a negative result is found, but clinical suspicion remains elevated or iliac vessel involvement is suspected, further testing is warranted.

The next test considered should be magnetic resonance imaging, which carries no radiation exposure risk to the fetus (1,2,5). If there is no MRI availability, and suspicion is high, other modalities including pulsed dopplers, computed tomography or even empiric treatment may be warranted. Finally, if symptoms persist, consider repeating compression ultrasound in 3–7 days (10).

Laboratory evaluation for DVT or pulmonary embolism (PE) is difficult in the pregnant patient. Commonly, a D-dimer test will be ordered during the evaluation of VTE (17). In a non-pregnant individual, a negative D-dimer and negative compression ultrasound will rule out the presence of a DVT (10). However, in normal pregnancy, the D-dimer level is elevated, thus making this an unreliable test in the pregnant population (10).

Prompt evaluation for a PE is also critical in the outcome of an affected patient. Similar to DVT, the symptoms associated with PE are often appreciated in normal pregnancies. These symptoms may include tachypnea, tachycardia, intermittent dyspnea, chest pain and hemoptysis (2). Initially, consideration should be given to obtaining a compression ultrasound, as often times a DVT is found in the presence of a PE (2,10). A high index of suspicion for PE is appropriate since a missed diagnosis may be lethal.

When a PE is suspected, various diagnostic tools may be useful in making an accurate diagnosis. A chest X-ray may not show a definitive PE, but will help rule out other pathologic conditions such as pneumonia; a chest X-ray transmits minimal radiation exposure to mother and fetus (1). If an electrocardiogram (EKG) is ordered, signs of right ventricular strain may be seen in the presence of a PE. After the chest X-ray is obtained, or if clinical suspicion is high and there is a desire to bypass the chest X-ray, either ventilation-perfusion (V/Q) scan or chest computed tomographic (CT) angiography are the next modalities of choice. CT-angiography is often preferred and if ordered first line, it may help confirm the diagnosis of PE in addition to help make an accurate alternative diagnosis if a PE is not found (1,5,8). A V/Q scan yields less radiation exposure than the CT angiography (1,5,8). Patients should be warned about the radiation exposure to breast tissue during CT-angio and V/Q scan, however in a potentially lethal situation, risks must be weighed against benefits (1,5).

Treatment

Anticoagulation is the standard treatment of VTE. VTE during pregnancy is usually treated with unfractionated heparin (UFH) or low-molecular-weight heparin (LMWH). Both UFH and LMWH do not cross the placenta (18–20). UFH and LMWH offer no teratogenic effects to the fetus (18–20). UFH and LMWH are both considered safe during pregnancy and breastfeeding and treatment is generally indicated with any pregnant patient who is diagnosed with a VTE.

LMWH is generally considered to have fewer complications than UFH (2,3,18). Complications seen with the heparin compounds include bleeding, reduced bone mineral density and heparin-induced thrombocytopenia (HIT). All of the previous mentioned adverse effects occur with less frequency with LMWH when compared to UFH. LMWH also has a longer half-life and a more predictable dose response (2,5,18). Consideration should be given to patients with renal insufficiency when deciding between UFH and LMWH. LMWH is mainly excreted through the renal system, where UFH is excreted through both the renal and hepatic systems (2,13). Generally, a glomerular filtration rate of < 30 mL/min warrants UFH use over LMWH (21).

Warfarin is a vitamin K antagonist that is often used for long-term anticoagulation. Warfarin is generally contraindicated during pregnancy since it crosses the placenta. The concern is for warfarin embryopathy, and exposure between 6 and 12 weeks gestation could have potentially lethal effects (5,13,18). The most common manifestations of warfarin embryopathy include nasal hypoplasia and epiphyseal stippling (18). Other potential effects of warfarin exposure in utero include problems with limb hypoplasia, abnormal neurodevelopment and fetal coagulopathy (18). Women who are being treated with warfarin and contemplating pregnancy should typically be switched to UFH or LMWH prior to conception (5,18). Although warfarin may cross into breast milk, the amount is miniscule and it is considered safe to breast feed while taking warfarin (13,18).

One exception to warfarin use during pregnancy may be women who have mechanical heart valves and therefore high risk of thrombosis. The American College of Chest Physicians suggests using LMWH or UFH until the 13th week, thus decreasing the risk of warfarin embryopathy. After the 13th week, patients may be switched back to warfarin and subsequently resume UFH or LMWH close to delivery (18). Another acceptable approach for women who are on long-term warfarin is continuing the warfarin while attempting pregnancy with frequent pregnancy tests, ultimately switching to UFH or LMWH when a positive pregnancy result is achieved (18).

The initiation of therapy for a newly diagnosed VTE should be with either adjusted subcutaneous LWMH or adjusted dose UFH using an intravenous bolus and continuous infusion (1,5,18). If using UFH, the activated partial thromboplastin time (aPTT) should be followed to a therapeutic range (18). UFH may be considered for initial therapy if imminent delivery or surgery is a possibility. Otherwise, patients may be started on LMWH with plans for discharge from the hospital once anticoagulation has been established. It is important to note that both LMWH and UFH should be given at therapeutic doses in the event of an acute VTE. Anticoagulation should be continued until at least 6 weeks postpartum and for duration of 6 months for total therapy (18).

In rare situations, anticoagulation may be contraindicated. This would be the case with certain comorbidities such as HIT. An inferior vena cava filter may be considered as a preventive measure to protect against development of PE. In cases of HIT or if a heparin allergy exists, a pentasaccharide medication called fondaparinux may be considered for treatment. Danaparoid is another alternative, but is currently unavailable in the United States (5,18).

If an immediate life-threatening or potentially limb-threatening VTE is encountered, there is limited evidence that thrombolytics could be used. Potential safety concerns include risk of placental abruption, labor or fetal demise. If possible, immediate delivery should be delayed if thrombolytics are employed (1,5,18).

Considerations at Delivery

Special care with anticoagulation at the time of delivery must be considered. For patients who are treated with LMWH, the longer half-life may interfere with the ability to safely administer regional anesthesia depending on when the patients last dose of LMWH was given. The fact that LMWH is not readily reversible also must be considered; administration of LMWH prior to labor or delivery may result in safety concerns that would preclude the use of an epidural or spinal anesthetics. It is therefore often an accepted practice to switch a patient from LMWH to UFH at 36 weeks gestation. UFH has a shorter half-life, and, if needed, can be reversed with protamine sulfate.

It may also be prudent to consider scheduling an induction of labor after 39 weeks gestation in order to manage anticoagulation and reduce the risk of complications with regional anesthesia (5). If anticoagulation is interrupted for delivery, pneumatic compression stockings should be considered while the patient is in the hospital until anticoagulation can be resumed.

After delivery, anticoagulation should be resumed if clinically indicated. Many variables may influence the timing of when to restart anticoagulation therapy. The route of delivery, amount and control of postpartum bleeding and type of anesthesia used during delivery all should be considered prior to restarting anticoagulation. It is reasonable to restart LMWH 12 hours after delivery or removal of epidural catheter (1,5). Warfarin may be considered in the postpartum period, but it must be bridged with LMWH or UFH accordingly. LMWH or UFH should be started simultaneously with warfarin after delivery; labs that should be followed to ensure therapeutic levels for warfarin include a prothrombin time international normalized ration (INR) (22). Several days may be required to achieve therapeutic levels for warfarin, so if a patient desires to stay on LMWH or UFH for the duration of anticoagulation therapy that is a reasonable approach (1,5,18).

Thromboprophylaxis

As with anything in obstetrics and gynecology, prevention is the best medicine. Although many risk factors exist for the development of a VTE during pregnancy, some risk factors may carry more weight than others. Many guidelines have been established for anticoagulation thromboprophylaxis in pregnancy. Due to the early physiologic change of pregnancy, if anticoagulation therapy is warranted, early initiation of therapy is the best practice (5,18,21).

One broad category of patients to consider for anticoagulation is the cohort who has a personal history of VTE. As stated earlier, history of previous VTE seems to be the single most important risk factor for subsequent VTE. It is prudent to consider prophylactic doses of LMWH or UFH in those individuals with a previous VTE during pregnancy. The one exception may be women who had a VTE in the presence of a transient risk factor that no longer remains (5,18). Since the postpartum period seems to convey a greater risk of VTE, if a woman has had a previous VTE, it is generally recommended she receive anticoagulation therapy postpartum (5,18).

The other broad category of Ob/Gyn patients who may need thromboprophylaxis include women who possess risk factors for VTE during pregnancy, but do not have a personal history of VTE. In this group, the specific risk factor may drive the use of anticoagulation. Specifically, the presence and degree of thrombophilia, amount of immobilization, family history of VTE and obesity all must be considered. High-risk thrombophilias that typically require anticoagulation include antithrombin deficiency, individuals who are double heterozygous for both prothrombin G20210A mutation and factor V Leiden, factor V Leiden homozygous status, or prothrombin G 20210A homozygous status (5,9,12).

Since the risk of VTE seems to be higher in the postpartum period, thromboprophylaxis should be considered based on risk factors. At minimum, pneumatic compression stockings should be considered for patients immediately after vaginal delivery or cesarean section while these patients are in the hospital and temporarily immobile. Although routine thromboprophylaxis is not recommended after cesarean delivery, the American College of Clinical Pharmacy (ACCP) recommends all patients having a cesarean delivery receive a risk assessment for VTE done (18).

Other Considerations

There may be some evidence that suggests that a DVT during pregnancy increases the risk of a preterm delivery (23). It is possible that the risk factors associated with the development of a VTE during pregnancy influence other complications of pregnancy. Complications that are encountered during pregnancy, which that are also associated with thrombophilias include intrauterine growth restriction, preeclampsia, placental abruption, or fetal loss (12,15,16). Fetal antenatal surveillance may be indicated during prenatal care when these conditions are encountered (11,12).

Long-term consequences may arise from the development of VTE. After the postpartum period, sequelae such as venous stasis syndrome, post-thrombotic syndrome, chronic venous stasis and stasis dermatitis can be seen (24). Post-thrombotic syndrome can be seen in 25–50% of non-pregnant individuals with a VTE and may be higher in the pregnant population (8). One strategy for prevention of this complication includes the use of compression stockings (8).

Concluding Remarks

In pregnancy, the single most important risk factor for a new VTE remains a history of prior VTE. A missed diagnosis may have lethal consequences, so if a VTE is suspected, expeditious evaluation is warranted. Upon diagnosis, LMWH and UFH are the accepted treatments. The timing of anticoagulation at delivery needs to be approached carefully, mainly due to the risks with regional anesthesia and postpartum hemorrhage. After delivery, the postpartum period remains the highest risk timeframe for VTE and thromboprophylaxis should be considered in high risk patients. If a VTE is diagnosed, therapy should be continued for a minimum of 6 weeks postpartum and ideally for 6 months after the diagnosis of the VTE is made.

References

1. Marik, P. E. (2010). "Venous thromboembolism in pregnancy." *Clin Chest Med* 31(4): 731–740.
2. Marshall, A. L. (2014). "Diagnosis, treatment, and prevention of venous thromboembolism in pregnancy." *Postgrad Med* 126(7): 25–34.
3. Krivak, T. C. and K. K. Zorn (2007). "Venous thromboembolism in obstetrics and gynecology." *Obstet Gynecol* 109(3): 761–777.
4. Heit, J. A., C. E. Kobbervig, A. H. James, T. M. Petterson, K. R. Bailey and L. J. Melton, 3rd (2005). "Trends in the incidence of venous thromboembolism during pregnancy or postpartum: A 30-year population-based study." *Ann Intern Med* 143(10): 697–706.
5. James A. (2011). ACOG Practice Bulletin 123: Thromboembolism in Pregnancy. *Obstetrics and Gynecology* 118 (3): 718–29.
6. Rudolph L.K. Virchow. (1998). *Thrombosis and Emboli.* Translated by Axel C Matzdorff and William R. Bell. Canton, MA: Science History Publications/USA.
7. Mackman, N. (2012). "New insights into the mechanisms of venous thrombosis." *J Clin Invest* 122(7): 2331–2336.
8. Barco, S., M. Nijkeuter and S. Middeldorp (2013). "Pregnancy and venous thromboembolism." *Semin Thromb Hemost* 39(5): 549–558.

9. Silver R, and Lockwood C. (2016). "Thrombosis, thrombophilia, and thromboembolism." *Clin Updates Women Health Care* XV (3): 5–19.

10. Chunilal, S. D. and S. M. Bates (2009). "Venous thromboembolism in pregnancy: Diagnosis, management and prevention." *Thromb Haemost* 101(3): 428–438.

11. James, A. H. (2008). "Thromboembolism in pregnancy: Recurrence risks, prevention and management." *Curr Opin Obstet Gynecol* 20(6): 550–556.

12. ACOG Practice Bulletin 138: Inherited Thrombophilias in Pregnancy. *Obstet Gynecol* 2013. 122(3): 706–717.

13. Greer, I. A. (2015). "Clinical practice. Pregnancy complicated by venous thrombosis." *N Engl J Med* 373(6): 540–547.

14. Stedman TL. (2000). *Stedman's Medical Dictionary*: New York: Lipincott Williams & Wilkins;.

15. Miyakis S, Lockshin MD, Atsumi T, Branch DW, Brey RL, Cervera R, Derksen RHWM, de Groot PG, Koike T, Meroni PL, Reber G, Shoenfeld Y, Tincani A, Vlachoyiannopoulos PG, and Krilis SA. (2006). International consensus statement on an update of the classification criteria for defintie antiphospholipid syndrome (APS). *J Thromb Haemost* 4: 295–306.

16. ACOG Practice Bulletin 132: Antiphospholipid syndrome. *Obstet Gynecol*, 2012; 120 (6): 1514–1521.

17. Chan, W. S. (2010). "Venous thromboembolism in pregnancy." *Expert Rev Cardiovasc Ther* 8(12): 1731–1740.

18. Bates, S. M., I. A. Greer, I. Pabinger, S. Sofaer and J. Hirsh (2008). "Venous thromboembolism, thrombophilia, antithrombotic therapy, and pregnancy: American College of Chest Physicians Evidence-Based Clinical Practice Guidelines (8th Edition)." *Chest* 133(6 Suppl): 844s–886s.

19. Bagaria, S. J. and V. B. Bagaria (2011). "Strategies for diagnosis and prevention of venous thromboembolism during pregnancy." *J Pregnancy* 2011: 206858.

20. Gherman, R. B., T. M. Goodwin, B. Leung, J. D. Byrne, R. Hethumumi and M. Montoro (1999). "Incidence, clinical characteristics, and timing of objectively diagnosed venous thromboembolism during pregnancy." *Obstet Gynecol* 94(5 Pt 1): 730–734.

21. Bates, S. M., S. Middeldorp, M. Rodger, A. H. James and I. Greer (2016). "Guidance for the treatment and prevention of obstetric-associated venous thromboembolism." *J Thromb Thrombolysis* 41(1): 92–128.

22. Chappell, JC., G. Dickinson, M.I. Mitchell, H. Haber, Y. Jin and E.D. Lobo (2012). "Evaluation of methods for achieving stable INR in healthy subjects during a multiple-dose warfarin study." *Eur J Clin Pharmacol* 68: 239–247.

23. Heit, J. A. (2006). "The epidemiology of venous thromboembolism in the community: implications for prevention and management." *J Thromb Thrombol* 21(1): 23–29.

24. Ben-Joseph, R., A. Levy, A. Wiznitzer, G. Holcberg, M. Mazor and E. Sheiner (2009). "Pregnancy outcome of patients following deep venous thrombosis." *J Matern Fetal Neonatal Med* 22(4): 332–336.

Disability in Pregnancy

Gwinnett M. Ladson, Kimberly R. Looney, and Sonia Jackson

Introduction

The Americans with Disabilities Act (ADA) of 1990 defines disability as a physical or mental impairment that substantially limits one or more major life activities. Up to 12% of reproductive age women have a physical, mental or sensory disability. Fifty-one percent of these disabilities are physical disabilities, according to the US Census supplement.

Actions not permissible under the ADA include denying goods or services because a person has a disability; offering unequal or separate benefits or segregated services; using eligibility or criteria or standards to screen out people with disabilities; and setting unnecessary rules that deny equal opportunity and excluding service animals.

Approximately one in every five women in the United States, with a prevalence of 11.7% among women of reproductive age, report that they have a disabling condition described as having difficulty with functional activities, activities of daily living, use of an assertive aid such as a wheelchair or crutches, or limitations in the ability to work at a job or around the house.[1]

Before the late twentieth century, people with disabilities were frequently isolated and marginalized in society. In 1990, the ADA was passed, increasing attention to the right of people with disabilities and prohibiting discrimination against people with disabilities in employment, transportation, public accommodation, communications, and governmental activities. Despite these efforts toward independence and inclusion in society, women with physical disabilities still face substantial barriers when trying to access health care. Both patients with and without insurance frequently express difficulty in accessing care secondary to difficulty with transportation, limited provider availability, lack of providers, acceptance of Medicaid patients, limited physical access to and within practitioners' offices, inconvenient hours of operation, communication barriers, and difficulties with diagnostic and other medical equipment that does not accommodate them.[2] Other barriers women face in access to health care face include physical conditions such as spinal cord injury (SCI), rheumatoid arthritis (RA), and multiple sclerosis (MS), leading to higher rates of abortion, miscarriages, cesarean sections, and lower usage of contraception.[3]

SCI, RA, and MS have low prevalence rates but are more common in the reproductive age group. Women with these physical conditions who become pregnant face similar issues and concerns as pregnant women without disabilities, but problems such as weight gain, fatigue, fluid retention, bladder dysfunction, and urinary tract infections, may be more serious.[1] An increased risk of adverse pregnancy outcomes is present in women with these physical conditions. These outcomes include, but are not limited to, increased rates of preterm births, low birth weight, and fetal growth restriction.[2] Due to the complications associated with these physical conditions that can affect pregnancy, pregnancy management in women with these physical conditions should include preconception counseling.[1]

Scope of the Problem

The most common causes of disability among women aged 18 or older are physical limitations attributable to arthritis or rheumatism, back or spine problems, and heart problems. Disability does not mean sickness. Women with disabilities face educational and economic barriers and unmet health needs. The main reasons are limited availability of providers and limited provider accessibility.[3]

The Title III ADA states "no individual shall be discriminated against on the basis of disability in the full and equal enjoyment of the goods, services, facilities, privileges, advantages of any public place of public accommodation."[4] It also mandates providing reasonable accommodations for workers with disabilities. In the original ADA, pregnancy-related conditions were often not considered disabilities.[5]

Sociodemographic analysis of women with disabilities show that they are more likely to be African American, have lower educational attainment, be unemployed (or earn lower wages when employed), live alone, live in urban areas, or live in poverty.[6] African Americans and American Indian/Alaskan Natives have the highest disability rates. These women, in addition to their disabilities, experience racism, gender discrimination, and disregard.

Physicians caring for disabled women must perform pelvic examinations in a way that assures patient access, safety, and comfort. Adjustable tables that lower to the standard wheelchair height of 19 or 20 inches facilitate access for the examination. Handrails on either side of the table enhance safety and allow independent movement up or down the table. Alternative stirrups, particular padded boot stirrups, increase comfort for women with limited range of motion of the lower extremities. An assistant should attend each examination and when necessary, manually support lower extremities. Individually assistance with adduction/abduction and flexion/extension positioning may be indicated.

Barriers to health care procurement include difficulty with transportation, limited provider availability, limited physical accessibility to health care facilities, and difficulty with diagnostic and other medical equipment that does not accommodate people with a physical disability. Facilities should have access in all areas including disabled parking with clear signage posted at an appropriate height for drivers to see. Accessibility improvement for hospital or clinical departments include dropped reception desks, automatic doors, wide doorways, and tactile buttons at a height accessible for wheelchair users. Assistance should be provided, when needed or desired, to escort patients to other areas of the clinic or hospital especially if in a wheelchair or traveling long corridors. Wheelchairs should be maintained near entrances. Appropriate space for wheelchair users to pull up alongside seated companions should be provided. Flexible seating should also include furniture styled with and without armrests. To ensure confidentiality, separate cubicles should be used.

Selected Specific Disabilities

In the following section, the specific disabilities of SCI, RA, and MS are discussed in depth as example disabilities. The large number of different disabilities that affect pregnant women make it appropriate for clinicians to review the literature on specific disabilities for additional insight when caring for pregnant women with these issues.

Spinal Cord Injury

In women of childbearing age, SCI is usually a result of trauma such as motor vehicle accidents, falls down stairs, diving into shallow water and less commonly gunshot, or stab wounds. The result of the transection of the spinal cord is either paralysis of the lower extremities (paraplegia) or all four extremities (quadriplegia). Acute transection produces a flaccid paralysis and loss of sensation below the lesion. Initially the patient's condition is characterized by hypotension, bradycardia, and EKG abnormalities. The chronic state that follows is characterized by potential muscle rigidity, spasm, anemia, and recurrent urinary tract infections.

Women with SCI ideally should have preconceptual counseling. A thorough discussion includes possible medical complications during pregnancy and delivery and the impact on any preexisting co-morbidities should be reviewed. A preconception evaluation of the patient's renal, urologic, and pulmonary status should be performed. Delivery in a tertiary care center should be considered if the general obstetrician is not familiar with possible complications or there is a likelihood of a preterm delivery. Women with lesions above T6 or a high likelihood of autonomic hyperreflexia should be cared for in a setting with physicians familiar and experienced with taking care of this condition.

The majority of women with spinal cord injuries do not have problems with fertility.[6] The presence of a spinal cord injuries is not a contraindication to pregnancy. According to the National Spinal Cord Injury Statistical Center, there are approximately 52,000 women living with SCI in the United States with another 2,400 surviving acute traumatic injuries each year.[6] Data is limited on pregnancy outcome among women with SCI, but outcomes are generally favorable for mother and neonate.[7] The pregnant woman who presents to the emergency department with SCI should receive sedation and anesthesia, as needed, and should have adequate diagnostic and therapeutic procedures performed to ensure her safety and recovery.[8]

Women with SCI have pregnancies complicated by an increased number of urinary tract infections, including asymptomatic bacteria, anemia, and venous thrombosis. Increased bladder spasms, incontinence, and changes in normal urologic management occur in 9–25% of patients.[9,10] Obstetric outcomes include increased preterm birth, increased cesarean birth, increased infant low birth weights, and unrecognized labor.

Two serious and life-threatening complications are associated with SCI. A transection injury above T10 causes impairment and compromise of the cough reflex. This increases the risk for pneumonitis. Pulmonary impairment may also lead to requirements for ventilation support in late pregnancy and possibly while in labor. The second complication involves women with lesions above T5–T6 who are at risk for autonomic dysreflexia (hyperreflexia).

Autonomic Hyperreflexia

The most significant medical complication to which SCI patients are susceptible is autonomic hyperreflexia. Autonomic hyperreflexia (sometimes called dysreflexia) was first described by Head in 1917. It consists of pilomotor erection, excessive sweating, facial flushing, dilated pupils, sweating, severe headache, bradycardia, and severe paroxysmal hypertension.[11] Increased blood pressure can result in loss of consciousness and seizures if the stimulus is not removed. Inciting factors include stimulation of the skin below the cord lesion, bladder distension, fecal impaction, rectal examination, genital stimulation, or contraction of a hollow viscus including the gut and the uterus; these may bring about massive stimulus of the sympathetic nervous system.

Autonomic hyperreflexia occurs in up to 85% of patients with lesions above T5–T6.[12,13] Cases have been reported in the antepartum, intrapartum, and postpartum time periods.

Autonomic hyperreflexia is a syndrome of uncontrolled sympathetic discharge. Splanchnic vasoconstriction of the injury occurs above T5–T6. This response is usually secondary to noxious stimulation and could occur during a cervical or rectal exam, during labor and urinary catheterization. The resultant sympathetic stimulation can be life-threatening. Symptoms include throbbing headache, blurred vision, dangerous hypertension, facial flushing, sweating, and general apprehension.

Autonomic hyperreflexia can be treated by removal of the noxious stimulus, pharmacologic therapy, and regional and general anesthesia. Labetalol or Nifedipine can be used to control blood pressure. A consensus has developed that the most effective preventative and therapeutic approach for autonomic hyperreflexia in labor is regional anesthesia. The most common technique is continuous epidural anesthesia.[14–16]

Data on the risk of hypertensive disorders of pregnancy with SCI is unclear. Women with SCI above T5 have significantly lower baseline systolic blood pressure than women with lower lesions. It may be difficult to distinguish preeclampsia from autonomic hyperreflexia. An important distinction is that the hypertension of autonomic hyperreflexia occurs during contractions and returns to normal between them, whereas hypertension of preeclampsia is unrelated to uterine contractions.

Epidural anesthesia early in labor is recommended to decrease the occurrence of autonomic dysreflexia. Continuous monitoring of vital signs, blood pressure management, is indicated throughout intrapartum management. Cesarean section is performed for obstetrical indications. Breastfeeding is possible in women with SCI.

Decubitus Ulcers

Persons with SCI are considered to be at increased risk for development of decubitus ulcers when anemic.[12]

Decubitus ulcers are a preventable complication of SCI and should be equally preventable in pregnancy.[13] Weight gain in pregnancy may cause women to need a larger wheelchair to prevent abrasions and pressure sores.

Labor and Delivery Issues

The rate of preterm labor delivery may be slightly higher in women with SCI. The concern of an unattended delivery could be great and, therefore, close surveillance for preterm labor is warranted. Women with spinal cord injuries above T6 should be questioned about symptoms of intermittent "gas pains," abdominal tightening, and pelvic pressure during prenatal visits since they may not sense classic labor pain.

Cesarean section should be performed for obstetrical indications. The finding of a contracted pelvis, however, will be more common in patients with a long-standing injury resulting in pelvic deformation.

Vaginal delivery is a common cause of bladder dysfunction. Care should be taken in the SCI patient to avoid urine retention to prevent deterioration of bladder function and to minimize the risk of urinary tract infection and autonomic hyperreflexia.

Urinary Tract Infections

Asymptomatic bacteria during pregnancy increases the risk of pyelonephritis. Pyelonephritis itself causes a higher risk of sepsis and acute respiratory distress syndrome. Most cases of pyelonephritis can be prevented by treatment of asymptomatic bacteria. Pregnant SCI women are at risk for urinary tract infection due to incomplete bladder emptying. The presence of foreign bodies such as catheters contribute to bacteruria. It is reasonable to obtain frequent urine surveillance cultures and attempt to eradicate bacteria.

Sexual Issues

Modesty, discretion, and uneasiness may cause some providers to have difficulty initiating discussions about sexual concerns of women with SCI.[17] Although increased information regarding sexual issues of women with SCI now exists, society and some health care providers may still perceive these women as asexual, weaker, and passive. Fertility following SCI returns to normal after a temporary period of amenorrhea. Interestingly, there is generally more literature regarding effects of SCI on pregnancy than on sexuality issues such as body image, orgasm, sexual function, and self-esteem. It is important to support women in their adjustment of SCI and to acknowledge and view sexuality counseling as necessary.

Contraception for SCI

Women with SCI may retain fertility therefore appropriate contraception should be discussed and prescribed unless contraindicated. Some concern may exist regarding increased risk of venous thromboembolism when hormonal contraceptives containing estrogens are considered when the patient has limited mobility.

Rheumatoid Arthritis

Women are affected with RA three times more often than men. RA is an autoimmune inflammatory arthritis with a prevalence of one percent worldwide. Numerous studies show that 50–75% of RA patients demonstrate improvement in their disease,[18] but worsening may occur. It has been reported that when symptoms of RA improve during pregnancy they generally return or worsen 3–4 months postpartum. Pregnancy outcomes in women with RA are generally good; no obvious adverse effects of RA pregnancy outcome, including preterm labor, are known. Rheumatoid nodules, composed of a local proliferation of small vessels, histocytes, fibroblasts, and other cells, are present in 20–30% of the affected patients.

RA is a debilitating disease involving chronic inflammatory arthritis of the synovial joints. It has an incidence of 2.5–7 per 10,000 per year and a prevalence of approximately one percent in the adult US population. As with most autoimmune conditions, it is more common in women than in men with a ratio of 2–3 female to one male. The most common initial symptoms are morning stiffness, pain, and swelling of peripheral joints. Fatigue, weakness, weight loss, and malaise can also be common findings. The disease primarily involves the joints of the wrists, knees, shoulders, and metacarpophalangeal joints. In an erosive arthritis that usually follows a slowly progressive course marked by exacerbations and remissions. It can cause serious and severe joint destruction leading to permanent disability. Criteria for classification of RA are seen in Box 52.1.

For a majority of patients, the improvement begins in the first trimester, when the patient notices less joint stiffness and pain.[19] Peak improvement occurs in the second and third trimesters. Although an overall improvement of symptoms occur, the clinical course of RA in pregnancy is characterized by short-term fluctuations in symptoms. Most, but not all patients who experience an improvement in RA during pregnancy have similar symptoms in subsequent pregnancies. No lab or clinical features predict improvement of RA in pregnancy. In some patients, the disease worsens. Nearly three-quarters of patients with improvement will suffer a relapse in the first postpartum months.[19,20]

The mechanism by which pregnancy favorably affects RA is unknown. Plasma cortisol, rising during pregnancy and peaking at term, was initially thought to be the source of the amelioration of RA.[18] Some studies suggest estrogen or estrogens and progesterone favorably affect arthritis.[20]

About 15–25% of pregnancies in women with RA end in miscarriage, which is consistent with the normal population of women.[21]

Box 52.1 Criteria for classification of rheumatoid arthritis

Criteria	Definition
1. Arthritis of hand joints	At least one area swollen in a wrist, MCP or PIP joint
2. Arthritis of three or more joint areas	Soft tissue observed by a physician in at least three joint areas concurrently having had soft tissue swelling or fluid (not bony overgrowth alone). The 14 possible areas are right or left PIP, MCP, wrist, elbow, knee, ankle, and MTP joints.
3. Morning stiffness	Stiffness in and around the joints during morning, lasting at least one hour before maximal improvement.
4. Radiographic changes	Inclusive but not limited to osteoarthritis changes are radiographic changes typical of rheumatoid arthritis on posteroanterior hand and wrist radiographs. This will include erosions or unequivocal bony decalcification localized in or most marked contiguous to the involved joints.
5. Rheumatoid nodules	Rheumatoid nodules are internal nodules, over bony bulges or extensor surfaces or in juxta articular regions observed by a physician.
6. Serum rheumatoid	Abnormal amounts of serum rheumatoid factor by any method for which the result has been positive in <5% of normal control subjects.
7. Symmetric arthritis	Simultaneous involvement of the same joint areas (as defined in #2) on both sides of the body. Bilateral of certain joints is acceptable (bilateral involvement of PIPs, MCPs, or MTPs is acceptable without absolute symmetry).

For classification purposes, a patient shall be said to have RA if he/she has satisfied at least four of these seven criteria. Criteria 1 through 3 and 7 must have been present for at least 6 weeks. Patients with two clinical diagnoses are not excluded. Designation as classic, definite, or probable rheumatoid arthritis is *not* to be made.

Abbreviations: MCP, metacarpophalangeal joint; MTP, metatarsophalangeal joint; PIP, proximal interphalangeal joint.

A woman with RA should have a preconception visit to discuss the state of her disease and to reduce or change maintenance medications so as to avoid fetal risks. Routine prenatal care is usually sufficient; patients with persistent symptoms may, however, require more attention and care by a rheumatologist. Rest is an important part of the management. Physical therapy may be helpful in those patients whose disease does not improve with pregnancy. Vaginal delivery is not precluded in those patients with severe hip disease or hip replacement, although the obstetrician should prepare the labor and delivery team to assist with leg placement given the limitations of the patient's hips and legs during delivery.

If at all possible, an attempt should be made to manage RA with acetaminophen and low-dose glucocorticoids. Patients who conceive on other medications may need medication changes. Concerning medications include methotrexate and leflunomide, which are both teratogenic and associated with fetal death.

Contraception for RA

All forms of reversible contraception are appropriate. Some may improve symptoms.

Breastfeeding

Breastfeeding is not contraindicated. Pikwer et al. reported a significant reduction in the risk of subsequent arthritis in women who breastfed for more than 12 months.[22] Low-dose prednisone (less than 20 mg/day) is considered safe while breastfeeding.

Multiple Sclerosis

MS is an autoimmune disorder that leads to demyelization of the white matter of the brain. Demyelization results from T-cell mediated autoimmune destruction of oligodendrocytes that synthesize myelin. Two-thirds of individuals with MS are women of childbearing age. The majority of cases are considered relapsing and remitting. Flare rates have been reported to decline during pregnancy, especially during the third trimester and increase transiently during the postpartum period.

There are four different types of multiple sclerosis[23]:

1. Relapsing-remitting MS accounts for 85% of the affected individuals.
2. Secondary progressive MS is a relapsing-remitting disease that begins to pursue a progressive downhill course after each relapse.

3. Primary progressive MS accounts for 15% of cases. It is characterized by gradual progression of disability from the time of initial diagnosis.
4. Progressive-relapsing MS refers to primary progressive MS with apparent relapses.

Common presenting symptoms include weakness of one or both lower extremities, visual complaints, and loss of coordination.

Flares during pregnancy often decline, most markedly in the third trimester[23] and increase transiently during the first three months postpartum. Postpartum flares can be severe and occur in almost 30 percent of women within 3 months.[23] Pregnancy in MS does not appear to adversely affect the long-term course of the disease and may decrease the risk of conversion from a relapsing remitting to a progressive one.[24]

The effect of MS on pregnancy outcome includes increased risk of fetal growth restriction, antenatal hospitalization, and cesarean delivery.

Concluding Remarks

Women with disabilities identify with a disability culture similar to cultural identities of other minority groups. Attitudinal barriers exist between women with disabilities and health care providers.[25]

Other barriers are barriers of assumption. It should not be assumed that the disability exclusively defines the patient's health care needs as she cannot make medical decisions. In addition, physicians must not assume that a woman with physical or intellectual disabilities cannot give informed consent or parent a child.[25]

Providers should become familiar with resources available to care for women with special disabilities and anticipate special needs, if required, of equipment and assistance needed to perform gynecological and obstetrical examinations.

Women with physical disabilities have the same women's health care needs as all women. As with women without disabilities, women with disabilities do desire pregnancy and a healthy outcome. A disabled woman can experience pregnancy as a rewarding experience even though she is faced with misperceptions when pregnant with her disability. Disabled women are met with many social biases when pregnant and often assumed to be considered high-risk pregnancies or even presumed to be in need of extra genetic counseling.[26]

Health care providers are encouraged to improve their knowledge in regard to preconception counseling, antepartum care, postpartum care, and most importantly attitudes in regard to women with disabilities who desire pregnancy. Providers and their staff are also encouraged to respect the expertise that each individual patient has acquired in the process of managing her disability. The development of local advocacy to support health equity for women with disabilities is appropriate.

References

1. JM Thierry. The importance of preconception care for women with disabilities. *Matern Child Health J* 2006 Sep;10(5 Suppl):S175–6. Epub 2006 Jul 19. No abstract available.
2. SC Smeltzer. Pregnancy in women with physical disabilities. *J Obstet Gynecol Neonatal Nurs* 2007 Jan–Feb;36(1):88–96. Review. Erratum in: *J Obstet Gynecol Neonatal Nurs* 2007 Mar–Apr;36(2):table of contents. Dosage error in article text.
3. M Redshaw, R Malouf, H Gao, R Gray. Women with disability: The experience of maternity care during pregnancy, labour and birth and the postnatal period. *BMC Pregnancy Childbirth* 2013 Sep 13;13:174. doi: 10.1186/1471-2393-13-174.
4. Americans with Disabilities Act of 1990 (ADA, P.L. 101-226).
5. R Jackson, S Gardner, M Torres. My obstetrician got me fired. *Obstet Gynecol* 2015 Aug;126(2):250–54.
6. A multicenter study of women's self-reported reproductive health after spinal cord injury. *Arch Phys Med Rehab* 1999; 80: 1420–8.
7. R Turk, M Turk, V Assejev. The female paraplegic and mother-child relations. *Paraplegia* 1983 Jun;21(3):186–91.
8. E Baker, D Cardenas. Pregnancy and spinal cord injured women. *J Arch Phys Med Rehabil* 1966;77:501–7.
9. MB Wanner, CJ Rageth, GA Zach. Pregnancy and autonomic hyperreflexia to patients with spinal cord injury. *Paraplegia* 1987; 25: 482–90.
10. MJ Aminoff. Urologic disorders in pregnancy. *Am J Obstet Gynecol* 1978; 132: 325–35.
11. H Head, , G Riddoch. The automatic bladder, excessive sweating and some other reflex conditions in gross injuries of the spinal cord. *Brain* 1917; 40: 188–263.
12. M Nath, J Vivian, W Cherry. Autonomic hyperreflexia in pregnancy and labor: A case report. *Am J Obstet Gynecol* 134: 390–2.

13. AG Timomey, PJ Shaw. Urological outcome in female patients with spinal cord injury, the effectiveness of intermittent catherization. *Paraplegia* 1990 Nov; 28: 556–63.
14. JA McGregor, J Meeuwsen, Autonomic hyperreflexia: A mortal danger for spinal cord-damaged women in labor. *Am J Obstet Gynecol* 1985 Feb 1;151(3):330–3.
15. R Lindan, E Lehler, A Freehafer, AM Lyons, H Colretta, Further experience with Nifrdipine in the treatment of autonomic dysreflexia. *Asia Bull* 1986;4:10–15.
16. SS Porter. Anesthesic management of the patient with spinal cord injury. *Kansas Med* 1988 Nov: 299–304.
17. S Charlifue,M Gerhart. Sexual issues of women with spinal cord injuries. *Paraplegia* 1992;30:192–9.
18. PS Hench. The ameliorating effect of pregnancy on chronic atrophic (infectious) rheumatoid arthritis, fibrosis and intermittent hydrarthritis. *Proc Mayo Clin* 1938;13:161.
19. RH Persellini. The effect of pregnancy on rheumatoid arthritis. *Bull Rheum Dis* 1977;27:922.
20. M Ostenen, G Husby. A prospective clinical study of the effect of pregnancy on rheumatoid arthritis and ankylosing spondylitis. *Arthritis Rheum* 1983;26:1155.
21. D Kaplan. Fetal wastage in patients with rheumatoid arthritis. *J Rheumatol* 1987;13:857.
22. M Pikwer, U Bergstrom, JA Nilsson, et al. Breast feeding, but not use of oral contraceptives, is associated with a reduced risk of rheumatoid arthritis. *Ann Rheum Dis* 2009 Apr;68(4):526–30.
23. S Vukusic, M Hutchinson, M Hours, T Moreau, P Cortinovis-Tourniaire, et al. Pregnancy and multiple sclerosis (the PRIMS study): Clinical predictors of post-partum relapse. *Brain* 2004 Jun; 127(Pt 6):1353–60.
24. B Runmarker, O Andersen. Pregnancy is associated with a lower risk of onset and a better prognosis in multiple sclerosis. *Brain* 1995 Feb; 118 (Pt 1):253–61.
25. American College of Obstetricians and Gynecologist. Access to reproductive healthcare for women with disabilities. In *Special Issues in Women's Health*. Washington, DC: ACOG; 2005, pp. 39–59.
26. EE Andrews. Pregnancy with a physical disability: One' psychologist's journey. American Psychological Association. *Spotlight on Disability* Newsletter, Dec 2011. Retrieved online from www.apa.org/pi/disability/resources/publications/newsletter/2011/12/pregnancy-disability.aspx. Accessed March 10, 2016.

The History of Obstetrics

George H. Davis

Introduction

Obstetrics (ŏb-stĕt'rĭks): The branch of medicine that deals with the care of women during pregnancy, childbirth, and the recuperative period following delivery.[1] The science of midwifery.[2]

The origins of the term *obstetrics* as a noun is relatively modern, dating to the early nineteenth century and owing its derivation from the adjective "obstetrical," first appearing in the literature in the mid-eighteenth century.[3] The term is derived from the Latin: *ob-* in front of, facing, *stet* combining form of the verb *stare* to stand, and *-trix* a woman. In other words, the term means a woman who stands in front of, or more simply, a midwife. This is understandable since childbirth, until very recently in the fifty thousand centuries of human existence, has been the province of women, and mostly lay women. Witkowski, in his classic work of 1887 *Histoire des Accouchements chez tous les Peuples*[4] (*History of Deliveries in All Peoples*), provides descriptions and illustrations of obstetrical practice throughout the known world at that time. Virtually without exception, the attendants are women (Figures 53.1 and 53.2).

The Beginnings

The dawn of obstetrical practice is shrouded in mystery. In prehistory, some women must have become more adept at facilitating childbirth and passed their knowledge orally through the generations. With the advent of recorded history, women were excluded from education and so little was written down. A very early written reference is found in the Hebrew Bible.[5] Hippocrates (460–370BC) appears to have had little, if any, understanding of normal midwifery practice.[6]

The first real source books for obstetrics and gynecology are attributed to Soranus of Ephysis (circa AD 98–138). His books on the diseases of women and reproductive anatomy became the standard texts on the subject for the next 1,500 years. At least one English translation is available today.[7] Soranus described podalic version, breech delivery, and care of the newborn. His observations in the field of gynecology almost certainly took advantage of earlier forms of the vaginal speculum.

The Middle Ages

During the Middle Ages, the art of medicine was more advanced in the Arab world than in Europe. The writings of two Arabian obstetricians, Avicena of Bokhara, near the Caspian Sea, and Albucasis of Cordova, Spain, both from the late tenth and early eleventh centuries AD, describe forceps deliveries. Some historians have tried to say that portions of these writings imply possible conservative extractions. The illustrations and diagrams within Albucasis quickly reveal, however, that these forceps, with their fixed articulations and multiple teeth, could not have been used on a living child. These instruments were not dissimilar to the destructive examples uncovered at Pompeii and were undoubtedly used for the extraction of the dead fetus.

Since manuscripts were rare and very expensive, it is doubtful that the lay midwives would have had access to these documents, especially since they were written in Latin. The first real advance in general codification of obstetrical practice came with the invention of the printing press circa 1440. In 1513 Eucharius Rösslin published *Rosengarten*, the first known printed treatise on midwifery. It was little more than a translation of Soranus's text from the Latin into German for the benefit of the local midwives over whom he had charge. Over the next several decades, it was translated into many different languages including Dutch (1516), French (1536), and eventually English (1540) by Richard Jonas. The English translation was issued with the better known title *The Byrth of Mankynde*.[8]

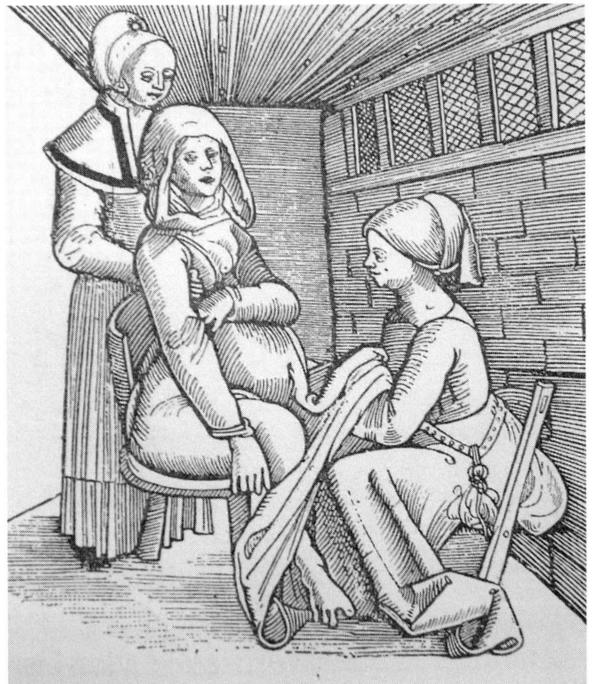

Figure 53.1 Midwifery delivery utilizing a birthing stool.

Five years later, it was reissued as a "newly set furth, corrected and augmented" version by Thomas Raynold, phisition, changing the title. *The Woman's Boke* by Thomas Raynod was a revision of these previous works, and yet another revision appeared in English in 1637 under the title of *The Expert Midwife*.[9] These two books remained the mainstay of obstetrical practice until at least the end of the seventeenth century, but it is worth noting the basis for all of these books was the work of Soranus from the second century AD.

The Renaissance

Even with the wider availability of obstetrical texts, accoucheurs were still encumbered with a very poor understanding of anatomy, in general, and especially of the female genital tract, in particular. This was because of a continued reliance on the writings and teachings of Galen (129 to c. 216 AD). Galen's teachings in anatomy were based on dissection of monkeys and pigs and most of his descriptions of female pelvic anatomy were erroneous.

Galenic anatomy was held as gospel until at least 1543 when Vesalius published *De humani corporis fabrica*.[10] The anatomic drawings of Vesalius were not widely accepted; Vesalius was forced to give up his post at Padua and return to his native Belgium due to his "heresy."

Human anatomical dissection is known to have been done by Greek physicians as early as the third century BC, but this practice was widely discouraged during the Roman era. Arabic physicians held prominence for the next 500 years. There are accounts of human dissection by these physicians. Although Shari'ah law does not specifically proscribe human dissection, the precepts of Islamic faith strongly discourage it. Throughout Europe, the practice was either discouraged or outlawed, in some counties until as late as the sixteenth century.

We owe most of the credit for a departure from taboos against human dissection to the artistic community of the Renaissance. It was these men who undertook the most serious study of human anatomy. And while most were concerned with the musculature and bone structure, a few, most notably Leonardo da Vinci (1452–1519), carried this study to the internal organs of the body.[11] Two of his most famous sketches depict with accuracy the female pelvic anatomy and the gravid uterus.

Vesalius's classic work of 1543, *De humani corporis fabrica*, is a monumental work encompassing seven volumes. It provided the first extensive look at female pelvic anatomy based on human dissection, He demonstrated the uterus as a single, pear-shaped organ, but the drawing suggests a sub-septate conformation. Given that this is a common variation, it is quite possible that this was what he found in the single reproductive aged woman he studied.

When Vesalius was run out of town, he was succeeded by his disciples. One former student, Gabrielle Fallopio (1523–1562), continued his mentor's practice of human dissection and became the first to provide a clear description of the uterus, tubes, and ovaries along with their associated ligaments and vascular supply. His name lives on eponymously in the Fallopian tubes. He was also the first to provide an accurate description of the vagina and the placenta.

Scipione Mercurio (1540–1616) wrote the first compendium of midwifery for Italian midwives. In it he covers prenatal care, management of difficult labors, and post-partum care of both the mother and the baby. Mercurio was among the first to advocate cesarean delivery for those women with a contracted pelvis. He even claimed to have seen two women who survived the operation.

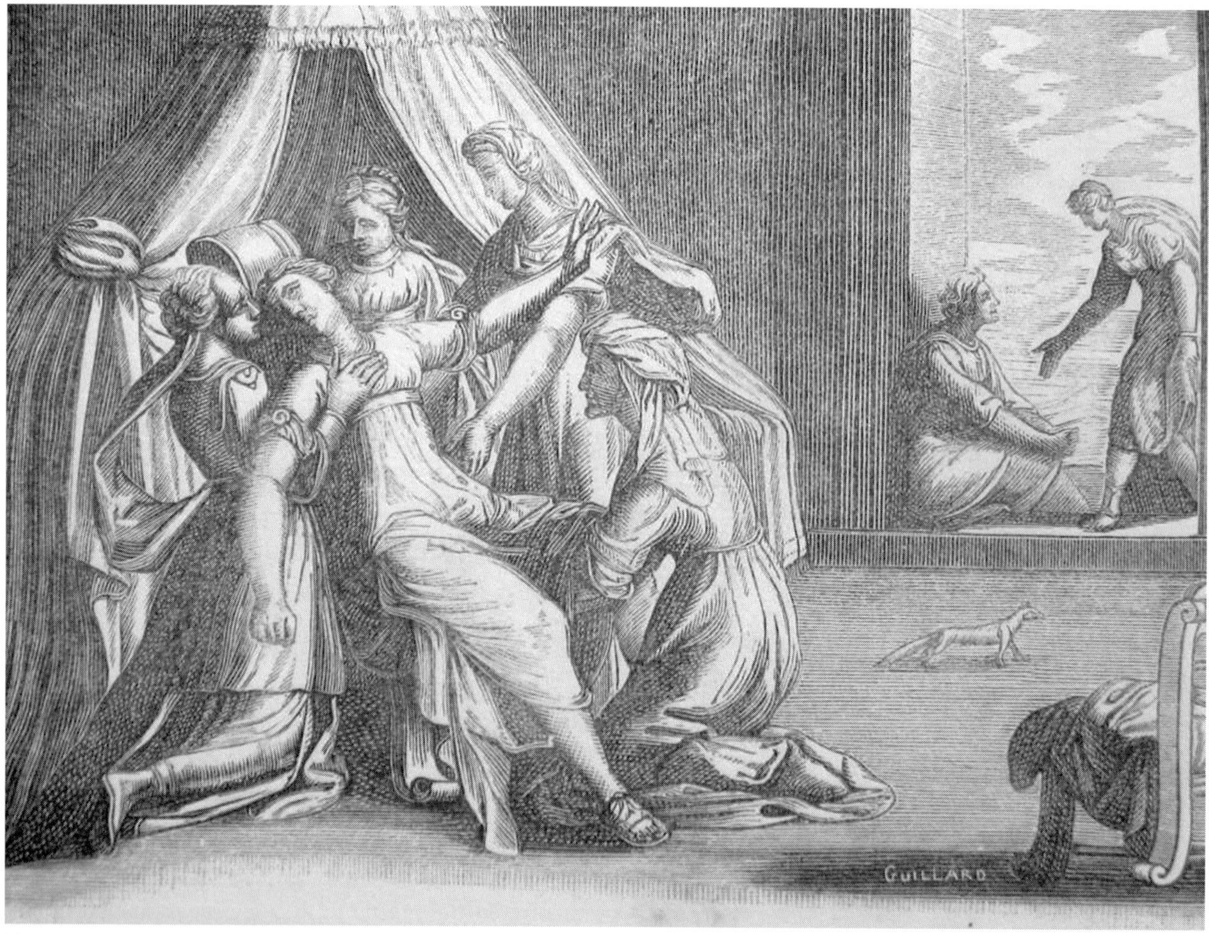

Figure 53.2 The birth of Helen of Troy.

William Hunter, coming after the Renaissance, published the best known atlas of pregnancy, *The Anatomy of the Human Gravid Uterus*, in 1774. An example from his text is seen in Figure 53.3.

The Hôtel-Dieu

The Hôtel-Dieu was founded in 651 and was the first hospital to be opened in Paris. It is now the oldest hospital in the world that is still in operation and is believed to house the first hospital wing anywhere dedicated as a lying-in ward for pregnant women.

In the 1500s, conditions were deplorable by today's standards. Its 1,200 beds were always overflowing with a daily census that often exceeded 2,000. Bed sharing was typical, with two patients to a bed commonplace. It was not unusual to find the living and the dead side by side. Mortality rates were in the realm of 20%, which was not surprising given the lack of sanitation. Until more modern times, there was an entrance right on the River Seine where boats could pull up to discharge patients. The river, at that time, was largely a sewage discharge canal and a constant source of infection. This was the institution that became a major source of education for midwives and surgeons of the era. (The institution is seen in Figure 53.4.)

In the hierarchy of the day, on the lowest rung were the barber-surgeons. These men were basically nothing more than skilled technicians. Above them were the master surgeons. These were educated men who jealously guarded their station through their organization, the College de Saint Come. Ironically, these master surgeons relegated most of the procedures, however, to the barber-surgeons as they considered most of the commonplace operations, including obstetrical interventions, to be beneath their dignity. At the top were the physicians, men with a formal

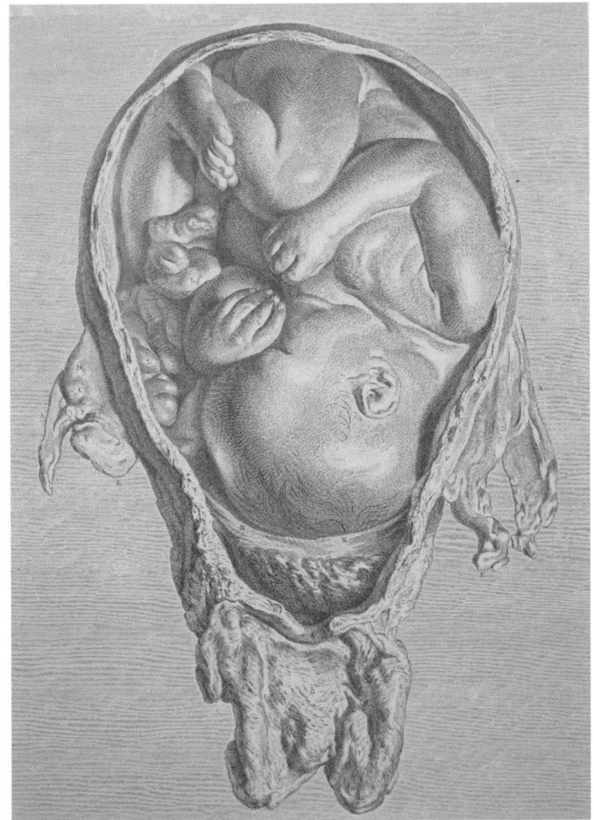

Figure 53.3 Placenta previa.

medical education for whom any invasion of the body was an anathema. The physicians directed the medical care with the master surgeons and barber-surgeons doing their bidding.

It was at the Hôtel-Dieu that Ambrose Paré (1510–1590) arrived when he was twenty-three years old. Starting as an apprentice barber-surgeon, he gained exposure to all aspects of surgery, including obstetrical interventions. He served three years as the resident surgeon amassing a wealth of experience. He then joined the army. As a result of his military service, he gained a reputation for both his skill and compassion. He was then elevated to the status of surgeon to the king, serving both Francis I and Henri II.

It was during this extended period of military service that the College de Saint Come, desirous of having such a pre-eminent surgeon in their midst (and probably to curry the favor of the king), invited him to sit for examination as a physician. Since Paré did not know Latin, accommodations were made, turning it essentially into a farce.[12] Today Paré is considered the father of modern surgery.

Paré wrote a number of books. In one particular volume (1549), he addressed the technique of internal podalic version, advocating its use in difficult deliveries, obstetrical hemorrhage, and placenta previa. Obstetrical forceps were yet to be invented. While breech delivery was well known and while internal version had previously been described, advocating its liberal use to speed up the delivery process no doubt saved many lives.

Louyse Bourgeois (1563–1626) was a French woman of at least upper middle class background as she had been taught to read and write. In 1684, at the age of twenty-one, she married Martin Boursier, an army surgeon, and quickly made the acquaintance of Ambrose Paré. She demonstrated an interest in midwifery and became Paré's most famous pupil. The lore of midwifery was still being handed down, to large extent, by tradition. She, however, studied the writings of Paré and undertook a much more systematic approach to learning the art. Being possessed of superior talent, skill, and intellect, she then sought to improve her station and reputation. She passed the certifying exam in 1598 and almost immediately began to attract clients among the wealthy.

In 1601 the young wife of Henry IV became pregnant. Bourgeois was appointed as the royal midwife in place of many rival midwives in the region.[13] Bourgeois became the first midwife to write a book on midwifery for midwives. Her first book, published in 1609, had a title two dozen words in length and is best known by its initial word, *Observations*. It quickly became a best seller as much for her vivid descriptions of the court intrigue surrounding the royal births as for its practical advice.[14] It was rapidly translated into many of the major European languages and remained the bible for lay midwives for the next century.

Bourgeois was able to provide sound practical advice for midwives in many areas including general advice, the management of normal labor, podalic version with breech extraction, ligation of the umbilical cord, and umbilical cord prolapse. Together with subsequent volumes published in 1617, 1626, and 1634, she elevated the craft of midwifery to a profession worthy of respect among physicians and barber-surgeons. The advice was structured with the goal to ensure that all women receive sound, appropriate, and compassionate care during childbirth.[15]

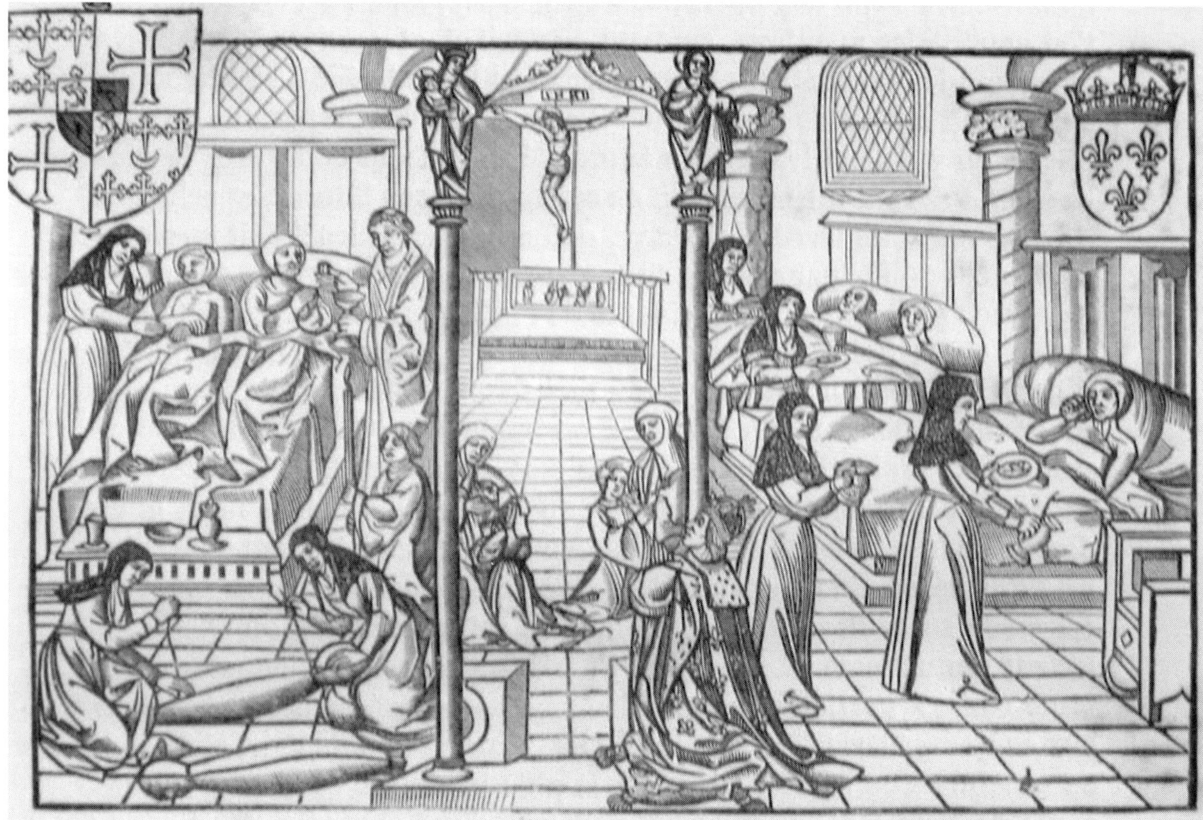

Figure 53.4 The interior of the Hôtel-Dieu.

François Mauriceau (1637–1709) was, without question, the most prominent obstetrician of the seventeenth century. He is known today as the father of modern obstetrics. After studying at the Hôtel-Dieu, at the age of only thirty-one, he published his seminal work *Traité des Maladies des Femmes Grosses et Accouchées* upon which his reputation rests to this day. His was first the original text on midwifery since that of Soranus. It likely did more to elevate the practice of obstetrics than any other effort to that time. The frontpiece of his book is seen in Figure 53.5.

Seminal among his instructions was the revision of how to do a breech delivery in which he advised bringing both arms down (in contrast to the teachings of Paré), placing a finger in the mouth to flex the head and bracing the neck with the opposite hand while an assistant held the already delivered body. This technique, which bears his name (Mauriceau-Smellie-Veit maneuver, or simply the Mauriceau maneuver), is still the way we deliver breeches today. His book was based on practical experience and the advice was realistic. He was also among the first to suture perineal lacerations, which went against all of the practical advice of the day.

Together with many of his colleagues at the Hôtel-Dieu, Mauriceau succeeding in making midwifery something that was worthy of, and within the province of, competent male surgeons. When Louis XIV called in Mauriceau's colleague Jules Clement to attend the delivery of his mistress in 1670, rather than a midwife, it gave credence and widespread recognition to the movement to make childbirth more scientific.

The Chamberlens and Their Legacy

The story of the Chamberlen family and the invention of the obstetrical forceps is a fascinating one, full of mystery and intrigue. The information is discussed in detail by Walter Radcliffe in *The Secret Instrument* from 1947.[16] His other major work is *Milestones in Midwifery.*[17]

Doctor William Chamberlen was a French Hugenot who fled religious wars in France. He fled

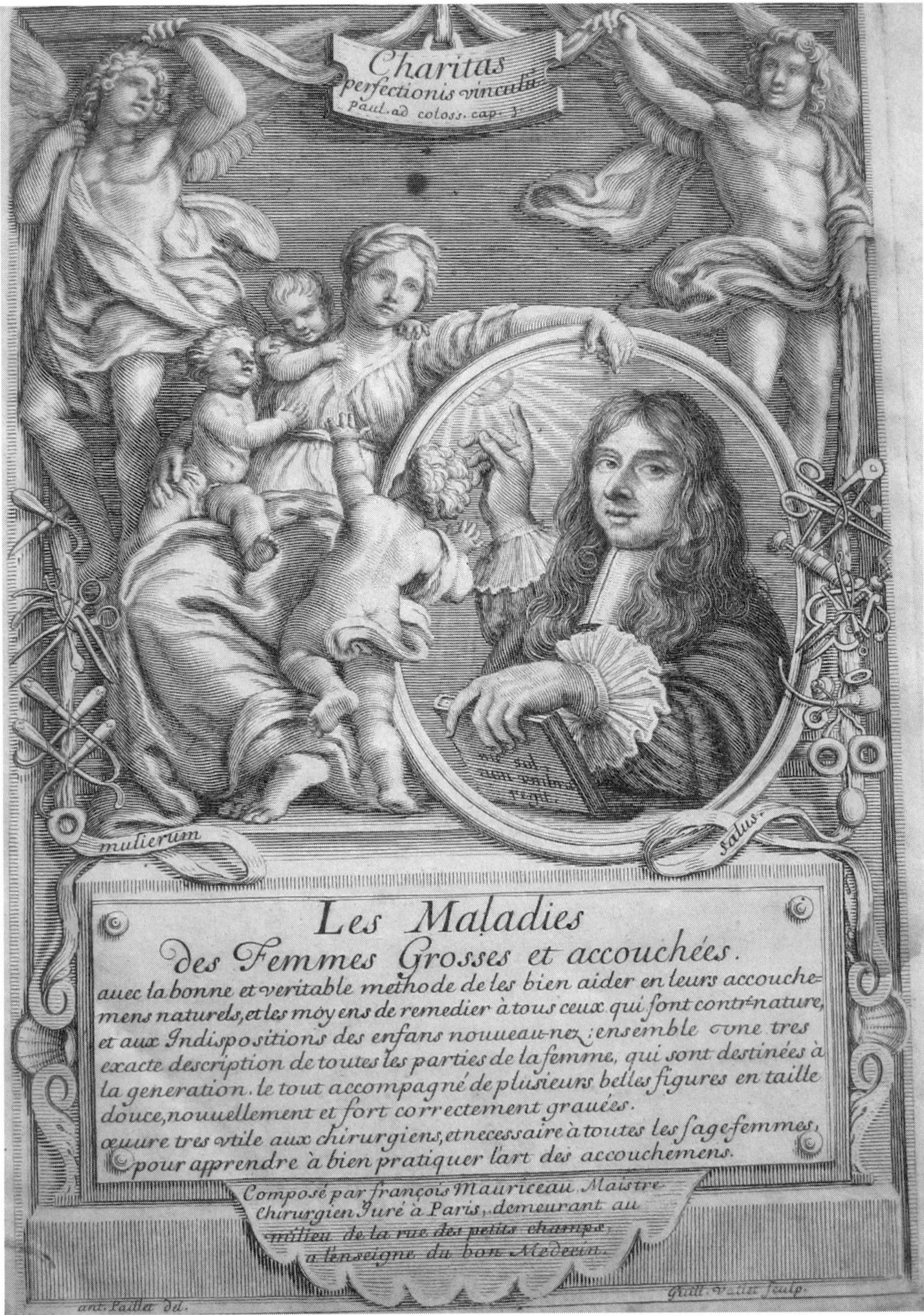

Figure 53.5 Frontispiece from Mauriceau (second edition, 1675).

to England with his wife and children in 1569. By all accounts, it was this family that developed the first pair of articulated obstetrical forceps, an instrument expressly designed for the delivery of a live-born infant. These forceps are seen in Figure 53.6.

William Chamberlen established a midwifery practice in Southampton and later moved to London. He was joined in this practice by his two sons, both of whom were named Peter. The Peters enjoyed widespread success. Although we will never know the exact

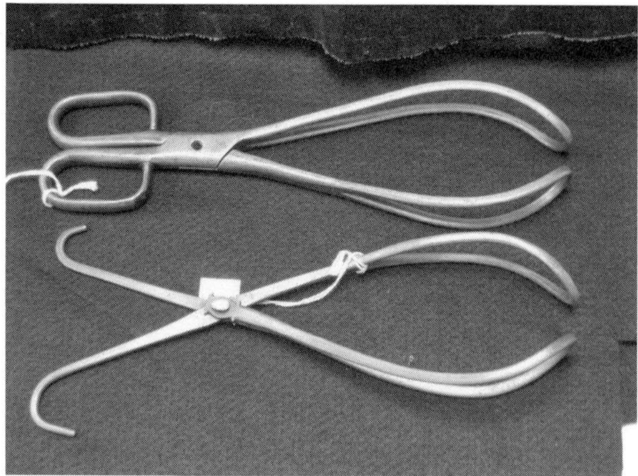

Figure 53.6 Chamberlen forceps.
(Courtesy of The Mütter Museum.)

story of how the forceps were conceived and invented, it is generally agreed that they were likely the brainchild of Peter the elder and served to further his reputation. Unfortunately, the Peters were frequently in trouble with the Royal College of Physicians for exceeding the limits of medical care generally ascribed to barber-surgeons. Peter the elder was actually imprisoned for a while, and his release was secured only by the intercession of the queen through the Archbishop of Canterbury.

Peter the younger had eight children, among them a son also named Peter. It was determined that this third Peter should get a formal medical education. He was sent off to Heidelberg and then to Padua where he received his doctor of medicine diploma at age eighteen. He returned to London and managed to become qualified as a doctor at both Oxford and Cambridge by the time his was twenty. He became a fellow of the Royal College of Physicians in 1628 at the age of twenty-seven.

Peter's son Hugh Chamberlen (1664–1728) became the fourth generation in the family to practice midwifery utilizing the family secret. He, like his father, earned his medical degree and also inherited the family penchant for getting trouble. The last two lines of an anonymous poem, circulated before Hugh Chamberlen escaped to the continent to avoid creditors, reads: "To give you his character truly compleat/He's a Doctor, Projector, Man-midwife and Cheat."[18]

To his credit, however, he was one of the few physicians who stayed in London through the Great Plague of 1665, and since he lived in a court just off the Old Bailey, he must have been right in the middle of the plague.

Hugh Chamberlen is perhaps best known for his attempt to sell the family secret to the French. When he approached Jules Clement in 1670 with request for 10,000 Crowns, he was not immediately dismissed out of hand. Rather, François Mauriceau agreed to put him to the test at the Hôtel-Dieu. The patient given for the demonstration was a rachitic dwarf whose pelvis was so small and deformed that a vaginal delivery by any means would have been impossible. Nevertheless, Hugh Chamberlen assured everyone that he could have her delivered within fifteen minutes. Three hours, later he admitted failure and left without having sold the secret.

Although unsuccessful in his attempts to sell the secret of the forceps, Hugh Chamberlen did return with a copy of Mauriceau's book, which he translated into English. Chamberlen credited the authorship to Mauriceau but added a preface in which he makes public that he and his family are in possession of "a Way to deliver Women in this Case, without any prejudice to them or their Infants."[19] He also added in his own criticisms and comments in the margins of the text throughout. This book went through no less than eight editions in English and remained a best-seller for almost a century. Hugh Chamberlain made more from the sale of this book in English than Mauriceau ever did in French. In fact, Mauriceau complained that Chamberlain had made £30,000, a figure that seems unlikely given that it would be roughly equivalent to $2 million today.

The fifth generation of Chamberlens, Hugh's son Hugh junior and two of his nephews, Chamberlen Walker and Middleton Walker, were the last Chamberlens to practice the art of midwifery and to share in the family secret. By the end of the careers, the secret had been revealed. Middleton Walker is credited with inventing the English lock, a modification that persists in many types of forceps to this day.

In 1813 the original Chamberlen forceps were discovered under the floorboards at Woodham Mortimer Hall in Essex. This is the home where both Hugh Chamberlen and his father Peter had resided.

It is not entirely known how the obstetrical forceps made their way into the armamentarium of practicing physicians, but there are many clues. It is known that Hugh Chamberlen sold some idea, probably that of the vectis, to Rogen van Roonhuysen, head of the council that governed the practice of midwifery. He, in turn, shared it with few of his closest council members. This council was charged with examining and licensing all those physicians wishing to practice midwifery. Over the next fifty to sixty years, anyone passing their examination was required to purchase the forceps, at great expense and under a vow of secrecy, before being granted a license to actually practice obstetrics.

The dawn of the golden age for obstetrical forceps really began with the introduction of Smellie's short forceps in England (1745) and Leveret's forceps, with their pelvic curve, in France (1747). From that point, and for the next two centuries, forceps designs proliferated, both throughout Europe and North America. Each design offered its own purported advantage and/or purpose. But from a practical standpoint, the basic design of the obstetrical forceps has not changed since Smellie and Leveret.

Sir Kedarnath Das was an Indian obstetrician and Professor of Obstetrics and Gynecology and Principal of the Carmichael Medical College in Calcutta. In 1929 he published a book on obstetrical forceps in which he described every known type of obstetrical forceps at that time in chronologic order.[20] He lists more 550 designs. Since this book was published, a number of other nineteenth-century models have come to light and, with the addition of twentieth-century designs; the total now stands closer to 700 unique styles.

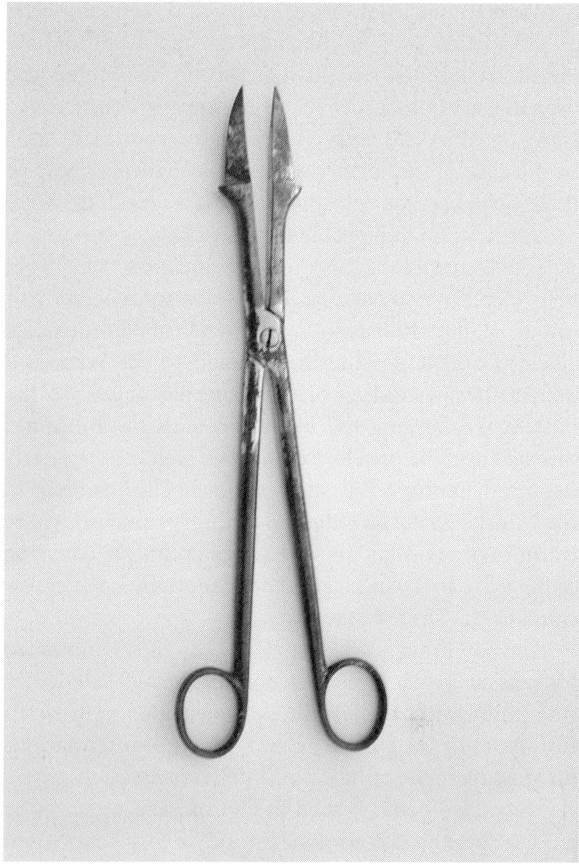

Figure 53.7 Smellie scissors used to incise fetal cranium; sharp edges are lateral.

Fetal destructive procedures

Destructive operations, referred to euphemistically as embryotomy, and destructive instruments have been a part of obstetrical care going back to biblical times. Destructive obstetrical instruments were recovered from the excavation of Pompeii, buried when Vesuvius erupted in AD 79. Instructions and indications for their proper use can be found in all manner of texts from Soranus to the twentieth century. The safety of pregnancy in this modern era has allowed both physicians and the public to forget that it was less than a century ago when pregnancy was more feared by women than embraced.

Active intervention has always been needed in cases of dissonance in fetal size and maternal pelvis to avoid maternal and or fetal death while trying to get the baby out. It was often said in the sixteenth to nineteenth centuries that if the doctor came, either the mother or the baby or both would die. Figures 53.7 and 53.8 are illustrations of instruments used in fetal destructive procedures.

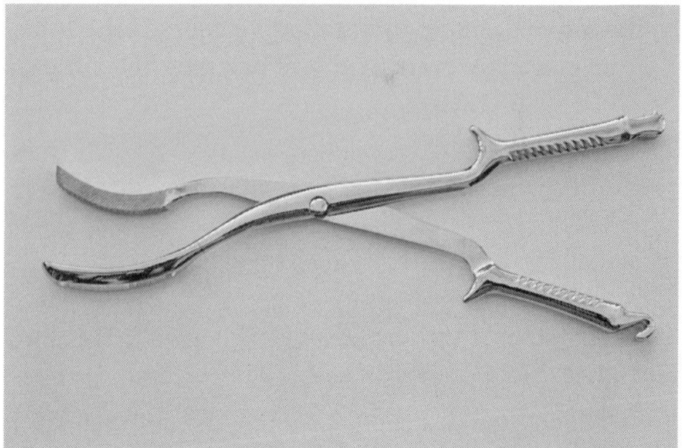

Figure 53.8 Illustration of cranioclast used to crush fetal head.

Safe cesarean delivery did not come about until the twentieth century. The common obstetrical practice, even into the early twentieth century, for indications such as fetal macrosomia, fetal demise, fetal malformations, malpresentation, and cephalopelvic disproportion was to decompress the head of any infant that could not fit through the mother's pelvis and then to use hooks, crochets, or crushing instruments to bring out the dead fetus. This was also frequently done in the case of malformations such as hydrocephaly or if the head became entrapped during a breech delivery.

Another major problem was rickets, a disease of defective mineralization or calcification of bones before epiphyseal closure. This is due to deficiency or impaired metabolism of vitamin D, phosphorus, or calcium and it potentially can lead to fractures and deformities, including of the maternal pelvis. In the past, it was among the most common of childhood diseases and the problem continued well into the early twentieth century. It is still a major health problem in the Middle East, secondary to malnutrition and where traditional women's dress requires complete covering of the skin. By 1945, rickets had essentially been eradicated in the United States.[21,22]

In 1839 Franz Carl Naegele (1778–1851) published his classic work, *The Obliquely Contracted Pelvis*.[23] In this publication he described, the various malformation types of the female pelvis with recommendations on management of labor and delivery in each case.[24] A contracted pelvis is seen in Figure 53.9.

One other less common historic disease bears mentioning as a cause of fetal descructive intervention during pregancy, as well as a major contributor to maternal mortality. Pott's disease, or spinal tuberculosis, is caused by vascular dissemination of the tuberculosis infection to the lower thoracic and lumbar vertebrae. The infection produced a severe kyphosis bringing the rib cage down to the pelvic brim and reducing the abdominal capacity. It also frequently led to severe spondylosis and paraplegia. Spinal abscesses were common.[25]

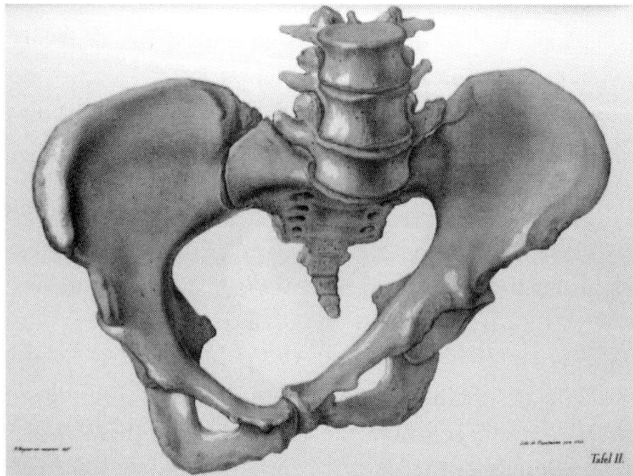

Figure 53.9 Obliquely contracted (rachitic) pelvis.

Cesarean Delivery

Abdominal delivery has its roots in antiquity with cultural references dating as far back as about 1000 BC in China and 320 BC in India. From Virgil's Aeneas to Shakespear's Macduff, poets have described individuals as having been "untimely ripped" from their mother's womb. In antiquity, abdominal delivery was almost always done as a post-mortem event, becoming more popular with the advent of Christianity so that the baby could be baptized. Neither Hippocrates nor Soranus make any mention of abdominal delivery.

Although origins of the term "Caesarean" are somewhat murky, the prevailing wisdom suggests that it is derived either from the Latin *caesus*, meaning cutting. While the first recorded use of the term "cesarean" delivery did not appear until 1581, it seems likely that the term antedates Gaius Julius Caesar (100–44 BC). We know that Julius Caesar could not have been born that way as his mother lived for many years afterward and abdominal delivery was universally fatal at that time. It was almost universally referred to as the caesarean operation until Jaqcues Guillimeau (of the Hôtel-Dieu) first used the term "section" in 1598. Understanding the derivation of the term "cesarean," however, it is more correct to use "section" by itself or the term "cesarean delivery."

The first recorded cesarean performed on a living woman appears in *Traité Nouveau de l'Hystérotomotokie ou l'Enfantement Césaerien,* published by Francois Rousett, in 1581.[26] He reports that some eighty-two years earlier, around the year 1500, a swine-gelder by the name of Jacob Nufer had sought the assistance of no less than thirteen mid-wives and two lithotomists for his wife's labor. When all were unsuccessful, he sought permission from the church and local authorities to perform an abdominal delivery. Having received these consents, he "invited the timid to retire" and all but two of the mid-wives and the two lithotomists excused themselves. With their assistance, and being in possession of very sharp instruments, he quickly opened his wife's abdomen, who delivered a healthy living child. The child is reported to have lived to the age of seventy-seven and his wife, having fully recovered, went on the have five more children including a set of twins, all delivered vaginally.[26]

Given that it wasn't recorded until eighty-two years after the fact, and given that his wife both lived and went on to have more children, there is some doubt about the validity of the claim. It has been suggested that, if indeed this were a true event, it was likely an abdominal pregnancy. Regardless, Rousset went on to advocate cesarean on the living. Although is appears than he had never done one, or seen one for that matter, he reported on fourteen successful cases, including one woman who had had six. These reports seem unlikely.[26]

The first authenticated case of cesarean on a living woman occurred on April 21, 1610. The woman apparently had a severe diastasis recti and the gravid uterus had protruded through this deviation in the abdominal wall. Covered only by a thin layer of skin, Jeremias Trautmann, assisted by two mid-wives and in the presence of the Archbishop of Saxony and Professor Stennert of the university, delivered a living child. The abdominal wall was sutured but the uterus was not. The patient died twenty-five days later.[27]

The profound maternal mortality rate associated with cesarean deliveries continued until the end of the nineteenth century. In Great Britain and Ireland, maternal mortality associated with abdominal delivery for the year 1865 was 85%. In Paris, during the ninety years ending in 1876, there was not a single successful outcome.[28] Hugh Hodge, of pessary and forceps fame, reviewed the world experience with cesarean in his 1864 textbook, *The Principles and Practice of Obstetrics.* He reported about 80% mortality. He wisely noted that the best outcomes occurred when the section was performed before the onset of labor (or early in labor) and before rupture of the membranes. Unfortunately, he still strongly advised against suturing of the uterus.[29] This was the common wisdom for at least the preceding two centuries, as it was felt that the uterus would quickly involute and heal itself and that suture material would only serve as a nidus for infection. The end result was that many patients died from hemorrhage and even more from sepsis.

The first real advance toward safe cesarean came in 1882 when Max Sänger advocated closing the uterine wall. Though he did this only once himself, he documented the experience from frontier outposts in America. Of the seventeen cesareans reported, all closed with silver wire suture, and eight of the mothers survived.[30] This approach has a major impact on maternal loss from hemorrhage but sepsis was still a big problem.

The latter half of the nineteenth century saw an evolving understanding of germ theory. In the pre-antibiotic era, obstetricians lacked methods to combat infection. In 1876, Porro introduced the concept of doing a supracervical hysterectomy at the time of abdominal delivery in an effort to remove the offending nidus for infection. In 1907, Frank introduced the concept of extraperitoneal section, where the bladder is moved away from the lower uterine segment and the peritoneal cavity is *not* entered. Five years later, Krönig postulated that the major advantage of the extraperitoneal approach was that it placed the uterine opening in the lower uterine segment. This low-segment vertical incision was introduced in the United States by Beck in 1919 and popularized by DeLee in 1922. Four years later, in 1926, a Scottish obstetrician, John Martin Munro Kerr, recommended the low transverse incision that is the most commonly used approach today.

Apart from the major advances in surgical technique, three other major contributors to the safe cesarean we enjoy today are noteworthy. In 1846, ether was introduced for use in surgery, including cesarean. One year later, chloroform was introduced. Chloroform also became popular for the pain of childbirth when it became known that Queen Victoria had used it during the births of her last two children in 1853 and 1857. Second was the availability of safe blood transfusion after World War I and third, the introduction of antibiotic therapy after World War II.

Puerperal Sepsis

It had long been known that disease could be spread from individual to individual or from noxious substances but the mechanism by which this happened was not at all understood. Among his other teachings, Galen had advanced the "miasma theory" or the idea that disease was passed by bad air. In the 1546 publication, *De Contagione et Contagiosis Morbis*, Girolamo Fracastoro proposed what is now known as the "germ theory," the idea that disease, and especially endemic disease, was spread by tiny particles or "spores." It was still another century before Anton van Leeuwenhoek first identified microscopic organisms.

In 1841 Edward Rigby Jr. published his work *A System of Midwifery.* This work is most notable for a single paragraph in which he states that the contagious nature of peurperal fever had been amply proved at the Vienna Hospital. There is no evidence that he actually knew Semmelweis who would have still been a medical student at that time and in the process of formulating his ideas. Although Rigby may have foreshadowed Semmelweis, he definitely caught the attention of Oliver Wendell Holmes, Sr. (1809–1894, father of Oliver Wendell Holmes, Jr., the jurist and Supreme Court justice), In 1843 Oliver Wendell Holmes, Sr. delivered an address in Boston citing the work of Rigby and many others to prove that puerperal sepsis was contagious.[31]

Holmes was so thorough and logical that it seems incredulous anyone would have failed to accept his argument. But he was still early in his career and without an academic appointment so when such notable authorities as Charles Meigs (1792–1869), and others, attacked him violently, controversy arose. Meigs was arguably one of the profession's most disagreeable and obstinate members, denouncing everything new, including anesthesia.

Holmes published his paper in a local journal that had a small circulation, one that closed down soon after. As such, it did not make much of an impact. In 1855, after becoming a professor at Harvard, he republished the paper with a new introduction in which he addressed his critics.[32,33] It is also worth noting that Holmes was responsible for introducing the term "anesthesia."

During the twelve years in between Holmes's publications, Ignaz Semmelweis was busy in Vienna. In the six years leading up to his appointment as assistant to the professor (roughly equivalent to "Chief Resident") in 1846, Semmelweis had noted that the maternal mortality rate in the physician-run clinic was double that of the clinic run by midwives (7.6% vs. 3.7%). In 1847 one of his colleagues cut himself with a scalpel during the autopsy of a woman who had died of childbirth fever. This colleague soon developed all of the same symptoms and died. Beginning in May of that year, he had all of the medical students begin washing their hands in chloride of lime solution. Almost immediately, the mortality rate in the physician ward dropped to that in the midwifery ward.

Never one for diplomacy, Semmelweis managed to alienate his professor and was not reappointed. He took a position in Budapest where he duplicated his results, bringing the mortality rate from puerperal sepsis down to under 1%. News of his success had spread throughout Europe and to the United States but he was often criticized for not having published his data. In 1861 he finally published his seminal work, *The Etiology, the Concept and the Prophylaxis of Childbed Fever.*[34] Despite his dramatic successes, many obstetricians still held to their old beliefs.

Semmelweis became more and more unstable mentally and offered a series of Open Letters, in which he severely criticized and insulted those who would not accept his assertions. There is great suspicion that he was now suffering from tertiary syphilis, a common affliction among obstetricians of the day as they would become infected while doing autopsies. In 1865 he was forcibly admitted to a mental hospital where he died from sepsis two weeks later, a consequence of injuries he sustained during his "arrest."

Pre-eclampsia

Pre-eclampsia is often referred to as the "disease of theories." When the Chicago Lying-In Hospital (founded 1895) was expanded, the architects placed several cement plaques along the colonnade. One was left blank for whoever discovered either the cause or the cure of pre-eclampsia. It is still blank.

Eclampsia was certainly known to exist prior to 400 BC. The *Coan Prognosis*, attributed to Hippocrates but probably written before his time, contains the statement, "In pregnancy, the onset of drowsy headaches with heaviness is bad; such cases are perhaps liable to some sort of fits at the same time."[35]

Beginning no later than the sixteenth century, and perhaps earlier, and continuing well toward the end of nineteenth century, it was felt that the best treatment for pre-eclampsia/eclampsia (also once called toxemia) was purging and bleeding. It was not until the sphygmomanometer was invented by Scipione Riva-Rocci in 1896 that the hypertensive nature of the disease became known. With this, the focus changed to trying to prevent the seizures and numerous agents. Intramuscular magnesium sulfate began in the early 1900s and by the 1920s had been supplanted by intravenous infusion.[36]

It was not until 1739 that Bossier de Sauvages made a distinction that the seizures of eclampsia were distinct from epilepsy, noting that eclamptic convulsions were cured by delivery while epileptic attacks were not. It would be another century before proteinuria was discovered. In November 1843, James Young Simpson (1811–1870), inventor of the Simpson forceps, and John Charles Lever (1811–1859) independently reported that proteinuria in pregnancy was specific to pre-eclampsia and this cleared following delivery.[37]

Concluding Remarks

From the middle of the nineteenth century to present day, obstetrical practice has been continuously influenced by research and critical observation to the point that every modern obstetrics and gynecology resident is well versed in the principle of evidenced-based medicine. Many noteworthy accomplishments did not occur until the twentieth century. Perhaps the greatest advance came with the introduction of prenatal care. Aside from general health advice, no medical care was typically provided to expectant women until the onset of labor or other symptoms until the early 1900s. In 1900, the maternal mortality rate in the United States was about 8.5%. One in 12 mothers died before, during or shortly after giving birth. With the advent of routine prenatal care in the 1930s, the rate dropped dramatically and steadily such that, by the 1950s, the rate had decreased by 99% to less than one-tenth of 1%.

Safe cesarean delivery, safe blood transfusion, and antibiotics were critical developments in the improvement of maternal mortality. The introduction of ergot alkaloids and oxytocin has helped to control postpartum hemorrhage. Epidurals have replaced general anesthesia and improved neonatal care has had a dramatic impact on perinatal mortality. Obstetrical care today bears little resemblance to what was practiced even fifty years ago. Today's expectant mother enters pregnancy fully confident that she and her baby will be fine. She is completely oblivious to how great the risks were less than a century ago and to how far we have come.

References

1. *The American Heritage® Stedman's Medical Dictionary*. Copyright © 2002, 2001, 1995 by Houghton Mifflin Company. Published by Houghton Mifflin Company.
2. *Online Etymology Dictionary*. © 2010 Douglas Harper.
3. Dictionary.com. Unabridged based on the *Random House Dictionary*. © Random House, Inc. 2016.
4. Witkowski GJ. *Histoire des Accouchements chez tous les Peuples*. Paris: G. Steinheil, 1887.
5. Genesis 35:16–18.
6. *The Aphorisms of Hippocrates*. Translation by Thomas Coar. London: AJ Valpy, 1822.
7. *Soranus' Gynecology*. Translated by Temkin O. © Johns Hopkins University Press, 1991.
8. Raynold T. *The Byrth of Mankynde*, 1514 (published 1545). New York: Gryphon Edition, 1994.
9. Reuff J. *The Expert Midwife*. London 1637. New York: Gryphon Edition, 1997.
10. Vesalius A. *De humani corporis fabrica*. Padua, 1543.
11. Radcliffe W. *Milestones in Midwifery*. Bristol: John Wright and Sons, 1967, p. 11.
12. Packard F. *The Life and Times of Ambroise Paré*. New York: Paul Hoeber, 1921, p. 53.
13. Bourgeois, Louyse. *Encyclopedia of World Biography*. Farmington Hills Michigan: The Gale Group. 2004.
14. Radcliffe W. *Milestones in Midwifery*. Bristol: John Wright and Sons, 1967, p. 22.
15. Dunn PM. Louise Bourgeois (1563–1636): royal midwife of France. *Arch Dis Child Fetal Neonatal Ed*. 2004;89.
16. Radcliffe W. *The Secret Instrument*. London: William Heinemann, 1947.
17. Radcliffe W. *Milestones in Midwifery and The Secret Instrument*. San Francisco: Norman Publishing, 1989.
18. Aveling JH. *The Chamberlens & the Midwifery Forceps*. London: J&A Churchill, 1882.
19. Mauriceau F. *The Diseases of Women with Child, and in the Child-Bed*. Translated by Chamberlen H. 7th edn. London: Cox & Clarke, 1736, p. xiv.
20. Das K. *Obstetrical Forceps*. Calcutta: The Art Press, 1929. Thackray Reprint. Leeds: Medical Museum Publishing, 1993.
21. Schwarz SM. Rickets. *Medscape, News and Information*, April 17, 2014.
22. Claerr J. The History of Rickets, Scurvy and Other Nutritional Diseases. *An Interesting Treatise on Human Stupidity*. Yahoo! Voices. February 6, 2008.
23. Naegele FC. *The Obliquely Contracted Pelvis*. Mainz: Victor von Zabern, 1839. 1939 Translated by Hellman AM and Musa G. New York: Gryphon Editions, 1939. Birmingham: Gryphon Editions, 1991.
24. Ibid. p. 34.
25. Yusuf N, Ali M, Ahmad Q, et al. Pregnancy in Pott's disease: a case report and review. *Bangladesh J Obstet Gynaecol* 2010; 25(1): 37–40.
26. Rousset F. *Traité Nouveau de l'Hystérotomotokie ou l'Enfantement Césaerien*. Paris, 1581.
27. De Costa C. *Hail Caesar*. Brisbane: Boolarong Press, 2008, pp. 28, 29.
28. Cunningham G, Gant N, Leveno K, et al., eds. *Williams Obstetrics*. 21st edn. New York: McGraw Hill, 2001, p. 560.
29. Hodge HL. *The Principles and Practice of Obstetrics*. Philadelphia: Blanchard and Lea, 1864, pp. 281–283.

30. Eastman NJ. The role of frontier America in the development of cesarean section. *Am J Obstet Gynecol.* 1932;24:919.

31. Radcliffe W. *Milestones in Midwifery*. Bristol: John Wright and Sons, 1967, p. 76.

32. Holmes OW. The contagiousness of puerperal fever. *New Engl Quart J Med Surgery.* 1843;1503–1530.

33. Reprinted in Medical Essays as *Puerperal Fever as a Private Pestilence* 1855. Harvard Classics, Vol 38, Part 5. 1909–1914.

34. Semmelweis IF. *The Etiology, the Concept and the Prophylaxis of Childbed Fever*. English translation by Murphy FP in *Medical Classics* 5–8 (1941), pp. 339–773. Birmingham: Gryphon Edition, 1990.

35. Hippocrates. The Medical Works of Hippocrates. *Coan Prognosis* XXXI, no. 523. English translation by Chadwick J, Mann WN. Oxford: Blackwell Scientific, 1950.

36. Bell MJ. A Historical overview of preeclampsia-eclampsia. *J Obstet Gynecol Neonatal Nurs*. 2010; 39(5):510–518.

37. Radcliffe W. *Milestones in Midwifery*. Bristol: John Wright and Sons. 1967, p. 82.

Index